■ Social Injustice and Public Health

Social Injustice and Public Health

SECOND EDITION

EDITED BY

Barry S. Levy

Victor W. Sidel

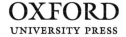

OXFORD
UNIVERSITY PRESS

OXFORD

UNIVERSITY PRESS

Oxford University Press is a department of the University of Oxford.
It furthers the University's objective of excellence in research, scholarship,
and education by publishing worldwide.

Oxford   New York
Auckland   Cape Town   Dar es Salaam   Hong Kong   Karachi
Kuala Lumpur   Madrid   Melbourne   Mexico City   Nairobi
New Delhi   Shanghai   Taipei   Toronto

With offices in
Argentina   Austria   Brazil   Chile   Czech Republic   France   Greece
Guatemala   Hungary   Italy   Japan   Poland   Portugal   Singapore
South Korea   Switzerland   Thailand   Turkey   Ukraine   Vietnam

Oxford is a registered trademark of Oxford University Press in the UK and certain other countries.

Published in the United States of America by
Oxford University Press
198 Madison Avenue, New York, NY 10016

Library of Congress Cataloging-in-Publication Data
Social injustice and public health/edited by Barry S. Levy, Victor W. Sidel.—2nd ed.
     p. ; cm.
Includes bibliographical references and index.
ISBN 978–0–19–993922–0 (pbk. : alk. paper)—ISBN 978–0–19–932478–1 (uPDF ebook)—
ISBN 978–0–19–932479–8 (epub ebook)
I. Levy, Barry S.   II. Sidel, Victor W.
[DNLM: 1. Social Medicine. 2. Public Health. 3. Social Justice. WA 31]
RA418
362.1′042—dc23
2013004942

9 8 7 6 5 4 3 2 1
Printed in the United States of America
on acid-free paper

Dedicated to health workers throughout the world committed to ending social injustice.

■ CONTENTS

Nothing is more basic to public health philosophy than social justice. The philosophy of science is based on the search for truth, an attempt to break down the walls of ignorance, and a desire to understand. The philosophy of medicine includes all of this, but is particularly concerned with applying truth to an individual patient seeking help. In contrast, the philosophy of public health is concerned with applying truth to everyone. It is therefore based on a search for social justice—a burden that drives the daily work of public health practitioners. While success is often possible with an individual patient, it is elusive and relative in public health.

Except for smallpox eradication, public health, in a sense, always falls short. We in public health make progress with individual diseases or at particular times or with specific populations, only to look up from our work and become overwhelmed by the millions of other people victimized in some way by social injustice.

Some people argue that "social injustice" is a soft subject, and, therefore, almost unscientific. Not at all. The consequences of social injustice are readily found in hard statistics. They are seen in the disparities in measures of life expectancy, premature mortality, preventable cancers and other chronic diseases, and infectious diseases—all of which are described in this fine book. These disparities are not the only consequences of social injustice, but they provide ways to identify, describe, measure, and understand social injustice.

The descriptions in this book of social injustice and its health consequences stimulate thinking on how to respond to social injustice. We public health workers must be constantly alert and must improve surveillance systems to collect, analyze, and interpret appropriate data. But this is not enough. We must use data analysis and interpretation to develop responses that not only minimize the consequences of social injustice, but also attempt to reduce—and ultimately eliminate—social injustice. It is not enough to identify poverty as the most important determinant of poor health—as dose-related as are blood pressure and cigarette consumption in eroding health. We must assume the responsibility of addressing poverty directly. Likewise, for the plethora of other forms of social injustice chronicled in this book, our voices must be heard and our actions must make a difference.

A final burden: Many people will not agree with public health workers that social injustice compromises health and quality of life. There are even some people who, with no qualms whatsoever, would continue slavery, poverty, and injustice—perhaps to maintain their status and advantage in society. As Archbishop Desmond

Tutu has said, "It's very difficult to wake up someone who is pretending to be asleep." Nevertheless, we should try to sound the alarm, even for these people.

Other people may ignore the problems of social injustice because of lack of thought or analysis. They actually *are* asleep. Lance Armstrong lost his medals, much money, and his reputation when it was determined that he had used banned performance-enhancing substances during his cycling career. He said in an interview that it was scary for him to realize that, at the time that he used these substances, he felt no guilt, no shame, and no sense that he was cheating or that his actions were unjust towards others. His change in attitude resulted from a system that awakened him. To promote social justice, we need to develop systems to awaken people. We need to educate and promote empathy, especially in young people. And we need to make clear the ethical dimensions of social injustice.

In his book *The Lucifer Effect: Understanding How Good People Turn Evil*, Philip Zimbardo asserts that it is not the "bad apples" but rather the "bad barrels" that often corrupt good people—making it easy for them to ignore what is ethically correct. He also asserts that "good barrels" can improve the behavior of people.

This book is a "good barrel" to reduce social injustice and to improve public health.

—William H. Foege

Social injustice underlies many public health problems throughout the world. It is manifested in many ways, ranging from various forms of overt discrimination to wide gaps between the "haves" and "have-nots" within countries and between high-income and low-income countries. It leads to higher rates of disease, injury, disability, and premature death. Public health workers and students need to understand social injustice in order to address these problems.

This book offers a comprehensive approach to understanding social injustice and its impact on public health. Part I explores the nature of social injustice and its adverse effects on public health. Part II describes in detail how the health of 10 specific population groups is affected by social injustice. Part III explores how social injustice affects 10 aspects of public health. Part IV provides an action agenda for what needs to be done to prevent social injustice and to minimize its impact on health.

This book arose from our experiences and our observations of the ways in which social injustice underlies public health problems. We have also edited the books *War and Public Health* and *Terrorism and Public Health*, in which we identified social injustice as a principal cause—and a major consequence—of war and terrorism. Likewise, this book examines social injustice as a principal cause and a major consequence of many public health problems.

We developed this book in order to facilitate a better understanding of the relationships between social injustice and public health, promote education and research on these subjects, and stimulate work to reduce social injustice and to minimize its impact on health and well-being.

B.S.L. and V.W.S
Sherborn, Massachusetts
The Bronx, New York
December 2012

■ ACKNOWLEDGMENTS

Developing the second edition of *Social Injustice and Public Health* has involved the skills and resources of many people, to whom we are profoundly grateful.

We thank all of the contributors who wrote chapters and textboxes that reflect their expertise and insights. Their commitment to social justice and to public health is evident in their work and their contributions to this book.

We express our deep appreciation to Heather McStowe for her excellent work in preparing multiple drafts of the manuscript and coordinating communication with contributors. We also thank Deyanira Acevedo for secretarial support.

We greatly appreciate the guidance, assistance, and support of Chad Zimmerman, Kurt Roediger, Maura Roessner, Nicholas Liu, and others at Oxford University Press and J. Ramprasad at Newgen Knowledge Works Pvt. Ltd.

Finally, we express our gratitude and love to Nancy Levy and Ruth Sidel for their continuing inspiration, encouragement, and support.

■ CONTRIBUTORS

Carol Easley Allen, PhD, RN
Twin Solutions LLC
Huntsville, AL
callen1946@gmail.com

Myron Allukian Jr., DDS, MPH
Oral Health Consultant
Boston, MA
myalluk@aol.com

Lisa Arangua, MPP
Senior Research Analyst
Department of Family Medicine
David Geffen School of Medicine
University of California, Los Angeles
Los Angeles, CA
LArangua@mednet.ucla.edu

Robert E. Aronson, DrPH, MPH
Associate Professor and Director
Public Health Program
Taylor University
Upland, IN
raronson@taylor.edu

Ruth Bell, PhD
Senior Research Fellow
Department of Epidemiology and
  Public Health
University College London
London
United Kingdom
r.bell@ucl.ac.uk

Talia Mae Bettcher, PhD
Professor and Chair
Department of Philosophy
California State University, Los
  Angeles
Los Angeles, CA
tbettch@calstatela.edu

Kathryn Bolles, MPH
Senior Director
Emergency Health and Nutrition
Save the Children
Washington, DC
kbolles@savechildren.org

Angie Brasington, MSPH
Community Health and Social
  Change Advisor
Department of Health and Nutrition,
  International Programs
Save the Children
Washington, DC
abrasington@savechildren.org

Paula Braveman, MD, MPH
Professor of Family and Community
  Medicine
Director, Center on Social Disparities
  in Health
University of California, San
  Francisco
San Francisco, CA
braveman@fcm.ucsf.edu

Joseph E. Brenner, MA
Co-Director
Center for Policy Analysis on Trade
    and Health (CPATH)
San Francisco, CA
jebrenner@cpath.org

J. Larry Brown, PhD
Faculty Member Emeritus
Harvard School of Public Health
Boston, MA
brown.jlarry@gmail.com

Colin D. Butler, BMed, MSc, PhD
Discipline of Public Health
Faculty of Health
University of Canberra
Canberra, Australia
colin.butler@canberra.edu.au

Arthur M. Chen, MD
Senior Fellow
Asian Health Services
Oakland, CA
achen61255@yahoo.com

Haejoo Chung, RPh, MS, PhD
Assistant Professor and Chair
Department of Healthcare
    Management
College of Health Sciences
Korea University
Seoul, Republic of Korea
hpolicy@korea.ac.kr

Sarah DeGue, PhD
Behavioral Scientist
Division of Violence Prevention
National Center for Injury Prevention
    and Control
Centers for Disease Control and
    Prevention
Atlanta, GA
sdegue@cdc.gov

Ernest Drucker, PhD
John Jay College of Criminal Justice
City University of New York
Mailman School of Public Health
Columbia University
New York, NY
emdrucker@earthlink.net

Cheryl E. Easley, PhD, RN
Twin Solutions LLC
Harvest, AL
ce6501@gmail.com

William W. Eaton
Harold and Sylvia Halpert Professor
    and Chair
Department of Mental Health
Johns Hopkins Bloomberg School of
    Public Health
Baltimore, MD
weaton@jhsph.edu

Carroll L. Estes, PhD
Professor Emerita
Department of Social and Behavioral
    Sciences
Founder and Former Director
Institute for Health & Aging
School of Nursing
University of California, San
    Francisco
San Francisco, CA
carroll.estes@gmail.com

Paul E. Farmer, MD, PhD
Kolokotrones University Professor
Harvard University
Co-Founder
Partners in Health
Boston, MA
paul_farmer@hms.harvard.edu

Oliver Fein, MD
Professor of Clinical Medicine and
  Public Health
Associate Dean
Departments of Medicine and Public
  Health
Weill Cornell Medical College
New York, NY
ofein@med.cornell.edu

Henry A. Freedman, LLB,
  Hon Dr Law
Executive Director
National Center for Law and
  Economic Justice
New York, NY
freedman@nclej.org

Sarita Fritzler, BA
Program Coordinator
Emergency Health and Nutrition
Save the Children
Washington, DC
sfritzler@savechildren.org

H. Jack Geiger, MD, MSciHyg
Arthur C. Logan Professor of
  Community Medicine Emeritus
CUNY Medical School
City College of New York
New York, NY
jgeiger@igc.org

Lillian Gelberg, MD, MSPH
Professor of Family Medicine and
  Professor of Public Health
David Geffen School of Medicine
University of California, Los Angeles
VA Greater Los Angeles Healthcare
  System
Los Angeles, CA
LGelberg@mednet.ucla.edu

Kay C. Goss, MA
President
World Disaster Management
Alexandria, VA
kay.goss@post.harvard.edu

Robert M. Gould, MD
Associate Adjunct Professor
Department of Obstetric, Gynecology,
  and Reproductive Sciences
UCSF School of Medicine
President
Physicians for Social Responsibility
San Francisco, CA
rmgould1@yahoo.com

Nora Ellen Groce, PhD
Professor and Leonard Cheshire
  Chair
Director
Leonard Cheshire Disability &
  Inclusive Development Centre
Department of Epidemiology and
  Public Health
University College London
London
United Kingdom
nora.groce@ucl.ac.uk

Sofia Gruskin, JD, MIA
Director
Program on Global Health and
  Human Rights
Institute for Global Health
University of Southern California
Adjunct Professor of Global Health
Harvard School of Public Health
Los Angeles, CA
gruskin@usc.edu

John W. Hatch, PhD
Emeritus Professor
Department of Health Behavior
University of North Carolina
Chapel Hill, NC
jhatch5505@yahoo.com

David U. Himmelstein, MD
Professor of Public Health
CUNY School of Public Health
New York, NY
dhimmels@hunter.cuny.edu

Alice M. Horowitz, PhD
Research Associate Professor
School of Public Health
University of Maryland
College Park, MD
ahorowit@umd.edu

Vincent Iacopino, MD, PhD
Senior Medical Advisor
Physicians for Human Rights
Cambridge, MA
Adjunct Professor of Medicine
University of Minnesota Medical
    School
Minneapolis, MN
viacopino@phrusa.org

Kay A. Johnson, MPH, EdM
Lecturer of Health Policy
School of Public Health and Health
    Services
George Washington University
kay.johnson@johnsongci.com

Richard Jolly, MA, PhD
Professor
Institute of Development Studies
University of Sussex
Brighton
United Kingdom
R.Jolly@ids.ac.uk

Micheal A. Kemp, PhD, CEM
Faculty Chair
School of Public Service Leadership
Capella University
Minneapolis, MN 55402
micheal.kemp@capella.edu

Omar Khan, MD, MHS
Medical Director
Center for Community Health
    & Eugene du Pont Preventive
    Medicine and Rehabilitation
    Institute
Director, Global Health Track
Department of Family & Community
    Medicine
Christiana Care Heath System
Wilmington, DE
okhan@med.upenn.edu

Andrea Kidd Taylor, DrPH, MSPH
Lecturer, Health Policy and
    Management Department
Morgan State University School of
    Community Health & Policy
Baltimore, MD
akiddtay@gmail.com

Nancy Krieger, PhD
Professor of Social Epidemiology
Department of Social and Behavioral
    Sciences
Harvard School of Public Health
Boston, MA
nkrieger@hsph.harvard.edu

Linda Young Landesman,
    DrPH, MSW
Landesman Consulting
Rye Brook, NY
Clinical Assistant Professor
Public Health Practice Program
University of Massachusetts, Amherst
lindalandesman@aol.com

Robert S. Lawrence, MD
Center for a Livable Future Professor
Professor of Environmental Health
    Sciences, Health Policy, and
    International Health
Johns Hopkins Bloomberg School of
    Public Health
Baltimore, MD
rlawrenc@jhsph.edu

Barry S. Levy, MD, MPH
Adjunct Professor of Public Health
Department of Public Health and
    Community Medicine
Tufts University School of Medicine
Sherborn, MA
blevy@igc.org

David MKI Liu, MD, JD, PhD
Consolidated Tribal Health Center
Redwood Valley, CA
k.liu.hpha@gmail.com

Emilia Lombardi, PhD
Assistant Professor
Health Promotion and Education/
    Public Health
Baldwin Wallace University
Berea, OH
elombard@bw.edu

Kay Lovelace, PhD, MPH
Associate Professor
Department of Public Health
    Education
University of North Carolina at
    Greensboro
Greensboro, NC
klovelace@uncg.edu

Gina Maranto
Director
Ecosystem Science and Policy
Graduate Program Coordinator
Environmental Science and Policy
The Leonard and Jayne Abess Center
University of Miami
Coral Gables, FL
glmaranto@gmail.com

Michael Marmot MD, PhD, FRCP
Professor
Institute of Health Equity
University College
London
United Kingdom
m.marmot@ucl.ac.uk

Porter McConnell
Policy and Advocacy Manager, Aid
    Effectiveness
Oxfam America
Washington, DC
m.porter.mcconnell@gmail.com

Anthony J. McMichael, MBBS, PhD
Professor of Population Health
National Centre for Epidemiology &
    Population Health
Australian National University
Canberra
Australia
tony.mcmichael@anu.edu.au

James A. Mercy, PhD
Special Advisor for Global Activities
Division of Violence Prevention
National Center for Injury Prevention
    and Control
Centers for Disease Control and
    Prevention
Atlanta, GA
JMercy@cdc.gov

Joia S. Mukherjee, MD, MPH
Associate Professor
Department of Global Health and
    Social Medicine
Harvard Medical School
Chief Medical Officer
Partners in Health
Boston, MA
jmukherjee@pih.org

Carles Muntaner, MD, PhD
Professor
Bloomberg Faculty of Nursing
Dalla Lana School of Public Health
Department of Psychiatry
University of Toronto
Toronto
Canada
carles.muntaner@utoronto.ca

Linda Rae Murray, MD, MPH
Chief Medical Officer
Cook County Department of Public
    Health
Chicago, IL
lindarae.murray@gmail.com

K.M. Venkat Narayan, MD
Ruth and O.C. Hubert Chair of
    Global Health
Hubert Department of Global Health
Rollins School of Public Health
Emory University
Atlanta, GA
knaraya@emory.edu

Carmen Rita Nevarez, MD, MPH
Vice-President, External Relations
Director, Center for Health
    Leadership and Practice
Public Health Institute
Oakland, CA
crnevarez@phi.org

Edwin Ng, MSW
Dalla Lana School of Public Health
University of Toronto
Toronto
Canada
edwin.ng@utoronto.ca

Judy Norsigian
Executive Director
Our Bodies Ourselves
Cambridge, MA
judy@bwhbc.org

Raymond C. Offenheiser
President
Oxfam America
Boston, MA

Charlotte Phillips, MD
Chairperson
Brooklyn For Peace
Brooklyn, NY
c.phillips8@verizon.net

Alonzo L. Plough PhD, MPH
Director, Emergency Preparedness
    and Response
County of Los Angeles Department
    of Public Health
Los Angeles, CA
Clinical Professor of Health Services
University of Washington School
    of Public Health
aplough@ph.lacounty.gov

Sara Rosenbaum, JD
Harold and Jane Hirsh Professor
Department of Health Policy
School of Public Health and Health
    Services
George Washington University
Washington, DC
sarar@gwu.edu

Leonard S. Rubenstein, JD, LLM
Director, Program on Human Rights, Health and Conflict
Center for Public Health and Human Rights
Johns Hopkins Bloomberg School of Public Health
Baltimore, MD
lrubenst@jhsph.edu

Peggy Saika
President/Executive Director
Asian Americans/Pacific Islanders in Philanthropy
San Francisco, CA
peggy@aapip.org

William F. Schulz, DMin
President
Unitarian Universalist Service Committee
Cambridge, MA
Adjunct Professor of Public Administration
Wagner School of Public Service
New York University
bschulz@uusc.org

Ellen R. Shaffer, PhD, MPH
Co-Director
Center for Policy Analysis on Trade and Health (CPATH)
San Francisco, CA
ershaffer@gmail.com

Mark Sidel, JD
Doyle-Bascom Professor of Law and Public Affairs
University of Wisconsin Law School
Madison, WI
sidel@wisc.edu

Victor W. Sidel, MD
Distinguished University Professor of Social Medicine Emeritus
Montefiore Medical Center
Albert Einstein College of Medicine
Bronx, NY
Adjunct Professor of Public Health
Weill Cornell Medical College
New York, NY
vsidel@igc.org

Karen R. Siegel, MPH
PhD Candidate
Hubert Department of Global Health
Rollins School of Public Health
Nutrition and Health Sciences
Graduate Division of Biological and Biomedical Sciences
Laney Graduate School
Emory University
Atlanta, GA
karen.siegel@emory.edu

Gail Snetro-Plewman, MPH
Senior Africa Area Capacity Building Advisor for Health
Department of Health and Nutrition, International Programs
Save the Children
Johannesburg, South Africa
gsnetro@savechildren.org

Patrice Sutton, MPH
Research Scientist
Program on Reproductive Health and the Environment
University of California, San Francisco
Oakland, CA
suttonp@obgyn.ucsf.edu

Michael J. Toole, MBBS, BMedSc, DTM&H
Professor
Burnet Institute
Adjunct Professor
Department of Epidemiology and
  Preventive Medicine
Monash University
Melbourne
Australia
toole@burnet.edu.au

Bailus Walker, Jr., PhD, MPH
Professor
Department of Community and
  Family Medicine
Howard University School of
  Medicine
Washington, DC
bailusw@comcast.net

Steven P. Wallace, PhD
Chair and Professor
Department of Community Health
  Sciences
Associate Director
UCLA Center for Health Policy
  Research
UCLA Fielding School of Public
  Health
University of California, Los Angeles
Los Angeles, CA
swallace@ucla.edu

Peter Weiss, JD
Vice President
Center for Constitutional Rights
New York, NY
petweiss185@gmail.com

Tony L. Whitehead, PhD, MSHyg
Professor and Director
Cultural Systems Analysis Group
Anthropology Department
Affiliate Professor
Department of Behavioral and
  Community Health
University of Maryland
College Park, MD
tonywhitehead1122@gmail.com

Chloe A. Wong, BA
Oral Health Analyst
Boston, MA
Chloe.A.Wong@gmail.com

Steffie Woolhandler, MD, MPH, MA
Professor of Public Health
CUNY School of Public Health
New York, NY
swoolhan@hunter.cuny.edu

Derek Yach, MBChB, MPH
Senior Vice President
The Vitality Group
Chicago, IL
dyach@thevitalitygroup.com

PART I

Introduction

1 The Nature of Social Injustice and Its Impact on Public Health

■ BARRY S. LEVY AND VICTOR W. SIDEL

■ INTRODUCTION

Social injustice has a wide variety of manifestations:

- For children in urban slums and depressed rural areas, it means few teachers, crowded classrooms, functional illiteracy, and no development of marketable skills.
- For unemployed youth, it means a lower probability of getting a permanent job.
- For minority workers, it means reduced income, reduced opportunities for promotion, and increased exposure to on-the-job health and safety hazards.
- For women, it means increased risk of being violently attacked or sexually abused.
- For people forced to migrate within or between countries, it means profound stress and less security.
- For many people throughout the world, it means unsafe food and water, poor sanitation, substandard housing, environmental hazards, violation of their human rights, inadequate access to medical care and public health services, and illness, injury, and premature death that could have been prevented.

Social injustice creates conditions that adversely affect the health of individuals and communities. It denies individuals and groups equal opportunity to have their basic human needs met. It violates fundamental human rights.

We define *social injustice* in two ways. First, we define it as the denial or violation of human rights (economic, sociocultural, political, or civil rights) of specific populations or groups in society based on the erroneous perception of their inferiority by those with more power or influence. Populations or groups that suffer social injustice may be defined by racial or ethnic status, socioeconomic position, age, gender, sexual orientation, or other perceived population or group characteristics. These populations or groups are often negatively stereotyped and stigmatized and may be the targets of hate and violence. Part II (Chapters 2 to 11) is organized around this definition of social injustice, with each chapter focusing on a population or group whose health is adversely affected by social injustice.

Our second definition of social injustice is based on the Institute of Medicine's definition of *public health*: what we, as a society, collectively do to assure the conditions in which people can be healthy.[1] This second definition of social injustice refers to policies or actions that adversely affect the societal conditions in which people can be healthy. Although this type of social injustice is often community-wide, nationwide, or even global, the populations and groups described in our first definition of social injustice—especially poor, homeless, ill, injured, young, and old people as well as women and members of racial and ethnic minority groups—usually suffer more than others in the population as a result of these policies and actions. Examples of this form of social injustice include policies or actions that promote:

- War and other forms of violence
- Climate change
- Damage to the environment
- Corruption of government or culture
- Erosion of civil liberties and freedoms
- Restriction of education, research, and public discourse

Part III (Chapters 12 to 21) is organized around this definition of social injustice, with each chapter focusing on a different aspect of public health. Public health workers are committed to the principle that all people are entitled to being protected against hazards and unnecessary harm.[2]

Under either definition, social injustice represents a lack of fairness or equity—resulting usually from the structure of society or discrimination by individuals or groups. Among the roots of social injustice are:

- Poverty and the socioeconomic gap between rich and poor people
- Maldistribution of resources in society
- Racism, sexism, ageism, and other forms of discrimination
- Weak laws—or weak enforcement of laws—protecting human rights
- Disenfranchisement of individuals and groups from the political process

It follows that concepts and definitions of social *justice* are based on justice, fairness, and equity (Box 1–1).

Social injustice leads to a wide range of adverse health consequences, as reflected by inequalities (disparities) within or between populations in health status and access to health services. Within the United States, there have been—and still are—many inequalities in health status, such as the following:

- In 2007, the infant mortality rate for infants born to African American, non-Hispanic mothers was almost three times that for infants born to Asian or Pacific Islander mothers.[3]
- In 2009–2010, among people age 20 and older, non-Hispanic blacks had a 50 percent rate of obesity, compared with 39 percent among Hispanics and 34 percent among non-Hispanic whites.[3]
- Women with lower levels of education and income as well as uninsured women, Latino women, and non-Hispanic black women are less likely to have access to family planning services.[3]
- A much higher percentage of Hispanics have had no health insurance coverage, compared with non-Hispanic blacks and non-Hispanic whites.

BOX 1-1 ■ Definitions and Concepts of Social Justice

While the focus of this book is social *injustice,* definitions and concepts of social *justice* are important to consider. Social justice means equity or fairness; it is an ethical concept based on principles of distributive justice[1]—the equitable societal distribution of valued goods and necessary burdens. Social justice applies the concept of distributive justice to the assets, privileges, and advantages that are present in society. It conforms to the principle that all people are equal. It is based on the belief that all people have "inalienable rights," as the U.S. Declaration of Independence stated. Social justice, which can be distinguished from legal justice and moral justice, is largely based on theories concerning the social contract, most of which are, in turn, based on the concepts that (a) governments are established for the benefit of members of populations, and (b) governments must provide for and protect the welfare of these populations—including upholding human rights.

Social justice is inextricably linked to public health. It is the philosophy on which public health is based.[2] Social justice means that all groups and individuals are entitled equally to important rights, such as health protection and minimal standards of income. Minimizing preventable illness, injury, and premature death is a goal of both public health and social justice. In a society, the extent to which social justice and equity are present correlates with health status of the population and reduction of health inequalities.[3] Health equity, a concept closely related to social justice, is the absence of systematic inequalities in health, or in the major social determinants of health, among groups at different levels in the social hierarchy in terms of wealth, power, and/or prestige.

Social justice is closely linked to human rights. The Universal Declaration of Human Rights (UDHR),[4] adopted by the United Nations General Assembly in 1948, consists of 30 articles that set forth rights to which all people are inherently entitled. It includes the right to a standard of living adequate for health and well-being. (The complete UDHR appears in the Appendix to this chapter.) The UDHR served as the foundation for the first two legally binding human rights documents of the United Nations: the International Covenant on Civil and Political Rights, and the International Covenant on Economic, Social, and Cultural Rights.[5] In the United States, civil and political rights are usually recognized as the most important human rights. However, in many other countries, economic, social, and cultural rights are recognized as most important, including the right to services to meet basic human needs, regardless of differences in economic status, class, gender, race, ethnicity, citizenship, religion, age, sexual orientation, disability, and health.

A widely accepted formulation for human rights is based on the writings of political philosopher John Rawls.[6] He asserted that everyone has an equal claim to basic rights and liberties, such as freedoms of thought, speech, association, and assembly; and that individuals should have not only the right to opportunities, but also an effectively equal chance as others of similar natural ability.

Box References

1. Braveman P, Gruskin S. Defining equity in health. *J Epidemiol Commun Health* 2003;57: 254–258.
2. Foege WH. Public health: Moving from debt to legacy (1986 presidential address). *Am J Pub Health* 1987;77:1276–1278.

3. Anderson LM, Scrimshaw SC, Fullilove MT, et al. The Community Guide's model for linking the social environment to health. *Am J Prev Med* 2003;24:12–20.
4. United Nations. Universal Declaration of Human Rights. Available at: http://www.un.org/en/documents/udhr/. Accessed January 3, 2013.
5. A call to action on the 50th anniversary of the Universal Declaration of Human Rights. *Health Hum Rights* 1998;3:7–18.
6. Rawls J. A theory of justice, Original edition. Cambridge, MA: Belknap Press of Harvard University Press, reissued 2005.

The Department of Health and Human Services through its Healthy People 2020 initiative has committed the United States to eliminating these and other health disparities.

Marked inequalities exist within countries. Over the course of U.S. history, for example, people of color have often been denied, by law, many opportunities. Even after the repeal of discriminatory laws and the adoption of laws banning discrimination, many opportunities have been denied to people of color by segregation and other practices (Chapter 3).

Marked inequalities also exist between countries (Chapter 21). For example, a female infant born today in Japan will live, on average, 86 years.[4] She will likely be fully vaccinated and will likely receive adequate nutrition and extensive education. If she becomes pregnant, she will receive adequate maternity care. If she develops chronic disease, she will likely receive excellent treatment and rehabilitation. If she becomes sick, she will likely receive medications valued at more than US$550. In contrast, a female infant born today in Sierra Leone will live, on average, 49 years.[4] She will not likely be immunized and will likely be underweight and malnourished. She will likely marry as a teenager and have five or more children, none of whom will be delivered by a trained birth attendant. One or more of her children will likely die during infancy. She will be at high risk of death during childbirth. If she becomes sick, she will likely receive medications valued at only a few dollars. If she develops a chronic disease, she likely will not have adequate treatment or rehabilitation. She will likely die prematurely of a preventable disease or injury.

Social injustice leads to increased rates of illness, injury, and premature death because of increased risk factors and decreased medical care and preventive services. People and communities affected by social injustice may have:

- Poorer nutrition, including less access to fruits, vegetables, and other healthful foods
- Greater exposure to unsafe water
- Greater contact with infectious disease agents
- Greater exposure to occupational and environmental hazards
- More frequent complications of chronic diseases
- More alcohol, tobacco, and drug abuse
- Less social support

- Greater physiological and immunological vulnerability to disease
- Less access to high-quality medical care and preventive services

The cause of disease is often a complex interplay of multiple factors, many of which are due to social injustice—including poverty, inadequate education, and inadequate health insurance. As a reflection of the association between poverty and many diseases, a former director of the National Cancer Institute declared that poverty is a carcinogen.[5]

Social injustice often occurs when those who control access to opportunities and resources block poor people, powerless people, and others from gaining fair and equitable access to these opportunities and resources. Social injustice enables those in the upper class to receive a disproportionate share of wealth and other resources while others may struggle to obtain the basic necessities of life.

Special circumstances may increase the level of social injustice. For example, a drought, flood, or other natural disaster that diminishes the availability of food supplies often affects some groups more than others, unless social or legal action is taken to prevent this disparity (see Box 18–2 in Chapter 18). War and other forms of armed conflict increase social injustice in many ways, including diverting resources from meeting basic human needs (see Box 17–1 in Chapter 17). However, major community emergencies may bring together people in ways that reduce social injustice.

The inequalities between rich and poor people within the United States and other countries and between rich and poor countries are greater than they have ever been. The gap in income between rich people and poor people is illustrated in Figure 1–1. In 2007, the wealthiest 61 million people (1 percent of the global population) had the same amount of income as the poorest 3.5 billion people (56 percent of the global population).[6] And rich people are getting richer, and poor people, poorer. Income inequality slows economic growth, causes health and social problems, and generates political instability.[6]

Market justice, which has created many of these inequalities, may be the primary roadblock to dramatically reducing preventable illness, injury, and premature death.[2] It has been asserted that market justice is a pervasive ideology that protects the most powerful people or the most numerous subgroup in a society from the burdens of collective action.[2] An important role for public health is to challenge market justice as fatally deficient in protecting the public's health and to advocate an ethic for protecting the public's health—giving highest priority to reducing illness, injury, and premature death and protecting all people against hazards.[2]

The global financial recession that began in 2008 exacerbated many inequalities and increased social injustice and its adverse effects on health. And, in 2010, as the United States began to emerge from recession, the top 1 percent of income-earners gained 93 percent of the additional income that accrued during the early recovery period. Joseph Stiglitz, a recipient of the Nobel Prize for

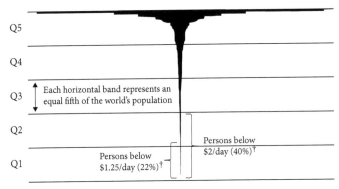

Figure 1-1 Global income distribution, by percentiles of the population in 2007 (or latest data available) in purchasing-power-parity (PPP) constant 2005 international dollars, according to the global accounting model. (*Source*: Ortiz I, Cummins M. Global inequality: Beyond the bottom billion—A rapid review of income distribution in 141 countries. New York: United Nations Children's Fund, 2011. Note: Persons below $2/day and $1.25/day based on: Chen S, Ravallion M. The developing world is poorer than we thought, but no less successful in the fight against poverty: Policy research working paper 4703. Washington, DC: World Bank, 2008.)

Economics, has asserted that because of economic and political inequalities, there is less equal opportunity and less fairness in the United States.[7] Globally, increasing unemployment, increasing commodity prices, and decreasing government spending indicate that income inequalities may worsen. And yet, the urgency for equitable economic policies has never been greater.[6]

▪ WHAT NEEDS TO BE DONE

Humanity, for the first time, has the technical capacity and the human and economic resources to address poverty, ill health, and human rights violations, as well as the social injustice that promotes these problems. Prevention or correction of most forms of social injustice requires individuals acting together in organizations or mass movements. A small group of individuals can—and often does—initiate progressive change. But it usually takes large numbers of people, with their diverse talents and commitments, to bring about significant progressive change through many different types of action: documenting problems, developing strategies and tactics, raising awareness among the general public, engaging in advocacy with policymakers, participating in rallies and demonstrations, raising and contributing money, and sometimes engaging in nonviolent forms of civil disobedience. And it takes both insiders, such as elected government officials, and outsiders, such as members of non-governmental educational and advocacy organizations, to reduce social injustice.[8]

As reflected in Part IV (Chapters 22 to 29), public health approaches need to be further developed and implemented to address social injustice. These approaches include:

- *Addressing social injustice in a human rights context*: The Universal Declaration of Human Rights (in the Appendix to this chapter) and the International Declaration of Health Rights (Box 25–1 in Chapter 25) provide a foundation for reducing, and ultimately eliminating, social injustice (Chapter 22).
- *Promoting social justice by public health policies, programs, and services*: Public health departments and other government bodies at the local, state, national, and international level can reduce social injustice and promote social justice (Chapter 23). Scientific evidence plays an important role in developing these policies, programs, and services (Box 1–2).
- *Strengthening communities and the roles of individuals in community life*: Communities—as well as civil-society organizations and individuals within communities—can play vital roles in addressing social injustice and its impact on public health (Chapter 24).
- *Promoting social justice through education in public health*: Schools of public health and educational programs in public health can promote social justice in many ways, including featuring social justice in their curricula (Chapter 25).
- *Researching critical questions on social justice and public health*: Systematic research approaches can better document social injustice, identify its underlying causes, and help point the way to reducing social injustice and its impact on public health (Chapter 26).
- *Protecting human rights through national and international laws*: National and international laws can be strengthened and better implemented to protect human rights and promote social justice (Chapter 27).
- *Promoting social justice through social movements*: Progress towards social justice often requires broad social movements (Chapter 28).
- *Promoting equitable and sustainable human development*: Progress toward social justice requires actions to promote human development, including making equity an economic priority (Chapter 29). International organizations (such as United Nations agencies and the World Bank), governments and bilateral aid organizations, international non-governmental organizations (Box 29–1 in Chapter 29), foundations (Box 29–2 in Chapter 29), and other organizations have important roles to play in promoting and supporting human development.

The Healthy People 2020 initiative in the United States and the United Nations' Millennium Development Goals (MDGs) initiative provide frameworks for making and monitoring progress in reducing social injustice as it affects public health. The MDGs include eradicating extreme poverty and hunger; promoting gender equality and empowering women; reducing childhood mortality; improving

---

BOX 1-2 ■ Science and Social Justice

Omar Khan and David MKI Liu

Social justice has been inextricably linked to public health in concept for many years. Unfortunately, it has not been consistently linked to public health in practice—perhaps due to scientific purism or to excessive reliance on "evidence-based public health." Social justice is seen too often simply as an idealistic concept.

How can public health incorporate both science and social justice when these two seem to be informed by different sets of governing principles?

Requiring a certain level of scientific evidence before acting can threaten both public health and social justice. Human rights issues provide some insight. Was slavery in the United States a public health issue? Today we would say, "Most certainly!" But in the mid-1800s, the scientific evidence to link social justice and public health was not as clear as it is now. Still, common sense dictated that social injustice would adversely affect health.

Daily public health practice needs to be based on a balance of social justice and scientific evidence—in defining, evaluating, controlling, and preventing problems. This balance can be achieved by recognizing that social justice is simply the milieu, or context, in which all public health activities function. At the same time, public health workers depend on science for performing these activities. We, as public health workers, need to harmonize science and social justice if we are not only to do things right, but also choose to do the right things.

We need to develop a set of philosophical and practical mental models that allow us to denounce social injustice without pondering whether it is "scientific"—or not—to do so. We suggest, below, four ways of developing and evaluating these mental models. These models could be used to assess public health policies—considering both their scientific basis and their relationships to social justice (and human rights).

1. *International human rights law, both directly in the Right to Health and indirectly in associated rights.*

The Right to Health, according to the World Health Organization (WHO), is "the right of everyone to the enjoyment of the highest attainable standard of physical and mental health"—defined as a "state of complete physical, mental, and social well-being, and not merely the absence of disease or infirmity."[1] The Right to Health is a broad human right, including or linked to rights related to housing, education, nutrition, employment, and environment. Sources of this right include (a) United Nations General Assembly resolutions; (b) decisions of the International Court of Justice and other similar bodies, such as the courts of the Organization of American States and the European Union; and (c) decisions of U.S. courts and other national courts in interpreting international law. In addition to supplying means of assessing social justice, international human rights law can also promote implementation of interventions based on social injustice—since human rights law has potential power over governments and non-state actors.[2]

2. *The rights described in the Universal Declaration of Human Rights, the WHO Constitution, the International Covenant on Civil and Political Rights, and other instruments of international law.*

These instruments, beginning with the Universal Declaration of Human Rights in 1948, have defined human rights, including rights related to health, education, housing, income, political participation, and a clean and healthy environment. As with scientific evidence, these rights have evolved—and continue to evolve— over time. And the vast majority of public health workers are familiar with, and accept, these instruments of international law. (See Chapter 27.)

3. The work of the WHO Commission on Social Determinants of Health (CSDH).[3]

The CSDH has demonstrated that social injustice increases morbidity and mortality. Its work relies on an extensive body of scientific literature on the linkage between social determinants of health and health disparities—and the mechanisms of this linkage. Of critical importance, the CSDH has demonstrated how social injustice and its resultant health outcomes represent a direct violation of human rights. (See Chapters 2 and 22.) The CSDH has recommended that practitioners "measure the problem, evaluate action, expand the knowledge base, develop a workforce that is trained in the social determinants of health, and raise public awareness about the social determinants of health."[3] Research is extending the CSDH analyses and recommendations.

4. The work of professional organizations.[4]

Organizations of public health workers can help to assess social injustice and develop and implement policy resolutions to address social injustice. The interplay between evidence-based public health and social justice is complex, but necessary for public health workers to address. Concepts and principles of international law enable public health workers to understand and to reconcile science and social justice in order to promote and protect the public's health.

Box References

1. World Health Organization. Constitution of the World Health Organization. Geneva: WHO, 1946. Available at: http://apps.who.int/gb/bd/PDF/bd47/EN/constitution-en.pdf. Accessed on July 10, 2012.
2. Venkatapuram S, Bell R, Marmot M. The right to sutures: Social epidemiology, human rights, and social justice. *Health and Human Rights* 2010;12:3–16.
3. Commission on Social Determinants of Health. Closing the gap in a generation: Health equity through action on the social determinants of health. Final Report of the Commission on Social Determinants of Health. Geneva: World Health Organization, 2008. Available at http://www.who.int/social_determinants/thecommission/finalreport/en/index.html Accessed on March 18, 2013.
4. Khan OA, Liu K, Lichtveld M, Bancroft E. Synergism of science and social justice. *Am J Publ Health* 2012;102:388–389.

maternal and reproductive health; combating HIV/AIDS, malaria, and other infectious diseases; ensuring environmental sustainability; and establishing a global partnership for development. (See Table 21–7 in Chapter 21, and Chapter 29.)

We believe that the ultimate remedy for social injustice and its adverse effects on health lies in the development, adoption, and implementation of policies and programs that promote social justice and protect individuals and communities from social injustice. Therefore, we believe that advocacy for these policies and programs is the most critical component of an agenda for social justice and public health. Ultimately, what is needed to reduce social injustice is the popular and political will to address its root causes. Primary goals of public health are to help develop this popular and political will and to use it to help reduce social injustice.

■ REFERENCES

1. Institute of Medicine. The future of public health. Washington, DC: National Academy Press, 1988.
2. Beauchamp DE. Public health as social justice (invited paper). *J Inquiry* 1976;XII:3–13.
3. U.S. Department of Health and Human Services. Healthy People 2020: Access to health services. Available at: http://www.healthypeople.gov/2020/topicsobjectives2020/overview.aspx?topicid=1. Accessed December 21, 2012.
4. The World Bank. Life expectancy at birth, female (years). Available at: http://data.worldbank.org/indicator/SP.DYN.LE00.FE.IN. Accessed January 3, 2013.
5. Broder S. Progress and challenges in the National Cancer Program. In: Brugge J, Curran T, Harlow E, McCormick F, eds. Origins of human cancer: A comprehensive review. Plainview, NY: Cold Spring Harbor Laboratory Press, 1991:27–33.
6. Ortiz I, Cummins M. Global inequality: Beyond the bottom billion—A rapid review of income distribution in 141 countries. New York: United Nations Children's Fund, 2011.
7. Stiglitz JE. The price of inequality: How today's divided society endangers our future. New York: W. W. Norton, 2012.
8. Dreier P. The 100 greatest Americans of the 20th century: A social justice hall of fame. New York: Nation Books, 2012.

■ APPENDIX TO CHAPTER 1: UNIVERSAL DECLARATION OF HUMAN RIGHTS

On December 10, 1948, the General Assembly of the United Nations adopted and proclaimed the Universal Declaration of Human Rights, the full text of which appears below. It then called upon all member countries to publicize the text of the Declaration and "to cause it to be disseminated, displayed, read and expounded principally in schools and other educational institutions, without distinction based on the political status of countries or territories."

Preamble

Whereas recognition of the inherent dignity and of the equal and inalienable rights of all members of the human family is the foundation of freedom, justice and peace in the world,

Whereas disregard and contempt for human rights have resulted in barbarous acts which have outraged the conscience of mankind, and the advent of a world in which human beings shall enjoy freedom of speech and belief and freedom from fear and want has been proclaimed as the highest aspiration of the common people,

Whereas it is essential, if man is not to be compelled to have recourse, as a last resort, to rebellion against tyranny and oppression, that human rights should be protected by the rule of law,

Whereas it is essential to promote the development of friendly relations between nations,

Whereas the peoples of the United Nations have in the Charter reaffirmed their faith in fundamental human rights, in the dignity and worth of the human person and in the equal rights of men and women and have determined to promote social progress and better standards of life in larger freedom,

Whereas Member States have pledged themselves to achieve, in co-operation with the United Nations, the promotion of universal respect for and observance of human rights and fundamental freedoms,

Whereas a common understanding of these rights and freedoms is of the greatest importance for the full realization of this pledge,

Now, therefore, the General Assembly proclaims this Universal Declaration of Human Rights as a common standard of achievement for all peoples and all nations, to the end that every individual and every organ of society, keeping this Declaration constantly in mind, shall strive by teaching and education to promote respect for these rights and freedoms and by progressive measures, national and international, to secure their universal and effective recognition and observance, both among the peoples of Member States themselves and among the peoples of territories under their jurisdiction.

Article 1

All human beings are born free and equal in dignity and rights. They are endowed with reason and conscience and should act towards one another in a spirit of brotherhood.

Article 2

Everyone is entitled to all the rights and freedoms set forth in this Declaration, without distinction of any kind, such as race, color, sex, language, religion, political or other opinion, national or social origin, property, birth or other status. Furthermore, no distinction shall be made on the basis of the political, jurisdictional or international status of the country or territory to which a person belongs, whether it be independent, trust, non-self-governing or under any other limitation of sovereignty.

Article 3

Everyone has the right to life, liberty and security of person.

Article 4

No one shall be held in slavery or servitude; slavery and the slave trade shall be prohibited in all their forms.

Article 5

No one shall be subjected to torture or to cruel, inhuman or degrading treatment or punishment.

Article 6

Everyone has the right to recognition everywhere as a person before the law.

Article 7

All are equal before the law and are entitled without any discrimination to equal protection of the law. All are entitled to equal protection against any discrimination in violation of this Declaration and against any incitement to such discrimination.

Article 8

Everyone has the right to an effective remedy by the competent national tribunals for acts violating the fundamental rights granted him by the constitution or by law.

Article 9

No one shall be subjected to arbitrary arrest, detention or exile.

Article 10

Everyone is entitled in full equality to a fair and public hearing by an independent and impartial tribunal, in the determination of his rights and obligations and of any criminal charge against him.

Article 11

(1) Everyone charged with a penal offence has the right to be presumed innocent until proved guilty according to law in a public trial at which he has had all the guarantees necessary for his defense. (2) No one shall be held guilty of any penal offence on account of any act or omission which did not constitute a penal offence, under national or international law, at the time when it was committed nor shall a heavier penalty be imposed than the one that was applicable at the time the penal offence was committed.

Article 12

No one shall be subjected to arbitrary interference with his privacy, family, home or correspondence, nor to attacks upon his honor and reputation. Everyone has the right to the protection of the law against such interference or attacks.

Article 13

(1) Everyone has the right to freedom of movement and residence within the borders of each state. (2) Everyone has the right to leave any country, including his own, and to return to his country.

Article 14

(1) Everyone has the right to seek and to enjoy in other countries asylum from persecution. (2) This right may not be invoked in the case of prosecutions genuinely arising from non-political crimes or from acts contrary to the purposes and principles of the United Nations.

Article 15

(1) Everyone has the right to a nationality. (2) No one shall be arbitrarily deprived of his nationality nor denied the right to change his nationality.

Article 16

(1) Men and women of full age, without any limitation due to race, nationality or religion, have the right to marry and to found a family. They are entitled to equal rights as to marriage, during marriage and at its dissolution. (2) Marriage shall be entered into only with the free and full consent of the intending spouses. (3) The family is the natural and fundamental group unit of society and is entitled to protection by society and the State.

Article 17

(1) Everyone has the right to own property alone as well as in association with others. (2) No one shall be arbitrarily deprived of his property.

Article 18

Everyone has the right to freedom of thought, conscience and religion; this right includes freedom to change his religion or belief, and freedom, either alone or in community with others and in public or private, to manifest his religion or belief in teaching, practice, worship and observance.

Article 19

Everyone has the right to freedom of opinion and expression; this right includes freedom to hold opinions without interference and to seek, receive and impart information and ideas through any media and regardless of frontiers.

Article 20

(1) Everyone has the right to freedom of peaceful assembly and association. (2) No one may be compelled to belong to an association.

Article 21

(1) Everyone has the right to take part in the government of his country, directly or through freely chosen representatives. (2) Everyone has the right to equal access to public service in his country. (3) The will of the people shall be the basis of the authority of government; this shall be expressed in periodic and genuine elections which shall be by universal and equal suffrage and shall be held by secret vote or by equivalent free voting procedures.

Article 22

Everyone, as a member of society, has the right to social security and is entitled to realization, through national effort and international co-operation and in accordance with the organization and resources of each State, of the economic, social and cultural rights indispensable for his dignity and the free development of his personality.

Article 23

(1) Everyone has the right to work, to free choice of employment, to just and favorable conditions of work and to protection against unemployment. (2) Everyone, without any discrimination, has the right to equal pay for equal work. (3) Everyone who works has the right to just and favorable remuneration ensuring for himself and his family an existence worthy of human dignity, and supplemented, if necessary, by other means of social protection. (4) Everyone has the right to form and to join trade unions for the protection of his interests.

Article 24

Everyone has the right to rest and leisure, including reasonable limitation of working hours and periodic holidays with pay.

Article 25

(1) Everyone has the right to a standard of living adequate for the health and well-being of himself and of his family, including food, clothing, housing and medical care and necessary social services, and the right to security in the event of unemployment, sickness, disability, widowhood, old age or other lack of livelihood in circumstances beyond his control. (2) Motherhood and childhood are entitled to special care and assistance. All children, whether born in or out of wedlock, shall enjoy the same social protection.

Article 26

(1) Everyone has the right to education. Education shall be free, at least in the elementary and fundamental stages. Elementary education shall be compulsory. Technical and professional education shall be made generally available and higher education shall be equally accessible to all on the basis of merit. (2) Education shall be directed to the full development of the human personality and to the strengthening of respect for human rights and fundamental freedoms. It shall promote understanding, tolerance and friendship among all nations, racial or religious groups, and shall further the activities of the United Nations for the maintenance of peace. (3) Parents have a prior right to choose the kind of education that shall be given to their children.

Article 27

(1) Everyone has the right freely to participate in the cultural life of the community, to enjoy the arts and to share in scientific advancement and its benefits. (2) Everyone has the right to the protection of the moral and material interests resulting from any scientific, literary or artistic production of which he is the author.

Article 28

Everyone is entitled to a social and international order in which the rights and freedoms set forth in this Declaration can be fully realized.

Article 29

(1) Everyone has duties to the community in which alone the free and full development of his personality is possible. (2) In the exercise of his rights and freedoms, everyone shall be subject only to such limitations as are determined by law solely for the purpose of securing due recognition and respect for the rights and freedoms of others and of meeting the just requirements of morality, public order and the general welfare in a democratic society. (3) These rights and freedoms may in no case be exercised contrary to the purposes and principles of the United Nations.

Article 30

Nothing in this Declaration may be interpreted as implying for any State, group or person any right to engage in any activity or to perform any act aimed at the destruction of any of the rights and freedoms set forth herein.

PART II

How Social Injustice Affects the Health of Specific Population Groups

2 Socioeconomically Disadvantaged People

■ MICHAEL MARMOT AND RUTH BELL

▓ INTRODUCTION

In many of the rich countries of the world, social inequalities in health have been increasing. This has happened at the same time as overall health has improved. National data from England and Wales have shown that although life expectancy improved for each social class between the 1970s and the late 1990s, it improved most for those initially in the highest social class.[1] As a result, the gap in life expectancy between the bottom and top social classes increased. And inequalities in life expectancy have continued to widen in Great Britain in the 2000s[1-3] (Figure 2–1). Similar changes have occurred in many European countries.[4-6] Widening socioeconomic inequalities in life expectancy have also occurred in the United States[7-10] (Figure 2–2).

Why is this relevant to social injustice? If differences in health among social groups were an inevitable consequence of the stratification that comes from living in different social groups, we might comment on it, but we might not regard it as unjust. But as overall health improves, inequalities in health can change—even during a relatively short period of time. Such inequalities are therefore unlikely to be inevitable. If they are not inevitable and if we can do something about them, they *are* unjust.[11]

Inequality in the conditions under which people live and work translates into inequalities in health. Inequality in these circumstances is unjust. To take action against the circumstances that determine ill health, we need a better understanding of what they are and how they come about.

▓ SOCIOECONOMIC DISADVANTAGE IS MORE THAN LOW INCOME

One could equate "socioeconomic disadvantage" with poverty and poverty with lack of money. Socioeconomic disadvantage does indeed imply lack of money, but it also implies more. One cannot understand the relation between socioeconomic disadvantage and health by focusing solely on money or material disadvantage. Other disadvantages are associated with socioeconomic position, and these are crucial for health. Amartya Sen, an Indian economist who won the 1998 Nobel Prize in Economic Science for his contributions to welfare

(a)

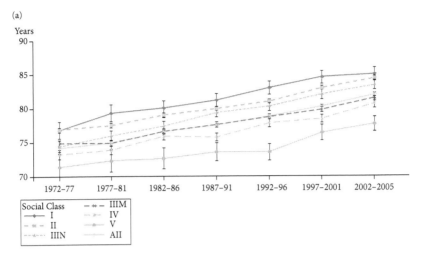

(b)

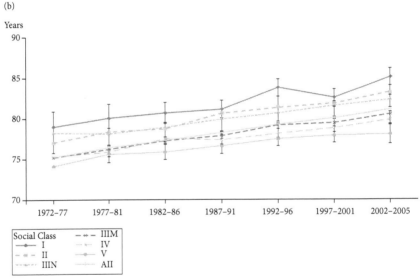

Figure 2-1 Trends in life expectancy at birth by social class, (a) males and (b) females, England and Wales, 1972–2005. Note: IIIN and IIIM are occupational classifications: N = Non-manual and M = Manual. (*Source*: Office for National Statistics. Trends in life expectancy by social class 1972–2005. London: Office for National Statistics, 2007.)

economics and social choice theory and for his interest in the problems of society's poorest members, was a pioneer in the use of the concept of *capabilities*. He observed that it is not so much what one has that is important, but rather what one can do with what one has.[12] Social inequalities in health may be a consequence of inequalities in capabilities.

In considering socioeconomic disadvantage or poverty, there is no sharp dividing line between "the poor" and "the non-poor." Many countries set a

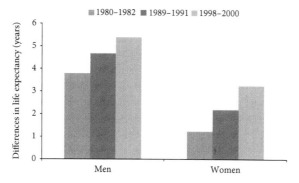

Figure 2-2 Inequalities in life expectancy at birth between the least-deprived and the most-deprived areas, United States, 1980–2000. (*Source*: Singh GK, Siahpush M. Widening socioeconomic inequalities in U.S. life expectancy, 1980–2000. *Int J Epidemiol* 2006;35: 969–979.)

threshold level of income for "poverty." Below it, people are considered to be poor, and above it, not poor. A fixed threshold is useful insofar as one can then calculate the prevalence of poverty and make comparisons over time and among countries. However, a limitation of using a fixed threshold is that there are degrees of socioeconomic disadvantage. Similarly, there are degrees of social inequalities in health—the lower one's social position, the higher one's risk of ill health.

To understand the important, but not comprehensive, role played by money in generating inequalities in health, consider these two crucial distinctions: (a) The importance of income for health depends on how much—or how little—money individuals or populations have, as described below. (b) Income or wealth of individuals has to be distinguished from income or wealth of populations.

■ INCOME MATTERS IF YOU HAVE LITTLE OF IT

If individuals or populations have little money, a small increase may make a big difference. Internationally, at low incomes, there is a strong association between per-capita gross national product (GNP) and life expectancy—much of it due to the inverse association between GNP and infant and child mortality. For example, in Sierra Leone, the mortality of children under age 5 is about 192 per 1,000 live births. This contrasts with Sweden and Japan, where the infant mortality rate and the under-5 child mortality rate are each approximately 3 per 1,000 live births.[13] Extreme poverty is related to extreme bad health. The disparities in health between rich and poor countries represent a gross abuse of human rights (Chapter 22).[14] However, this situation can be changed; investment in public services and poverty relief in poor countries leads to a major improvement in health.[15]

The remainder of this chapter addresses socioeconomic differences in health within the richer countries of the world.

■ WITHOUT MATERIAL DEPRIVATION, ABSOLUTE INCOME MATTERS LESS

Among richer countries, differences in absolute income appear to be less important than among poorer countries. Among richer countries, there is no relationship between national income, as measured by gross domestic product per capita (GDP*) and life expectancy (Table 2–1).[13] For example, although the United States ranks sixth in per-capita GDP—behind Qatar, Luxembourg, the United Arab Emirates, Norway, and Singapore—it ranks 35th in life expectancy among countries.[16] People in Greece, Malta, Cyprus, and Portugal—all countries with a per-capita GDP less than $30,000—have a longer average life expectancy than people in the United States. Portugal, with a per-capita GDP of about $21,000, has a longer life expectancy than the United States, which has nearly twice the national income of Portugal. Once a country has solved its basic material conditions for good health, more money does not necessarily buy better health.[17]

TABLE 2–1 *Life Expectancy at Birth and Per-Capita Gross Domestic Product (GDP) in Constant International Dollars, Adjusted for Purchasing Power, Selected Countries*

Country	Life Expectancy at Birth (2011)	Per Capita GDP (2009)
Japan	83.4	$29,692
Switzerland	82.3	36,954
Australia	81.9	34,259
Italy	81.9	26,578
Israel	81.6	25,474
France	81.5	29,578
Sweden	81.4	32,314
Spain	81.4	27,066
Norway	81.1	47,676
Singapore	81.1	45,978
Canada	81.0	34,567
Netherlands	80.7	36,358
New Zealand	80.7	24,706
Ireland	80.6	36,278
Germany	80.4	32,255
United Kingdom	80.2	32,147
Greece	79.9	26,482
Malta	79.6	21,987
Cyprus	79.6	25,759
Portugal	79.5	21,370
Costa Rica	79.3	10,085
Cuba	79.1	Not available
United States	78.5	41,761

(*Source:* United Nations Development Programme, International Human Development Indicators. Available at: http://hdrstats.undp.org/en/indicators/default.html. Accessed on October 10, 2012.)

* Gross domestic product is adjusted for purchasing power in order to make the "meaning" of a dollar comparable among countries.

Life expectancy in Costa Rica (79.3 years) is higher than in the United States (78.5 years), despite Costa Ricans having one-fourth the purchasing power of Americans. Cuba is another example of a low-income country that has achieved higher life expectancy (79.1 years) than the United States.

All of the countries listed in Table 2–1 have low infant and child mortality rates—an indication that none of them has the severe material deprivation seen in such poor countries as Sierra Leone. In the United States, for example, infant mortality is about 7 per 1,000 live births.[7]

Nevertheless, socioeconomic disadvantage continues to adversely affect health in the United States and other rich countries. While there are relatively small differences in infant mortality rate by socioeconomic disadvantage in these countries, there are substantial differences in life expectancy between socioeconomic groups. For example, there is a 7.3-year gap in life expectancy between the lowest and highest social classes in England and Wales (Figure 2–1). Measures of ill health in these countries also show a socioeconomic gradient. For example, in England, with increasing age, there is a stepwise association between low wealth and poor health (Figure 2–3)[18]; the lower one's wealth, the worse is one's health. For all groups, ill health increases with age; however, the level of ill health for those in the top quintile of wealth in the 70–74 age group is less (they are healthier) than the level of ill health for those in the bottom quintile in the 50–54 age group. If one substituted income for wealth in Figure 2–3, one would obtain similar findings.

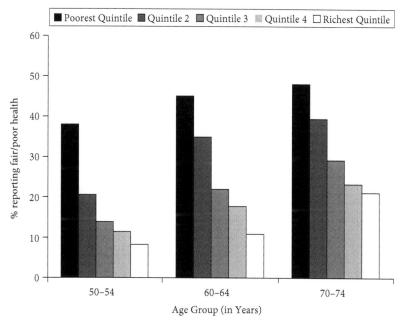

Figure 2–3 Self-reported health, by total wealth quintile. (*Source*: The English Longitudinal Study of Ageing. University College London and the Institute for Fiscal Studies.)

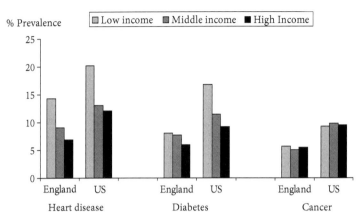

Figure 2-4 Health differences between England and the United States, 55- to 64-year-olds, by level of income. (*Source*: Banks J, Marmot M, Oldfield Z, Smith JP. Disease and disadvantage in the United States and in England. *JAMA* 2006;295:2037–2045.)

A study comparing the health of men and women age 55 to 64 in the United States and England demonstrated the social gradient in health in both countries and showed higher illness rates in the United States than in England at every point along the scale of income (Figure 2–4) or education.[19] The largest difference was in diabetes, with U.S. rates twice as high as those in England (Figure 2–4).

There appears to be a paradox: Among the rich countries, national income is not related to health or life expectancy. However, within a rich country, there is a strong relationship between measures of socioeconomic status and health. Therefore, in rich countries, where the problems of absolute material deprivation have been solved, it is not so much absolute level of income or wealth that matters for health. What matters is a person's position within the social hierarchy. Let us examine which features of socioeconomic position are important for health.

▨ AT HIGHER LEVELS OF INCOME, RELATIVE POSITION REMAINS IMPORTANT

A focus on the "haves" and "have-nots" leads to concern with those toward the bottom of any hierarchy or with those who are socially excluded. The social gradient in health, however, runs all the way from the top to the bottom of society. The Whitehall studies of British civil servants* found a social gradient in health and disease, in which those second from the top had worse health than those at the top.[20,21] One could not describe those second from the top

---

* The first Whitehall study, of 17,530 civil servants, examined their mortality recorded over 10 years according to employment grade. Whitehall II studied social and occupational influences on health and illness. The Whitehall II cohort comprised 10,308 civil servants (men and women) 35 to 55 years of age working in the London offices of 20 Whitehall departments from 1985 to 1988. The study continues to investigate the determinants of health.

as socioeconomically disadvantaged, yet the social gradient in health includes them. This phenomenon is not confined to British civil servants. In Sweden, for example, men with a doctoral degree had a lower mortality rate than those with a master's degree or professional qualification, even after adjusting for income.[22]

■ THE IMPACT OF SOCIAL INJUSTICE ON THE SOCIOECONOMICALLY DISADVANTAGED

"Modern" Impoverishment

Over the past 100 years, life in poverty in richer countries has changed. For example, in the early 20th century, "poverty" in Great Britain meant living in damp, cold, crowded houses, with poor sanitation, unclean water, and lack of nutrition. It meant working in dusty, hazardous workplaces in physically demanding occupations. These living and working conditions explained the high mortality rate of children and the high incidence of chronic respiratory disease in adults. This is no longer the typical picture of poverty in Great Britain. For example, a lower-status civil servant in Great Britain said about her earlier work:[17]

> I went to the typing pool, and sat there typing documents. Which was absolutely soul destroying. The fact that we could eat sweets and smoke was absolute heaven, but we were not allowed to talk.

About her life after retirement, although she had a "reasonable" occupational pension, but not the resources to engage in a meaningful retirement, she said:

> I've got used to my own company.... I do find the week-ends a bugger.... I've got no incentive.... I sit and read the paper...and breakfast at 10:30. If you sit watching TV in the afternoon...I'm at rock bottom.

Her statements demonstrate what "poverty" means for people not at the bottom of the social hierarchy. For those closer to the bottom, there may be no work and no social isolation—but life in disordered circumstances.

A young man living in an impoverished neighborhood in the north of England said:[17]

> I trust my work mates more than my close mates. I've experienced what they've done with each other, I've watched as they've slagged each other off to me and I think, you know, I'll not say anything to this guy 'cos he'll go and tell him, so I just keep it hush hush, I don't tell 'em much.

> I'd never trust anyone else, not in this area. A lot are drug dealers who would rob you, it's as simple as that, they would do anything to get in your house. They would backstab you. They will just turn around and rob you.

How do the circumstances of impoverished lives lead to poor health when people have enough to eat, do not drink contaminated water, have adequate shelter, and are not dying very much of infectious disease?

Early Life

David Barker, a physician and clinical epidemiologist, has demonstrated the importance of early life for the risk of diseases in adulthood. He described the long-term effects of exposure during a critical period of development. He showed that height and thinness of children at birth and at 1 year of age predict diabetes, hypertension, and heart disease in adulthood[23]—presumably due to maternal and child malnutrition, which, in turn, are likely to be associated with low social position of mothers. He and his colleagues showed that thinness at birth* and low social position in adulthood were associated with an increased risk of heart disease; adult socioeconomic position was more strongly related to heart disease if people had also had a low birthweight.[24]

There are at least two other ways in which social and environmental circumstances, starting in childhood, can affect one's adult risk of disease: (a) the pathway effect, and (b) the accumulation of advantage and disadvantage. The pathway effect emphasizes that it is not the circumstances of early life *per se* that increase risk of disease in adulthood, but rather that circumstances in childhood shape trajectories throughout life, leading to circumstances in adulthood that affect adult risk. Concerning accumulation of disadvantage, the effects of poor nutrition, infections, and psychosocial exposures at different points in life may accumulate to increase the risk of disease in adulthood.[25] The strong association between education and disease in adulthood may reflect both pathway and cumulative effects. Indeed, in order to understand the impact of socioeconomic disadvantage on adult disease, circumstances throughout the entire life span need to be considered.[26–28]

One way to understand the effects of early life is to study adult height. In the Whitehall studies, taller height in men was associated with higher employment grade.[29] On average, men in the top employment grades were 5 cm taller than men in the bottom grades. A similar pattern is present in the United States.[30] Heights of individuals are clearly related to genetic inheritance. Heights of groups, however, are far more likely to be related to nutritional status at birth, during childhood, and during adolescence—all of which are associated with socioeconomic circumstances.

In the Whitehall studies, short height was a strong predictor of adult coronary heart disease.[31,32] The additive effects of short height and adult social position on increasing the risk of coronary heart disease suggest that social circumstances of both childhood and adulthood make important contributions to risk of adult disease.

Medical Care

Equity in health care can be viewed as equal access for equal need. In theory, lack of utilization of health care could be related to lack of access or, conversely,

---

* Thinness at birth is assessed by measures of length from crown to heel and birthweight.

to personal disinclination to use health care that cannot be attributed to lack of access.[33] "Inequity" is a reasonable description of lack of access that results from circumstances beyond an individual's control. However, since disinclination to use health care can also be attributed to social, cultural, or educational barriers, utilization of health care can reasonably be used as a proxy for lack of access.

When considering social inequities in health care as a contributor to social inequalities in health, there is a striking contrast between Great Britain and the United States. In Great Britain, the entire population has access to the National Health Service, which provides care independent of ability to pay. In the U.S. system, over 49 million people do not have health insurance[34] and, therefore, have less access to health care.* With access to Medicare starting at age 65, differential access is markedly reduced in older people. Generalizations like these do not reveal the patterns of inequity in relation to need that occur. Equity of access in theory differs from equity of access in practice.

In Great Britain, the pattern of access in relation to need is a mixed picture[35]— partly due to problems in defining "need." If need for health care is defined as "capacity to benefit from that care," then people with terminal cancers may have no "need" for curative treatment since they have no capacity to benefit from it. In contrast, people with less advanced cancers have the capacity to benefit from health care and, therefore, have greater "need" for health care. In practice, health status is taken as a measure of need.

In Great Britain, most studies show that people of lower socioeconomic status (SES) have higher rates of health service utilization than people of higher SES. But they have greater need. When adjusted for need, the results seem to depend on the type of need. Use of general practitioner services is broadly equitable. For emergency hospital admissions, people of lower SES seem to have rates proportional to need. For elective procedures and those involving preventive care, people of lower SES are underserved, according to an article published in 2007.[35] An article that was published in 2012, which analyzed reforms of the British National Health Service between 2000 and 2009, reported no substantial improvement in socioeconomic equity in use of hospital-based services.[36]

Health care access by income level has been reviewed comprehensively by the U.S. Agency for Healthcare Research and Quality.[37] It found that the lower the income, the less satisfactory is entry to the health care system, as reflected by: (a) no or inadequate health insurance, (b) no specific source of ongoing care, and/or (c) difficulties in obtaining care. It also found that low income is associated with (a) reports of poor communication with health care personnel, and (b) less likelihood of having had blood pressure or serum cholesterol checked as part of preventive health care.

Disparities in health care may appear to be greater in the United States than in Great Britain. In both countries, however, there are large socioeconomic differences in health, which cannot easily be attributed to lack of access to high-quality

* The number of people in the United States without health insurance and less access to health care will decrease with the implementation of the Patient Protection and Affordable Care Act.

medical care since these differences are seen for both onset of new disease and treatment of existing disease. Where inequities in health care exist, they are a further cause of morbidity among people with low SES.

Lifestyle and Its Effects

It is common to refer to the diseases that affect people in rich countries as "diseases of affluence" and, in turn, attribute them to lifestyle factors, such as smoking, poor diet, and sedentary habits. This is misleading for two reasons. First, the major causes of morbidity and mortality in rich countries affect socioeconomically disadvantaged people to a greater extent than they affect those who are more affluent. Second, to think of lifestyle as something freely chosen provides little insight into why relevant health behaviors follow a social gradient.

How much of the social gradient in health and disease does "lifestyle" explain? And why should there even be a social gradient in lifestyle? Consider cigarette smoking, which becomes much more prevalent as one descends the social hierarchy.[38] In studies of British civil servants, smoking accounted for about one-fourth of the social gradient in coronary heart disease.[39,40] Explanations for the social gradient in smoking have been unsatisfactory. It has been suggested that people of low SES are more oriented to the present than the future, and hence are less likely to take actions that will lead to future health benefits—although it is unclear why this should be. Smoking by women can be associated with problems in their lives due to precarious social and economic circumstances.[41,42]

Smoking cigarettes makes no economic sense because it costs the smoker money and leads to worse health. In contrast, the cost of food may help explain the high rate of obesity among low-income people because eating energy-dense food may be a less expensive way to consume adequate calories. In the United States, there is an inverse association between the energy density of foods (in calories per kilogram) and energy cost (per calorie); that is, cheaper foods have more calories per weight. However, food items with high energy density usually have high levels of fat and added sugar.[43] Given that lower income means, among other things, lower expenditure on food, this pattern may help explain the link between low SES and obesity. The association between low SES and obesity is stronger among women than among men,[44] possibly because body weight is under stronger cognitive control in women with higher SES. The quality of diet is important in other ways. For example, higher SES is associated with greater consumption of fruits and vegetables, which reduces the risk of several diseases.

A contributor to SES differences in obesity is differences in level of physical activity. Higher SES is associated with more frequent participation in leisure-time physical activity.[45,46]

The Circumstances in Which People Live and Work

Employment and working conditions are important determinants of health status.[47] Unemployment, especially if it is long-term, is associated with increased risks of physical and mental disorders.[47] In Europe, the unemployment rate is higher among those with lower levels of educational attainment.[48] Insecure, precarious, and temporary employment conditions adversely affect health.[49-51]

Working environments are also important for health[52] and may play an important role in generating inequalities in health.[40] Associated with increased risk of cardiovascular disease are (a) jobs characterized by high psychological demand and low control, and (b) jobs that entail high effort and low rewards in terms of esteem, career opportunities, and financial remuneration. These aspects of work may be important links between SES and disease.[53] Psychosocial characteristics of work are related not only to cardiovascular disease,[54] but also to sickness absence, mental and physical functioning, mental illness, and musculoskeletal disorders.[55-58]

Socioeconomic characteristics of residential areas are associated with the health status of residents of these areas, even after taking into account individual characteristics.[59-63] Part of the explanation for this association appears to be social cohesion of neighborhoods.[64,65]

Physical exposures are also important. Lower SES means worse housing quality in ways that may damage health.[66] In addition to worse working and housing conditions, lower-income people are more likely to be exposed to residential crowding, hazardous wastes, ambient and indoor air pollutants, adverse water quality, and ambient noise.[67]

The Effects of the Economic Downturn

Following the global financial crisis and recession, unemployment in the United States and the United Kingdom increased from about 5 percent in early 2008 to about 8 percent in 2012.[68] Data from previous recessions indicates that economic downturns are associated with increased rates of suicide and attempted suicide, depression and other mental health problems, increased incidence of tuberculosis and HIV infection, and possibly other long-term effects on health.[69] For example, in England, between the start of the financial crisis in 2008 and 2010, there were 846 more suicides among men and 155 more among women than would have been expected based on historical trends.[70] Regions with the largest increases in unemployment experienced the largest increases in suicides.[70] The economic downturn in the United Kingdom since 2008 and austerity measures implemented in response to the debt crisis are likely to exacerbate health inequalities.[69] Low income, poor housing, and less favorable employment and working conditions contribute to poor health of socioeconomically disadvantaged people.[71] The health status of various groups in the population is a good indicator of how well macroeconomic and social policies are serving society.

Policy responses to economic problems in Europe have resulted in tightening public expenditures. Yet a body of evidence brought together by the European Review of Social Determinants of Health and the Health Divide shows that investment in the social determinants of health, including early child development, active labor market policies, social protection, housing, and the environment, will mitigate the adverse effects of the economic downturn on populations.[72] For example, an analysis of the historical association between social spending in 18 European countries and population health outcomes demonstrated an inverse association between social welfare spending and overall mortality.[73] Further modeling of the results showed that each additional $100 increase (adjusted for purchasing power parity) in social spending (including for health care) was associated with a 1.2 percent decrease in all-cause mortality.[73]

■ ROOT CAUSES AND UNDERLYING ISSUES

Social stratification, which is present in all societies, means unequal access to resources, unequal privileges, and unequal self-esteem. But current levels of social inequalities in health are not inevitable.

Fundamental human needs can be placed in the following interrelated categories: (a) health and its determinants, (b) autonomy or control over one's life, (c) opportunities for full social participation, (d) respect and self-respect, and (e) participation in culture.[17,74] Failure to meet needs for autonomy and social participation adversely affects health. Although social hierarchies are universal, the degree of inequality in meeting these needs varies and can constitute social injustice. This approach is closely linked to Amartya Sen's concept of "capabilities" or "freedoms."[75] Capabilities and freedoms are fundamental to health.

It is tempting to think that marked social and economic inequalities are due to unbridled markets seen in advanced capitalist countries. Indeed, there is evidence to support the view that income inequalities are not only tolerated, but also encouraged, in some capitalist countries more than in others. But it is not accurate to attribute these inequalities solely to markets. However, much of the accumulation of great wealth can be attributed to distortions of markets, such as monopolies.

The degree of income inequalities among the rich countries varies widely. According to data recorded by the World Bank, the top 10 percent of households in Japan, Sweden, the Netherlands, Norway, and Canada received less than 25 percent of total income, but in the United States and the United Kingdom they received almost 30 percent. And income differentials are growing in both countries.[76-79] Income inequalities were smaller within rich countries than within poor countries, such as Paraguay, Sierra Leone, and even Costa Rica, which has good health indicators (Table 2–2).[80] (See Figure 1–1 in Chapter 1.)

TABLE 2-2 *Percentage Share of Income Distribution of Top and Bottom 10 Percent of Households*

Country (Survey Year)	Bottom 10%	Top 10%
Japan (1993)	4.8	22
Sweden (2000)	3.6	22
Netherlands (1999)	2.5	23
Norway (2000)	3.9	23
Canada (2000)	2.6	25
France (1995)	2.8	25
Switzerland (2000)	2.9	26
Greece (2000)	2.5	26
Italy (2000)	2.3	27
United Kingdom (1999)	2.1	29
United States (2000)	1.9	30
Sierra Leone (2003)	2.6	34
Dominican Republic (2010)	1.8	36
Costa Rica (2009)	1.2	40
Paraguay (2010)	1.0	41

(Adapted from: The World Bank, World development indicators 2012. Washington, DC: The World Bank, 2012.)

There has been a vigorous debate as to whether income inequalities, *per se*, lead to worse health.[81-83] We do not need to review the arguments here to note that increasing income inequalities indicate increasing divisions in society. These are likely to be fundamental drivers of inequality in access to resources. In other words, inequality in income is likely to be correlated with inequality in meeting needs. Such inequalities are not inevitable but are, in part, a consequence of decisions taken as to how a society's economic and social affairs are organized.

There is a view that, for a society to be affluent, its wealth-producers have to be motivated to generate wealth—without being hampered by progressive taxation or other perceived restrictions. From this perspective, increasing economic inequalities are acceptable side effects, even if they lead to health inequalities. The view that growing income inequalities aid economic growth has been seriously questioned.[84] And it has been characterized as a myth convenient to the interests of those who benefit from inequalities.[85]

There is a case to be made that growing income and social inequalities damage social cohesion,[86] adversely affecting not only socioeconomically disadvantaged people, but everyone in society. A society that is more socially cohesive is likely to be a healthier society.

Concurrent with increased income inequalities is increasing geographic segregation of affluence and poverty, especially in the United States.[84] Increasingly, poor people live in neighborhoods with a high proportion of poor households, and affluent people live in neighborhoods that are exclusively affluent. Such residential segregation generally means services of low quality, more crime, and more civil disruption in poorer neighborhoods than in wealthier areas. In the United Kingdom, affluence and poverty also tend to be spatially segregated, and there is an increasing concentration of wealthy families in wealthy areas, and poor families in poor areas.[87,88]

Another fundamental cause of inequalities is disparities in education. Inequalities affecting today's adults are passed on via today's children to tomorrow's adults.[17] Disadvantage starts before birth and accumulates throughout life.[71] For example, parents' educational attainment is associated with their children's educational attainment, and parents' level of education is highly correlated with their children's literacy levels.[89] The higher the level of parents' education, the better their children perform (Figure 2–5).[90] The slope of this association varies; for example, it is much shallower in Sweden than it is in the United States. Family background matters, but so does the general environment of the country. Development of literacy is influenced by family background, quality of schools, and social capital of the area in which a person lives.[90] Robert Putnam, a professor of public policy at Harvard, defined *social capital* as "the connections among individuals—social networks and the norms of reciprocity and trustworthiness that arise from them."[86] In sum, various measures of education are strongly related to health.

Figure 2–5 presents a mechanism by which socioeconomic disadvantage is passed down from one generation to another. The degree of the intergenerational transmission varies among countries; for example, it is less in Sweden than in the United States.

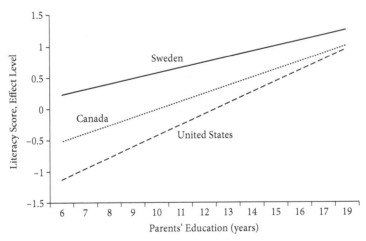

Figure 2–5 Literacy scores of people age 16 to 25, according to level of education of their parents, in the United States, Canada, and Sweden. (Adapted from: Willms JD. Statistics Canada: inequalities in literacy skills among youth in Canada and the United States. International Adult Literacy Survey No. 6, Reference period: September 1999. Adapted from Figure A Statistics Canada information is used with the permission of the Minister of Industry, as Minister responsible for Statistics Canada. Information on the availability of the wide range of data from Statistics Canada can be obtained from Statistics Canada's Regional Offices at http://www.statcan.ca, or its toll-free number, 800-263-1136.)

■ WHAT NEEDS TO BE DONE

Every society has a social hierarchy—even hunter-gatherer societies, which have been thought to be relatively egalitarian.[91] Societies with more complex forms of social organization have clearer hierarchies than others. Social hierarchies cannot be abolished. And history does not generate much enthusiasm for the type of communist governments in Central and Eastern Europe during the 20th century. The health records of these countries demonstrate that, during the 1970s and 1980s, these countries failed to meet human needs on a grand scale.[92,93]

Levels of health status and inequalities in health vary over time within countries and among countries. This gives reason to believe that health inequalities are not inevitable. But reducing health inequalities is challenging. Political will at the highest level is crucial, and a comprehensive set of policies involving multiple sectors is needed.[71,72]

Within the United Kingdom a series of initiatives have ensured that addressing health inequalities is a government priority. In 1997, the government initiated an independent inquiry into inequalities in health. (One of us, M.M., was a member of the scientific advisory group of that inquiry.[94]) The group concluded that health inequalities result from wider social and economic inequalities in society. It therefore recommended fundamental changes in societal attitudes to inequalities. Its 39 recommendations, only two of which were related to health care, included monitoring inequalities in health, evaluating the impact of policies and other measures to reduce health inequalities, increasing employment opportunities, and reducing poverty among women of childbearing age, expectant mothers, young children, and older people by increasing in-kind or cash benefits. It also recommended improving the provision and availability of healthy food, exercise facilities, and nicotine-replacement therapy for former smokers in economic need. The government implemented many of these recommendations.[95] It also made reduction in child poverty a major goal and established a new program focused on early child development.

In 2008, the U.K. government commissioned a strategic review of health inequalities, to take into account new evidence and the changing social and economic context. The review was chaired by one of us, M.M., and was known as the Marmot Review.[71] One aim of the review was to consider how the recommendations of the global Commission on Social Determinants of Health (CSDH) could be translated into the U.K. context.[96] The policy recommendations in the Marmot Review were organized under the following six policy objectives:[71]

1. Give every child the best start in life.
2. Enable all children, young people, and adults to maximize their capabilities and have control over their lives.
3. Create fair employment and good work for all.
4. Ensure a healthy standard of living for all.
5. Create and develop healthy and sustainable places and communities.
6. Strengthen the role and impact of ill health prevention.

The Marmot Review was well received by the central government and by local government authorities. In 2012, the Health and Social Care Act in England mandated unprecedented legal duties concerning health inequalities for the Secretary of State for Health, the National Health Service Commissioning Board, and, at the local level, Clinical Commissioning Groups.* These groups are required to integrate provision of health services in local areas with other health-related services and social care services. Local health and well-being boards have been established to ensure delivery of these services. Local officials are developing strategies, based on local needs, based on the six broad policy recommendations of the Marmot Review.

▇ CONCLUSION

Inequalities in health relate fundamentally to inequalities in society. Overall health and inequalities in health in a population are indicators of how successful a society is in meeting the needs of its members. There is no reason to believe that the health of today's disadvantaged groups could not improve, were that socioeconomic disadvantage to be relieved.

The fact that socioeconomic disadvantage is not relieved is a matter of social injustice. This is not to call for egalitarianism in the sense of everyone being the same—a hopeless and undesirable goal. It is, however, to suggest that society may benefit if our set of social arrangements were to move towards a situation where control over one's life and full social participation are more equitably distributed. Governments can help this occur by the way they channel resources to improve the conditions under which people live and work and in which our children develop and older people thrive.

▇ REFERENCES

1. Office for National Statistics. Trends in life expectancy by social class 1972–2005. London: ONS, 2007.
2. Office for National Statistics. Statistical bulletin: Trends in life expectancy by the National Statistics Socio-economic Classification 1982–2006. London: ONS, 2011.
3. Shaw M, Davey SG, Dorling D. Health inequalities and New Labour: How the promises compare with real progress. *BMJ* 2005;330:1016–1021.
4. Steingrimsdottir OA, Naess O, Moe JO, et al. Trends in life expectancy by education in Norway 1961–2009. *Eur J Epidemiol* 2012;27:163–171.
5. Tarkiainen L, Martikainen P, Laaksonen M, Valkonen T. Trends in life expectancy by income from 1988 to 2007: Decomposition by age and cause of death. *J Epidemiol Community Health* 2012;66:573–578.
6. Mackenbach JP, Bos V, Andersen O et al. Widening socioeconomic inequalities in mortality in six Western European countries. *Int J Epidemiol* 2003;32:830–837.

* Clinical Commissioning Groups are groups of general practitioners who, since April 2013, are responsible for designing local health services in England. They work with patients and health care professionals and in partnership with local communities and local government authorities.

7. National Center for Health Statistics. Health, United States, 2011: With special feature on socioeconomic status and health. Hyattsville, MD: National Center for Health Statistics, 2012.

8. Singh GK, Siahpush M. Widening socioeconomic inequalities in U.S. life expectancy, 1980–2000. *Int J Epidemiol* 2006;35:969–979.

9. Crimmins EM, Saito Y. Trends in healthy life expectancy in the United States, 1970–1990: Gender, racial, and educational differences. *Soc Sci Med* 2001;52:1629–1641.

10. Olshansky SJ, Antonucci T, Berkman L, et al. Differences in life expectancy due to race and educational differences are widening, and many may not catch up. *Health Aff (Millwood)* 2012;31:1803–1813.

11. Marmot M. Do inequalities matter? In: Daniels N, Kennedy B, Kawachi I, eds. Is inequality bad for our health? Boston: Beacon Press, 2000.

12. Sen A. Inequality reexamined. Oxford, England: Oxford University Press, 1992.

13. United Nations Development Programme. International human development indicators. 2012. Available at: http://hdrstats.undp.org/en/indicators/default.html. Accessed on October 10, 2012.

14. Farmer P. Pathologies of power: Health, human rights, and the new war on the poor. Berkeley, CA: University of California Press, 2003.

15. Anand S, Ravallion M. Human development in poor countries: On the role of private incomes and public services. *Journal of Economic Perspectives* 1993;7:133–150.

16. United Nations Development Programme. International human development indicators. 2011. Available at: http://hdrstats.undp.org/en/indicators/default.html. Accessed on October 10, 2012.

17. Marmot M. Status syndrome. London: Bloomsbury, 2004.

18. Marmot M, Banks J, Blundell R, et al. Health, wealth and lifestyles of the older population in England. The 2002 English longitudinal study of ageing. London: Institute for Fiscal Studies, 2003.

19. Banks J, Marmot M, Oldfield Z, Smith JP. Disease and disadvantage in the United States and in England. *JAMA* 2006;295:2037–2045.

20. Marmot MG, Shipley MJ. Do socioeconomic differences in mortality persist after retirement? 25-year follow up of civil servants from the first Whitehall study. *BMJ* 1996;313:1177–1180.

21. Marmot MG, Ryff C, Bumpass L, et al. Social inequalities in health: Next questions and converging evidence. *Soc Sci Med* 1997;44:901–910.

22. Erikson R. Why do graduates live longer? In: Jonsson JO, Mills C, eds. Cradle to grave: Life-course change in modern Sweden. Durham, England: Sociology Press, 2001.

23. Barker DJP. Mothers, babies and health in later life. Edinburgh, Scotland: Churchill Livingtone, 1998.

24. Barker D, Forsen T, Uutela A, et al. Size at birth and resilience to effects of poor living conditions in adult life: Longitudinal study. *BMJ* 2001;323:1273–1276.

25. Power C, Hertzman C. Social and biological pathways linking early life and adult disease. *Br Med Bull* 1997;53:210–221.

26. Kuh D, Ben-Shlomo Y. A life course approach to chronic disease epidemiology. 2nd ed. New York: Oxford University Press, 2004.

27. Kuh D, Hardy R. A life course approach to women's health. New York: Oxford University Press, 2003.

28. Davey Smith G (ed.). Health inequalities: Lifecourse approaches. Bristol, England: The Policy Press, 2003.

29. Marmot MG, Davey Smith G, Stansfeld SA, et al. Health inequalities among British civil servants: The Whitehall II study. *Lancet* 1991;337:1387–1393.
30. Komlos J, Baur M. From the tallest to (one of) the fattest: The enigmatic fate of the American population in the 20th century. *Economics and Human Biology* 2004;2:57–74.
31. Marmot MG, Shipley MJ, Rose G. Inequalities in death—Specific explanations of a general pattern. *Lancet* 1984;323:1003–1006.
32. Marmot M, Shipley M, Brunner E, Hemingway H. Relative contribution of early life and adult socioeconomic factors to adult morbidity in the WII [Whitehall II] study. *J Epidemiol Community Health* 2001;55:301–307.
33. Dixon A, Le Grand J, Henderson J, et al. Is the NHS equitable? A review of the evidence. London: The London School of Economics and Political Science. LSE Health and Social Care Discussion Paper Number 11, 2003.
34. Kaiser Commission on Medicaid and the Uninsured. Five facts about the uninsured. Washington DC: Kaiser Family Foundation, 2011.
35. Dixon A, Le GJ, Henderson J, et al. Is the British National Health Service equitable? The evidence on socioeconomic differences in utilization. *J Health Serv Res Policy* 2007;12:104–109.
36. Cookson R, Laudicella M, Li DP, Dusheiko M. Effects of the Blair/Brown NHS reforms on socioeconomic equity in health care. *J Health Serv Res Policy* 2012;17 (Suppl 1):55–63.
37. US Department of Health and Human Services. National healthcare disparities report. Rockville, MD: Agency for Healthcare Research and Quality, 2003.
38. Jarvis MJ, Wardle J. Social patterning of individual health behaviours: The case of cigarette smoking. In: Marmot MG, Wilkinson RG, eds. The Social Determinants of Health. Oxford, England: Oxford University Press, 1999:240–255.
39. van Rossum CTM, Shipley MJ, Van de Mheen H, et al. Employment grade differences in cause specific mortality. A 25-year follow up of civil servants from the first Whitehall study. *J Epidemiol Community Health* 2000;54:178–184.
40. Marmot M, Bosma H, Hemingway H, et al. Contribution of job control and other risk factors to social variations in coronary heart disease incidence. Whitehall II study. *Lancet* 1997;350:235–239.
41. Graham H, Hunt K. Socio-economic influences on women's smoking status in adulthood: Insights from the West Scotland Twenty-07 study. *Health Bulletin* 1998;56: 757–765.
42. Graham H. Hardship and health in women's lives. London: Harvester Wheatsheaf, 1993.
43. Drewnowski A, Specter SE. Poverty and obesity: The role of energy density and energy costs. *Am J Clin Nutr* 2004;79:6–16.
44. National Obesity Observatory. Adult obesity and socioeconomic status: Factsheet. 2012. Available at: http://www.noo.org.uk/uploads/doc/vid_16966_AdultSocio econSep2012.pdf. Accessed on October 10, 2012.
45. Marmot MG, Davey Smith G, Stansfeld SA, et al. Health inequalities among British civil servants: The Whitehall II study. *Lancet* 1991;337:1387–1393.
46. Joint Health Surveys Unit. Health survey for England, 1994. London: The Stationery Office, 1996.
47. Siegrist J, Benach J, McKnight A, et al. Final report of Task Group 2 for the strategic review of health inequalities in England: Employment arrangements, work conditions and health inequalities. London: Institute of Health Equity, 2009.

48. European Commission. Eurostat online database. 2012. Available at: http://epp.eurostat.ec.europa.eu/portal/page/portal/statistics/search_database.

49. Ferrie JE, Shipley MJ, Stansfeld SA, Marmot MG. Effects of chronic job insecurity and change in job security on self reported health, minor psychiatric morbidity, physiological measures, and health related behaviours in British civil servants: The Whitehall II study. *J Epidemiol Community Health* 2002;56:450–454.

50. Virtanen P, Vahtera J, Kivimaki M, et al. Employment security and health. *J Epidemiol Community Health* 2002;56:569–574.

51. Virtanen M, Kivimaki M, Joensuu M, et al. Temporary employment and health: A review. *Int J Epidemiol* 2005;34:610–622.

52. Marmot M, Siegrist J, Theorell T, Feeney A. Health and the psychosocial environment at work. In: Marmot M, Wilkinson RG, eds. Social Determinants of Health. Oxford, England: Oxford University Press, 1999:105–131.

53. Siegrist J, Marmot M. Health inequalities and the psychosocial environment—Two scientific challenges. *Social Science and Medicine* 2004;58:1463–1473.

54. Kivimaki M, Nyberg ST, Batty GD, et al. Job strain as a risk factor for coronary heart disease: A collaborative meta-analysis of individual participant data. *Lancet* 2012; doi:10.1016/S0140-6736(12)60994-5.

55. North F, Syme SL, Feeney A, et al. Explaining socioeconomic differences in sickness absence: The Whitehall II study. *BMJ* 1993;306:361–366.

56. Stansfeld S, Bosma H, Hemingway H, Marmot M. Psychosocial work characteristics and social support as predictors of SF-36 functioning: The Whitehall II study. *Psychosom Med* 1998;60:247–255.

57. Stansfeld SA, Fuhrer R, Head J, et al. Work and psychiatric disorder in the Whitehall II study. *J Psychosom Res* 1997;43:73–81.

58. Hemingway H, Shipley M, Stansfeld S, et al. Are risk factors for atherothrombotic disease associated with back pain sickness absence? The Whitehall II study. *J Epidemiol Community Health* 1999;53:197–203.

59. Marmot M. Inequalities in Health. *N Engl J Med* 2001;345:134–136.

60. Diez-Roux AV, Nieto FJ, Muntaner C, et al. Neighborhood environments and coronary heart disease: A multilevel analysis. *Am J Epidemiol* 1997;146:48–63.

61. MacIntyre S, Ellaway A, Cummins S. Place effects on health: How can we conceptualise, operationalise and measure them? *Soc Sci Med* 2002;55:125–139.

62. Diez-Roux A. Bringing context back into epidemiology: Variables and fallacies in multi-level analysis. *Am J Public Health* 1998;88:216–222.

63. Stafford M, Bartley M, Mitchell R, Marmot M. Characteristics of individuals and characteristics of areas: Investigating their influence on health in the Whitehall II study. *Health and Place* 2001;7:117–129.

64. Stafford M, Bartley M, Boreham R, et al. Neighbourhood social cohesion and health: Investigating associations and possible mechanisms. In: Morgan A, Swann C, eds. Social capital and health: Issues of definition, measurement and links to health. London: Health Development Agency, 2004:111–131.

65. Sampson RJ, Raudenbush SW, Earls F. Neighborhoods and violent crime: A multilevel study of collective efficacy. *Science* 1997;277:916–924.

66. Blane D, Mitchell R, Bartley M. The "inverse housing law" and respiratory health. *J Epidemiol Community Health* 2000;54:745–749.

67. Evans GW, Kantrowitz E. Socioeconomic status and health: The potential role of environmental risk exposure. *Annu Rev Public Health* 2002;23:303–331.

68. Office for National Statistics. International comparisons of employment and unemployment rates. 2012. Available at: http://www.ons.gov.uk/ons/publications/re-reference-tables.html?edition=tcm%3A77-222482. Accessed on October 10, 2012.

69. Institute of Health Equity. The impact of the economic downturn and policy changes on health inequalities in London. London: UCL Institute of Health Equity, 2012.

70. Barr B, Taylor-Robinson D, Scott-Samuel A, et al. Suicides associated with the 2008–2010 economic recession in England: Time trend analysis. *BMJ* 2012;345:e5142.

71. UCL Institute of Health Equity. Fair society, healthy lives (the Marmot review). London: Institute of Health Equity, 2010. Available at: http://www.instituteofhealthequity.org/projects/fair-society-healthy-lives-the-marmot-review. Accessed on October 10, 2012.

72. Marmot M, Allen J, Bell R, et al. WHO European review of social determinants of health and the health divide. *Lancet* 2012;380:1011–1029.

73. Stuckler D, Basu S, McKee M. Budget crises, health, and social welfare programmes. *BMJ* 2010;340:c3311.

74. Sennett R. Respect in a world of inequality. New York: W.W. Norton and Co., 2003.

75. Sen A. Development as freedom. New York: Alfred A. Knopf, 1999.

76. Saez E. Striking it richer: The evolution of top incomes in the United States (update with 2007 estimates). Berkeley, CA: UC Berkeley Institute for Research on Labor and Employment, 2009.

77. Hills J, Brewer M, Jenkins S, et al. An anatomy of economic inequality in the UK: Report of the National Equality Panel. London: Her Majesty's Government, 2010.

78. Organisation for Economic Co-operation and Development. Growing unequal? Income distribution and poverty in OECD countries. Paris: OECD, 2008.

79. Department of Work and Pensions. Households below average income: An analysis of the income distribution 1994/95–2009/10. Available at: http://research.dwp.gov.uk/asd/hbai/hbai2011/pdf_files/full_hbai12.pdf. Accessed on October 10, 2012.

80. World Bank. World development indicators 2012. Available at: http://issuu.com/world.bank.publications/docs/9780821389850. Accessed on October 10, 2012.

81. Wilkinson RG. Unhealthy societies: The afflictions of inequality. 1st ed. London: Routledge, 1996.

82. Wilkinson RG, Pickett KE. The spirit level: Why more equal societies almost always do better. London: Allen Lane, 2009.

83. Deaton A. Health, inequality, and economic development. *Journal of Economic Literature* 2003;41:113–158.

84. Kawachi I, Kennedy BP. The health of nations: Why inequality is harmful to your health. New York: The New Press, 2002.

85. Galbraith JK. The culture of contentment. 1st ed. London: Sinclair-Stevenson, 1992.

86. Putnam R. Bowling alone: The collapse and revival of American community. New York: Simon and Schuster, 2000.

87. Dorling D, Rigby J, Wheeler B, et al. Poverty, wealth and place in Britain 1968 to 2005. York, England: Joseph Rowntree Foundation, 2007.

88. Fenton A. Housing benefit reform and the spatial segregation of low-income households in London, 2011. Available at: http://www.cchpr.landecon.cam.ac.uk/outputs/detail.asp?Outp utID=240. Accessed on October 10, 2012.

89. Willms JD. Quality and inequality in children's literacy: The effects of families, schools and communities. In: Keating D, Hertzman C, eds. Developmental health and the

wealth of nations: Social, biological, and educational dynamics. New York: Guilford Press, 1999:72–93.

90. Willms JD. Inequalities in literacy skills among youth in Canada and the United States. (International Adult Literacy Survey No 6). Ottawa: Human Resources Development Canada and National Literacy Secretariat, 1999.

91. Erdal D, Whiten A. Egalitarianism and Machiavellian intelligence in human evolution. In: Mellars P, Gibson K, eds. Modelling the early human mind. Cambridge, England: McDonald Cambridge, 1996.

92. Bobak M, Marmot MG. East-West mortality divide and its potential explanations: Proposed research agenda. *BMJ* 1996;312:421–425.

93. Bobak M, Pikhart H, Rose R, et al. Socioeconomic factors, material inequalities, and perceived control in self-rated health: Cross-sectional data from seven post-communist countries. *Soc Sci Med* 2000;51:1343–1350.

94. Acheson D. Inequalities in health: Report of an independent inquiry. London: Her Majesty's Stationery Office, 1998.

95. Exworthy M, Stuart M, Blane D, Marmot M. Tackling health inequalities since the Acheson inquiry. Bristol, England: The Policy Press, 2003.

96. Marmot M, Friel S, Bell R, et al. Closing the gap in a generation: Health equity through action on the social determinants of health. *Lancet* 2008;372:1661–1669.

3 Racial and Ethnic Minorities

■ CAROL EASLEY ALLEN AND
CHERYL E. EASLEY

▓ INTRODUCTION

More than one-third of the people in the United States identify themselves as members of racial or ethnic minorities.[1,*] Many Americans who are members of these minority groups confront complex, historical, multifaceted disparities as they navigate the U.S. health care system, as documented by an extensive review by the Institute of Medicine.[2] In many instances, racial and ethnic minorities receive a lower quality of care than others. Many Americans do not receive the care that they need—or they receive it too late or without due consideration of their preferences and values. Or they receive care that causes them harm.[2,3]

The U.S. health care system often provides services inefficiently and unevenly, so that some people receive worse care than others. These disparities may be due to a variety of factors, including differences in access to care, provider bias, poor provider–patient communication, and poor health literacy.[3] Although the focus of this chapter is on racial and ethnic minorities in the United States, the concerns and solutions presented apply to racial and ethnic minorities in many other countries.

In every year since 2003, the Agency for Healthcare Research and Quality (AHRQ) has reported on progress in reducing disparities and improving quality in health care.[3,4] The Centers for Disease Control and Prevention (CDC) annually publishes an analysis of recent trends and ongoing variations in health disparities and inequalities in selected social and health indicators.[5] The federal Office of Management and Budget established guidelines in 1997 to collect and present data on race and Hispanic origin. These guidelines were first used in the 2000 U.S. census.

The concept of race reflects self-identification by people according to the race or races with which they closely identify. Racial categories are sociopolitical constructs. They are not based on science. Race and Hispanic origin are treated as separate and distinct concepts in census data. (See Box 3–1.)

---

* The term *racial and ethnic minorities*, as used in this chapter, includes any of the nonwhite racial or ethnic groups in the United States as well as people of Hispanic origin; blacks regardless of country of origin (African Americans); American Indians and Alaska Natives; Asians and Pacific Islanders; Native Hawaiians and other Pacific Islanders; and Hispanics (Latinos). The terms *Hispanic* and *Latino* are used interchangeably, as are the terms *black* and *African-American*, with the recognition that not all blacks in the United States are African American, such as Haitian Americans, Jamaican Americans, and people from African countries. The terms *white* and *Caucasian* are also equivalent.

BOX 3-1 ■ **Racial and Ethnic Definitions in the U.S. Census**

The following definitions were used in the 2010 U.S. Census:

White
A person having origins in any of the original peoples of Europe, the Middle East, or North Africa, including people who indicate their race as "White" or report on entries such as Irish, German, Italian, Lebanese, Arab, Moroccan, or Caucasian.

Black or African American
A person having origins in any of the black racial groups of Africa, including, for example, people who indicate their race as "Black, African-Am., or Negro" or report on entries such as African American, Kenyan, Nigerian, or Haitian.

American Indian and Alaska Native
A person having origins in any of the original people of North and South America (including Central America) who maintains tribal affiliation or community attachment, including people who indicated their race as "American Indian or Alaska Native" or reported their enrolled or principal tribe, such as Navajo, Blackfeet, Inupiat, Yup'ik, or Central American Indian groups or South American Indian groups.

Asian
A person having origins in any of the original people of the Far East, Southeast Asia, or the Indian subcontinent, including, for example, Cambodia, China, India, Japan, Korea, Malaysia, Pakistan, the Philippine Islands, Thailand, and Vietnam. It includes people who indicated their race as "Asian" or reported entries such as Asian Indian, Chinese, Filipino, Korean, Japanese, Vietnamese, and Other Asian or reported other Asian responses.

Native Hawaiian and Other Pacific Islander
Includes people who have origins in any of the original peoples of Hawaii, Guam, Samoa, or other Pacific Islands, including people who indicated their race as "Pacific Islander" or who reported entries such as Native Hawaiian, Guamanian or Chamorro, Samoan, and Other Pacific Islander or provided other detailed Pacific Islander responses.

Some Other Race
This category includes all other responses not included in the White, Black or African American, American Indian or Alaska Native, Asian, and Native Hawaiian or Other Pacific Islander race categories, including those reporting entries such as multiracial, mixed, interracial, or a Hispanic or Latino group.

In the 2000 census, respondents were given for the first time the option to identify themselves as belonging to more than one racial group. Given this change, the 2000 and the 2010 census data on race are not directly comparable to previous U.S. census data.[1,2]

Hispanic or Latino
"Hispanic" or "Latino" refers to a person of Cuban, Mexican, Puerto Rican, South or Central American, or other Spanish culture or origin regardless of race. Origin

can be viewed as heritage, nationality group, lineage, or country of birth of the person or person's parents, or ancestors before a person's arrival in the United States. A person who identifies his or her origin as Spanish can be of any race.[1]

Box References

1. Centers for Disease Control and Prevention. Health disparities & inequalities report, 2011. Atlanta, GA: U.S. Department of Health and Human Services, 2011. Available at: http://www.cdc.gov/mmwr/pdf/other/su6001.pdf. Accessed August 29, 2012.
2. U.S. Census Bureau. Overview of race and Hispanic origin, 2010. Washington, DC: U.S. Census Bureau, 2011.

In mid-2012, the U.S. population was distributed in the following racial and ethnic categories: white, 80 percent; black, 13 percent; Asian, 4.4 percent; American Indian and Alaska Native, 1.0 percent; Native Hawaiian and Other Pacific Islander, 0.2 percent; and, by a 2007 estimate, people identifying themselves as of two or more races, 1.6 percent. Persons of Hispanic origin, who may be of any race or ethnic group, were 15 percent of the population.[6]

African Americans and Non-American Blacks in the United States

Black Americans, including both African Americans and non-American blacks, include a rich diversity of cultural groups. Most have descended from the more than four million enslaved persons stolen from Africa, but some are descendants of blacks who were free in this country before the arrival of the *Mayflower* in 1620. The end of slavery in the United States in 1865 was followed by the enactment of laws that disfranchised blacks and imposed racial segregation. Despite advances in civil rights since the 1960s, blacks continue to experience racism throughout the United States. Black migrants now come to the United States from many places in Africa, the Caribbean, Europe, and elsewhere.

Black Americans live in every region of the country, with most (55 percent) living in the South. Over half of blacks live in urban areas that are adversely affected by conditions of poverty—overcrowding, inadequate housing, poor public education, and crime.[7,8]

Latinos

Latinos, with a diverse population, have overtaken blacks as the largest minority group in the United States. Subgroups are distinguished by their place of origin, length of time in the United States, income level, family size, educational attainment, and the degree to which members of the subgroup speak

Spanish, English, or both.[9] Shared aspects among Hispanic groups include language and emphasis on the extended family. Hispanics tend to be younger than non-Hispanics; however, Cubans, a subgroup, have a higher proportion of older people.[9,10] Mexicans are the largest Hispanic subgroup (63 percent), followed by Puerto Ricans (9.2 percent), Cubans (3.5 percent), Salvadorans (3.3 percent), and Dominicans (2.8 percent); the remaining 18 percent are people of Central and South America in origin or other Hispanic or Latino origins. Hispanic communities are geographically concentrated in southwestern states from Texas to California.[11]

Asian Americans

Asian Americans, the fastest growing segment of the U.S. population, are a diverse group, claiming descent from 28 countries in the Far East and Southeast Asia. Most Asian Americans were born in other countries. Although some groups have long histories in this country, others, especially some Southeast Asians, are relatively recent arrivals. Asian Americans are prevalent at the extremes of the socioeconomic spectrum and at the extremes of health status.[12] They have the highest rate of college graduation, and their median income is higher than that of the overall population. However, 12 percent of Asian Americans live in poverty, compared to 10 percent of all Americans.[13] The Hmong, the Khmer, Laotians, Chinese-Vietnamese, and Vietnamese are at increased risk of extreme poverty and poor health status.

Native Hawaiians and Other Pacific Islanders

Native Hawaiians and Other Pacific Islanders have descended from the original peoples of Hawaii, Guam, Samoa, and other Pacific islands. Although the Hawaiian islands are the best known of the Pacific islands, there are many other islands with political or historical ties to the United States in both the North Pacific and South Pacific.[14]

Native Hawaiians and Other Pacific Islanders compose only about 0.2 percent of the U.S. population, with approximately one-third of them under age 18. Until 2000, they were grouped with Asians under the category "Asian-Americans/ Pacific Islanders," in which demographic trends and health needs of Pacific Islanders were often hidden.[15] Native Hawaiians and Other Pacific Islanders compare poorly with most other ethnic groups in per-capita and median household income, education, employment, and access to affordable housing.[16] Native Hawaiians have had to fight to retain their language, culture, and lands. They are working to (a) achieve congressional recognition of their status as indigenous to the Hawaiian Islands, and (b) establish a government-to-government relationship with the United States.[16]

Native Americans

There are 569 federally recognized and 100 state-recognized American Indian and Alaska Native tribes, in addition to an unknown number of tribes that are not recognized—each with its own culture and beliefs. The unique relationships between the tribes and the federal government derive from wars more than two centuries ago and subsequent treaties that recognize the tribes as sovereign entities. While the histories of these tribes vary according to the timing and nature of their encounters with Europeans, common features of these encounters include the introduction of infectious diseases into tribal populations, ecological alterations of tribal land, forced relocation, genocidal violence, social and cultural devastation, and poverty.[17]

Although the Indian Health Service is designated by the federal government to fulfill its legal and treaty obligation to provide health services for American Indians and Alaska Natives, inadequate funding has limited their access to care. Other adverse effects on their health status are due to their geographic isolation, cultural insensitivity of health care providers, and inadequate access to safe water and sanitation.[18] These groups have high rates of poverty, low rates of high-school graduation, high unemployment, and limited coverage by private health insurance. Comprehensive health care for those residing in urban areas is often limited. In some instances, tribes, with federal financial support, have arranged for the provision of their own health care. For example, Alaska Natives receive their health care through Alaska Native health organizations, established by the Alaska Natives themselves and partially funded by the Indian Health Service.

▪ THE IMPACT OF SOCIAL INJUSTICE ON THE HEALTH OF RACIAL AND ETHNIC MINORITIES

African Americans and Non-American Blacks in the United States

Despite overall decreases, the infant mortality rate among blacks has remained at double—or more than double—the rate among whites for many years. The death rate from HIV/AIDS among African Americans is more than seven times that for Caucasian Americans.[4,19,20] Black men and women experience higher morbidity and mortality rates for many diseases, such as diabetes, coronary heart disease, and stroke.[21,22] Although cancer rates have declined for both whites and blacks, blacks continue to have increased death rates for all of the common types of cancer. And for all types of cancer combined, blacks experience a 25 percent higher death rate than whites. For example, black men are more likely to die from prostate cancer than men of any other racial or ethnic group.[23-27] While racial minorities as a whole suffer disproportionately from sexually transmitted infections, blacks—especially young black women—have higher rates of chlamydia infection and gonorrhea than any other groups. The highest rates of syphilis occur in black males.[28] Blacks have a 51 percent higher obesity rate than whites.[29]

Latinos

An estimated 3.1 million Hispanics suffer from arthritis. Prevalence rates in Hispanic subgroups range from 12 percent in Cuban Americans to 22 percent in Puerto Ricans. At least 20 percent of Hispanics experience adverse effects from arthritis, such as limitation of activities. Hispanics have the second highest obesity rate in the United States, and their prevalence rate for diabetes is 50 percent higher than for whites. Hispanics represent approximately 16 percent of the U.S. population, but, in 2009, accounted for 20 percent of all new HIV infections. Puerto Ricans have a relatively high prevalence of asthma. Mexican Americans suffer disproportionately from diabetes. Contributing factors for poorer health outcomes among Hispanics include language and cultural barriers, including poor communication with health care providers; lack of access to preventive care; and lack of health insurance.[22,26,29-32]

Asian Americans

While Asian-American women have the highest life expectancy of any group in the United States, this parameter varies among Asian subgroups. Asian Americans are at increased risk of cancer, heart disease, stroke, unintentional injuries, and diabetes. They have high prevalence of chronic obstructive pulmonary disease (and smoking), tuberculosis, liver disease, and HIV/AIDS.[12,28] Many Asian Americans hesitate to access health care due to fear of deportation, cultural and language barriers, and lack of health insurance.[28] Discrimination contributes significantly to poorer health among Asian Americans.[13,33]

Native Hawaiians and Other Pacific Islanders

Native Hawaiians and Other Pacific Islanders experience poorer health overall than the total U.S. population, with high rates of smoking and alcohol consumption and the highest rates of obesity of any group. They are consequently at increased risk for heart disease, cancer, stroke, diabetes, and unintentional injuries. They are also at increased risk for hepatitis B, tuberculosis, infant mortality, and HIV/AIDS. They are less likely to be covered by private health insurance. They have inadequate access to cancer prevention programs.[34]

Native Americans

Compared with other racial and ethnic groups, Native Americans (including, but not limited to, Alaska Natives) are more likely to die from cancer, unintentional injuries, diabetes, stroke, teenage pregnancy, chronic liver disease (including cirrhosis), heart disorders, and suicide. More than 23 percent smoke, and about 20 percent are binge drinkers.[13,35,36] In 2008, their infant mortality rate was 60 percent higher than that of whites, and their mortality rate for sudden infant death syndrome (SIDS) was 70 percent higher.[37] The average suicide rate among Alaska Natives is more than twice that of others, with two-thirds of these deaths occurring in persons under age 29. The suicide rate for Alaska Native men in the 20- to 29-year-old age group is 155 per 100,000.[36]

■ HEALTH ISSUES FOR SPECIFIC GROUPS

Women

One-third of U.S. women self-identify as belonging to a racial or ethnic minority group. These women continue to fare worse than white women in terms of life expectancy (except for Asian-American women), health status, and disability. Areas of marked disparity include heart disease, diabetes, breast cancer mortality, hypertension, lupus erythematosus, and HIV/AIDS. Asian and Hispanic women have lower rates of receiving mammograms and pap tests. Disparities are widening between black and other women in maternal mortality ratio and the proportion of breast cancers diagnosed at an advanced stage.[35,38-39] (See also Chapter 4.)

Children and Adolescents

Food-insecure families eat food of lower quality, use emergency food sources more, and have more anxiety about their food supply. About 17 percent of children in the United States—about 16 million—live in a food-insecure household, unable to consistently access nutritious and adequate amounts of food necessary for a healthy life.[40] (See Chapter 14.)

Minority children and adolescents have many more health burdens than their non-minority counterparts. Black children have been less likely to receive all recommended vaccinations than white children. And they have higher rates of visiting hospital emergency departments for asthma. The birth rate for Hispanic adolescents is three times that of non-Hispanic whites. Black and Mexican American children have significantly higher percentages of untreated cavities (dental caries) than white children. American Indian and Alaska Native infants die from SIDS at nearly 2.5 times the rate of white infants. And people in some groups have markedly increased HIV infection rates, such as black males age 13 to 29 who have sex with men.[3,31,41-43]

In sum, racial and ethnic health disparities among children in the United States are extensive, pervasive, and persistent—in lower overall health status and quality of health care, less access to health care and use of health services (including preventive services), worse adolescent health, increased rates of chronic diseases, and more special health care needs. Children in all racial and ethnic minority groups have substantially greater rates than white children for many parameters, including all-cause mortality, drowning, acute lymphoblastic leukemia, and mortality after congenital heart defect surgery. They have an earlier median age at death for Down syndrome and congenital heart defects.[44] (See also Chapter 5.)

Older People

In 2011, there were about 37 million U.S. residents age 65 and older. The life expectancy for men at age 65 was 17.6 years; for women, it was 20.3 years.[45] Compared with previous generations, older people now are more racially diverse and better educated, and they have less poverty and more income. Older people born in 1946 or later now work more than older people of earlier generations, perhaps due to economic necessity or desire for social contact, intellectual challenge, or a sense of value. For many older people, housing presents a cost burden, with older people, on average, spending more than 30 percent of their incomes on housing and utilities. Some experience overcrowding in multigenerational households.[46]

Inequalities persist for older people who are racial and ethnic minorities. For example, older African Americans report having fewer financial resources than other older people. Among older people, households headed by blacks have a net worth that is only about one-third that of households headed by whites. Older women who are racial and ethnic minorities are more likely to live in poverty than their white counterparts.[46]

Health disparities are present for racial and ethnic minority groups at all ages, but older adults may experience the effects of these gaps more dramatically than any other age group.[45] Numbers of Hispanic and immigrant older people are likely to increase in the coming decades. Currently, many of them experience poorer health outcomes than their white counterparts. Older people who are not fluent in English are nearly 50 percent more likely to become disabled after age 65. Older people who are members of minority groups experience higher rates of obesity, stroke, Alzheimer's disease, and limitations in activities of daily living—and they have reduced access to a variety of health services.[47] (See also Chapters 8 and 15.)

Non-Hispanic black older people have an increased rate of hypertension, and several other groups of older people are at increased risk of diabetes and related complications.[46] Older people of racial and ethnic minorities have decreased access to clinical preventive services, such as pneumococcal and influenza vaccinations, breast and colorectal cancer screening, and screening for hyperglycemia (high blood glucose), hypercholesterolemia, and osteoporosis.[48] (See also Chapter 6.)

Men

Men of color are less healthy than other men. Although life expectancy for black males has improved compared with white males, blacks males still have the lowest life expectancy of any group. Between 2000 and 2009, overall life expectancy at birth in the United States increased by 1.9 years for males and 1.6 years for females. The gap in life expectancy between males and females narrowed from 5.2 years in 2000 to 4.9 years in 2009. During this period, life expectancy also narrowed between blacks and whites. In 2000, life expectancy at birth for whites was 5.5 years longer than for blacks; by 2009, this difference had narrowed to 4.3 years.[49]

While cancer of the prostate is by far the most prevalent cancer in men in the United States, more men die from lung cancer than any other type of cancer—and black men have an especially high mortality rate for lung cancer. Colorectal cancer is the third most prevalent cancer in men, and it affects minority men at a disproportionately high rate. Asian males have lower cancer screening rates than all other groups. Disparities in HIV infection continue to widen between African American, Hispanic, and American Indian/Alaska Native men, and their white counterparts.[50-57] (See also Chapters 13 and 15.)

Men of color are more likely than white men to be poor, less educated, and unemployed. They are more likely to experience the detrimental effects of residential segregation and other socioeconomic problems associated with poor health. Black and Latino men are less likely than white men to see a physician, even when they are in poor health. Non-elderly black and Latino men are less likely than white men to have health insurance. Men of color, regardless of their insurance status, are less likely to receive timely health care services for diseases that require prompt attention, such as leg amputation for impaired circulation and radical surgery for cancer.

Economic marginalization and unemployment are more frequent among men of color, contributing to adverse physical and mental health. Occupational hazards, low-wage jobs, poor educational opportunities, discrimination, and poor housing frequently add to economic stressors of minority men.

Immigrants

Immigrants to the United States are a large and growing segment of the population. Except for some groups of Asians, immigrants have low rates of high school graduation, tend to work in service occupations, and often live in poverty. In 2009, the rate of lack of health insurance for native-born citizens was 13 percent, while among non-citizens—classified as temporary workers, foreign students, permanent residents, and undocumented persons—it was 44 percent. Additional barriers to their access to health care include limited proficiency in English, fear of risk of deportation, and state and federal policies. Immigrants often suffer from inadequate prenatal care, lack of a regular source of health care, inadequate immunizations, and a variety of infectious diseases.[58,59] (See also Box 22–1 in Chapter 22.)

■ ENVIRONMENTAL QUALITY

Disparities in the exposure of racial and ethnic minority groups to unsafe or unhealthy environments have been reported for decades. Hazards of concern have included air and water contaminants, toxic chemicals, and unhealthful and unsafe work and home environments. These concerns led to the environmental justice movement, which is based on the tenet that no group should bear a disproportionate share of the adverse effects of unhealthy environments. (See also Chapters 18 and 19.)

Most people living in neighborhoods with hazardous waste facilities are people of color.[60] The residence of children in low-income areas is associated with exposure to environmental pollutants.[61]

The proportion of inadequate housing units in the United States is about 5 percent. Women are 20 percent more likely to live in inadequate housing than men. In 2009, non-Hispanic blacks had the highest rates of living in inadequate housing, followed by Hispanics, American Indians/Alaska Natives, and Asian/Pacific Islanders.[62] (See also Box 18–1 in Chapter 18.)

Social injustice is evident in the differential implementation of environmental regulations and other policies that are designed to protect communities, such as cleaning up toxic waste sites and prosecuting violators of environmental laws and regulations. Unequal protection, favoring white communities over communities of color, occurs whether the community is wealthy or poor.[63]

■ ACCESS TO AND QUALITY OF HEALTH CARE

Disparities in access to and quality of health care may be due to inadequate or no insurance coverage, no regular source of care, inadequate financial resources, legal or structural barriers, language and cultural barriers, deficiencies in the health care financing system, scarcity or maldistribution of health care providers, lack of diversity and lack of cultural competence among health care providers, geographic isolation, and inadequate support services, such as child care and transportation. These problems are more likely to affect racial and ethnic minorities.[64,65] Members of racial or ethnic minority groups are more likely than whites to live in poverty, and, except for some Asian subgroups, less likely to have finished high school. More than others, low-income people have poor health and die prematurely.[3] (See also Chapter 12.)

Over time, there has been no significant change in most of the disparities in access to and quality of care tracked by AHRQ for Asians, Hispanics, African Americans, and American Indians and Alaska Natives. (Changes in the format for data collection and small numbers have made assessment of disparities for Native Hawaiians and Other Pacific Islanders difficult.) While there have been some improvements for all minority groups, for most there have also been areas where disparities have widened.[3] Health care providers for patients from racial and ethnic minority groups report barriers to their obtaining access to high-quality subspecialty care and services, diagnostic procedures, and elective hospital admission.[66]

In all six domains of quality defined by the Institute of Medicine—safe, timely, effective, efficient, patient-centered, and equitable—there have been significant disparities between care for people in racial and ethnic minority groups and care for others.[64] Patients from these groups also receive lower quality interpersonal care than do white patients.[66]

▪ ROOT CAUSES AND UNDERLYING ISSUES

Racial Discrimination

Many white people have no awareness of their privileged status. Although many admit that disparities exist, they attribute them to lack of ambition or initiative by minorities rather than structural favoritism for white people, which has always been an integral part of U.S. society. As David Wellman, Professor of Community Studies at the University of California, Santa Cruz, and co-author of a textbook on racial discrimination, has stated: "You don't need to be a racist to promote qualities that are race-conscious. Most whites don't see white as a race. Like a fish in water, they don't think about whiteness because it's so beneficial to them."[67]

Three types of racism have been described by Camara Jones, a former professor at the Harvard School of Public Health.[68]

Institutionalized racism, "differential access to the goods, services, and opportunities of society by race," is structured into norms, customs, and sometimes the laws of a society. It occurs in both (a) material conditions, such as lack of equal access to quality education, sound housing, gainful employment, and adequate health care; and (b) access to power, such as differential access to information, resources, and voice (voting rights, representation in government, and control of the media). The historical association between socioeconomic status and race in the United States is perpetuated by contemporary structural arrangements.

Personally mediated racism, what many people mean by "racism," is prejudice and discrimination—assumptions about others based on race and actions toward others according to race. It may be intentional or unintentional and may include acts of commission or omission. It may be demonstrated as lack of respect, suspicion, avoidance, devaluation, scapegoating, or dehumanization. Condoned by societal norms and maintained by structural barriers, it is manifested in everyday customs of interaction, such as poor service in a department store or police brutality.

Internalized racism occurs when members of a stigmatized race accept negative messages about themselves and engage in devaluation of themselves and others of their race—leading to hopelessness, resignation, and helplessness.

Poverty, Income, and Wealth/Assets

The official poverty rate in the United States in 2010 was 15.1 percent, a 0.9 percent increase from the previous year—the third consecutive annual increase. There were an estimated 46.2 million people living in poverty, with all ethnic groups, except Asian Americans, showing annual increases in their poverty rates. This was the highest U.S. poverty rate since 1993, and the number of people in poverty in 2010 was the largest in the 52 years in which poverty estimates have been published.[69] The numbers of children in poverty has increased.[70] Between 2009 and 2010, as the poverty rate increased, median household income decreased. Since 2007, median household income has decreased by 6.4 percent.

Although income disparities between minority groups and others are substantial and widening, even more important are disparities in wealth. More than 33 percent of non-white households in the United States do not have any wealth at all, compared with 12 percent of white households.[71]

Although social policies in the United States for asset development have, since the 1800s, been beneficial to whites and disadvantageous to minorities, the discriminatory impacts of these policies have accumulated over time. Three of these policies, whose discriminatory effects persist, are the Homestead Act of 1862, the G.I. Bill of 1944, and a series of federal government initiatives designed to facilitate home ownership in the 1940s and 1950s. Racial discrimination and segregation inherent in the implementation of these policies provided opportunities for asset development among whites that were denied to blacks and other ethnic minorities. And the more recent policy of *redlining* by banks—designating a residential area for preferential or prejudicial treatment based on race or ethnicity—continues to discriminate against blacks and other minorities.[71]

Today, institutional policies related to asset development favor those with incomes of $50,000 or more, who receive approximately 90 percent of the benefits from tax deductions or tax "breaks." These deductions are actually tax expenditures that include tax credits, preferential tax rates, tax deferrals, and exclusions from taxation. Such deductions represent approximately 50 percent of direct federal expenditures. The largest of these tax expenditures, which help rich people to accumulate financial and real assets, are in the areas of home ownership, retirement accounts, and preferential treatment of gains from investments. The housing tax exemption policy, for example, provides those who are not poor with substantial subsidies that assist them to become homeowners, while the overwhelming majority of the housing subsidies for the poor, such as through Section 8 of the Housing Code, rental vouchers, and public housing, enable them only to rent housing—not to own homes.[71-73]

Social Exclusion

The concept of social exclusion arose out of dissatisfaction with definitions of poverty based entirely on income. Persons can experience social exclusion resulting from their membership in a variety of groups that suffer discrimination due to race, ethnicity, religion, sexual orientation, HIV status, and other factors.[74] Exclusionary processes operate in economic, political, social, and cultural dimensions and at societal levels ranging from individual to global. These processes create a continuum of inclusion/exclusion that involves unjust distribution of resources and access to rights that are required for the achievement of health. Measurement of social exclusion and its relationship to health is sometimes challenged, since those most excluded—marginalized people—are least likely to be counted.[75]

Geographical Location and Residence Patterns

Segregated residential location has been linked to poor health since Louis Villerme described the differential risks of premature deaths in affluent and poor neighborhoods in Paris in 1817.[76] While the social support derived from living within one's ethnic community may be beneficial, damaging conditions of poverty, if present, adversely affect the health of all community residents.[77] Although residential segregation by race declined between 2000 and 2010, black and Hispanic Americans continue to live in segregated communities that tend to be of low socioeconomic status. It is possible that health disparities may largely be a function of residential segregation—the separate and unequal neighborhoods in which most minorities and whites reside, irrespective of their socioeconomic status. In general, minority neighborhoods, compared with white neighborhoods, have significantly poorer health care facilities that are staffed by less competent physicians, higher environmental exposures, and built environments that are less healthful—all of which contribute to poorer health outcomes.[78-83]

Two mechanisms link health disparities and residential segregation: (a) exposure to health risks, and (b) access to resources. Minorities residing in segregated neighborhoods live in a health "riskscape." Characteristics of the built environment, such as billboards advertising tobacco, liquor stores, and easy access to crack cocaine, place communities at risk.[77,84-86]

Residential segregation also reduces access, not only to essential health care services, but also to other resources that lead to good health, such as constructive social networks and access to nutrient-rich food.[87-91]

Compared to adults living in urban areas, adults living in rural areas receive fewer health care services, are more likely to engage in risky health-related behaviors, and experience higher rates of chronic diseases and limitations of activity. A larger proportion of rural than urban adults report having fair-to-poor physical and mental health status. In addition, chronic diseases such as arthritis, asthma, chronic obstructive pulmonary disease, diabetes, cardiac disorders, hypertension, and mental disorders are more common among rural than urban residents.[92]

Employment Status and Occupational Health Issues

In spite of increases in government spending to address these issues, disparities among demographic groups persist. Resulting problems among poor Americans and racial and ethnic minorities include disproportionately higher rates of disease, fewer treatment options, and less access to care. As unemployment increases, especially among racial and ethnic minorities, existing disparities among these groups increase.[22] Unemployment can lower a person's motivation and can lead to physical and mental disorders. There are disproportionately higher rates of injury and disease among workers of color. (See Chapter 19.)

Health Literacy

The average American adult reads at the eighth- to ninth-grade level, whereas most health education and information materials are written above the tenth-grade level. Health literacy—the ability to read, understand, and act on health information—is a stronger predictor of health status than one's age, income, employment status, educational level, or racial or ethnic group. Health literacy problems affect a disproportionate number of racial and ethnic minorities and immigrants, especially those who speak English as a second language.[62] Low health literacy results in higher health care costs, problems with self-management of health care, and increased risk of hospitalization.[93]

Specific Implications of Social Injustice for Racial and Ethnic Minorities

The same problems that contribute to discriminatory practices in society at large also adversely affect the experience of minorities in their encounters with the health care system. These problems include individual and institutional racism in health care and the legal, regulatory, financial, and political environments in which health care decisions are made and implemented. All of these factors can deny social justice to minorities who seek health care.

The health inequities that exist in every nation are largely due to the social injustice that leads to unequal access to societal resources. These inequities are caused by unjust social arrangements that often discriminate against minority groups.[94] The health status of disadvantaged minorities is extremely sensitive to economic, social, and political factors. Whether a country is rich or poor, better health is associated with higher social position.

In important ways, the health inequities in a country may be seen as a barometer of its citizens' experiences of social justice and human rights. Health equity should not be seen only as a societal goal, but also as a measure of social justice.[94]

▓ **WHAT NEEDS TO BE DONE**

Ensuring Cultural Competence Among Health Professionals and Institutions

An expert panel appointed by Physicians for Human Rights has made 24 policy recommendations to address racial and ethnic disparities in the quality of medical care, based on a comprehensive survey of peer-reviewed medical literature.[95] These recommendations include the following:

- The federal government should create an Office of Health Disparities, within the Office of Civil Rights of the Department of Health and Human Services, to determine if health disparities are the products of discrimination and to take appropriate action.
- The federal government should collect data from health plans on race, ethnicity, and primary language of members to assure analysis of data on racial and ethnic disparities and to provide resources to agencies addressing racial and ethnic health disparities.
- National professional organizations, educational institutions, accrediting bodies, and health care provider associations should take appropriate action to assure that health professionals are educated on health disparities and cultural competence, and these competencies should be evaluated for licensure and individual and institutional credentialing purposes.
- Research should be performed on interactions between health care providers and patients, providers' attitudes and behaviors related to race and ethnicity, disparities in care within health care systems, and interventions to eliminate disparities.

Cultural competence and language sensitivity are important aspects of public health measures to eliminate health disparities among population groups. (We encourage public health workers to use resources such as our chapter entitled "Practicing Cultural Competence" in *Mastering Public Health: Essential Skills for Effective Practice.*[96])

Increasing Recruitment and Retention of Minority Youth into Health Professions

The history of health professional education has been characterized by segregation and denial of access for racial and ethnic minorities. Under-representation in the health care work force of African Americans, Hispanics, American

Indians and Alaska Natives, and some subgroups of Asians and Pacific Islanders contributes to the persistence of disparities in health status and access to care.

Three principles are critical to solving this situation:

- Change in the culture of the health professions schools
- Exploration of new and non-traditional paths for the health professions
- High-level commitment to diversity

Specific strategies for progress include making sure that the educational needs of minority and low-income students are being met from kindergarten through grade 12, financially supporting more students with scholarships (as opposed to student loans), reaching beyond traditional applicant pools, reducing dependency on standardized tests for admission to professional schools, and intervening at the college and graduate school levels through such strategies as targeted recruiting, mentoring and support for students, and engaging community advocates.[97,98]

Addressing Health Literacy

Minority and immigrant groups are more likely to have low health literacy. A variety of approaches are available to mitigate this. For example, the Ask Me 3 campaign, developed from the National Patient Safety Foundation,[99] teaches patients to ask their health care providers three simple, but essential, questions in each interaction: "What is my main problem?" "What do I need to do?" "Why is it important for me to do this?" Another approach is using Newest Vital Sign, a bilingual screening tool that can be administered in 3 minutes in a clinical setting and is as effective as more complex tools to assess health literacy.[100,101] More broadly, public health workers should advocate for better public education for poor and minority children, whose overall literacy skills are often deficient.

Developing Policies and Initiating Action to Reduce Poverty

Reducing poverty requires a multifaceted approach. Public health workers can assist in many ways, such as monitoring health outcomes related to poverty and educating health care providers on how poverty affects health. Health workers should collaborate with workers in other sectors to address poverty-related issues concerning food, housing, community safety, employment, health care, and social, economic, and political participation. Policies should be strengthened to ensure that all children, irrespective of ethnicity, residential location, or socioeconomic status, receive adequate education.

Community-based interventions, designed for specific community contexts, can help reduce poverty and improve health outcomes. These interventions should build on community assets, such as engaging local residents in bridging cultural gaps,[102] and should support capacity-building in minority communities by both the public and private sectors. Capacity-building includes improving access to capital, such as with loans to small businesses; education of minority groups in business management; and improving transportation systems for people to commute to work. Capacity-building in health includes increasing the numbers of minority physicians, nurses, and other health professionals; and providing health education to minority group members so they can assume greater responsibility for their own health and serve as health resources to other community members.

Residential segregation, unless forced, is not inherently bad. Indeed, many ethnic minorities prefer to live in neighborhoods of their own race. However, public policy should remove barriers that often prevent minorities from buying houses in choice neighborhoods.

All people should have access to gainful employment and a guaranteed minimum wage. Unemployment benefits should be set at levels that prevent individuals and families from drifting into poverty. Job training programs can help prevent unemployment and underemployment.[94]

Public and private mechanisms, such as credit unions and credit counseling programs, can help reduce indebtedness among poor people. Low-income households should have access to the same institutional mechanisms, incentives, and subsidies that those who are not poor have, such as employer-matched pension plans, payroll-deduction savings programs, and prudent mortgage-financed home purchases. Since they do not frequently own their own homes, poor people generally do not receive tax deductions for mortgage interest; even if they are homeowners, they typically receive lower rates of return when they sell their homes. Ironically, the main federal social welfare program to which poor people have access, Temporary Assistance for Needy Families (TANF), discourages their saving money because it sets asset limits above which benefits are denied.

Matched savings accounts—known as Individual Development Accounts (IDAs)—enable low-income families to save enough money for a down payment on a home, pay for post-secondary education, or obtain start-up capital for a small business. There are more than 500 community-based asset-building programs in 49 states, with over 20,000 account-holding beneficiaries. These programs stimulate saving, facilitate use of IDAs for the purchase of assets expected to have high returns, and increase future-oriented thinking.[103,104] A study found that 28 percent of matched withdrawals from the IDAs were used to purchase homes, 23 percent to start businesses, 21 percent for post-secondary education; and 18 percent for home repair. Acquiring assets enabled participants to improve their outlook and helped them to focus on long-term planning.[105]

Addressing Racial Discrimination

Just as racial discrimination takes many forms, so measures to end it need to be multifaceted. Public health workers should assess the living conditions of racial and ethnic minorities so they can implement measures to reduce any adverse health effects of racial discrimination. Specific interventions may include raising public awareness of discrimination, advocating for clients and communities, and ensuring that health services have published policies that are implemented to forbid discrimination.

Government agencies can improve health opportunities of people in racially segregated communities by stimulating public and private investment. In low-income communities, incentives for improving food options, eliminating environmental degradation, and reducing concentrations of poverty by implementing smart housing and transportation policies will not only improve health but will also likely save money.[77] Public health workers can help to assess and improve these policies.

Performing Research

Comprehensive research is needed on the roots and effects of racial and ethnic discrimination on the impact of individual and institutional racism on health. Surveillance systems should be developed to obtain data on the determinants and distribution of physical, mental, social, and environmental health outcomes due to racial and ethnic disparities. Data collection should account for the diversity of minority subgroups. Research should be enhanced by the inclusion of data on such issues as residential segregation, occupational health problems, employment discrimination, individual exposure to discrimination and related coping mechanisms, physiological effects of racism and discrimination, and behaviors of health care providers that contribute to disparities. Research on the relationship between race/ethnicity and occupational health and safety should be performed and used to facilitate policy changes to reduce the increased occupational health risks faced by workers of color.[106] Researchers need to be sensitive to racial and ethnic-group perspectives on genetic research with respect to handling of human tissue, confidentiality, and the appropriateness of various types of questions; for example, questions to family members should be phrased to protect the confidentiality of all affected family members.[107]

Considering New Concepts of Health and Social Justice

Valuable insights into understanding health as a human right and the intersection of health and social justice can be learned from a variety of sources, such as the book *Health Justice* by Sridhar Venkatapuram, in which he proposes that health is a capability, founded in biology, exposures, behavior, and social conditions.[108] Drawing on various disciplines including social epidemiology and distributive justice, he provides fresh perspectives on how "health" can be defined and how the related roles and responsibilities of individuals and societies can be understood. He conceptualizes health as the ability to be and do things that make up a minimally good, flourishing, and non-humiliating life. The assertion of the capability for health as a human right gives rise to an obligation for nation-states and policymakers to develop and maintain the social and environmental conditions within which people can make choices for health. Broadly understood, this right includes not only such things as clean air and water, but also the facilitation of health literacy, as well as access to an acceptable range of preventive and therapeutic health services.[108]

■ CONCLUSION

The most important immediate action in response to social injustice against racial and ethnic minorities that leads to disparate health outcomes is the equitable provision of health care. We must enact legislation that ensures better quality of and access to health care through the provision of health care for all people in an atmosphere of acceptance and respect.

Initiatives that address the specific areas of health disparities for ethnic minorities should be promoted, including the collection of data on barriers to equitable care and the monitoring of progress toward the elimination of health disparities. Additional recommendations, from the Institute of Medicine report *Unequal Treatment*,[2] include the following:

- Increase awareness of disparities among the general public, among key stakeholders (such as health care agencies and organizations, third-party payers, and state and local health departments), and among health care providers
- Integrate cross-cultural topics into the education of all health professionals
- Provide patient education on how to access health care and participate in health care planning
- Use evidence-based guidelines to promote consistency of and equity in health care, with financial incentives to ensure evidence-based practice
- Structure payment systems that ensure adequate services to minorities and that eliminate incentives for health care providers that promote disparities—and instead implement health care financing arrangements that discourage fragmented care, inadequate standards of care, and inadequate services to racial and ethnic minorities
- Provide sufficient resources to the Office of Civil Rights of the Department of Health and Human Services to enforce civil rights laws

Eliminating racial and ethnic health disparities will require attention not only to its immediate consequences, but also to the many contextual issues that have caused and now perpetuate its devastating effects. Health workers should collaborate with people in other disciplines, the business community, the general public, and minority groups to reach an effective and sustainable resolution to these problems.

▨ REFERENCES

1. U.S. Census Bureau. Overview of race and Hispanic origin, 2010. Washington, DC: U.S. Census Bureau, 2011.
2. Smedley BD, Stith AY, Nelson AR, eds. Unequal treatment: Confronting racial and ethnic disparities. Washington, DC: National Academies Press, 2003.
3. Agency for Healthcare Research and Quality. National health care disparities report. Rockville, MD: AHRQ, 2012. Available at: http://www.ahrq.gov/qual/nhdr11/nhdr11. pdf. Accessed September 21, 2012.
4. Agency for Healthcare Research and Quality. National health care quality report. Rockville, MD: AHRQ, 2012. Available at: http://www.ahrq.gov/qual/nhqr11/nhqr11. pdf. Accessed September 21, 2012.
5. Centers for Disease Control and Prevention. Health disparities and inequalities report, 2011. Atlanta, GA: U.S. Department of Health and Human Services, 2011. Available at: http://www.cdc.gov/mmwr/pdf/other/su6001.pdf. Accessed August 29, 2012.
6. IndexMundi. United States demographics profile 2012. Available at: http://www. indexmundi.com/united_states/demographics_profile.html. Accessed August 29, 2012.
7. Office of Minority Health and Health Disparities. Black or African American populations. Atlanta, GA: Centers for Disease Control and Prevention. Available at: http://www. cdc.gov/minorityhealth/populations/REMP/black.html. Accessed August 29, 2012.
8. U.S. Census Bureau. The black population: 2010 census briefs. Washington, DC: U.S. Census Bureau, 2011.
9. Rodriguez-Trias H, Bracho A, Gil RM, et al. Eliminating health disparities: Conversations with Latinos. Santa Cruz, CA: ETR Associates, 2003.
10. Office of Minority Health and Health Disparities. Hispanic or Latino populations. Atlanta, GA: Centers for Disease Control and Prevention. Available at: http://www.cdc. gov/omhd/Populations/HL/HL.htm. Accessed August 29, 2012.
11. Office of Minority Health and Health Equity. Hispanic/Latino heritage. Available at: http//www.cdc.gov/minority health. Accessed August 28, 2012.
12. Centers for Disease Control and Prevention. Observances—May, Asian American & Pacific Islander Heritage Month. CDC, 2012. Available at: http://www.cdc.gov/ minorityhealth/observances/AAPI.html. Accessed August 27, 2012.
13. Office of Minority Health. Asian American/Pacific Islander profile. Available at: http:// minorityhealth.hhs.gov/templates/content.aspx?ID=3005. Accessed August 27, 2012.
14. Aiu P, Blaisdell K, Pretrick EK, et al. Eliminating health disparities: Conversations with Pacific Islanders. Santa Cruz, CA: ETR Associates, 2004.
15. Grieco E. The Native Hawaiian and Other Pacific Islander population: 2000: Census 2000 brief. Washington, DC: U.S. Department of Commerce, Economics and Statistics Administration, U.S. Census Bureau, 2001.
16. Lai E, Arguelles D. Native Hawaiians and Pacific Islander Americans: Asian nation. Available at: http://www.asian-nation.org/hawaiian-pacific.shtml. Accessed August 27, 2012.
17. Olsen B. Culture, colonization, and policy making: Issues in Native American health. Presented at the Symposium in the Politics of Race, Culture, and Health, Ithaca College, Ithaca, NY, November 13 and 14, 2003.
18. Office of Minority Health. American Indian/Alaska Native profile. Available at: http:// minorityhealth.hhs.gov/template/browser.aspx?lvl=38lvlid=26. Accessed August 27, 2012.

19. American Public Health Association. Health disparities primer: Get the facts: Health disparities. Available at: www.apha.org. Accessed August 28, 2010.

20. Henry J. Kaiser Family Foundation. Fact sheet: The HIV/AIDS epidemic in the United States, December 2012. Available at: http://www.kff.org/hivaids/upload/3029-13.pdf. Accessed March 6, 2013.

21. Centers for Disease Control and Prevention. Fact sheet: Health disparities in coronary heart disease and stroke. Available at: http://www.cdc.gov/stroke/prevention.htm. Accessed August 28, 2012.

22. HealthReform.gov. Health disparities: A case for closing the gap. Available at: http//www.healthreform.gov. Accessed August 29, 2012.

23. National Cancer Institute. Researchers find biological factors that may drive prostate tumor aggressiveness in African-American men. Bethesda, MD: National Cancer Institute, 2008.

24. Centers for Disease Control and Prevention. Cancer rates by race and ethnicity. Atlanta, GA: U.S. Department of Health and Human Services. Available at: http://www.cdc.gov/cancer/dcpc/data/index.htm. Accessed August 29, 2012.

25. Centers for Disease Control and Prevention. Colorectal cancer rates by race and ethnicity. Atlanta, GA: U.S. Department of Health and Human Services. Available at: http://www.cdc.gov/cancer/dcpc/data/index.htm. Accessed August 29, 2012.

26. Centers for Disease Control and Prevention. HPV-associated cancers rates by race and ethnicity. Atlanta, GA: U.S. Department of Health and Human Services. Available at: http://www.cdc.gov/ccncer/dcpc/data/index.htm. Accessed August 29, 2012.

27. Centers for Disease Control and Prevention. Prostate cancer rates by race and ethnicity. Atlanta, GA: U.S. Department of Health and Human Services. Available at: http://www.cdc.gov/cancer/dcpc/data/index.htm. Accessed August 29, 2012.

28. Centers for Disease Control and Prevention. Chlamydia and gonorrhea—Two most commonly reported infectious diseases in the United States. Atlanta, GA: U.S. Department of Health and Human Services. Available at: http://www.cdc.gov/nchhstp/Default.htm. Accessed August 29, 2012.

29. Centers for Disease Control and Prevention. Differences in prevalence of obesity among black, white, and Hispanic adults—United States, 2006–2008. *MMWR* 2009;58:740–744.

30. Centers for Disease Control and Prevention. Prevalence of doctor-diagnosed arthritis and arthritis-attributable effects among Hispanic adults, by Hispanic subgroup—United States, 2002, 2003, 2006, and 2009. *MMWR* 2011;60:167–171.

31. National Council of State Legislatures. Disparities in health. Available at: http://www.ncsl.org/issues-research/health/health-disparities-overview.aspx. Accessed August 29, 2012.

32. Office of Minority Health and Health Equity. Hispanic/Latino heritage. Available at: http//www.cdc.gov/minority health. Accessed August 28, 2012.

33 . Nadimpalli SB, Hutchinson MK. An integrative review of relationships between discrimination and Asian American health. *J Nurs Scholarsh* 2012;44:125–135.

34 . Office of Minority Health. Native Hawaiian and Other Pacific Islander profile. Available at: http://minorityhealth.hhs.gov/templates/browse.aspx?lvl+2&lvlid=71. Accessed August 27, 2012.

35. James CV, Salganifcoff A, Thomas M, et al. Putting women's health care disparities on the map: Examining racial and ethnic disparities at the state level. Menlo Park, CA: Kaiser Family Foundation, 2009. Available at: http://www.edfoxphd.com/women_first.pdf . Accessed March 6, 2013.

36. Craig J, Hull-Jilly D. Characteristics of suicide among Alaska Native and Alaska Non-Native People, 2003–2008. State of Alaska Epidemiology Bulletin, Recommendations and Reports, 2012. Available at: http://www.epi.alaska.gov/bulletins/docs/rr2012_01.pdf. Accessed on August 29, 2012.

37. Office of Minority Health. Infant mortality of American Indians/Alaska Natives. Available at: http://minorityhealth.hhs.gov/templates/content.aspx?ID=3038. Accessed on August 27, 2012.

38. Agency for Healthcare Research and Quality. Health care for minority women: Recent findings. AHRQ, 2010. Available at: http://www.ahrq.gov/research/minority.htm. Accessed August 28, 2012.

39. Mead H, Cartwright-Smith L, Jones K, et al. Racial and ethnic disparities in U.S. health care: A chartbook. Commonwealth Fund, 2008. Available at: http://www.commonwealthfund.org/~/meia/File. Accessed August 28, 2012.

40. Feeding America. Impact of hunger. Available at: http://feedingamerica.org/hunger-in-america/impact-of-hunger.aspx. Accessed August 31, 2012.

41. Centers for Disease Control and Prevention. Fact sheet: Health disparities in adolescent pregnancy and childbirth. Atlanta, GA: U.S. Department of Health and Human Services. Available at: http://www.cdc.gov/teenpregnancy/. Accessed August 29, 2012.

42. Centers for Disease Control and Prevention. Untreated dental caries (cavities) in children ages 2–19, United States. Available at: http://www.cdc.gov/Features/dsUntreated-CavitiesKids/. Accessed August 29, 2012.

43. National Center for HIV/AIDS, Viral Hepatitis, STD, and TB Prevention. Division of Adolescent and School Health. HIV and young men who have sex with men. Available at: http://www.cdc.gov/healthyyouth/sexualbehaviors/pdf/hiv_factsheet_ymsm.pdf. Accessed August 29, 2012.

44. Flores G. Racial and ethnic disparities in the health and health care of children. *Pediatrics* 2010;125:979–1020.

45. Centers for Disease Control and Prevention, Merck Company Foundation. The state of aging and health in America, 2007. Available at: http://www.cdc.gov/aging and http://www.merck.com/cr. Accessed August 27, 2012.

46. Federal Interagency Forum on Aging Related Statistics. Older Americans, 2012. Accessed at http://www.agingstats.gov/Main_Site/Data/2012_Documents/docs/EntireChartbook.pdf. Accessed August 27, 2012.

47. LeadingAge. Special needs of older minorities. LeadingAge, 2011. Available at: http://www.leadingage.org/Article.aspx?id=303. Accessed August 31, 2012.

48. Centers for Disease Control and Prevention, Administration on Aging, Agency for Healthcare Research and Quality, and Centers for Medicare and Medicaid Services. Enhancing use of clinical preventive services among older persons. AARP, 2011. Available at: http://www.cdc.gov/aging and http://www.aarp.org/healthpros. Accessed August 31, 2012.

49. National Center for Health Statistics. Health, United States, 2011: With special feature on socioeconomic status and health. Hyattsville, MD: NCHS, 2012.

50. Centers for Disease Control and Prevention. 10 top cancers in men. Available at: http://www.cdc.gov/Features/dsmentop10cancers/. Accessed August 29, 2012.

51. Centers for Disease Control and Prevention. Prostate cancers rates by race and ethnicity. Atlanta, GA: U.S. Department of Health and Human Services. Available at: http://www.cdc.gov/cancer/lung/statistics/race.htm. Accessed August 29, 2012.

52. Centers for Disease Control and Prevention. Lung cancers rates by race and ethnicity. Atlanta, GA: U.S. Department of Health and Human Services. Available at: http://www.cdc.gov/cancer/lung/statistics/race.htm. Accessed August 29, 2012.

53. Centers for Disease Control and Prevention. Colorectal cancer rates by race and ethnicity. Atlanta, GA: U.S. Department of Health and Human Services. Available at: http://www.cdc.gov/cancer/colorectal/statistics/race.htm. Accessed August 29, 2012.

54. National Cancer Institute. Cancer health disparities. Available at: http://www.cancer.gov/cancertopics/factsheet/disparities/cancer-health-disparities. Accessed August 29, 2012.

55. Centers for Disease Control and Prevention. Diagnoses of HIV infection and AIDS in the United States and dependent areas, 2009. HIV Surveillance Report No. 21. Atlanta, GA: U.S. Department of Health and Human Services, 2011a. Available at: http://www.cdc.gov/hiv/surveillance/resources/reports/2009report/index.htm.   Accessed December 1, 2011.

56. Centers for Disease Control and Prevention. HIV among Latinos. Atlanta, GA: U.S. Department of Health and Human Services, 2011. Available at: http://www.cdc.gov/hiv/latinos/index.htm. Accessed January 30, 2012.

57. Centers for Disease Control and Prevention. Fact sheet: Health disparities HIV infection. Atlanta, GA: U.S. Department of Health and Human Services. Available at: http://www.cdc.gov/minorityhealth/reports/CHDIR11/FactSheets/HIV.pdf Accessed August 29, 2012.

58. Derose KP, Escarce JJ, Lurie N. Immigrants and health care: Sources of vulnerability. *Health Aff* 2007;26:1258–1268. Available at: http://content.healthaffairs.org/content/26/5/1258.full.html. Accessed on August 28, 2012.

59. Footracer KG. Immigrant health care in the United States: What ails our system. *JAAPA* 2009. Available at: http://www.jaapa.com/immigrant-health-care-in-the-united-states-what-ails-our-system/article/130524/. Accessed August 28, 2012.

60. Bullard RD, Mohai P, Saha R, et al. Toxic wastes and race at twenty, 1987–2007: A report prepared for the United Church of Christ Justice & Witness Ministries, 2007. Available at: http://www.ucc.org/assets/pdfs/toxic.20.pdf. Accessed August 30, 2012.

61. Dilworth-Bart JE, Moore CF. Mercy mercy me: Social injustice and the prevention of environmental pollutant exposures among ethnic minority and poor children. *Child Dev* 2006;77:247–265.

62. Raymond J, Wheeler W, Brown MJ. Inadequate and unhealthy housing, 2007–2009. *MMWR* 2011;60:21–27. Available at: http://www.cdc.gov/mmwr/preview/mmwrhtml/su6001a4.htm?s_cid=su6001a4_w. Accessed August 31, 2012.

63. Bullard RD. Dumping in Dixie: Race, class, and environmental quality. Boulder, CO: Westview Press, 2000.

64. Mead H, Cartwright-Smith L, Jones K, et al. Racial and ethnic disparities in U.S. health care: A chartbook. Commonwealth Fund, 2008. Available at: http://www.commonwealthfund.org/Publications/Chartbooks/2008/Mar/Racial-and-Ethnic-Disparities-in-U-S—Health-Care—A-Chartbook.aspx. Accessed August 28, 2012.

65. News Medical. Disparities in access to health care. Available at:http://www.news-medical.net/health/Disparities-in-Access-to-Health-Care.aspx. Accessed August 29, 2012.

66. Cooper LA, Beach MC, Johnson RL, Thomas SI. Delving below the surface: Understanding how race and ethnicity influence relationships in health care. *JGIM* 2006;21:S21–S27. Available at: http://www.ncbi.nlm.nih.gov/pubmed/16405705. Accessed August 27, 2012.

67. Lehrman S. Colorblind racism. AlterNet. Available at: http://www.alternet.org/story/16792/colorblind_racism?paging=off. Accessed September 1, 2012.

68. Jones CP. Levels of racism: A theoretic framework and a gardener's tale. *Am J Public Health* 2002;90:1212–1215.

69. U.S. Census Bureau. Income, poverty and health insurance in the United States: 2010—highlights. U.S. Census Bureau, 2012. Available at: http://www.census.gov/hhes/www/poverty/data/incpovhlth/2010/highlights.html. Accessed August 27, 2012.

70. DeNavas-Walt C, Proctor BD, Smith JC. Income, poverty, and health insurance coverage in the United States: 2010. U.S. Census Bureau, 2011. Available at: http://www.census.gov/prod/2011pubs/p60-239.pdf. Accessed August 31, 2012.

71. Bailey J. Assets, the poor and democracy. Unpublished paper presented at the American Academy of Religion annual meeting, Atlanta, GA., November 24, 2003.

72. Sherraden M. Assets and the poor: Implications for individual accounts and Social Security. Invited testimony to the President's Commission on Social Security, Washington, DC, October 18, 2002.

73. Howard C. The hidden welfare state: Tax expenditures and social policy in the United States. Princeton, NJ: Princeton University Press, 1997.

74. Governance and Social Development Resource Centre. Social exclusion. Available at: http://www.gsdrc.org/go/topic-guides/social-exclusion/introduction. Accessed August 30, 2012.

75. Social Exclusion Knowledge Network. Understanding and tackling social exclusion. WHO Commission on Social Determinants of Health, 2008. Available at: Accessed on August 30, 2012.

76. Amick BC, Levine S, Tarlov AR, Walsh DC. Introduction. In: Society and health. New York: Oxford University Press, 1995.

77. LaVeist, TA, Gaskin D, Trujillo, AJ. Segregated spaces: The effects of racial segregation on health inequalities. Washington DC: Joint Center for Political and Economic Studies, 2011.

78. Kramer MR, Hogue CR. Is segregation bad for your health? *Epidemiol Rev* 2009;31: 178–194.

79. Williams DR, Jackson PB. Social sources of racial health disparities. *Health Aff* 2005;24: 325–334.

80. Gaskin DJ, Dinwiddie GY, Chan KS, McCleary RR. Residential segregation and the availability of primary care physicians. Available at: http://onlinelibrary.wiley.com/doi/10.1111/j.1475-6773.2012.01417.x/abstract. Accessed August 30, 2012.

81. Landrine H, Corral I. Separate and unequal: Residential segregation and black health disparities. *Ethn Dis* 2009;19:179–184.

82. Walton E. Residential segregation and birth weight among racial and ethnic minorities in the United States. *J Health Soc Behav* 2009;50:427–442.

83. Williams DR, Collins C. Racial residential segregation: A fundamental cause of racial disparities in health. *Public Health Rep* 2001;116:104–116.

84. Luke D, Esmundo E, Bloom Y (2000) Smoke signs: Patterns of tobacco billboard advertising in a metropolitan region. *Tobacco Control* 2000;9:16–23.

85. LaVeist TA, Wallace J. Health risk and inequitable distribution of liquor stores in African American neighborhoods. *Soc Sci Med* 2000;51:613–617.

86. Lillie-Blanton M, Anthony JC, Schuster CR. Probing the meaning of racial/ethnic group comparisons in crack cocaine smoking. *JAMA* 1993;269:993–997.

87. Small ML. Neighborhood institutions as resource brokers: Childcare centers, inter-organizational ties, and resource access among the poor. *Social Problems* 2006;53: 274–292.

88. Small ML, Jacobs EM, Massengill RP. Why organizational ties matter for neighborhood effects: Resource access through childcare centers. *Social Forces* 2008;87:387–414.

89. Gordon C, Purciel-Hill M, Ghai NR, et al. Measuring food deserts in New York City's low-income neighborhoods. *Health Place* 2011;17:696–700.

90. Larsen K, Gilliland J. A farmers' market in a food desert: Evaluating impacts on the price and availability of healthy food. *Health Place* 2009;15:1158–1162.

91. Powell L, Slater S, Mirtcheva D, et al. Food store availability and neighborhood characteristics in the United States. *Prevent Med* 2007;44:189–195.

92. Community Partnerships for Older Adults. Health status: Disadvantaged groups and health status. Available at: http://www.partnershipsforolderadults.org/resources/levelthree.aspx?sectionGUID=dd373056-ff83-412b-b6eb-5c34ddda125e. Accessed August 31, 2012.

93. Institute of Medicine. Health literacy: A prescription to end confusion. Washington, DC: National Academies Press, 2004.

94. Evans T, Whitehead M, Wirth M, et al. Challenging inequities in health: From ethics to action: Summary. New York: Rockefeller Foundation, 2001.

95. Panel on Racial and Ethnic Disparities in Medical Care Convened by Physicians for Human Rights. The right to equal treatment: An action plan to end racial and ethnic disparities in clinical diagnosis and treatment in the United States. Available at: http://www.paeaonline.org/index.php?ht=a/GetDocumentAction/i/135605. Accessed September 1, 2012.

96. Allen CE, Easley CE. Practicing cultural competence. In: Levy BS, Gaufin JR, eds. Mastering public health: Essential skills for effective practice. New York: Oxford University Press, 2012:102–127.

97. Grumbach K, Mendoza R. Disparities in human resources: Addressing the lack of diversity in the health professions. *Health Aff* 2008;27:413–422.

98. Sullivan Commission. Missing Persons: Minorities in the health professions. A report of the Sullivan Commission on diversity in the health care workforce. 2006. Available at: http://health-equity.pitt.edu/40/1/Sullivan_Final_Report_000.pdf. Accessed August 27, 2012.

99. National Patient Safety Foundation. Ask me 3. Available at: http://www.npsf.org/for-healthcare-professionals/programs/ask-me-3/. Accessed September 1, 2012.

100. Pfizer Corp. The Newest Vital Sign: A new health literacy assessment tool for health care providers. Available at: http://www.pfizerhealthliteracy.com/physicians-providers/NewestVitalSign.aspx. Accessed August 30, 2012.

101. Shah LC, West P, Bremmeyr, Savoy-Moore RT. Health literacy instrument in family medicine: The "Newest Vital Sign" ease of use and correlates. Available at: http://www.jabfm.org/content/23/2/195.full. Accessed August 30, 2012.

102. Policy Link. Reducing health disparities through a focus on communities. Oakland, CA: Policy Link, 2002.

103. Wilkerson R, Marmot M, eds. The solid facts: Social determinants of health. 2nd ed. Copenhagen, Denmark: World Health Organization, 2003.

104. Bailey J. Assets, the poor and democracy. Unpublished paper presented at the American Academy of Religion annual meeting, Atlanta, GA, November 24, 2003.

105. Schreiner M, Clancy M, Sherraden M. Final report: Saving performance in the American dream demonstration, a national demonstration of individual development accounts. St. Louis, MO: Center for Social Development, Washington University in St. Louis, 2002.

106. Murray LR. Sick and tired of being sick and tired: Scientific evidence, methods, and research implications for racial and ethnic disparities in occupational health. *Am J Public Health* 2003;93:221–225.

107. Bird ME, ed. Eliminating health disparities: Conversations with American Indians and Alaska Natives. Santa Cruz, CA: ETR Associates, 2002.

108. Venkatapuram S. Health justice: An argument from the capabilities approach. Cambridge, United Kingdom: Polity Press, 2011.

4 Women

■ GINA MARANTO AND JUDY NORSIGIAN

■ INTRODUCTION

Consider two photographs from the "Arab spring" in Egypt: One, in early 2011, shows a little girl in a red sweater standing tall atop the shoulders of a grizzled, plaid-shirted man, possibly her father, amidst a crowd in Tahrir Square in Cairo. One of her hands grasps a tricolor flag; the other hand is raised in a fist, pumping against a hazy blue sky. Her mouth is open, mid-chant. She is a petite representative of her gender: for months, women, whether in traditional hijab or Western attire, participated in protests against President Hosni Mubarak and helped bring about the end of his regime.[1]

However, as demonstrated by the other photograph, in late 2011, women's presence in the public demonstrations was fraught with danger. In this photograph, five Egyptian army soldiers clad in camouflage, flak jackets, and visored helmets surround a woman, whom they are dragging across a littered tarmac. Her black abaya has been pulled over her head, exposing her bare midriff and bright turquoise brassiere. The other soldiers wear jackboots, except for one who wears beige hightop sneakers—his raised left foot is about to stomp on the woman's stomach.

These counterpoised images illustrate the realities of the status of women globally. In recent years, in some places, great strides have been made in overcoming ingrained biases and political and economic barriers to women's health and well-being (Figures 4–1 and 4–2). And, sometimes, in these same places, backlash against such gains has been swift and pronounced—even though public health and international policy experts agree that "empowering women, including their ability to achieve desired family size, is the most important driver of modern development efforts."[2]

Two of the eight Millennium Development Goals (MDGs) (Table 21–7 in Chapter 21; and Chapter 29) specifically pertain to women: Goal 3 is "Promote gender equality and empower women," and Goal 5 is "Improve maternal and reproductive health." The remaining MDGs are related to women, who—with children—are disproportionately impacted by poverty and environmental degradation, including climate change.[3,4] According to a 2012 assessment of progress toward the MDGs since 2008, equal girls' enrollment in primary school globally, a central component of Goal 3, has either already been met or is expected to be met by 2015 in all regions except Oceania.[5] However, except in Eastern Asia, Latin America, and the Caucasus and Central Asia, the trends are discouraging in terms of women's share of paid employment. And in all regions, the level of women's representation in national legislatures suggests that the goal of gender equality will not be met by 2015.[5]

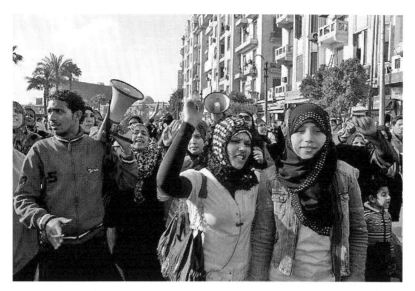

Figure 4–1 A women's rights protest in Egypt in March 2011. (*Source:* Al Jazeera English at http://www.flickr.com/photos/aljazeeraenglish/5509250057/.)

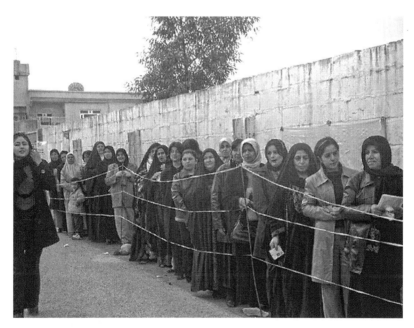

Figure 4–2 Iraqi women waiting to vote in election in January 2005. (*Source:* Photo courtesy of U.S. Embassy, Baghdad.)

▩ GENDER EQUITY

On the basis of the Gender Inequality Index, the global condition of women is deficient. This parameter evolved from the Human Development Index, which recognizes that, because Gross Domestic Product is an insufficient measure of development, human well-being must also be considered.[6] Encompassing three broad categories (women's health, empowerment, and the labor market), the Gender Inequality Index is based on rates of maternal mortality, adolescent fertility, parliamentary representation, educational attainment at the secondary level and higher, and participation in the workforce. An index of 0 (zero) represents full equality with men, and an index of 1, almost total inequality. A 2011 report that tabulated the index for 195 countries found a world average ratio of 0.49 (49 percent), but also large disparities in ratios between the Global North (such as 0.31 for Europe) and the Global South (such as 0.61 for sub-Saharan Africa). The report identified reproductive health (maternal mortality and adolescent fertility) as the main contributor to gender inequality—and also to health disparities among countries. In this category, sub-Saharan Africa fared worst (an index of 0.73), with South Asia, the Arab states, and Latin America and the Caribbean following closely behind.[7]

Gender inequality is associated with a range of health and psychological impacts, some of which are intertwined. Low- and middle-income nations have appropriately focused on key public health goals, such as controlling infectious diseases and improving the health of childbearing women and their children. However, these countries should also focus on women's mental health, which is adversely affected by gender inequality.[8] And poor mental health contributes to the incidence of several chronic diseases and sexually transmitted infections, including HIV.[9]

▩ FAMILY PLANNING AND RELATED ISSUES

Family planning continues to be critical for health and economic development. It is essential for achieving all eight MDGs. Where women have access to contraception and can choose the timing and number of their children, it can have impacts on areas beyond reproductive health. In many countries where family planning is implemented, malnutrition decreases, girls stay in school longer, women can work without interruptions for pregnancies and gain greater equality in the workforce, and the economy becomes stronger.[10] Spacing out births enables young children to have a better chance of surviving.[11,12] Contraception also lessens maternal mortality by (a) lowering rates of both legal and illegal abortion, and, (b) especially in countries where poor women have little access to prenatal care, eliminating their exposure to the risks associated with pregnancy.[2] In addition, by preventing births in HIV-positive women, contraception prevents HIV infections in children.[13]

Although family planning can achieve reductions in population growth at a relatively low cost,[14] it is critical that services are organized in a non-coercive fashion and with a real choice of methods. There are still unethical examples of coercion, such as the recent provision of Depo-Provera to Ethiopian women entering Israel.[15]

Despite advances in family planning over the past 50 years, there is still extensive unmet need, which the United Nations Population Division defines as women of reproductive age, who are married or in a union, and are fecund, not using contraception, and report that they do not want any more children or wish to delay the next child.[16]

"The level of unmet need for family planning varies from 2 percent in France to 46 percent in Samoa," and the poorest countries have the most unmet need: In 2011 in these countries, almost one-fourth of women of childbearing age who were married or in a union lacked access to modern methods of family planning, such as sterilization, birth control pills, implantable or injectable birth control, intrauterine devices, condoms, and vaginal barriers.[16]

Factors that determine contraception use include geographic proximity (most important), cost to the user (including money and other costs, such as transport and time away from work), and psychosocial barriers.[17] Adequate counseling and an array of birth control choices, including barrier methods such as the female condom, are also important to enabling women to make the best choices for themselves and their families. An additional barrier to hormonal birth control in the United States is the requirement for a prescription, which is not required in many other countries. Many obstetricians and gynecologists now recommend having oral contraceptives available over the counter, although some women's advocates want to be sure that drospirenone-containing oral contraceptives are excluded, given their problematic safety profile in comparison to other oral contraceptives.[18-20]

ABORTION

Abortion to eliminate unwanted pregnancies continues to be a contested issue in many countries, including the United States, where it was a key issue in 2012 election campaigns. The Republican Party platform featured several abortion-related planks, including support for appointments of "pro-life" judges, a call for a permanent "ban [on] all federal funding and subsidies for abortion and health care plans that include abortion coverage," and opposition to the use of taxpayer dollars "to promote or perform abortion or fund organizations which perform or advocate it." The platform also saluted "the many States that have passed laws for informed consent, mandatory waiting periods prior to an abortion, and health-protective clinic regulation."[21] In addition, in the year before the election, anti-abortion legislators engaged in a concerted effort to restrict women's access to abortion. In 2011, 19 states enacted 80 abortion restrictions, compared to 23 enacted in 2010.[22]

Laws against abortion do not reduce its incidence. Instead, they *increase* the number of abortions outside legitimate clinical settings and, consequently, the numbers of medical complications and deaths. Although the number of induced abortions in the United States decreased from 45.6 million in 1995 to 41.6 million in 2003, this decrease was largely attributable to fewer legal abortions—and from 2003 to 2008, the decline ceased.[23] For 2008, analysis of data suggested that, at least in low-income countries, more abortions were performed under unsafe conditions—often extralegally—than under safe ones.[24,25]

Because it is difficult to gain accurate information about abortion rates in countries where the practice is banned or stigmatized or where medical care is delivered in remote locations, it is difficult to estimate mortality from poorly performed abortions. However, the World Health Organization estimated that there had been 66,500 deaths globally due to unsafe abortions in 2003—fewer than 60 in high-income countries, and the vast majority in sub-Saharan Africa.[26]

Activist women's groups have in recent years launched initiatives to expand access to safe abortion (Figure 4–3). For example, Women on Waves provides medical abortions onboard a ship that anchors offshore from countries where abortion is illegal. It also operates an extensive website, which includes information on safe-abortion hotlines globally, instructions on the use of the drugs mifepristone and misoprostol to induce abortion before the 12th week of gestation, and links to websites where women can buy abortion pills online.[27]

The Internet can be a source of erroneous health information. It can be used by governments for oppression. However, the Internet can also significantly enhance women's ability to gain power by enabling them to (a) "construct counterpublics and [gain] new forms of access to deliberation and decision making," and

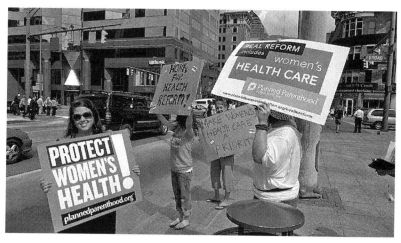

Figure 4–3 Planned Parenthood volunteers demonstrating for women's health protection and health insurance reform in Columbus, Ohio, in August 2009. (*Source:* ProgressOhio at http://www.flickr.com/photos/65312697@N00/3812663670.)

(b) counter male-dominated public discourse transnationally.[28] As occurred during the Arab Spring, the Internet provides women with new opportunities for engaging in political speech and for organizing politically.[29]

▪ INFERTILITY AND ASSISTED REPRODUCTION

Since the birth of the first "test-tube" baby in 1978, the global proliferation of technologies that enable scientists to manipulate sperm, eggs, and embryos has enabled millions of infertile women and couples to have biologically related children. An estimated 5 million infants have been born as a result of assisted reproductive technologies (ARTs), which include *in vitro* fertilization (IVF), artificial insemination, and intracytoplasmic sperm injection (ICSI).[30]

ARTs have allowed couples who might otherwise never have been able to reproduce to form families—including same-sex couples. Their use has led to many ethical, legal, and sociological dilemmas. Concerns about ARTs have included:

- Potential long-term adverse health effects to children born via assisted reproduction[31]
- Effects on families of keeping secrets from their offspring about their origins[32]
- Psychological adjustment of children raised in non-traditional families[33]
- The property status of eggs, sperm, and embryos[34]
- The high rate of twin and triplet births from IVF, with attendant health risks to mothers and offspring[35]
- Equity of access, especially in countries without national health programs[36]

In the United States, activists concerned about the inability of people to pay for expensive infertility treatments have lobbied legislatures to mandate that health insurance companies cover them, although this does not help Americans who lack such insurance (48.6 million in 2011).[37,38] However, in 2012, only 15 states had laws requiring insurers to either cover, or offer coverage for, diagnostic procedures and treatment for infertility, and only three of these states—California, Louisiana, and New York—allowed insurers to exclude IVF procedures.[39]

Assisted reproduction often involves third parties, including men who provide sperm (anonymously or not), women who provide eggs (egg donors), and women who gestate fetuses that may or may not have a genetic relationship to them (surrogates). All such third-party arrangements have been legally contested multiple times.

In industrialized countries, bioethics experts and women's rights groups have widely debated issues regarding egg harvesting, especially from young women.[40] Of special concern has been whether or not young women, who are actively recruited by clinics—often by advertisements in college newspapers—receive adequate information about potential risks of the procedure,[41] such as the frequent off-label use of Lupron™ (leuprolide acetate). For example, some young women develop chronic inflammation of their ovaries and may, as a result, become infertile.[42] And it is still uncertain whether or not the procedure of egg harvesting might increase the risk of ovarian cancer.[43,44]

The only national registry in the United States that is now tracking the health of all people engaged with ARTs is the Infertility Family Research Registry (IFRR) at the Dartmouth Hitchcock Medical Center (www.ifrr-registry.org). Participation in it is entirely voluntary. (Compliance with clinical-practice guidelines for ARTs, promulgated by the American Society of Reproductive Medicine, is also entirely voluntary.) The vast majority of fertility centers have done very little to promote awareness of this important registry, despite repeated requests to post a simple placard next to IFRR brochures in their waiting rooms.[45] Consequently, the claims of the infertility industry about the long-term safety of ARTs should be regarded with some skepticism, as data on ART safety are not comprehensive and, in most countries, neither egg donors nor children born with the assistance of ARTs have been tracked.[46–48]

The ways in which market forces shape the supposedly voluntary process in which sperm and eggs are obtained by the highly profitable infertility industry—estimated as a $3 billion-per-year enterprise in the United States—have been extensively scrutinized.[49] The industry perpetuates gender stereotypes, racism, and unscientific notions of inheritance through such practices as (a) paying women of certain races and body types more for eggs—a practice that contradicts industry claims that women are being compensated for time and effort, rather than for their biological material; and (b) creating catalogs of sperm donors according to their height, financial status, and educational level—none of which are directly heritable.[50,51] This practice has disquieting echoes:

> In this market, race and ethnicity are biologized, as in references to Asian eggs or Jewish sperm, and it is one of the primary sorting mechanisms in donor catalogs, along with hair and eye color. This routinized reinscription of race at the genetic and cellular level in donation programs, which…medicalized organizations offer [as] a veneer of scientific credibility to such claims, is worrisome given our eugenic history.[52]

Further ethical discussion has centered on the emerging trend of seeking young women's eggs not for purposes of infertility treatment, but rather for use in creating clones by a technique known as *somatic-cell nuclear transfer* (SCNT). Such clones are vital for stem-cell research. Proponents argue that the risk of complications from ovarian stimulation and egg harvesting in the IVF setting is low, and therefore, if researchers use the same procedures to obtain eggs for SCNT, it does "not warrant undue concern."[53] But established risks in the context of infertility clinics cannot be assumed to equal the risks for women involved in egg harvesting for stem-cell research—in part because these two groups of women could have different demographic characteristics, which could affect outcomes.[54] "In addition, egg harvesting [for SCNT] is taking place in a research climate marked by conflicts of interest, the misleading use of language to describe research goals, and a commercial push that may lead to the exploitation of women."[55] As a result, there have been calls for an international moratorium on egg harvesting for SCNT, including by a coalition of women's rights and pro-choice groups under the banner "Hands Off Our Ovaries."[56]

Although most women in developing countries do not have access to ARTs, infertility clinics catering largely to an international clientele have been established in Korea, countries in South Asia and Southeast Asia, and a few major cities in Central and South America.[57] Advertising widely on the Internet, these clinics represent *reproductive tourism*, cross-border reproductive health care that is a part of the global trend in *medical tourism*—although women who participate have experiences that are far more stressful than those of the average tourist. Reproductive tourism has grown exponentially since 2000, and an estimated 11,000 to 14,000 people in the European Union alone travel outside their home countries to access ART services.[58,59] They do so for multiple reasons, mainly to avoid long waiting times for service from national health programs in their home countries, or to access procedures that (a) are banned in their home countries, or (b) they cannot access because of their marital status or sexual orientation.[60]

India has become the "surrogacy capital" of the world. Since surrogacy was legalized there in 2002, a multimillion-dollar surrogacy industry has grown. Clinics typically recruit poor (often illiterate) women, many of whom have not previously had any medical care at all. These clinics pay them a small percentage of the fees collected from clients, who often deal with brokers in their home countries before travelling to these clinics.[61] Activist groups in India and elsewhere have supported restrictions on surrogacy clinics—such as requirements that clinics report to a national registry.[62] They also note the profound power imbalance between clients, who are often well-to-do residents of industrialized countries, and gestational mothers, who often come from the poorest and least educated classes.[63]

▨ HIV/AIDS

As of late 2010, there were 34 million people infected with HIV—almost half of them female; in sub-Saharan Africa, 59 percent were female, and in the Caribbean, 53 percent.[64] In the United States, 25 percent of the 1.1 million people infected are women.[65] African-American women account for 57 percent of new cases in the United States, 40 percent of them 13 to 29 years of age.[66] Of particular concern in many urban areas are homeless young women, among whom *survival sex*—that is, sex performed for money, food, or shelter—is prevalent. Survival sex is associated not only with an increased chance of contracting sexually transmitted infections (STIs) and HIV, but also increased drug use, suicide, unplanned pregnancy, and victimization.[67]

Many social factors increase the vulnerability of women to HIV infection, especially in low-income countries, but also in impoverished communities in high-income countries.[68] These include "gender disparities, poverty, cultural and sexual norms, lack of education, and violence. Biological factors also make women vulnerable to HIV infection, including hormonal changes, vaginal microbial ecology and physiology, and a higher prevalence of sexually transmitted infections than men."[69] In countries where gender disparities deprive women of the ability to work in the mainstream labor force, pressing economic circumstances may lead them to sex work or to migrate in search of work, sometimes under coerced conditions. (See Box 21–1 in Chapter 21.)

HIV-infected women who are pregnant risk transmitting the virus to their off-spring, although, in 2007, only about one-third of all pregnant women infected with HIV received medication to prevent such transmission.[70]

HIV/AIDS has devastating consequences for women. A cascading effect may begin when the male head of the household becomes infected, limiting his ability to work and requiring female relatives, often including grandmothers and daughters, to care for him. Household income decreases, and children are forced to leave school and find whatever work they can—for young girls, this often means sex work, exposing them to HIV. When parents die of HIV/AIDS or its complications, children are forced to leave their homes and live on the street.[71]

■ WAR, VIOLENCE, AND FORCED MIGRATION

War and other forms of armed conflict have profound effects on women and their families (Figure 4–4). "Coercive sex, sexual violence, and [sexually

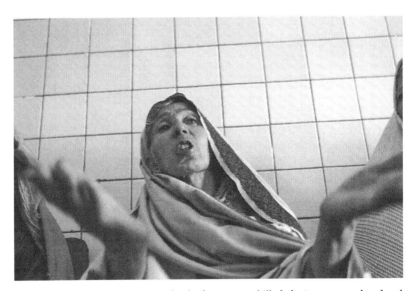

Figure 4-4 A 45-year-old woman who had two sons killed during war and a daughter injured by a bomb at their home cries during her therapy session at a mental health hospital in Kabul, Afghanistan. Due to the tragedies suffered by the women, many have developed mental health problems, including anxiety, depression, and other related disorders. (*Source:* AP Photo/Silvia Izquierdo.)

transmitted infections] are magnified and accelerated by armed conflict"[71]—such as in the civil war in the Democratic Republic of the Congo (DRC), which has been financed by trade in "blood minerals," such as coltan, which is used in cell phones, laptops, and other electronic devices.[72] Since 1998, five million people have died during this war, which has displaced 2.2 million people internally and many others in neighboring countries.[73] Women and children in refugee camps throughout the region have been threatened by armed groups of men on a regular basis.[74] (See Chapter 11 and Box 17–1 in Chapter 17.)

DRC troops and rebel soldiers have institutionalized rape as a weapon of war.[75] Women's and human rights groups have raised awareness of and support for the plight of the hundreds of thousands of women and girls who have been raped during this war. Sexual violence has profound psychological consequences and causes genital lesions, traumatic fistulae, fractured and severed limbs, unwanted pregnancies, and sexually transmitted infections, including HIV. In addition, rape victims are ostracized and abandoned by their families and communities.[76] (See Chapter 17.)

Similar violence against women is occurring globally. The United Nations Special Rapporteur on violence against women has, since 2007, visited more than 24 countries[77] to (a) investigate and report on all forms of such violence in civil, cultural, economic, political, and social spheres; (b) recommend measures for eliminating it; and (c) seek remedies for victims.[78] In 2011, the United Nations General Assembly adopted Resolution 65/187, Intensification of Efforts to Eliminate All Forms of Violence Against Women. It affirmed the General Assembly's deep concern about pervasive violence against women and girls in its many forms globally and "the need to intensify efforts to prevent and eliminate all forms of violence against women and girls."[79]

▓ AGING

The aging of the population globally, coupled with mass migration of people—due to war, economic conditions, and environmental threats—is creating new issues for women and altering family structures. In places like the Philippines and Central America, which younger women leave for prolonged periods or permanently for household and childcare work in Europe, the Middle East, and the United States, female relatives left behind face added burdens caring for children and aging parents.[80]

As the population ages in any given country, the proportion of women increases, although women consigned to household work have no pensions or retirement savings. This problem affects both developed and developing countries, as poverty, emigration, and changing cultural norms eliminate family support systems for older people. (See Chapter 6.)

In the absence of pensions, women in developing countries are often poorer in old age than men. For example, in cities in China, poverty rates among older women are four times higher than among older men. In India, 60 percent of older women have no valuable assets, compared to 30 percent of older men."[81]

▨ CLIMATE CHANGE

Climate change is also likely to have major impacts on women. The Fourth Assessment Report of the Intergovernmental Panel on Climate Change recognizes that gender roles and gender relations influence vulnerability and people's capacity to adapt to climate change. Especially vulnerable are rural women in developing countries, who are often dependent on natural resources for their livelihoods, do most of the agricultural work, and bear responsibility for collecting water and fuel. Climate change is likely to adversely affect these women's lives in many ways.[82] Shifting monsoon and storm patterns will impact agriculture and water availability in both rural areas and cities. While people can adapt, cultural and social norms that dictate who does what work could make any adaptations especially difficult for these women. Gender equality must be considered in plans that address climate change so that women receive the necessary financial and technological support.[83] (See Chapter 18.)

▨ WHAT NEEDS TO BE DONE

There is much that needs to be done to address the many social injustice issues that adversely affect the health of women. (See Boxes 4–1 and 4–2) This section provides some suggestions concerning issues of highest priority.

Gender Equity

As Nyaradzayi Gumbonzvanda, now with the World YWCA, has advocated, to advance the discourse on gender relations and to achieve gender equity, we need to have a larger conceptual framework for women's issues that links empowerment of women, women's rights, and mainstreaming in all social spaces.[84] Challenges include "top-down" development strategies that fail to recognize gender inequities, ingrained patriarchies, and the special needs of women and children.[84] One approach, albeit controversial, to foster gender equity would be ratification by the United States and many other countries of the Convention on the Elimination of All Forms of Discrimination Against Women (CEDAW), an international convention adopted by the United Nations General Assembly in 1979 and ratified by more than 50 countries. Using a rights framework, it could provide throughout the world a coherent foundation for a comprehensive policy to enhance the well-being of women and girls.[8]

BOX 4-1   ■   Our Bodies Ourselves

Our Bodies Ourselves (OBOS), also known as the Boston Women's Health Book Collective, is a global nonprofit, public interest organization based in Cambridge, Massachusetts. OBOS promotes accurate, evidence-based information on girls' and women's reproductive health and sexuality, and addresses the social, economic, and political conditions that affect health care access and quality of care. It advances health and human rights within a framework of values shaped by women's voices and a commitment to self-determination and equality. OBOS's landmark publication, *Our Bodies, Ourselves*, first published in 1971, has been translated and adapted into 25 languages by women's groups around the world.

Beginning in 1970 with the publication of the first edition of *Our Bodies, Ourselves*, OBOS has inspired the Women's Health Movement by:

- Producing books that make accurate health and medical information accessible to a broad audience by weaving women's stories into a framework of practical, clearly written text
- Identifying and collaborating with exemplary individuals and organizations that provide services, generate research and policy analysis, and organize for social change
- Inspiring and empowering women to become engaged in the political aspects of sustaining good health for themselves and their communities

OBOS helped to introduce the following key concepts into the public discourse on women's health:

- Women, as informed health consumers, are catalysts for social change.
- Women can become their own health experts, especially through discussing issues of health and sexuality with each other.
- Health consumers have a right to know about controversies concerning medical practices and about where consensus among medical experts may be developing.
- Women compose the largest segment of health workers, health consumers, and health decision-makers for their families and communities, but are under-represented in positions of influence and policymaking.
- A pathology/disease approach to normal life events—such as birthing, menopause, aging, and death—is not an effective way in which to consider health or structure a health care system.

During the past several years, OBOS has:

- Published the ninth edition of *Our Bodies, Ourselves* (*Our Bodies, Ourselves: Pregnancy and Birth*) and *Our Bodies, Ourselves: Menopause*
- Produced *De Camino a la Maternidad*, a Spanish-language resource on pregnancy and childbirth, as well as *Promotoras de Salud*, a peer health-educator training guide based on *Nuestros Cuerpos, Nuestras Vidas*, the Spanish-language adaptation of *Our Bodies, Ourselves*
- Facilitated translation/adaptation projects in other countries
- Developed and maintained the Women's Health Information Resource Center, the companion website for its books

- Distributed more than 3,000 books and materials free of charge worldwide
- Acted as a key voice in policy, advocacy, and educational work related to women's health through its Public Voice and Action program

In 2012, OBOS launched its "Our Bodies, Our Votes" campaign, a nonpartisan program to alert younger women to political attacks on reproductive health services, especially contraception and abortion. Its press release quoted Marcia Angell, M.D., former editor-in-chief of the *New England Journal of Medicine*, who said: "Requiring doctors to perform procedures that are not medically indicated, or to provide false information about medical evidence, violates women's rights and leaves doctors with an untenable dilemma: Violate state law, or betray their professional obligations to patients."

More information is available at: http://www.ourbodiesourselves.org.

Family Planning and Related Issues

In the United States, oral contraceptives should be provided over the counter (without a physician's prescription being necessary). The Women's Health Practice and Research Network of the American College of Clinical Pharmacy has advocated for this change, citing ample evidence that women are able to

---

BOX 4-2 ◼ Engagement of Men in Gender-Based Violence Prevention

Men are increasingly engaged in gender-based-violence prevention with athletic coaches, law enforcement personnel, military service members, fathers in church and school groups, and others providing leadership. The following are some examples.

White Ribbon Day is a statewide campaign in Massachusetts. One day in March each year, men speak out to promote safety and respect in all relationships and to change societal attitudes and beliefs that perpetuate gender-based violence. (More information is available at http://whiteribbonday.janedoe.org/.)

Voice Male magazine chronicles changes that men have undergone, men's work in challenging male violence, and men's ongoing exploration of their interior lives. It honors men's and women's contributions to promoting gender equality. (More information is available at http://voicemalemagazine.org/.)

The Mentors in Violence Prevention (MVP) Model is a gender-violence, bullying, and school-violence approach to prevention that encourages young men and women from all backgrounds to provide leadership in their schools and communities. Training in the MVP Model consists of role-plays to allow students to construct and practice responses to harassment, abuse, or violence. (More information is available at http://www.mvpnational.org and http://www.mvpstrategies.net.)

MenEngage is a global alliance of non-governmental organizations and United Nations agencies that encourages men to help build gender equality and help improve men's and women's health. It works to transform pervasive gender inequalities through public policy and collaboration with the Women's Rights Movement. (More information is available at http://www.menengage.org.)

self-screen for major contraindications to oral contraceptives, and that pharmacists in the community could help women choose appropriate hormonal contraception.[85] The American College of Obstetricians and Gynecologists has also supported over-the-counter access for oral contraceptives.[86]

In low-income countries, a variety of family planning services and contraceptives, including barrier methods that prevent HIV/STI transmission, should be made accessible, available, and affordable to all women, a goal that many foundations and professional organizations have supported. For example, Melinda Gates, of the Bill & Melinda Gates Foundation, has advocated for women to have access to modern contraceptives. She has said, "(G)overnment leaders who used to think family planning was just a health issue or just a women's issue are now asking how they can help build a national program. They are beginning to understand that providing access to contraceptives is a cost-effective way to foster economic growth."[87]

Abortion

In the United States, activists in public health, women's rights, and human rights should persuade federal and state legislators to reverse many of the draconian measures that have impeded women's access to safe abortion services. The Hyde Amendment, which the Congress first passed in 1976, barred the use of federal funds to pay for abortions. It has since been the most significant assault on poor women's access to abortion. The current version of the Hyde Amendment, passed in 1997, allows federal funding for abortion in cases of rape and incest and when a pregnant woman's life is threatened by "physical disorder, physical injury, or physical illness, including a life-endangering physical condition caused by or arising from the pregnancy itself."

Examples of state laws that should be reviewed include: vaginal-probe ultrasound examinations for women considering abortion; mandated abortion counseling that provides inaccurate or misleading information (such as asserting that having an abortion increases a woman's risk of breast cancer); and "personhood amendments" that aim to give full legal rights to a fertilized egg—effectively making illegal most forms of hormonal contraception, including birth control pills, and raising barriers to terminating pregnancy. Public health advocates should insist that non-governmental organizations that receive funding from the U.S. government can, with funds from other sources, continue to perform or promote awareness of abortion services in other countries.

HIV/AIDS

In all countries, all men and women should be educated and informed about HIV/AIDS as well as other STIs, including how to negotiate safe sex. A multifaceted approach should include making female and male condoms accessible to everyone in ways that do not stigmatize; further developing methods of protection initiated by women, such as microbicides[88,89]; and studying the influence of hormones on the progression of disease and responses to treatment.[69] Developing countries and funding agencies should support:

- Prevention programs that are designed to reach diverse groups of people and encourage them to be tested[90]
- Increased research on vaccines
- Wider access to antiretroviral drugs and to clinical care[91]
- Prevention of HIV infections among children[92]
- Measures to end discrimination and violence against people with HIV/AIDS[93]

▨ REFERENCES

1. Khamis S. The Arab "feminist" spring? *Feminist Studies* 2011;37:692–695,748.
2. Cates W Jr. Family planning: The essential link to achieving all eight Millennium Development Goals. *Contraception* 2010;81:460–461.
3. Denton F. Climate change vulnerability, impacts, and adaptation: Why does gender matter? *Gender & Development* 2002;10:10–20.
4. Cannon T. Gender and climate hazards in Bangladesh. *Gender & Development* 2002;10: 45–50.
5. Statistics Division, Department of Economic and Social Affairs, United Nations. Millennium Development Goals: 2012 progress chart. Available at: http://www.un.org/millenniumgoals/pdf/2012_Progress_E.pdf Accessed December 13, 2012.
6. United Nations Development Programme. About human development. Available at: http://hdr.undp.org/en/humandev/. Accessed December 13, 2012.
7. United Nations Development Programme. Human development reports, Gender Inequality Index (GII). Available at: http://hdr.undp.org/en/statistics/gii/. Accessed December 13, 2012.
8. Sianko N. Gender equality and women's mental health: What's on the agenda? *Am J Orthopsychiatry* 2011;81:167–171.
9. Prince M, Patel V, Saxena S, et al. Global mental health 1: No health without mental health. *Lancet* 2007;370:859–877.
10. FHI 360. Women's voices, women's lives: The impact of family planning: Executive summary. Available at: http://www.fhi360.org/en/RH/Pubs/wsp/synthesis/ExecSum.htm. Accessed December 20, 2012.
11. Park CB. The place of child-spacing as a factor in infant mortality: A recursive model. *Am J Public Health* 1986;76:995–999.
12. Alam N. Birth spacing and infant and early childhood mortality in a high fertility area of Bangladesh: Age-dependent and interactive effects. *J Biosoc Sci* 1995;27:393–404.
13. Hladik W, Stover J, Esiru G, et al. The contribution of family planning towards the prevention of vertical HIV transmission in Uganda. *PLoS ONE* 2009;4:e7691. doi:10.1371/journal.pone.0007691.
14. Speidel JJ, Weiss DC, Ethelston SA, Gilbert SM. Family planning and reproductive health: The link to environmental preservation. *Population and Environment* 2007;28: 247–258.
15. Yardai E. An inconveivable (sic) crime. Haaretz, November 12, 2012. Available at: http://www.haaretz.com/opinion/israel-s-ethiopians-suffer-different-planned-parenthood.premium-1.484110. Accessed December 19, 2012.

16. United Nations Population Division. World contraceptive use 2011. Available at: http://www.un.org/esa/population/publications/contraceptive2011/wallchart_front.pdf. Accessed December 13, 2012.

17. Hanson K, Kumaranayake L, Thomas I. Ends versus means: The role of markets in expanding access to contraceptives. *Health Policy Plan* 2001;16:125–136.

18. Grindlay K, Burns B, Grossman D. Prescription requirements and over-the-counter access to oral contraceptives: A global review. *Contraception* 2012;[in press]. doi: 10.1016/j.contraception.2012.11.021.

19. Sidney S, Cheetham TC, Connell FA, et al. Recent combined hormonal contraceptives (CHCs) and the risk of thromboembolism and other cardiovascular events in new users. *Contraception* 2013;87:93–100.

20. National Research Center for Women & Families. Letter to Dr. Hamburg, FDA Commissioner, on the review of drospirenone (DRSP)-based oral contraceptives, March 9, 2012. Available at: http://center4research.org/public-policy/letters-to-government-officials/letter-to-fda-commissioner-yaz-drospirenone-contraceptives/. Accessed January 2, 2013.

21. Republican National Committee. Republican Party platform 2012. Available at: http://www.gop.com/wp-content/uploads/2012/08/2012GOPPlatform.pdf. Accessed December 14, 2012.

22. Guttmacher Institute. Laws affecting reproductive health and rights: State trends at midyear, 2011. Available at: http://www.guttmacher.org/statecenter/updates/2011/statetrends22011.html. Accessed December 14, 2012.

23. Sedgh G, Singh S, Shah IH, et al. Induced abortion: Incidence and trends worldwide from 1995 to 2008. *Lancet* 2012;379:625–632.

24. World Health Organization. Unsafe abortion: Global and regional estimates of the incidence of unsafe abortion and associated mortality in 2008. Available at: http://whqlibdoc.who.int/publications/2011/9789241501118_eng.pdf. Accessed December 19, 2012.

25. Shah I, Åhman E. Unsafe abortion: Global and regional incidence, trends, consequences, and challenges. *J Obstet Gynaecol Can* 2009;31:1149–1158.

26. World Health Organization. Unsafe abortion: Global and regional estimates of the incidence of unsafe abortion and associated mortality in 2003. Available at: http://whqlibdoc.who.int/publications/2007/9789241596121_eng.pdf. Accessed December 13, 2012.

27. Women on Waves. Available at: http://www.womenonwaves.org. Accessed on December 31, 2012.

28. Bohman J. Expanding dialogue: The Internet, the public sphere and prospects for transnational democracy. *Sociological Review* 2004;52:131–155. doi: 10.1111/j.1467-954X.2004.00477.x.

29. Newsom V, Lengel L. Arab women, social media, and the Arab spring: Applying the framework of digital reflexivity to analyze gender and online activism. *Journal of International Women's Studies* 2012;13:31–46.

30. European Society of Human Reproduction and Embryology. *ART Fact Sheet*. Available at: http://www.eshre.eu/ESHRE/English/Guidelines-Legal/ART-fact-sheet/page.aspx/1061. Accessed December 19, 2012.

31. Hansen M, Kurinczuk J, Bower C, Webb, S. The risk of major birth defects after intracytoplasmic sperm injection and in vitro fertilization. *N Engl J Med* 2002;346:725–730.

32. Shenfield F, Steele SJ. What are the effects of anonymity and secrecy on the welfare of the child in gamete donation? *Hum Reprod* 1997;12:392–395.

33. Golombok S, Badger S. Children raised in mother-headed families from infancy: A follow-up of children of lesbian and single heterosexual mothers, at early adulthood. *Hum Reprod* 2010;25:150–157. doi: 10.1093/humrep/dep345.

34. Pennings G. What are the ownership rights for gametes and embryos? Advance directives and the disposition of cryopreserved gametes and embryos. *Hum Reprod* 2000;15:979–986. doi: 10.1093/humrep/15.5.979.

35. Roberts SA, McGowan L, Hirst M, et al. Reducing the incidence of twins from IVF treatments: Predictive modeling from a retrospective cohort. *Hum Reprod* 2011;26: 569–575.

36. Pennings G, de Wert F, Shenfield J, et al. ESHRE Task Force on Ethics and Law 14: Equity of access to assisted reproductive technology. *Hum Reprod* 2008;23:772–774.

37. U.S. Census Bureau. Income, poverty and health insurance coverage in the United States: 2011. Available at: http://www.census.gov/newsroom/releases/archives/income_wealth/cb12-172.html. Accessed December 19, 2012.

38. Shanley ML, Asch A. Involuntary childlessness, reproductive technology, and social justice: The medical mask on social illness. *Signs: Journal of Women in Culture and Society* 2009;34:851–874.

39. National Conference of State Legislatures. State laws related to insurance coverage for infertility treatment. Available at: http://www.ncsl.org/issues-research/health/insuranc e-coverage-for-infertility-laws.aspx. Accessed December 19, 2012.

40. Bercovici M. Biotechnology beyond the embryo: Science, ethics, and responsible regulation of egg donation to protect women's rights. *Women's Rights Law Reporter* 2008;29: 193–212.

41. Bodri D, Guillén J, Polo A, et al. Complications related to ovarian stimulation and oocyte retrieval in 4052 oocyte donor cycles. *Reproductive Biomedicine Online* (Reproductive Healthcare Limited) [serial online]. August 2008;17:237–243.

42. Maxwell K, Cholst I, Rosenwaks Z. The incidence of both serious and minor complications in young women undergoing oocyte donation. *Fertility and Sterility* 2008; 90:2165–2171.

43. Brinton LA, Lamb EJ, Moghissi KS, et al. Ovarian cancer risk associated with varying causes of infertility. *Fertility and Sterility* 2004;82:405–414.

44. Konishi I, Kuroda H, Mandai M. Gonadotropins and development of ovarian cancer. *Oncology* 1999;57(suppl 2):45–48.

45. Personal communications with the staff of the Infertility Family Research Registry, summer 2012.

46. Gender and Justice Program. Assisted reproductive technologies: Overview and perspective using a reproductive justice framework. Available at: http://www.geneticsandsociety.org/downloads/ART.pdf. Accessed December 31, 2012.

47. Elton C. Study: Why IVF is linked with cancer risk. Available at: http://www.time.com/time/health/article/0,8599,2004668,00.html. Accessed December 31, 2012.

48. Daily Mail Online. Expert warns of IVF time bomb. Available at: http://www.dailymail.co.uk/health/article-195627/Expert-warns-IVF-timebomb.html. Accessed December 20, 2012.

49. Spar D. The baby business: How money, science, and politics drive the commerce of conception. Cambridge, MA: Harvard Business School Press, 2006.

50. Daniels CR, Golden J. Procreative compounds: Popular eugenics, artificial insemination and the sperm banking industry. *Journal of Social History* 2004;38:5–27.

51. Almeling R. Gender and the value of bodily goods: Commodification in egg and sperm donation. *Law and Contemporary Problems* 2009;72:37–58.

52. Almeling R. Selling genes, selling gender: Egg agencies, sperm banks, and the medical market in genetic material. *American Sociological Review* 2007;72:319–340.

53. Ellison B, Melikera J. Assessing the risk of ovarian hyperstimulation syndrome in egg donation: Implications for human embryonic stem cell research. *American J Bioethics* 2011;11:22–30.

54. Bamford R. Reconsidering risk to women: Oocyte donation for human embryonic stem cell research. *Am J Bioethics* 2011;11:37–39.

55. Beeson D, Lippman A. Egg harvesting for stem cell research: Medical risks and ethical problems. *Reproductive BioMedicine Online* 2006;13:573–579. Available at: www.rbmonline.com/Article/2503. Accessed December 13, 2012.

56. Hands Off Our Ovaries. Hands off manifesto. Available at: http://www.handsoffourovaries.com/manifesto.htm. Accessed December 19, 2012.

57. Darnovsky M. Egg raffles and shadow markets: The fertility industry goes global and skirts laws. *Biopolitical Times* 2010. Available at: http://www.biopoliticaltimes.org/article.php?id=5125. Accessed December 19, 2012.

58. Shanks P. Struggling to control fertility tourism. *Biopolitical Times* 2010. Available at: http://www.biopoliticaltimes.org/article.php?id=5156. Accessed December 19, 2012.

59. Shenfield F, de Mouzon J, Pennings G, et al. Cross border reproductive care in six European countries. *Hum Reprod* 2010;25:1361–1368.

60. Ikemoto L. Reproductive tourism: Equality concerns in the global market for fertility services. Available at: http://prochoicealliance.org/files/Ikemoto_Reproductive_Tourism_Equality_Concerns_Book_Proof_final.pdf.Accessed December 31, 2012.

61. Pande A. Commercial surrogacy in India: Manufacturing a perfect mother-worker. *Signs: Journal of Women in Culture and Society* 2010;35:969–992.

62. Ministry of Health & Family Welfare, Government of India. Draft: Assisted reproductive technology (regulation) bill - 2010. Available at: http://www.scribd.com/doc/33533932/Art-Regulation-Draft-Bill1-India. Accessed December 19, 2012.

63. Rotabi K, Bromfield N. Intercountry adoption declines lead to new practices of surrogacy in Guatemala: Global human rights concerns in the context of violence and the era of advanced fertility technology. *Affilia* 2012;27:129–141.

64. UNAIDS. World AIDS Day report 2011. Available at: http://www.unaids.org/en/media/unaids/contentassets/documents/unaidspublication/2011/JC2216_WorldAIDSday_report_2011_en.pdf. Accessed December 14, 2012.

65. Centers for Disease Control and Prevention. HIV among women. Available at: http://www.cdc.gov/hiv/topics/women/index.htm. Accessed December 14, 2012.

66. Prejean J, Song R, Hernandez A, et al. Estimated HIV incidence in the United States, 2006–2009. *PLoS ONE* 2011;6: e17502. doi:10.1371/journal.pone.0017502.

67. Greene J, Ennett S, Ringwalt C. Prevalence and correlates of survival sex among runaway and homeless youth. *Am J Public Health* 1999;89:1406–1409.

68. Shannon K, Bright V, Gibson K, Tyndall MW. Sexual and drug-related vulnerabilities for HIV infection among women engaged in survival sex work in Vancouver, Canada. *Can J Public Health* 2007;98:465–469.

69. Quinn TC, Overbaugh J. HIV/AIDS in women: An expanding epidemic. *Science* 2005;308:1582–1583.

70. Women's Health Office. AIDS worldwide. Available at: http://www.womenshealth.gov/hiv-aids/aids-worldwide/#pubs. Accessed December 14, 2012.

71. Kamal Smith M. Gender, poverty, and intergenerational vulnerability to HIV/AIDS. Available at: http://hivaidsclearinghouse.unesco.org/search/resources/gender_vulnerability_hivaids.pdf. Accessed December 31, 2012.

72. International Peace Information Service. Supporting the war economy in the DRC: European companies and the coltan trade: Five case studies. Available at: http://www.grandslacs.net/doc/2343.pdf. Accessed December 20, 2012.

73. UNHCR: The UN Refugee Agency. UNHCR D.R. Congo Fact Sheet 30, September 2012. Available at: http://www.unhcr.org/4fab74189.pdf. Accessed December 20, 2012.

74. UNHCR: The UN Refugee Agency. UNHCR still concerned about security situation in camps near Goma. Available at: http://www.unhcr.org/50d049206.html. Accessed December 19, 2012.

75. Institute for Policy Studies. Stabilizing Congo. Available at: http://www.fpif.org/articles/stabilizing_congo. Accessed December 19, 2012.

76. VDAY.org. Why Congo? Congo is the most dangerous place on the planet to be a woman or a girl. Available at: http://drc.vday.org/why-congo. Accessed December 19, 2012.

77. UN Special Rapporteur on violence against women. Annual reports. Available at: http://www.ohchr.org/EN/Issues/Women/SRWomen/Pages/AnnualReports.aspx. Accessed December 20, 2012.

78. Office of the UN High Commissioner for Human Rights. Special Rapporteur on violence against women, its causes and consequences. Available at: http://www.ohchr.org/EN/Issues/Women/SRWomen/Pages/SRWomenIndex.aspx. Accessed December 20, 2012.

79. UN General Assembly. Resolution adopted by the General Assembly, 65/187. Intensification of efforts to eliminate all forms of violence against women. Available at: http://www.un.org/ga/search/view_doc.asp?symbol=A/RES/65/187. Accessed December 20, 2012.

80. Bastia T. Women's migration and the crisis of care: Grandmothers caring for grandchildren in urban Bolivia. *Gender & Development* 2009;17:389–401.

81. Kidd S. Equal pensions, equal rights: Achieving universal pension coverage for older women and men in developing countries, *Gender & Development* 2009;17:377–388.

82. Terry G. No climate justice without gender justice: An overview of the issues. *Gender & Development* 2009;17:5–18.

83. Women's Environment and Development Organization. Gender, climate change and human security lessons from Bangladesh, Ghana and Senegal. Available at: http://www.wedo.org/wp-content/uploads/hsn-study-final-may-20–2008.pdf. Accessed December 20, 2012.

84. Woodrow Wilson Center. Strategies for promoting gender equity in developing countries: Lessons, challenges, and opportunities. Available at: http://www.wilsoncenter.org/sites/default/files/Promoting%20Gender%20Equity%20in%20Developing%20Countries.pdf. Accessed December 20, 2012.

85. McIntosh J, Rafie S, Wasik M, et al. Changing oral contraceptives from prescription to over-the-counter status: An opinion statement of the Women's Health Practice and Research Network of the American College of Clinical Pharmacy. *Pharmacotherapy* 2011;31:424–437.

86. American College of Obstetricians and Gynecologists. Oral contraceptives OTC access. Available at: http://www.acog.org/About_ACOG/ACOG_Districts/District_II/Oral_Contraceptives_OTC. Accessed December 20, 2012.

87. Melinda Gates. 2011 International Conference on Family Planning. Available at: http://www.fpconference2011.org/2011/11/melinda-gates-2011-international-conference-on-family-planning/Accessed December 19, 2012.

88. WHO. Microbicides. Available at: http://www.who.int/hiv/topics/microbicides/microbicides/en/. Accessed December 20, 2012.

89. Global Campaign for Microbicides. Available at: http://www.global-campaign.org/EngDownload.htm. Accessed December 20, 2012.

90. UNAIDS. Reducing sexual transmission. Available at: http://www.unaids.org/en/targetsandcommitments/reducingsexualtransmission/. Accessed December 20, 2012.

91. UNAIDS. A decade of progress and sustained funding for HIV prevention research provides a pathway for ending AIDS. Available at: http://www.unaids.org/en/resources/presscentre/pressreleaseandstatementarchive/2012/july/20120723prresourcetraking/. Accessed December 20, 2012.

92. UNAIDS. Eliminating new HIV infections among children. Available at: http://www.unaids.org/en/targetsandcommitments/eliminatingnewhivinfectionamongchildren/. Accessed December 20, 2012.

93. UNAIDS. Eliminating stigma and discrimination. Available at: http://www.unaids.org/en/targetsandcommitments/eliminatingstigmaanddiscrimination/. Accessed December 20, 2012.

5 Children

■ SARA ROSENBAUM AND
KAY A. JOHNSON

■ INTRODUCTION

This chapter deals primarily with the impact of social injustice on children in the United States, emphasizing children's rights in a legal context.

International Standards

The United Nations Convention on the Rights of the Child (CRC) is an international treaty establishing the human rights of children, including the right to an education and health care and protection against execution and life imprisonment for crimes committed by those under age 18.[1] Although U.S. Secretary of State Madeline Albright signed the CRC in 1995, the U.S. Senate has not ratified it; as of 2012, the United States, Somalia, and South Sudan were the only United Nations member countries who had not done so.[2] The Senate's failure to ratify the treaty may reflect its concern that the CRC has the potential to preempt parental authority over children—although, paradoxically, a central provision is the right to be raised by, and have a relationship with, parents. The United States Supreme Court's rulings in 2005 and 2012 to strike down the death penalty and life imprisonment for children as unconstitutional has removed these issues as potential barriers to ratification.[3,4]

Children's Rights Under U.S. Law

The U.S. Constitution protects individuals who are recognized as legal *persons*. U.S. law does not recognize fetuses as *persons*. However, it gives government considerable powers to protect its interest in potential life—not only once a fetus becomes viable,[5] but also at the earliest stages of life, as illustrated by the debate over stem-cell research involving human embryos.[6] Children are recognized as legal *persons*; the U.S. Supreme Court has recognized that children possess certain constitutional rights independent from those of their parents.[7] However, children who have not reached the *age of legal majority* (the legally-defined age at which a person is considered an adult) under state law are restricted considerably in their legal autonomy on decisions concerning family living arrangements, education, and health care. Because children are not autonomous individuals, relying instead both economically and physically on adults, they lack full legal personhood under U.S. law. The Supreme Court has stated that the constitutional rights of children cannot be equated with those of adults because of the peculiar vulnerability of children; their inability to make critical decisions in an informed, mature manner; and the importance of the parental role in child rearing.[8]

The Supreme Court has recognized that states may restrict children's freedom to make important decisions for themselves because children lack the maturity and experience "to recognize and avoid choices that could be detrimental to them."[8] In general, children's rights are assigned to the parents or to the state *in loco parentis* ("in the place of a parent"). The Supreme Court has established parents' "liberty interest" in directing the education of their children.[9] Similarly, it accords considerable deference to a parent's substantive due process right to determine what is in a child's best interest and has declared that such parental rights are "fundamental."[10]

Although children are *persons* within the meaning of the Constitution and therefore must be accorded procedural and substantive due process, the Supreme Court has ruled that a state has no constitutional *duty of rescue*—that is, no duty to protect children from their parents, even when the state knows children's safety is at risk.[11] The Court stated that the 14th Amendment does not require states to protect individuals from violence between private individuals, but that instead it is meant to safeguard the liberty interests of private persons from state intrusion.[11] States have no affirmative duty to protect individuals from private violence; however, when states have limited individual autonomy, they have a duty to provide basic medical services to prisoners and a duty to protect those who have been involuntarily committed.[12]

Children have very limited rights to make their own medical decisions. "Informed consent" presumes that the individual giving consent is mature enough to understand a choice of treatment and its consequences. Many courts have held that children under the age of 18 do not have the intellectual or emotional capacity to make those decisions, and, consequently, their parents are given the discretion to consent to or refuse medical treatment for their children. The Supreme Court has also recognized that parental consent is not absolute and that states are required, in some instances, to provide procedural due process to children. For example, a parent does not have absolute discretion over a decision to institutionalize a child in a state facility, and commitment can be ordered only following an independent review procedure that meets standards of due process.[13]

Children have somewhat greater rights concerning abortion and reproductive health. Under rulings of the U.S. Supreme Court, states may constitutionally require that a minor receive parental consent for an abortion, but may not grant absolute veto power to a parent or guardian over such a decision and must provide a judicial bypass procedure.[14]

■ THE HEALTH NEEDS OF CHILDREN

Although a complex set of factors influences children's health, what children need to promote their optimal health is relatively straightforward.[15] Overall, children are healthier than adults. When acute or chronic health threats occur, their symptoms are generally milder and more easily treated. A small proportion of children suffer from serious illnesses, but their overall prevalence in children is lower than in adults.

Development is the most socially and biologically significant process of childhood. Children are not expected to be self-sufficient and productive in a grown-up sense; rather, society expects that they will develop and evolve toward productivity as they get older.[15] Utilitarian norms of functionality for adults, such as measures of employment or wages, have only a limited role in evaluating children's health needs. For children, the ability to engage in activities of daily living, school, and play/recreation are important measures of functionality.

Adult health problems may manifest as problems of physical or mental development in children. Because poor health in children tends to be expressed in developmental—rather than overt and diagnosable—terms, the health status and needs of children differ from those of adults.[15] For an infant or toddler, signposts of development might be the ability to roll over, use one's hands, walk, or talk. For any child or adolescent, developmental tasks include the ability to learn, pay attention, and engage in appropriate social interactions. When development goes wrong, the consequences can be long-lasting. Adverse childhood experiences (ACEs), such as abuse, neglect, violence, and other traumatic stressors, increase risk for adult health problems, such as heart disease, tobacco and alcohol abuse, depression, and unintended pregnancy.

Children in the United States are generally healthy. More than 80 percent are considered to be in "good to excellent health" by their parents and caregivers, and more than 95 percent are reported to have a regular source of health care.[16] In the United States and Western Europe, deaths among children are rare. Based on parental assessments in 2011, 2 percent of U.S. children were in fair to poor health.[16] This percentage is higher when others perform these assessments. And it is higher for children living in poverty and those without health insurance.[15] (See Box 5–1 concerning children in other high-income countries, and, at the end of this chapter, Box 5–2 on children in low-income countries.)

The U.S. infant mortality rate has been declining over several decades, reaching an historic low of 6.15 deaths per 1,000 live births in 2010.[17] The U.S. rate remains higher than that in other high-income countries, mainly due to high rates of pre-term births (less than 37 weeks' gestation) (Figure 5–1).[18] If the United States had Sweden's distribution of births by gestational age, nearly 8,000 infant deaths would be prevented annually.[19] The infant mortality rate is disproportionately high for African American and American Indian infants, mainly due to high rates of pre-term and low-birthweight births.[20] The black–white gap in infant mortality

BOX 5-1 ■ **How the United States Compares with Other High-Income Countries**

While social justice can be improved in almost all countries, they differ widely in how strongly they are committed to social justice. As a reflection of this difference, the rate of children living in poverty greatly differs among countries.

For example, in the United States in 2011, 20 percent of children were living in households whose income is below the federal poverty level.[1] During the economic boom of the 1990s, child poverty in the United States decreased, reaching a low of 15 percent in 2000. Since then, it has risen steadily. Government benefits, such as income transfer programs and food stamps, only reduce child poverty to a minimal extent. In contrast, France has national government programs that reduce the child poverty rate to 6.5 percent. France's family policy has included universal family allowance, job-protected maternity leave, free public preschool, and parental leave for serious childhood illness. In 11 countries surveyed, government programs reduce child poverty by at least 50 percent. In 2004, less than 6 percent of children in Denmark, Finland, Norway, and Sweden lived in poor households, and 7 to 9 percent of children were poor in Austria, the Netherlands, and Switzerland.[2]

Among high-income countries, the United States has the highest rate of child poverty for three reasons: First, governments of other high-income countries use tax systems relatively aggressively to reduce or prevent disparities. Americans, in contrast, have a *laissez-faire* approach to income differences, typically believing that income disparities reflect hard work and self-worth. This approach is reflected in the minimum wage in the United States, which is at a level that cannot lift full-time workers out of poverty—thereby increasing the need for supplemental forms of income, such as by the Earned Income Tax Credit and the Child Tax Credit.[3]

Second, taxes in the United States are unpopular, so much so that even with enormous deficits and unprecedented income disparities, political leaders generally resist calls for higher taxes on the wealthiest Americans. Between World War II and the 1970s, all Americans shared in rising incomes. Then incomes declined, and wealth became concentrated in fewer households. From 1979 to 2007, after-tax income for the wealthiest 1 percent of the population tripled, while the lowest 80 percent of the population saw their income only marginally increase or actually decline.[4] U.S. tax policy, while progressive, currently has only a moderate impact on income distribution. Between 2000 and 2010, the concentration of income among the wealthiest families in the United States rose to the highest level since the 1920s, with 20 percent of the nation's before-tax income concentrated in the highest 1 percent of households and 15 percent of income concentrated in the highest 0.5.[4] (See Box 28-1 in Chapter 28.) Wealth has a greater concentration, with the highest 1 percent holding 35 percent of wealth. In many other high-income countries, taxes are accepted as the price of civilization. Taxes are seen as holding society together and providing a moral defense against unacceptable disparities. In contrast, the United States has the lowest household tax burden among high-income countries. Except for the Earned Income Tax Credit for low-wage families, the United States has not used tax policy to reduce poverty. The Patient Protection and Affordable Care Act of 2010 also may reduce the impact of poverty through tax policy by providing tax credits to uninsured low- and middle-income households in order to make health insurance—a major protection against economic loss—affordable.

Third, the United States relies far more on "welfare programs" to reduce poverty than do other countries. Rather than developing categorical programs designed only for poor people, other countries typically rely far more on their progressive tax systems to temper economic extremes—with taxes levied at a higher rate on the wealthiest people and programs used to bolster incomes of otherwise impoverished households.

Box References

1. U.S. Census Bureau. Statistical abstract of the United States: 2012. Table 712. Available at: http://www.census.gov/compendia/statab/2012/tables/12s0712.pdf Accessed October 30, 2012 Also see: https://www.census.gov/hhes/www/poverty/data/index.html.
2. Gornick JC, Jantti M. Child poverty in comparative perspective: Assessing the role of family structure and parental education and employment. *LIS Working Paper Series No. 570.* September, 2011. Available at: http://www.lisdatacenter.org/wps/liswps/570.pdf. Accessed October 30, 2012.
3. Center on Budget and Policy Priorities. Studies show the Earned Income Tax Credit encourages work and success in school and reduces poverty. June 2012. Available at http://www.cbpp.org/cms/index.cfm?fa=view&id=3793. Accessed October 30, 2012.
4. Center on Budget and Policy Priorities. A guide to statistics on historical trends in income inequality, 2012. Available at http://www.cbpp.org/cms/index.cfm?fa=view&id=3629. Accessed October 30, 2012.

rate did not change significantly between 1990 and 2011, with the rate for black infants remaining more than twice that of white infants.[17] Other measures of child health have also shown positive trends. For example, in 2011, 90 percent of all U.S. children age 19 to 35 months of age had received the basic immunizations against preventable diseases.[21]

A significant proportion of the child population in the United States has a special health need, such as a severe disability or functional impairment.[15] (See Chapter 8.) The most widely used definition of *special needs*, developed by the U.S. Department of Health and Human Services, includes "chronic physical, developmental, behavioral, or emotional conditions [which] require health and related services of a type or amount beyond that required by children generally."[22] Using this definition, 15 percent of U.S. children under age 18 in 2009–2010 had a special need, and 20 percent of households had at least one child with a special need.[23] An estimated 20 percent of all children age 3 to 17 in the United States have at least one mental health problem.[24] Many of these problems are associated with unhealthy or risk-taking behaviors, such as drug addiction and alcoholism, an unhealthy diet, and unprotected sex.[15] Child and adolescent health problems should therefore be seen in a broad context. Their causes and contributing factors are often complex. And they are often concentrated in groups at especially high risk.

▪ THREATS TO CHILDREN'S HEALTH

To be healthy, children need access to regular, continuous, comprehensive health care that identifies problems in their growth and development at the earliest possible stage and provides supportive interaction with their parents.[25] Children

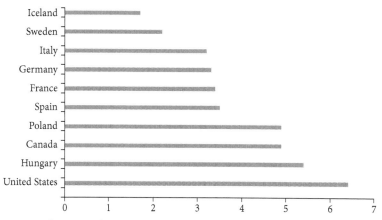

Figure 5–1 Infant mortality rates (per 1,000 live births), selected countries in the Organization for Economic Co-operation and Development, 2011. (*Source*: World Bank. World Bank indicators. Available at: http://data.worldbank.org/indicator/SP.DYN.IMRT. IN. Accessed January 4, 2013.)

need to be free from conditions—including community and social threats—that increase their risk of disease and diminish their potential and attainment. The first 1,000 days of child development, starting in pregnancy, are critical to life-time health and well-being.[26]

Poverty and Health

Among children, there is a strong association between low socioeconomic status (SES) and their poor health—an association that appears to exist in all stages of development and for almost all preventable disorders.[27] Therefore, SES may be the single most important determinant of child health and development. In the United States, about 20 percent of children live in poverty, and younger children are more likely to live in a poor family. In most parts of the country, an income that is at least twice the federal "poverty level" ($23,050 for a family of four in 2012) is necessary for ensuring adequate food, clothing, housing, and other basic needs. In 2010, family income below the "low-income" threshold adversely affected 44 percent of all children in the United States—and 64 percent of African American children, 63 percent of Native American children, and 63 percent of Latino children.[28] After accounting for food, rent assistance, and taxes, the proportion of children living in deep poverty has grown steadily since 1990, with the largest increases following the enactment of federal welfare reform legislation in 1996 and the economic downturn in 2008.

Poverty creates and maintains poor living conditions for children. Poverty threatens access to adequate food, shelter, health care,[29] child care, family time, and other aspects of daily life that make a child's environment safe and stable.

Poverty threatens the ability of families to invest in the necessities of daily life that promote a sense of well-being and stability. Inadequate income hampers families' ability to address adversity and threats to their health. Poverty is also associated with stress that robs children and adults of their health and deprives children of their parents as functional and strong caregivers.[30]

The worst form of childhood poverty in the United States may be the concentrated poverty found in poor urban communities, which have high rates of illness, disability, and death.

Environmental Health Threats

Children are especially vulnerable to environmental health threats. Young children are more likely to absorb more toxic substances, because they breathe faster and eat and drink more in proportion to their body weight than do adults. Young children play close to the ground and engage in more hand-to-mouth behavior, which increases their contact with toxic substances in soil, dust, and carpets. And children are often exposed to substances that cause asthma and other allergic disorders.

In at least 4 million households in the United States, children are exposed to lead.[31] Approximately one-quarter million children age 1 to 5 have blood lead levels (BLLs) above 5 micrograms per deciliter (µg/dL); African American young children who live in homes built before 1946 have the highest prevalence of elevated BLLs.[32] Poor children are more likely to have elevated BLLs than their non-poor counterparts. Children exposed to lead suffer intellectual impairment, even at 5 µg/dL and lower BLLs.

Hazardous waste is a danger to children. As of 2009, approximately 6 percent of children in the United States lived within 1 mile of a Superfund hazardous waste site that had not been cleaned up or had human health protective measures in place.[33] African American, Hispanic, Asian, and Native Hawaiian or Other Pacific Islander children, as well as poor children of any race/ethnicity, are disproportionately likely to live within 1 mile of a Superfund or a Corrective Action site with contaminated land.[34]

Poor air quality also is a threat to children. In 2009, approximately half of all children were residents of counties that exceeded officially acceptable air quality standards.[35] Air pollution triggers asthma attacks. In 2012, 7 million children in the United States had asthma.[36]

Elevated mercury levels, mainly due to its unregulated emission from coal-burning power plants, represent another hazard. An estimated 8 percent of women of childbearing age have levels of mercury higher than what the Environmental Protection Agency considers safe, due to consumption of fish contaminated with mercury. As a result, approximately 300,000 infants are at increased risk for neurodevelopmental deficits and learning disabilities.[37]

Poor water quality is another problem. Millions of children reside in areas without adequate water treatment and filtration systems or in areas served by public water systems that have had violations of health regulations.[38]

The presence of pesticides in food represents another health threat. In 2001, 19 percent of fruits, vegetables, and grains had detectable residues of organophosphate pesticides.[39]

Disparities in family income and in risk factors for poor health adversely affect millions of children in the United States. Children of low-income families are at increased risk for many preventable and treatable conditions, including diabetes, visual impairment, severe anemia, immunizable diseases, meningitis, lead-related disorders, and death from injuries and violence. They are more likely to be born prematurely, at low birthweight, and to mothers who received inadequate or no prenatal care. Adolescents of families at high risk are more likely to abuse alcohol and drugs, smoke cigarettes, engage in unsafe sex, and develop mental health problems, acquire sexually transmitted infections, and have unintended pregnancies and become single parents.[40]

▪ ROOT CAUSES AND UNDERLYING ISSUES

Numerous factors contribute to childhood poverty, including maldistribution of income, inadequate income-replacement policies, and inadequate government commitment to societal investments in families and children, such as paid maternity and parental leave, high-quality child care and education, and support for vulnerable families. These societal investments help strengthen families and communities, helping them to raise children who are healthy, ready to learn, and capable of the maximum possible growth and achievement.

The United States stands alone among 24 industrialized nations in its failure to guarantee paid parental leave with the birth of a child, and a family allowance/child dependency grant. The Patient Protection and Affordable Care Act of 2010 (ACA) establishes a near-universal system of health insurance coverage for all non-elderly Americans, including children. Through a combination of expanded coverage under Medicaid and the establishment of a subsidized health insurance market through state health insurance exchanges, the ACA is likely to reduce the number of uninsured children in the United States to 4.2 million.[41]

Maldistribution of Income

The income gap between rich and poor families in the United States is wider now than it has ever been, mainly due to three factors. First, education: Workers with limited education are increasingly relegated to low-wage jobs, disproportionately vulnerable to economic slowdowns and job layoffs, and likely to be chronically underemployed. Second, the failure of the government to intervene: The minimum wage has failed to keep pace with inflation. In 1970, minimum-wage workers could earn enough from full-time jobs to lift their families above the federal poverty level; by 2012—when the minimum wage was 64 percent of its 1968 peak, full-time work at the minimum wage left millions of families below the poverty level.[42] U.S. median family household income has steadily declined: In 2011, for example, it was 8 percent lower than in 2007.[43] Third, family composition: Approximately one-fourth of children live with only one parent, a fraction that has steadily increased in recent years. Between 1990 and 2008, the proportion of all U.S. births that were to unmarried women rose from 28 to 41 percent.[44] Among 21 high-income countries, the United States has the highest percentage of single-parent households (for children age 11, 13, and 15)—mainly due to greater social acceptability of divorce and births to unmarried women. Single parenthood usually predicts lower economic prospects for both parent and child.

Failure to Invest in the Neediest Families

Direct economic interventions aimed at infusing both cash and in-kind income into low-income families is critically important, given the market conditions that feed low-wage and poverty-level work and promote formation of families at risk for poverty. Child support collections help, but these are small relative to the number of low-income children living in single-parent families, mainly because of inadequate resources to aid in collection of child-support payments, and the low income of absent parents. Direct government economic transfers, both cash and in-kind, are critically important for households headed by a single parent and for low-wage workers generally, whether or not there is parental presence in the household.

There are several sources of economic cash transfer programs, including welfare assistance and income transfers based on the U.S. tax code. By far, the most important source of cash transfer has become the U.S. tax code, especially since the 1996 welfare reform legislation, which by 2000 had reduced the already-low number of people on welfare by nearly an additional 50 percent over peak levels in 1994.[45] It is notable that most families work after leaving welfare; two-thirds of low-income children live in households in which someone works.[46] Their jobs, however, are unstable, and their wages are low.

The Earned Income Tax Credit (EITC), which is available to low-income families under U.S. tax law, represents a critical source of family support. In 2010, as a result of improvements (some of which were temporary) in the EITC and the Child Tax Credit (CTC), changes in tax policy lifted some 9.2 million persons out of poverty, half of whom were children. Yet only about half of states supplement the EITC, for which the upper eligibility threshold for a single working parent with two children is about $40,000 in annual income.[47,48]

Some of the most critical income-transfer programs represent in-kind assistance, such as food stamps, housing assistance for rental housing, and health insurance. Housing and health care assistance are also available to—and heavily skewed toward—affluent families. In the United States, the value of the home mortgage deduction increases with the value of the home, without regard to family income. But poor people often face onerous housing costs. For example, in 2009, three-fourths of the poorest people who rented their homes faced severe housing burdens, and 56 percent of lower–middle-income renters were forced to use half or more of their incomes for housing and utilities.[49] In 2012, in no state could a person working full-time for the minimum wage afford the "Fair Market Rent" cost of a two-bedroom rental unit (as defined by the Department of Housing and Urban Development).[50]

As a result of the severe economic downturn that began in 2008, receipt of food stamps through the Supplemental Nutrition Assistance Program (SNAP) markedly increased. As of mid-2012, 47 million people were receiving food stamps. Yet about 30 percent of those eligible for food stamps do not receive them, and about 20 percent of Americans struggle with food hardship.[51]

The 1996 welfare reform legislation included new restrictions on the Supplemental Security Income (SSI) program, which provides cash assistance to children with severe disabilities.[52] As a result of restrictive criteria for determining disability, hundreds of thousands of children no longer receive SSI support.

Immigrant children have also been adversely affected by the 1996 welfare reform legislation. Recently arrived, legally resident children no longer qualify for either Medicaid or the State Child Health Insurance Program (CHIP). As of March 2011, only 22 states and the District of Columbia had adopted replacement programs for children barred from Medicaid and CHIP eligibility—and, in some cases, barred pregnant women from Medicaid eligibility.[53] In addition, an increasingly aggressive stance by the federal government toward immigrant families has elevated their already high concerns about the potential adverse impact on their U.S. legal status that could result from attempts to obtain cash assistance or medical or food assistance—even for eligible children born in the United States.

▪ WHAT NEEDS TO BE DONE

Improving the health of children in the United States means enabling all children to live under conditions that foster strong growth and development, rather than conditions that act as impediments. It is one thing to make the assertion that the government affords equal opportunity to all residents. But it is quite another to carefully, consciously, and affirmatively pursue the policies that make such assertions meaningful.

The United States has never provided adequate investment in community development. But circumstances have grown far worse recently due to structural poverty—the most serious economic crisis since the Great Depression—and increasing opposition to a greater role for government in assuring the health and well-being of all people.

Promoting child health includes favoring investments in those families who will most benefit from them. Tax-based economic supports for workers, such as the EITC, should be further broadened to ensure that all families who work can escape low income status. Programs for families who do not work because of illness or disability should be established—programs that combine economic supports with education and job training to promote self-sufficiency. Investments should be made in maternity-leave and parental-leave policies; education improvements, especially for low-income communities; and housing assistance.

Protection of children in all environments, including the home environment, is essential. Strong, stable, and loving parents represent important assets to children. Also important for children's health and well-being are child welfare programs aimed at (a) strengthening and supporting families through social investments, and (b) providing services to families under stress—including home visits to mothers, infants, and young children.

The Role of Health Workers

Given their knowledge and experience and respect accorded to them, physicians, nurses, and other health workers can have a substantial influence on the development of public policies concerning children. Whether the issue is building a playground, expanding public health insurance programs, raising the minimum wage, or investing in children and their families in other ways, health workers have important educational and advocacy roles to play. Therefore, health workers who wish to influence policy should have ongoing communication—individually or through their professional organizations—with government officials (and with representatives of relevant non-governmental organizations). Health workers should ensure that government officials see the conditions in which low-income children live, and personally monitor programs that are assisting these children and their families. And health workers should support political candidates who support programs and services for children. In addition, clinicians can make more personal investments, such as by accepting publicly insured children into their practices, volunteering at clinics serving low-income families, participating in community health outreach to identify children at high risk, promoting prevention and wellness activities in schools and child care programs, and investing time and energy in other ways that promote the health and well-being of children.

■ CONCLUSION

This chapter has reviewed factors that influence child health, especially the important role of social determinants. The well-being of children depends on many investments and protective factors, such as adequate family income, safe housing and neighborhoods, and children's caregivers whose lives are sufficiently supported so they can adequately nurture their children.

While most children lead healthy lives that are only punctuated by episodes of acute illness, many children experience significant disabilities and impairments that require ongoing investments to promote growth and development. Other children live in conditions of poverty associated with high stress, violence, and other forms of trauma.

In the United States, the most serious threat to children and their families is from poverty and its consequences—largely resulting from social policies that are less adequate than those of other countries. Health professionals and others can play critical roles in promoting social justice and the health of children by advocating for progressive social policies and personally investing time and energy in activities to promote children's health and well-being.

BOX 5-2 ■ Children in Low-Income Countries

Kathryn Bolles and Sarita Fritzler

Which Children Are at Risk?

Globally, nearly 7 million children under the age of 5 die from preventable causes such as pneumonia, diarrhea, newborn complications, malaria, and underlying malnutrition—despite the wide availability of effective interventions for low-resource settings that could save most of these lives.[1] Over 70 percent of child deaths occur in Africa and Southeast Asia, with children in sub-Saharan Africa being 16 times more likely to die than children in developed countries—largely due to the high prevalence of HIV/AIDS in this region.[2] In addition, high levels of absolute poverty (a daily income of US$1.25 or less) prevent families from having adequate food, housing, sanitation, safe drinking water, basic health care, and education.[3]

Within these countries, children from the poorest 20 percent of households are twice as likely to die as those from the richest 20 percent.[2] The poorest families live in the most rural areas, have less knowledge about healthy behaviors, and have little to no access to quality health services, such as vaccination or treatment for malaria. In addition to poverty, lack of education, distance from the health facilities, language barriers, caste, gender, and adverse consequences of armed conflict and disasters all decrease child survival.

What Have We Learned?

Addressing neonatal mortality is increasingly important to saving lives since the proportion of deaths that occur in the neonatal period (the first month of life) is increasing—representing over 40 percent of all under-5 deaths.[2,4] Life-saving interventions such as tetanus toxoid immunization during pregnancy, delivery by skilled birth attendants, and basic obstetrical services, including drying and keeping a baby warm ("kangaroo mother care") after birth, can save many newborn infants. In addition, programs that encourage exclusive breastfeeding for the first 6 months of life can prevent 13 percent of infant deaths.[5]

After the first month, the leading causes of death for children are largely preventable and treatable at very low cost. Pneumonia, the primary cause of death, annually kills 1.5 million children, although a course of life-saving antibiotics and preventable vaccines is available for less than US$1 per child.[1] Oral rehydration therapy (ORT), a simple solution of salt and sugar, prevents nearly 1 million deaths annually, and has reduced under-5 deaths due to diarrhea by half.[6]

Immunization campaigns protect against serious illness or death from diseases like measles, tetanus, and polio. For malaria, the availability of rapid diagnostic tests, mass mosquito net distribution, and indoor residual spraying has saved many children's lives. These solutions are simple and available, but challenges of access to care remain for those most in need.

A Life-Saving Approach That Works

The international community has learned how to save children's lives from these diseases at scale and at a low cost through a promising approach called *community case management* of childhood illnesses (CCM). CCM provides immediate, high-impact, and large-scale access to preventive and curative care by training and equipping health workers and volunteers from their own communities to reach those who live farthest from health facilities or are unable to use them. A cadre of community health workers (CHWs), given only 6 weeks of training and a few basic tools, could reduce global child mortality by an estimated 24 percent by treating sick children according to the guidelines of UNICEF and ministries of health.[7] In Pakistan, children with severe pneumonia who were treated with oral antibiotics by Lady Health Workers at home were more likely to recover than those who were referred to the nearest hospital.[8] CHWs are able to maintain their knowledge and clinical competencies several years after being trained, including integrating newer technologies such as the rapid-diagnostic tests for malaria.[9] Even in areas of low literacy, CHWs use pictorial algorithms to assess and treat illness. CCM, now in over 40 countries, has a strong evidence base and an increasing record of research and programming, including integrating treatment of acute malnutrition and some illnesses of newborn infants.[10]

Including CCM as part of the standard approach to addressing health needs in emergency situations could save many children's lives. In the midst of humanitarian crises caused by natural disasters or conflicts, children and their needs are often overlooked for the more immediate and visible responses of the emergency. Countries like Malawi, Haiti, and Mali are experiencing humanitarian crises—brought on by drought, political unrest, and natural disasters—which increase morbidity and mortality. In these humanitarian crises, CCM programs to prevent pneumonia, malaria, and diarrhea—using CHWs in the rural areas most affected—could save many lives. And CCM could transform the way the international community responds to emergencies.

Finishing the Unfinished Agenda

Although much progress has been made in reducing child mortality, much work remains.[11] More children's lives in developing countries and during humanitarian crises could be saved by applying available solutions at a large scale in areas with greatest need.

Box References

1. World Health Organization. Children: Reducing mortality. Available at: http://www.who.int/mediacentre/factsheets/fs178/en/index.html. Accessed on November 2, 2012.

2. UN Inter-Agency Group for Child Mortality Estimation. Levels and trends in child mortality, 1990–2011: Report 2012. Available at: http://www.unicef.org.uk/Documents/Publications/UNICEF_2012_IGME_child_mortality_report.pdf. Accessed on November 2, 2012.

3. Ravallion M, Chen S, Sangraula P. Dollar a day revisited. *The World Bank Economic Review* 2009;23:163–184.

4. Liu L, Johnson HL, Cousens S, et al. Global, regional, and national causes of child mortality: An updated systematic analysis for 2010 with time trends since 2000. *Lancet* 2012;379:2151–2161.

5. Black RE, Allen LH, Bhutta ZA, et al. Maternal and child undernutrition: Global and regional exposures and health consequences. *Lancet* 2008;371:243–260.

6. UNICEF/WHO. Diarrhea: Why children are still dying and what can be done. Geneva: World Health Organization, 2009.

7. Black R, Perry P. Community health workers: Key agents for saving children. State of the world's mothers. Westport, CT: Save the Children, 2011. Available at: http://www.savethechildren.org/atf/cf/%7B9def2ebe-10ae-432c-9bd0-df91d2eba74a%7D/SOWM2011_FULL_REPORT.pdf. Accessed on November 2, 2012.

8. Bari A, Sadruddin S, Khan A, et al. Community case management of severe pneumonia with oral amoxicillin in children aged 2–59 months in Haripur district, Pakistan: A cluster randomised trial. *Lancet* 2011:378:1796–1803.

9. CORE Group, Save the Children, BASIC, and MCHIP. Community case management essentials: Treating common childhood illnesses in the community: A guide for program managers. Washington, DC: CORE Group, Save the Children, BASIC and MCHIP, 2010.

10. UNICEF. Maternal and newborn health. State of the world's children. New York: UNICEF, 2009. Available at: http://www.unicef.org/sowc09/. Accessed on November 2, 2012.

11. Kenny C, Sumner A. More money or more development: What have the MDGs achieved? Working Paper 279, Center for Global Development, December 12, 2011. Available at: http://www.cgdev.org/files/1425806_file_Kenny_Sumner_MDGs_FINAL.pdf. Accessed on November 2, 2012.

■ REFERENCES

1. UN General Assembly Res. 44/25, U.N. GAOR, 44th Sess., Supp. No. 49, at 167 U.N. Doc. A/44/49 (1989).

2. United Nations Children's Fund. State of the world's children 2012: Children in an urban world. Available at http://www.unicef.org/sowc/files/SOWC_2012-Main_Report_EN_21Dec2011.pdf. Accessed November 16, 2012.

3. *Roper v. Simmons*, 125 S. Ct. 1833 (2005) (Holding that the death penalty for offenders under the age of 18 violates the 8th Amendment's prohibition of "cruel and unusual punishments").

4. Gavett G, Childress S. Supreme Court bans mandatory life terms for kids: What it means. Frontline, June 25, 2012. Available at: http://www.pbs.org/wgbh/pages/frontline/

criminal-justice/supreme-court-bans-mandatory-life-terms-for-kids-what-it-means/. Accessed November 16, 2012.

5. See *Roe v. Wade*, 410 U.S. 113 (1973) and *Planned Parenthood v. Casey*, 505 U.S. 833 (1992).

6. The Hastings Center. Stem cells. 2008. Available at: http://www.thehastingscenter.org/ Issues/Default.aspx?v=260&gclid=CLHbmOjaqLMCFQJx4AodAlUAZA. Accessed October 30, 2012.

7. See *In re Gault*, 387 U.S. 1 (1967) (Juvenile offender has procedural due-process rights); *Tinker v. Des Moines Indep. Cmty. Sch. Dist.*, 393 U.S. 503, 506 (1969) (Free speech right to wear armbands in school to protest war); *Brown v. Bd. of Educ.*, 347 U.S. 483 (1957) (14th Amendment applies to school children).

8. *Bellotti v. Baird*, 443 U.S. 622, 634, 635 (1979).

9. *Meyer v. Nebraska*, 262 U.S. 390 (1923) (Invalidation of state laws that prohibited teaching a class below the eighth grade in any other language other than English; Violation of parents' 14th Amendment liberty interest to control the education of their children); *Pierce v. Soc'y of Sisters*, 268 US 510 (1925) (State law requiring parents to enroll their children in public rather than private elementary schools struck down; Violation of parents' substantive due process rights to control education of their children); *Wisconsin v. Yoder*, 406 U.S. 205 (1972) (First and 14th Amendments allow parents the right to educate their children at home according to their faith; the Court held that state compulsory education law violated the constitutional rights of Amish parents to educate their children at home according to their religion).

10. *Troxel v. Granville*, 530 U.S. 57, 65 (2000) (State statute allowing "any person" to petition the court for visitation rights violated parents' substantive due process rights).

11. *DeShaney v. Winnebago County Dep't of Soc. Serv.*, 489 U.S. 189, 196 (1989).

12. *Estelle v. Gamble*, 429 U.S. 97 (1976) (States have a duty to provide basic medical services to prisoners); *Youngberg v. Romero*, 457 U.S. 307 (1982) (States have a duty to protect the involuntarily committed).

13. *Parham v. J.R.*, 442 U.S. 584 (1979).

14. *Bellotti v. Baird*, 443 U.S. 622, 643 (1979). See also *Planned Parenthood of Central Mo. v. Danforth*, 428 U.S. 52 (1976) and *Ohio v. Akron Ctr. for Reprod. Health*, 497 U.S. 502, 510–19 (1990).

15. Stein RE, Stanton B, Starfield B. How healthy are U.S. children? *JAMA* 2005;293: 1781–1783.

16. U.S. Department of Health and Human Services. Summary health statistics for U.S. children: National Health Interview Survey, 2011. DHHS publication no. (PHS)-2013–1582, December 2012. Available at: http://www.cdc.gov/nchs/data/series/sr_10/ sr10_254.pdf. Accessed November 6, 2012.

17. Hoyert DL, XU J. Deaths: Preliminary data for 2011. National Vital Statistics Reports. U.S. Department of Health and Human Services. October 10, 2012. Available at: http:// www.cdc.gov/nchs/data/nvsr/nvsr61/nvsr61_06.pdf. Accessed November 6, 2012.

18. March of Dimes; The Partnership for Maternal, Newborn, & Child Health; Save the Children; and World Health Organization. Howson CP, MV Kinney, JE Lawn, eds. Born too soon: The global action report on preterm birth. Geneva: World Health Organization, 2012. Available at: http://www.who.int/pmnch/media/news/2012/ 201204_borntoosoon-report.pdf. Accessed November 6, 2012.

19. MacDorman MF, Mathews TJ. Behind international rankings of infant mortality: How the United States compares with Europe. NCHS Data Brief No. 23. Hyattsville, MD: National Center for Health Statistics, 2009. Available at: http://www.cdc.gov/nchs/data/databriefs/db23.pdf. Accessed November 6, 2012.

20. MacDorman MF, Mathews TJ. Recent trends in infant mortality in the United States. NCHS Data Brief No. 9. Hyattsville, MD: National Center for Health Statistics, 2008. Available at: http://www.cdc.gov/nchs/data/databriefs/db09.pdf. Accessed November 6, 2012.

21. Centers for Disease Control and Prevention. National, state, and local area vaccination coverage among children aged 19–35 months, United States, 2011. *MMWR* 2012;61: 689–696. Available at: http://www.cdc.gov/mmwr/preview/mmwrhtml/mm6135a1.htm. Accessed October 30, 2012.

22. McPherson M, Arango R, Fox H, et al. A new definition of children with special health care needs. *Pediatrics* 1998;102:137–140.

23. Child and Adolescent Health Measurement Initiative (CAHMI). 2009–2010 national survey of children with special health care needs (NS-CSHCN). Available at: http://childhealthdata.org/docs/drc/200910-cshcn-sas-codebook_final_052912.pdf. Accessed November 6, 2012.

24. National Institute of Mental Health. Children's mental health statistics. 2010. Available at: http://www.nimh.nih.gov/statistics/index.shtml. Accessed October 30, 2012.

25. National Research Council and Institute of Medicine (IOM). From neurons to neighborhoods: The science of early childhood development. Washington, DC: National Academies Press, 2000. (Also see: From neurons to neighborhoods: An update. National Academies Press, 2012.)

26. Shonkoff JP. Leveraging the biology of adversity to address the roots of disparities in health and development. *Proc Natl Acad Sci* 2012;109(Suppl2):17302–17307.

27. Braveman P, Barclay C. Health disparities beginning in childhood: A life-course perspective. *Pediatrics* 2009;124(Suppl 3):S163–S175.

28. National Center for Children in Poverty. Low income children in the United States, 2010. New York: Columbia University, 2012. Available at: http://www.nccp.org/topics/childpoverty.html. Accessed October 30, 2012.

29. Rowland D. Health challenges facing the nation. Washington, DC: Joint Economic Committee, United States Congress, October 1, 2003.

30. American Academy of Pediatrics; Committee on Psychosocial Aspects of Child and Family Health; Committee on Early Childhood Adoption, and Dependent Care; and Section on Developmental and Behavioral Pediatrics. Policy statement: Early childhood adversity, toxic stress, and the role of the pediatrician: Translating developmental science into lifelong health. *Pediatrics* 2012;129:e224–e231. Available at: http://pediatrics.aappublications.org/content/129/1/e224.full.html. Accessed October 8, 2012.

31. U.S. Centers for Disease Control and Prevention. Lead. June 1, 2009. Available at: http://www.cdc.gov/nceh/lead/.Accessed October 30, 2012.

32. U.S. Centers for Disease Control and Prevention. Blood lead levels, United States, 1999–2002. *MMWR* 2005;54:513–516. Available at: http://www.cdc.gov/mmwr/preview/mmwrhtml/mm5420a5.htm.Accessed October 30, 2012.

33. U.S. Environmental Protection Agency. America's children and the environment (3rd edition), January, 2013. Available at http://epa.gov/opeedweb/children/index.html. Accessed March 8, 2013.

34. U.S. Environmental Protection Agency. America's children and the environment. 3rd edition. January, 2013. Available at: http://epa.gov/opeedweb/children/index.html. Accessed March 8, 2013.

35. U.S. Environmental Protection Agency. America's children and the environment. 3rd edition. January, 2013. Available at: http://epa.gov/opeedweb/children/index.html. Accessed March 8, 2013.

36. Centers for Disease Control and Prevention. Asthma fast stats. January 11, 2013. Available at: http://www.cdc.gov/nchs/fastats/asthma.htm. Accessed March 8, 2013.

37. Shore M. Out of control and close to home: Mercury pollution from power plants. Environmental Defense Fund. 2003. Available at: http://www.edf.org/sites/default/files/3370_mercuryPowerPlants.pdf. Accessed March 8, 2013.

38. Centers for Disease Control and Prevention. Drinking water. January 4, 2013. Available at: http://www.cdc.gov/healthywater/drinking/. Accessed March 8, 2013.

39. U.S. Environmental Protection Agency. Children are at greater risks from pesticide exposure. January 2002. Available at: http://www.epa.gov/opp00001/factsheets/kidpesticide.htm. Accessed October 30, 2012.

40. Healthy people.gov. Adolescent health. September, 2012. Available at: http://www.healthypeople.gov/2020/topicsobjectives2020/overview.aspx?topicid=2. Accessed October 30, 2012.

41. Kenney G, Buettgens M, Guyer J, Heberlein M. Improving coverage for children under health reform will require maintaining current eligibility standards for Medicaid and CHIP. *Health Affairs* 2011;30:122371–122381. Available at: http://content.healthaffairs.org/content/30/12/2371. Accessed November 6, 2012.

42. Alberti M. Individual minimum wage versus family poverty threshold: Remapping debate. April, 2012. Available at: http://www.remappingdebate.org/map-data-tool/individual-minimum-wage-versus-family-poverty-threshold. Accessed March 8, 2013.

43. DeNavas-Walt C, Proctor BD, Smith JC. Income, poverty, and health insurance coverage in the United States, 2011. Current population reports. Available at: http://www.census.gov/prod/2012pubs/p60-243.pdf. Accessed October 31, 2012.

44. U.S. Census Bureau. Statistical abstract of the United States, 2012. Table 1335. Available at: http://www.census.gov/compendia/statab/2012/tables/12s1337.pdf. Accessed October 31, 2012.

45. Schoeni RF, Blank RM. What has welfare reform accomplished? Impacts on welfare participation, employment, income, poverty, and family structure. Santa Monica, CA: RAND, 2000. Available at: http://www.dtic.mil/cgi-bin/GetTRDoc?AD=ADA376640. Accessed November 26, 2012.

46. Addy S, Wight VR. Basic facts about low income children in the United States, 2010. February 2012. Available at: http://www.nccp.org/publications/pdf/text_1049.pdf. Accessed October 31, 2012.

47. Center on Budget and Policy Priorities. Policy basics: State earned income tax credits. January 13, 2011. Available at: http://www.cbpp.org/cms/index.cfm?fa=view&id=2506. Accessed October 30, 2012.

48. Tax Policy Center. Taxation and the family: What is the earned income tax credit? June 22, 2011. Available at: http://www.taxpolicycenter.org/briefing-book/key-elements/family/eitc.cfm. AccessedMarch 8, 2013.

49. Alexander B, Baker K, Baldwin P, et al. America's rental housing: Meeting challenges, building on opportunities. Cambridge, MA: Joint Center for Housing Studies of

Harvard University, 2011. Available at: http://www.jchs.harvard.edu/sites/jchs.harvard.edu/files/americasrentalhousing-2011.pdf. Accessed November 6, 2012.

50. Rosenthal A. Paying rent on minimum wage. *New York Times*, May 30, 2012. Available at:http://takingnote.blogs.nytimes.com/2012/05/30/paying-rent-on-minimum-wage/. Accessed November 26, 2012.

51. Food Research and Action Center (FRAC). SNAP/Food stamp historic trends: 1998–2010. Available at: http://frac.org/federal-foodnutrition-programs/snapfood-stamps/historic-trends-1998–2008. Accessed October 31, 2012.

52. Committee of Ways and Means, U.S. House of Representatives. The Personal Responsibility and Work Opportunity Reconciliation Act and associated legislation. November 6, 1996 (*Public Law* 104–193, 104th Congress, 2nd Session). Available at: http://www.gpo.gov/fdsys/pkg/CPRT-104WPRT27305/html/CPRT-104WPRT27305.htm. Accessed November 6, 2012.

53. Fortunyk, Chaudry A. A comprehensive review of immigrant access to health and human services. (Report to HHS Office of Assistant Secretary for Planning and Evaluation). Washington, DC: Urban Institute, June 2011. Available at: http://aspe.hhs.gov/hsp/11/ImmigrantAccess/Review/index.pdf Accessed November 26, 2012.

6 Older People

■ CARROLL L. ESTES AND
STEVEN P. WALLACE

■ INTRODUCTION

Despite the growing academic and political interest in health equity and in social justice in health care, little attention has been paid to these issues as they relate to older people. Healthy People 2020, a program of the U.S. Department of Health and Human Services that provides evidence-based 10-year national objectives for improving the health of all Americans, has four overarching goals. One of these goals focuses on equity (eliminating health disparities), and two of them are particularly relevant to older people (longer and healthier lives, and promoting quality of life and healthy behaviors throughout the life course). Although many of the Healthy People 2020 targets focus on issues of concern to older persons and although age is identified as a possible source of disparities, health equity among age groups that include the elderly is not included as a priority topic. (This omission also occurred while the United Nations was declaring 1999 the "International Year of Older Persons" and developing a program called "Building a Society for all Ages,"[1] which links the status of older people to that of others in society.)

There is a burgeoning literature on disparities within the older population,[2,3] but there has been a decline during the past 40 years in attention given to ageism and inequities based on age. The growing popularity of trends such as "anti-aging" medicine and the continued blaming of older people for national deficits suggest that they are likely to face less equitable treatment because of their age in the future, unless social policies and political ideologies change.[4] Therefore, it is important to consider the inequities both *within* the older population and *between* the older and younger populations.

Eliminating inequities in the determinants of health care and health status for older people is an ethical imperative. However, it is also in society's social and material interests to promote conditions in which older people can be healthy. Many older people continue to contribute to their families and communities through very old age,[5] and as the "baby boom" generation ages, an even larger pool of older people with valuable skills and experiences will become important resources. If older people are not healthy, their ability to contribute to their communities declines, and the costs of their debilitating illnesses are borne by society.

■ THE GLOBAL CHALLENGE

Population aging is often thought of as a phenomenon of high-income countries, but it marks low-income countries as well. The number of older people (defined here as 60 years of age and older) was almost 900 million globally in 2011 and is projected to reach 2.4 billion by 2050. The older population is growing fastest in low-income countries, where currently almost two-thirds of all older people (590 million) now live. In high-income countries, the fastest growing age group is comprised of people age 80 and older.[6] In 2011, about half of the world's population age 65 and older lived in five countries: China, India, the United States, Japan, and Russia. Life expectancy at birth is over 80 years in 11 high-income countries, but remains below 50 in 25 African countries. Both the AIDS pandemic and development loans that require the privatization of health care have lowered life expectancy in many low-income countries.[7,8]

Increasing life expectancy is usually viewed as a societal achievement, but it is also seen as a socioeconomic burden of crisis proportions by adherents of "apocalyptic demography."[9] This view, common in the United States and elsewhere, assumes that aging populations will burden public policies to the point of creating disastrous social consequences. Some politicians and demographers have made dire warnings of impending national bankruptcy, under-investment in children, and the overwhelming of available family support systems.[10] This view scapegoats older people for political problems, such as budget deficits that reflect tax cuts and rising military spending.[11,12] Internationally, aging is not distinct from issues related to social integration, gender advancement, economic stability, or poverty. Societies need to recognize the potential benefits from ongoing contributions of older people.[13]

The aging of societies is mainly an issue of older women.[14] In all societies, women outlive men; by very old age, the female:male ratio is generally 2:1.[8] Women are caregivers for people of all ages, especially children and, increasingly, grandchildren. For example, in places where HIV/AIDS prevalence is high, older women are essential caregivers of their adult children and their orphaned grandchildren. Although unpaid, women's caregiving work generally ceases only when they are physically and mentally unable to provide it and in need of care themselves. As a result, older women throughout the world experience more economic deprivation and insecurity than do older men.[15] Older women are highly vulnerable to the government upheavals and restrictions of safety-net policies, especially in low-income countries.

"Building a Society for All Ages," the Second World Assembly on Ageing (2002), developed a framework for economic development and poverty reduction that emphasized the importance of active aging, intergenerational solidarity, and the necessity of high-income countries helping low-income countries. Participants at this conference discussed principles of justice that are used to legitimate social policies. The United States and other high-income countries have been supporting free-market policies that embody an individualistic principle of justice, based on a utilitarian philosophy in which maximizing the sum of individuals' health and wealth has been the primary goal—as reflected in regularly reported data on life expectancy and gross domestic product (GDP). These measures ignore the distribution of health and wealth, making them inadequate—even detrimental—to ensuring equal opportunities for all.[1]

One example of implementing increased attention to equity is the framework of the World Health Organization (WHO) for evaluating health systems. Its two health objectives—the "best attainable level" (goodness) and the "smallest feasible differences" among individuals and groups (fairness)—are applied across three key dimensions of health systems: (a) health outcomes, such as morbidity and mortality; (b) the responsiveness of the health care system, such as being treated with dignity and technically competent care; and (c) the financing of the system. Although not incorporated in the current United Nations documents on aging, such performance measures need to be applied to older people.[3]

■ THE IMPACT OF SOCIAL INJUSTICE ON THE HEALTH OF OLDER PEOPLE

Injustice among older people is well documented. Health status varies by race, ethnicity, income, and gender among older persons. Older African Americans have worse health than do older whites for all measures of health status, including disease, disability, and self-assessed health. Older Latinos have lower rates than non-Latino whites of some diseases, most notably coronary artery disease and stroke, but higher rates of diabetes and disability. Poverty is strongly associated with all measures of poor health in old age. And women have more chronic conditions and disability than do men, despite their longer life expectancy.[16,17] (See Chapters 2, 3, and 4.)

Self-assessed health status, a good predictor of death and disability as well as a good indicator of current health status,[18] follows social categories of inequality. Older people with the lowest income are more than twice as likely as older people with higher incomes to report reduced health status (Table 6–1). Latinos and non-Latino African Americans, and American Indians are almost twice as likely, and Asian Americans 50 percent more likely, to report reduced health status as are non-Latino whites. Women and men report similar levels of fair or poor health.

With the substantial reduction in deaths from acute infectious diseases during the past century, mortality is mostly due to chronic conditions that are most common in old age. Noncommunicable diseases, such as arthritis, hypertension, coronary artery disease, cerebrovascular disease, and cancer, are conditions that disproportionately affect older adults. (See Chapter 15.) The "epidemiological transition" from acute to chronic diseases has occurred in high-income countries and is occurring in low-income countries.[8] Many chronic diseases could be prevented or delayed by health promotion and disease prevention measures. The prevalence of chronic diseases varies by race, class, and gender. Chronic diseases, such as strokes and diabetes, are leading causes of death and disability. Diabetes, in particular, shows a striking association with race, income, and gender (Table 6–2). Older African Americans have more chronic conditions overall than older whites,

TABLE 6–1 *Age-Adjusted Percentages of Self-Assessed Health Status of Persons Age 65 and Older by Income, Race/Ethnicity, and Gender, United States, 2008–2010*

	Percent Reporting Fair/Poor Self-Assessed Health
Income	
Below poverty level: 0%–99% poverty level	42.8
Near-poor: 100%–199% poverty level	33.1
Non-poor: 200% & above poverty level	19.1
Race/Ethnicity	
Non-Latino white	21.6
Non-Latino African American	38.2
Latino	38.2
American Indian/Alaska Native	38.0
Asian	29.2
Gender	
Women	24.3
Men	24.9

(*Source:* Centers for Disease Control and Prevention. National Health Interview Survey, 2008–10. Atlanta, GA: CDC, 2012. From Health Data Interactive. Available at www.cdc.gov/nchs/hdi.htm. Accessed on November 14, 2012.)

and older women have more than older men.[17] Incontinence—especially among older women—is not a fatal condition, but is associated with social isolation and reduced quality of life.[19] While psychological distress is lower among older adults than younger adults, it is a leading cause of disability and is strongly associated with low income and female gender. And disability also varies by income, race/ethnicity, and gender (Table 6-1). (See also Chapters 8 and 16.)

TABLE 6–2 *Age-Adjusted Percentages of Persons Age 65 and Older with Chronic Conditions, by Income, Race/Ethnicity, and Gender, United States, 2008–2010*

	Stroke	Diabetes	Incontinence	Serious Psychological Distress	Needs Help with Activities of Daily Living**
Income					
Below poverty	10.9	29.2	25.0#	6.2	4.5#
Near-poor	10.7	23.0	25.5#	3.3	3.6#
Non-poor	7.1	19.8	18.1#	1.5	1.5#
Race/Ethnicity					
Non-Latino whites	8.0	18.9	29.6	2.2	6.2
African Americans*	11.4	31.2	26.1	2.2	11.5
Latinos	8.2	34.4	26.8	4.2	11.5
Gender					
Women	7.6	18.9	37.2	2.7	5.8
Men	9.2	24.5	18.6	1.8	8.0

* Non-Latino
**Needs help with personal care needs such as eating, bathing, dressing, or getting around inside the home.
(*Source*: Centers for Disease Control and Prevention. National Health Interview Survey, 2008–10. Atlanta, GA: CDC, 2012. From Health Data Interactive. Available at www.cdc.gov/nchs/hdi.htm. Accessed on November 14, 2012.)
Data not available from above; these data only from 2003 California Health Interview Survey, www.chis.ucla.edu.

Disability rates fell steadily in the late 20th century, but have declined less rapidly since 2000.[20] Declines in mortality may result in increased life expectancy, but those extra years may continue to be associated with high rates of disability, which can place additional demands on health care systems and communities. Increasing rates of obesity and diabetes, which are highest among racial/ethnic minorities and poor people, may account for some of this disability.

Inequities also exist in the access to health services by different groups of older persons. The same social and economic characteristics that are associated with worse health outcomes account for differences in the use of health services. Indicators of difficulty accessing needed care—such as not having a usual source of care, delaying or not obtaining prescriptions, and having a hard time understanding one's physician—are all higher among low-income and Latino older people, as illustrated with data from California (Table 6–3). Although most older people have a regular site for health care, about 10 percent of older and low-income Latinos do not. Poor older people are almost twice as likely to delay or skip obtaining needed medications (Table 6–3). Older people who are poor or members of racial/ethnic minority groups have more disease; their greater difficulty in obtaining health care represents the inequitable distribution of health care resources.

In addition to differences in receiving any health care, there are disparities among older people in the quality of care they receive. The Institute of Medicine has determined that racial and ethnic disparities in health care are independent of economic status, health insurance, and other factors.[21] Some of the differences in quality of care among older people are reflected in measures of satisfaction with care. Older African Americans have the lowest satisfaction rates; Latinos, intermediate rates; and whites, the highest rates (Table 6–4).

To summarize, inequities in health status, access to health care, and the quality of care received among different groups of older people are based on their social characteristics.

TABLE 6–3 *Percentage of People Age 65 and Older Reporting Access to Health Care Problems, by Income, Race/Ethnicity, and Gender, California, 2009*

	No Regular Source of Care	Delayed or Did Not Get Prescription Medicine	Hard Time Understanding Doctor
Income			
Below poverty	9.7	11.6	9.4
Near-poor	7.3	8.5	4.6
Non-poor	3.5	6.2	1.7
Race/Ethnicity			
Non-Latino whites	3.4	6.3	1.6
Non-Latino African Americans	3.5	7.9	2.8
Latinos	9.9	8.3	7.7
Gender			
Women	4.3	8.2	2.7
Men	5.9	6.3	3.8

(*Source:* 2009 California Health Interview Survey. Available at www.chis.ucla.edu. Accessed on November 14, 2012.)

TABLE 6-4 *Percentage of People Age 65 to 74 Who Are Very Satisfied with Care, United States, 2010*

	Follow-up Care	Ease of Access to Physician	Information from Physician	Physician's Concern for Overall Health
Race/Ethnicity				
Non-Latino whites	29.0	33.0	26.8	32.0
Non-Latino African Americans	15.4	22.0	17.2	20.9
Latinos	20.0	17.4	20.0	22.8
Gender				
Women	28.5	32.1	26.3	31.1
Men	26.1	30.0	24.9	29.7

(*Source:* Centers for Medicare and Medicaid Services [CMS]. The characteristics and perceptions of the Medicare population: Data from the 2010 Medicare Current Beneficiary Survey. Baltimore, MD: CMS, 2012.)

In addition to inequities within the older population, there is a continuing bias against older people as a group in several health-related dimensions. For example, there is much devaluing of older people by health professionals[22,23] and policymakers. Treatment decisions for older people are often influenced by their age—rather than the costs and benefits of treatment. Older people, for example, are less likely to receive recommendations for cancer treatments that could extend their lives than younger people, even when there is no medical reason to avoid those treatments. The pattern of under-treatment is exacerbated by the under-representation of older people in most clinical trials.[24] Some academics and politicians have even suggested that older people, such as those over age 80, should receive no curative treatments, regardless of their prognosis, because they have lived out their "natural" lives.[25]

Older people are often devalued in discussions of the costs of health and social programs that they use.[11] Some policymakers blame the rising costs of Medicare on older people, even though much medical treatment is driven by physician referral—not patient demand. In addition, the rapidly rising costs of prescription medications appear to be partly a function of manufacturer-induced demand (especially by direct advertising to consumers) for high-cost drugs—rather than use of new drugs that improve treatment of disease.[26]

The technology-intensive medical care system in the United States is increasingly inappropriate for the health challenges of older people, such as hearing impairment, injuries due to falls, incontinence, and social isolation, as well as end-of-life care.[19] These challenges do not usually require expensive tests, surgical interventions, or state-of-the-art technologies. An example is the current treatment pattern of older people with incontinence—frequently an embarrassing condition that contributes to social isolation and increases the risk for deconditioning, falls, and institutionalization. It is often erroneously seen as a "normal" part of growing old. Although behavioral therapy, including pelvic exercises, is the most effective treatment of the most common type of urinary incontinence,[27] drug therapy, surgery, and the use of adult diapers continue to be the most common forms of treatments. An estimated 8 percent of women age 60 and older have had surgery for incontinence.[28] An estimated $2 billion is spent annually in the United States for absorbent pads and related supplies.[29] Adult diapers and drugs produce significant profits for their manufacturers, creating incentives to promote these products; in contrast, behavioral therapy is time-consuming and not very profitable. As a result, many older people with incontinence do not receive adequate treatment for this condition.

▪ ROOT CAUSES AND UNDERLYING ISSUES

Among the underlying causes of social injustice affecting the health of older people are (a) poverty and inequalities associated with differences in socioeconomic status (SES) over the life course (the "graying" of the SES-health gradient), (b) the biomedicalization of aging, and (c) globalization.

The Graying of the Socioeconomic Status–Health Gradient

The association between health and poverty in all age groups also affects older people. The poor have reduced life expectancy, lower self-rated health status, increased morbidity and disability, and worse functional status.[19] SES, whether defined by income, education, employment, poverty, or wealth, is inversely associated with mortality in virtually all countries.[30,31] In addition, socioeconomic inequality, independent of economic status, is related to health status.[16] (See Chapter 2.)

There has been both political and academic discussion of the increasing economic inequality generated since 2000. While the rising tide of economic growth from 2000 to 2008 disproportionately benefited those with the highest incomes, the recession that started in 2008 especially hurt those with the lowest incomes. For example, in families with older adults in California, the consequences of cuts in government budgets for programs and services as well as reduced incomes have more heavily impacted households with annual incomes less than $50,000 (Table 6–5). Older people in these households were at least twice as likely to be

TABLE 6–5 *Response to Recession, by Registered Voters Age 60 and Older, California, 2012*

In Past Year	Income <$50,000	Income $50,000 or Higher
Very worried that family income will not be enough to meet living expenses	28%	12%
Had to reduce money spent on food	47%	18%
Had to reduce savings for retirement	44%	26%
Received or borrowed money	24%	10%

(*Source:* The SCAN Foundation/UCLA Center for Health Policy Research. 2012 Long-Term Care Issues poll. Available at http://www.healthpolicy.ucla.edu/pubs/files/scansurveyfindings-sep2012.pdf. Accessed on November 14, 2012.)

very worried that they would not have enough money to meet living expenses and, as a result, reduced spending on food and savings for retirement, and increased borrowing. These people are unlikely to recover financially.

The health status of older people is also impacted by their SES and health status throughout their life course.[32,33] Poverty and poor health during childhood may:

- Impact the health of people so that they are at greater risk of illness and disability later in life—a latent effect
- Set people on occupational or other pathways in which they are at greater risk of health-damaging exposures or other health-damaging situations later in life
- Lead to the accumulation of health-damaging impacts continually throughout life.

Therefore, when social injustice based on race/ethnicity, class, or gender early in life adversely affects one's health, access to quality health care, and life opportunities, it is likely to adversely affect one's health later in life.

Over the life course, three types of capital translate health disparities early in life to those later in life:

1. Human capital—knowledge and skills of individuals that influence employment, job satisfaction, and income. Local zoning, transportation, and financial institutions interact to segregate many neighborhoods by race and class, and the educational systems then reproduce these advantages and disadvantages.

2. Social capital—the types and density of ties among people that enhance social integration and support. This is fostered by both community resources and the type of education young people receive.

3. Personal capital—in lifestyle, sense of efficacy, and personal control, which has developed during younger adult years.[16] Interactions with the criminal justice system in low-income and minority communities and messages conveyed through the educational system help shape personal capital early in life.

Health disparities are influenced throughout the life course by the interactive effects of racism, sexism, discrimination based on social class, and ageism on human, social, and personal capital.[34-36] These disparities are significantly influenced by the institutional effects of race, government, the market, gender, and family structures.[35,37] Poverty in older women arises partly from "the family care penalty"—the economic and health costs to female caregivers for their substantial unpaid caregiving throughout their lives that affects their ability to develop their own human capital. Older women's Social Security benefits, for example, are often lower because government policy penalizes them for years out of the labor force for child-rearing or elder care. Older women's dependence on the government, including public health services, increases with aging, widowhood, divorce, and declining economic and health status.[38] Privatization of core public services and reduction of public pensions compound the gender disadvantages of earlier life and place older women at a higher risk for adverse health consequences. Health disparities by income, social class, gender, and race are reinforced by government policies concerning aging and retirement.[39]

The Biomedicalization of Aging

In Western countries (especially the United States), old age has often been equated with specific diseases or a general pathological state. The cultural aversion to aging and the veneration of youth have spawned negative attitudes toward older people that are sometimes internalized and manifested in personal low self-esteem, low self-efficacy, and low sense of control—all of which are risk factors for dependency, depression, and illness.[34] The problems of older people have been described as rooted in biology, placing the treatment of these problems in the realm of medicine. This biomedicalization of aging has facilitated the "commodification" (transformation into commodities) of the needs of older people, which has produced a high-cost—and highly profitable—"aging enterprise" and enlarged the medical-industrial complex.[40] As a result, the goal of producing medical goods and services has shifted from fulfilling human needs (basic shelter and nutrition) to monetary exchange and private profit—and, with it, increasing social inequality.

The biomedicalization of aging obscures the extent to which the health of older people can be improved by modifying social, economic, political, and environmental factors. Biological and genetic factors account for only 20 to 25 percent of successful aging, while behavioral, social, and environmental factors account for the rest.[41] Therefore, public health approaches to improving the health of older people focus on population-level interventions, rather than clinical approaches that focus on individuals.[19] These population-level approaches include (a) distributing wealth more equally; (b) increasing education opportunities; (c) providing adequate housing for all; (d) enhancing opportunities for meaningful human connections; (e) ensuring universal access to health care, including long-term care and rehabilitation; and (f) creating policies and community environments that promote healthful behaviors, such as eating a healthy diet and regularly performing physical exercise.[42]

Globalization

Growing old is increasingly viewed in a transnational context of international organizations and cross-border migration that creates new conditions and challenges for older people and their families. There is a growing tension between an individual country's policies on aging and those formulated by global organizations and institutions. Aging can no longer be viewed solely as a national issue.[7] (See Box 19–1 in Chapter 19.)

We believe that promotion of privatization and restructuring of the welfare state are parts of an intentional global strategy of capitalist financial organizations to get nations to divest themselves of public retirement benefit retirement programs and to adopt privatized pension and health schemes[43]—thereby increasing reliance on private capital markets for pensions and health insurance and creating new markets to generate profits in the provision of services. This neoliberal agenda is being promoted by policies and actions of the World Bank, the International Monetary Fund (IMF), the World Trade Organization (WTO) and its General Agreement on Trade in Services, and the North America Free Trade Agreement that threaten increasingly fragile welfare states.[44,45]

Globalization disempowers citizens within countries, while globally citizens' power is dwarfed by that of transnational organizations.[46] We believe that there needs to be a new form of politics for older people in the current global situation.[47] The World Social Forum and similar international programs offer a start in bringing together civil society organizations and individual people to build coalitions that advocate for human needs over international corporate and financial interests. Nevertheless, there are few organizations that are opposing the adverse social consequences of globalization that have a primary focus on older people. With few exceptions, older people in the United States are not engaged in movements for social justice at the global level. For example, the American Association of Retired Persons (AARP), which has more than 37 million members, engages globally in some issues related to aging, but not from a social justice perspective. Other organizations in the United States that have global interests in aging include professional and trade organizations that focus on promoting their own professional and business interests. The National Institute on Aging of the National Institutes of Health has a scientific interest in the demography and diseases of older people, but not in social justice issues.

In low-income countries, the marginalization of women occurs when government no longer protects subsistence activities. Women's economic participation is restricted with (a) the increase of self-regulating markets and privatization of farm land for cash crops, creating food insecurity; (b) the increase in out-of-pocket costs that accompanies privatization of health services; and (c) the decrease in government support for other vital services.[48] These forces encourage some women to move from low-income to high-income countries, where they find work as caregivers for children and older people, even as they rely on female relatives back home to care for their own children and aging parents.

■ WHAT NEEDS TO BE DONE

Given the cumulative lifetime disadvantage underlying much of the social injustice that affects the health of older people, much needs to be done to improve the distribution of health and health services among the current and future generations of older people. Addressing social injustice among older people requires public policies that reduce disparities—by race, ethnicity, income, and gender—in retirement income, quality of medical care, and community integration.

Raising political awareness is necessary to promote these policies. Because older people of color, older poor people, and older women tend to be disenfranchised from the political process,[49] it is important to increase policymakers' understanding about the health status, health care, and financial burdens of these groups of older people. Organizations that focus on race and ethnicity, poverty, and women's health need to advocate for these policies.

Policies that focus on structural factors, such as the organization and financing of medical care and the social environments where older people live, affect all people. Population-based interventions that potentially affect all older people, such as ensuring access to appropriate health care, may draw political support from others, including middle-class and politically influential people. Because patients' satisfaction with physicians is higher when they can choose physicians of the same ethnic group,[50] equity in medical care depends, in part, on the racial and ethnic composition of the physician workforce. Members of racial and ethnic minority groups need to be provided the tools and incentives to pursue careers in medical care.

Community-level changes can also promote health. Building large supermarkets in inner cities, for example, can increase the consumption of fruits and vegetables by low-income older people.[51] Economic-development or zoning policies that encourage such construction may help reduce disparities in nutrition and health. And providing older people with financial resources to obtain adequate housing, nutrition, and medical care can help reduce many of the financing, process-of-care, and health-status inequities that they experience.[52]

All of these types of policy changes will require broad coalitions of advocates. Policies that have substantially improved the distribution of resources to older people, such as Social Security and Medicare, were adopted when there were broad coalitions of advocates for them, including organized labor, citizen's groups, and health professionals.[53]

To improve equity and justice for the coming generations of older persons, we must address earlier phases of the life course. Public policy should encourage the payment of a living wage so that lifetime earnings can lead to Social Security and pension benefits that provide a reasonable income. Changes in tax policy, higher wages for top earners, and an increase in single-mother families have combined to create the highest level of economic inequality in the United States in over 40 years.[54] Policy changes can redistribute income and create employment and retirement measures that improve the lives of working-class people in old age. Racial and gender inequities in wages also need to be addressed, because these disparities generate lifelong disadvantages.

Incentives in the medical care system are needed to promote the most efficacious and least invasive ways of improving the health and quality of life of older people. Health care providers and financial mechanisms need to prioritize care for chronic conditions and, where appropriate, palliative care.

We need revolutionary thinking in which aging is viewed as a lifelong and society-wide phenomenon that permeates all social, economic, and cultural domains of life.[55] Influenced by health and aging research in the high-income countries and the U.S. paradigm of "successful" and "productive" aging,[56] the World Health Organization and the United Nations as a whole have adopted an objective of "active aging"—enhancing the quality of life of older people through activities and measures that increase health, participation, and security.[57]

There is a dual challenge of both implementing public health measures to achieve healthy aging and increasing access to affordable medical care.[58] Public health measures focus on assuring safety and security of family and home, housing, sanitation, food and economic security, and access to primary care and supportive social and rehabilitative care.

In high-income countries, the strategy of active aging focuses on improving the health of sedentary "couch potatoes." Overemphasis on active aging can draw attention and resources away from measures to overcome disparities of class, race, and gender throughout the life course[59] that, cumulatively, produce serious health disparities.[16] The active aging strategy risks blaming the victim while elevating productivity as the only acceptable parameter for assessing older people. For older women, active aging can easily be interpreted as there being no end to one's responsibility for unpaid caregiving—now recast as "productive" if rendered during old age.

In low-income countries, strategies should link public health and medical care with other sectors to address sanitation, housing, potable water, and other issues. Globally, older people and their advocates need to resist privatization of services and the biomedicalization of aging. Without such resistance, "prefabricated, selectively chosen, market- and technology-driven, externally monitored, and dependency-producing programs" may be imposed on older people—especially poor older people—in much of the world.[60]

In the poorest countries, where obtaining the basic necessities for survival supercedes all other needs, the consequences of social injustice against older people, the poor, and women are often life-threatening. Inequities between rich and poor countries in terms of trade and the impact of globalization serve to exacerbate internal inequities.

Fighting Back: Reclaiming Public Health and the State

Older people, women, minorities, and poor people have been largely absent from policy-making discussions at the World Bank against public pensions and at the World Trade Organization for the commercialization of care services. The major participants in these discussions have been governments from high-income countries, desiring to deregulate government provision of services; and corporations, wanting to expand into lucrative areas of work globally.[7,61] Major entities in the international provision of health services include health insurance companies, drug companies, and medical equipment suppliers.

Opponents of globalization have been mobilized in areas of human rights, ecology, women's rights, race and ethnic justice, and worker rights. Advocates for the right of older people are invisible, except for the formal positions in United Nations and WHO documents that offer little guidance or commitment to the goals of universal, collective, and social obligations enacted through government programs. Current United Nations and WHO activities are no match for those of the WTO, the International Monetary Fund, and the World Bank to privatize government provision of care and support for older people. The privatization of these services, known as *structural adjustment*, is now commonly inserted as a condition of development loans and debt relief to low-income countries.

Organizations representing older people need to link with larger organizations and forums working on a global justice agenda. The political activity among older people in some countries provides a platform upon which to build an age-integrated social movement for social change.[62,63] The merger of movements that oppose the worst abuses of globalization is essential, and the role of organizations of older people is pivotal, because older people have much to lose should there be widespread privatization of health services and retirement programs. An example of such a merger is that of Eastern European and Third World women working together on women's rights issues, in such collaborations as Women's Edge, the Association for Women in Development, the Center for Economic Justice, the InterAction/Commission on the Advancement of Women, and the Open Society Institute's Network Women's Program. In the former Soviet Union in 1991, declining women's participation in politics and their relegation to traditional women's work inspired the first independent Women's Forum, which adopted the platform that "democracy without women is no democracy." Forms of resistance and collective action are emerging in *submerged networks* (those without defined organizational structures), such as the Internet, and everyday forms of resistance, such as boycotts of certain products and business entities.[48]

Globalization does not inexorably lead to minimal levels of social protection.[64] We believe that the agenda for future work opposing the abuses of globalization consists of actions and activities that promote pro-welfare, social-protection, and full-employment policies.

Finally, policy changes must address the needs of older women who compose three-fourths of poor older people and receive a smaller proportion of every income source than older men. U.S. policies reduce the proportionate share of income for women in old age.[65] Their lower retirement income is linked to (a) wages for labor, which discriminate against women; (b) non-waged reproductive labor (largely women's unpaid caregiving work that is not treated or counted under Social Security policy as work, but counted as time outside the workforce); and (c) retirement policy that is based on women being permanently married to male breadwinners.[66]

CONCLUSION

Rights for older people must be defined as basic human rights. (See Chapter 22.) Social justice for older people must begin with the assertion of the human right to health, as established in the Universal Declaration of Human Rights (see Appendix to Chapter 1) and other international agreements. Social justice includes the human rights of older people as a group, as well as those of subgroups of older people who have suffered lifelong injustice. Working to reduce the SES-health gradient at all ages promotes justice for both current and future cohorts of older people. Promoting public health approaches to aging will reduce the biomedicalization of old age. Activists must denounce macro-economic adjustment policies and militarization of relationships among nations for their devastating effects on people's health and quality of life, and must demand ethical principles in politics and economics that support the needs of all people.[67]

REFERENCES

1. United Nations. Second World Assembly on Ageing adopts Madrid Plan of Action and Political Declaration. Second World Assembly on Ageing, Madrid, 2002.
2. Dunlop DD, Manheim LM, Song J, Chang RW. Gender and ethnic/racial disparities in health care utilization among older adults. *J Gerontol Soc Sci* 2002;57B:S221–S233.
3. Villa VM, Wallace SP. Diversity and aging: Implications for aging policy. In: Carmel S, Morse C, F Torres Gil, eds. Lessons on aging from three nations. New York: Baywood, 2007:91–102.
4. Walker A. The new ageism. *The Political Quarterly* 2012;83:812–819.
5. Wallace SP. Community formation as an activity of daily living—The case of Nicaraguan immigrant elderly. *J Aging Studies* 1992;6:365–383.
6. United Nations. World population prospects, the 2010 revision. New York: Department of Economic and Social Affairs, Population Division, 2011. Available at http://esa.un.org/wpp/other-information/faq.htm. Accessed on November 14, 2012.
7. Estes CL, Biggs S, Phillipson C. Ageing and globalization. In: Social theory, social policy and ageing: A critical introduction. London: Open University Press, 2003:102–121.
8. Kinsella K, He W. An aging world: 2008. Washington, DC: U.S. Census Bureau, International Population Reports, 2009. Available at https://www.census.gov/prod/2009pubs/p95-09-1.pdf. Accessed on November 14, 2012.
9. Robertson A. Beyond apocalyptic demography: Toward a moral economy of interdependence. In: Minkler M, Estes CL, eds. Critical gerontology: Perspectives from political and moral economy. Amityville, NY: Baywood Publishing Company, 1999:75–90.
10. Lamm RD. The moral imperative of limiting elderly health expenditures. In: Altman SH, Shactman DI, eds. Policies for an aging society. Baltimore, MD: Johns Hopkins University Press, 2002:199–216.
11. Binstock RH. Scapegoating the old: Intergenerational equity and age-based health care rationing. In: Williamson JB, Watts-Roy DM, Kingson ER, eds. The generational equity debate. New York: Columbia University Press, 1999:157–184.

12. Quadagno J. Social security and the myth of the entitlement "crisis." In: Williamson JB, Watts-Roy DM, Kingson ER, eds. The generational equity debate. New York: Columbia University Press, 1999:140–156.

13. Desai N. The world ageing situation. New York: United Nations, 2000.

14. Calasanti TM, Slenin KF. Gender, social inequalities and aging. Walnut Creek, CA: Alta Mira, 2001.

15. Estes CL. Social policy and aging: A critical perspective. Thousand Oaks, CA: Sage, 2001.

16. Wallace SP. Social determinants of health inequities and health care. In: Prohaska TR, Anderson LA, Binstock RH, eds. Public health for an aging society. Baltimore, MD: Johns Hopkins University Press, 2012:99–118.

17. Christensen K, Doblhammer G, Rau R, Vaupel JW. Ageing populations: The challenges ahead. *Lancet* 2009;374:1196–1208.

18. Idler EL and Kasl SV. Self-ratings of health: Do they also predict change in functional ability? *J Gerontol Ser B Psychol Sci Soc Sci* 1995;50:S344–S353.

19. Wallace SP. The public health perspective on aging. *Generations* 2005;29:5–10.

20. Freedman VA, Spillman BC, Andreski PM, et al. Trends in late-life activity limitations in the United States: An update from five national surveys. Demography 2012;DOI 10.1007/s13524-012-0167-z.

21. Smedley BD, Stith AY, Nelson AR, eds. Unequal treatment: Confronting racial and ethnic disparities in health care. Washington, DC: National Academy Press, 2003.

22. Kane RL. The future history of geriatrics: Geriatrics at the crossroads. *J Gerontol A Biol Sci Med Sci* 2002;57:M803–M805.

23. Reuben DB, Fullerton JT, Tschann JM, Croughan-Minihane M. Attitudes of beginning medical students toward older persons: A five-campus study. *J Am Geriatr Soc* 1995;43:1430–1436.

24. Muss HB. Older age—Not a barrier to cancer treatment. *N Engl J Med* 2001;345: 1128–1129.

25. Callahan D. Aged-based rationing of medical care. In: Williamson JB, Watts-Roy DM, Kingson ER, eds. The generational equity debate. New York: Columbia University Press, 1999:101–114.

26. Mintzes B. Advertising of prescription-only medicines to the public: Does evidence of benefit counterbalance harm? *Ann Rev Public Health* 2012;33:259–277.

27. Kafri R, Shames J, Raz M, Katz-Leurer M. Rehabilitation versus drug therapy for urge urinary incontinence: Long-term outcomes. *Int Urogynecol J* 2008;19:47–52.

28. Diokno AC, Burgio K, Fultz H, et al. Prevalence and outcomes of continence surgery in community dwelling women. *J Urol* 2003;170(2, Part 1):507–511.

29. Wagner TH, Subak LL. Talking about incontinence: The first step toward prevention and treatment. *JAMA* 2010;303:2184–2185.

30. Crystal S. America's old age crisis. New York: Basic Books, 1982.

31. Sen A. Why health equity? *Health Economics* 2002;11:659–666.

32. O'Rand A. Cumulative advantage theory in life course research. *Ann Rev Gerontol Geriatrics* 2003;22:14–30.

33. Ferraro KF, Shippee TP. Aging and cumulative inequality: How does inequality get under the skin? *Gerontologist* 2009;49:333–343.

34. Bytheway B. Ageism and age categorization. *Journal of Social Issues* 2005;61:361–374.

35. Dressel P, Minkler M, Yen I. Gender, race, class, and aging: Advances and opportunities. *Int J Health Serv* 1997;109:579–600.

36. Folbre N. The invisible heart: Economics and family values. New York: New York Press, 2001.

37. Estes CL. From gender to the political economy of ageing. *The European Journal of Social Quality* 2001;2:28–46.

38. Estes CL, Phillipson C. The globalization of capital, the welfare state and old age policy. *Int J Health Serv* 2002;32:279–297.

39. Wallace SP, Villa VM. Healthy, wealthy and wise? Challenges of income security for elders of color. In: Estes C, Rogne L, eds. Social insurance and social justice. New York: Springer, 2009:165–178.

40. Estes CL, Harrington C, Pellow D. The medical-industrial complex and the aging enterprise. In: Estes CL, ed. Social policy and aging. Thousand Oaks, CA: Sage, 2001: 165–186.

41. Pruchno RA, Wilson-Genderson M, Rose M, Cartwright F. Successful aging: Early influences and contemporary characteristics. *Gerontologist* 2010;50:821–833.

42. Northridge ME, Freeman L. Urban planning and health equity. *J Urban Health* 2011; 88:582–597.

43. Svihula J, Estes CL. Social Security privatization: The instituionalization of a social movement. In: Estes C, Rogne L, eds. Social insurance and social justice. New York: Springer, 2009:217–232.

44. Scholte JA. The sources of neoliberal globalization. Geneva: UN Research Institute for Social Development, 2005.

45. Spilimbergo A, Symansky S, Blanchard O, Cottarelli C. Fiscal policy for the crisis. IMF staff position note. Washington, DC: International Monetary Fund, 2008. Available at http://www.imf.org/external/pubs/ft/spn/2008/spn0801.pdf. Accessed on November 14, 2012.

46. Phillipson C, Estes CL, Portacolone E. Health and development: The role of international organizations in population ageing. In: Gatti A, Boggio A, eds. Health and development. New York: Palgrave Macmillan, 2009:155–167.

47. Phillipson C. Aging and globalization: Issues for critical gerontology and political economy. In: Baars J, Dannefer DD, Phillipson C, Walker A, eds. Aging, globalization and inequality: The new critical gerontology. New York: Baywood, 2006:43–59.

48. Mittelman JH, Tambe A. Global poverty and gender. In: Mittelman JH, ed. The globalization syndrome. Princeton, NJ: Princeton University Press, 2000:74–89.

49. Wallace SP, Villa VM. Caught in hostile cross-fire: Public policy and minority elderly in the United States. In: Minkler M, Estes CL, eds. Critical gerontology: Perspectives from political and moral economy. New York: Baywood, 1998:237–256.

50. Street Jr RL, O'Malley KJ, Cooper LA, Haidet P. Understanding concordance in patient–physician relationships: Personal and ethnic dimensions of shared identity. *Annals of Family Medicine* 2008;6:198–205.

51. Walker RE, Keane CR, Burke JG. Disparities and access to healthy food in the United States: A review of food deserts literature. *Health & Place* 2010;16:876–884.

52. Marmot M, Allen J, Bell R, Goldblatt P. Building of the global movement for health equity: From Santiago to Rio and beyond. *Lancet* 2012;379:181–188.

53. Wallace SP, Williamson JP, Lung RG, Powell LA. A lamb in wolf's clothing? The reality of senior power. In: Minkler M, Estes CL, eds. Critical perspectives in aging. Farmingdale, NY: Baywood, 1991:105–123.

54. McCall L, Percheski C. Income inequality: New trends and research directions. *Annual Review of Sociology* 2010;36:329–347.

55. United Nations. UN world ageing situation. New York, United Nations, 2000. Available at: https://unp.un.org/details.aspx?entry=E00182.

56. McLaughlin SJ, Connell CM, Heeringa SG, et al. Successful aging in the United States: Prevalence estimates from a national sample of older adults. *J Gerontol Ser B: Psychol Sci & Soc Sci* 2010;65B:216–226.

57. World Health Organization. Good health adds life to years: Global brief for World Health Day 2012. Geneva: WHO, 2012. Available at http://whqlibdoc.who.int/hq/2012/WHO_DCO_WHD_2012.2_eng.pdf. Accessed on November 14, 2012.

58. World Health Organization. Towards policy for health and ageing. Geneva: WHO, 2001. Available at http://www.who.int/mip/2003/other_documents/en/E%20AAE%20Towards%20Policy%20for%20Health%20and%20Ageing.pdf. Accessed on November 14, 2012.

59. Estes CL, Mahakian J, Weitz T. A political economy critique of productive aging. In: Estes C, ed. Social policy and aging: A critical perspective. Thousand Oaks, CA: Sage, 2001:187–199.

60. Banerji D. Report of the WHO Commission on Macroeconomics and Health: A critique. *Int J Health Serv* 2002;32:733–754.

61. Vincent J, Patterson G, Wale K. Politics and old age. Aldershot, Hampshire, England: Ashgate Books, 2002.

62. Walker A, Maltby A. Ageing Europe. Buckinghamshire, England: Open University Press, 1997.

63. Campbell AL, Binstock RH. Politics and aging in the United States. In: Binstock RH, George LK, eds. Handbook of aging and the social sciences. 7th ed. San Diego, CA: Academic Press, 2011:265–279.

64. Navarro V. Are pro-welfare state and full employment policies possible in the era of globalization? *Int J Health Serv* 2000;30:231–251.

65. Estes CL, O'Neill T, Hartmann H. Breaking the Social Security glass ceiling: A proposal to modernize women's benefits. Washington, DC: The National Committee to Preserve Social Security and Medicare Foundation, the National Organization of Women Foundation, and the Institute for Women's Policy Research, 2012.

66. Harrington-Meyer M. Making claims as workers or wives: The distribution of Social Security benefits. *American Sociological Review* 1996;61:449–465.

67. International Forum for the Defense of the Health of the People. Health as an essential human need, a right of citizenship, and public good: Health is possible and necessary. *Int J Health Serv* 2002;32:601–606.

7 Lesbian, Gay, Bisexual, and Transgender/Transsexual Individuals

■ EMILIA LOMBARDI AND
TALIA MAE BETTCHER

▨ INTRODUCTION

Liberty protects the person from unwarranted government intrusions into a dwelling or other private places. In our tradition the state is not omnipresent in the home. And there are other spheres of our lives and existence, outside the home, where the state should not be a dominant presence. Freedom extends beyond spatial bounds. Liberty presumes an autonomy of self that includes freedom of thought, belief, expression, and certain intimate conduct.[1]

With those words, written by Justice Anthony M. Kennedy in 2003, the U.S. Supreme Court removed legislation criminalizing same-gender sexual relations throughout the country—a major event in the history of lesbian, gay, bisexual, and transgender/transsexual (LGBT) men and women. This event makes it clear that consensual sexual relationships between adult, same-gender couples are not to be prohibited. Previous legislation was a major barrier for LGBT men and women. While it was not used directly against them very often, it restricted their activities in other situations, such as adoption and employment protection. The removal of legislation criminalizing same-gender sexual activity leads the way toward granting the lives of LGBT men and women greater legitimacy, and hence better health outcomes. However, there is still much to be done.

In general, LGBT people continue to be stigmatized and marginalized, both legally and culturally. This can affect their health in various ways:

- Stigma can impair health through direct acts of violence—even murder.
- It may affect an individual's psychology. For example, increased stress from stigma and internalized homophobia may lead to such behaviors as substance use or high-risk sex.
- Access to health and social services may be constrained. For example, organizations may fail to provide LGBT men and women specific services, may fail to demonstrate adequate LGBT sensitivity, or may even be overtly hostile to them.

While the Supreme Court ruling was clearly an important event, it masks complex issues found within LGBT populations. The ruling focuses specifically on sexual behavior among consenting adults. Transgender and transsexual people often experience discrimination based on gender presentation and identities rather than sexual/affectional orientations. Bisexual individuals continue to be represented, if at all, as indecisive and promiscuous, and bisexual men are often identified only as a sexually transmitted infection (STI) and/or HIV bridge between gay men and heterosexual women. Both gay men and lesbians experience discrimination based on their sexual orientation, such as lack of partner benefits. However, lesbians must also deal with sexism, such as in their lack of access to economic resources. In addition, many LGBT people also experience race- and/or class-based injustice that intertwines with LGBT-based injustice in complicated ways. Although progress has been made, these considerations make the promotion of social justice difficult because the failure to address the specific and multiple needs within LGBT communities may actually lead to the promotion of further injustice.

■ THE IMPACT OF SOCIAL INJUSTICE ON THE HEALTH OF LGBT MEN AND WOMEN

Violence

Stigma-based violence and the threat of violence can undermine the health and well-being of LGBT people. This situation is aggravated by the use of "blame-shifting" rhetoric to justify or excuse such violence. In 2012, for example, 63 murders of transgender people were reported throughout the world (12 in the United States).[2-6] Most of these murder victims were killed because of their "non-normative" gender presentations. Most were transgender women of color.

Transphobia (the hatred and intolerance people feel toward those who do not conform to traditional gender norms)—and perhaps LGBT phobia more generally—may not always be easily separable from race- and class-based injustice. For example, one of us (E.L.) found that African American men and women reported higher levels of transphobic life events than did others.[3]

Domestic violence among LGBT couples is much more a problem than some might suppose.[7] Domestic violence in LGBT relationships appears to occur as often as in heterosexual relationships. However, the myth of egalitarian same-gender relationships creates a barrier for those who experience domestic violence. Helping professionals often may not be able to distinguish victim from batterer. Most domestic violence workers assume that there is a heterosexual relationship and that the wife is the victim and the husband, the batterer. Therefore, many do not know how to respond to reports of same-gender domestic violence.[8] Most shelters admit only women, which leaves men with fewer resources.[9] In addition, many shelters do not acknowledge the gender of transsexual women and refuse services to them. Batterers might also use LGBT-based prejudice to control their victims or to further harass them by informing others about their LGBT identity.

Bullying due to one's sexual or gender expression is associated with suicide, depression, and substance use among young sexual- and gender-minority men and women.[10-12] Bullying has received greater social attention after several high-profile suicides. As a result, there has been a movement to implement legislation designed to address bullying, with 48 states currently having some form of anti-bullying legislation.[13] Legislation has also been created to address *cyber-bullying*, harassment that occurs over social media, such as Facebook. Reducing harassment during adolescence can be important in reducing health disparities later in life.

HIV/AIDS

HIV/AIDS remains a major health issue for many LGBT men and women. There has been a resurgence of HIV infection among men who have sex with men, especially among men of color.[14-19] In addition, the rate of HIV infection is high among transgender women (people who are assigned male at birth but have the gender identity and expression of women).[20-26]

Research on the health of LGBT individuals in areas other than HIV/AIDS is limited.[27,28] Depression and illicit substance use issues are especially important and are linked to HIV infection.[29,30]

In 2010, the federal government developed its HIV strategic plan[31] to (a) reduce new HIV infections, (b) increase access to care and improve health outcomes for people living with HIV, (c) reduce HIV-related disparities and health inequities, and (d) achieve a more coordinated national response to the HIV epidemic. This strategic plan provides federal, state, and local agencies with a template on how to reduce HIV infection and to improve HIV care. A significant aspect of the plan is its focus on targeting gay and bisexual men as well as transgender people. Leadership provided by the Obama administration has been important in highlighting HIV disparities in the United States and facilitating care for HIV-positive men and women.

Mental Health and Alcohol, Tobacco, and Other Drugs

Gay men and lesbians generally have higher rates of substance use and mental health disorders, which may be linked to societal discrimination.[32-34] (See Chapter 16.) Experiences of violence, harassment, and discriminatory events can significantly affect the mental health of gay men and lesbians.[35,36] In addition, factors relating to the hiding and concealment of identities, expectations of rejection, and internalized homophobia are specific stressors that LGB men and women experience.[37] The internalization of negative attitudes about their identity can also weigh heavily on their lives and cause them much distress.[38]

Focus groups conducted with lesbian, gay, bisexual, and *two-spirit people* (LGBT persons of Native American origin) indicate that hiding one's identity is unhealthy, especially when one hides one's identity from health care providers.[39] Internalized homophobia can interfere with HIV prevention measures.[40] Many LGBT people live under the assumption that they will experience negative sanctions if other people find out about them, and, as a result, many constantly evaluate whether actions or words may identify them as being LGBT.

Transgenderism and transsexuality, unlike homosexuality or bisexuality, are still listed in diagnostic manuals of the American Psychiatric Association as mental illnesses (referred to as "gender identity disorder" and "transvestic fetishism" in the current and recent editions of the *Diagnostic and Statistical Manual of Mental Disorders*).[41] Furthermore, many clinicians classify transsexualism among the psychotic disorders, such as schizophrenia,[42,43] even though transsexuals as a population are not more likely to have mental disorders than are non-transsexual men and women.[44] This problem is augmented by the existence of social policies that require individuals to obtain medical services before they are allowed to change/amend their legal documents (such as driver's licenses, passports, and birth certificates) and, therefore, require transgender/transsexual people to seek mental health services and be diagnosed with a mental disorder.

The psychological impact of LGBT-related social injustice can directly influence people's health. Gay men who conceal their sexual identity may have worse health outcomes, such as increased incidence of cancer and infectious diseases. For gay men who are HIV-positive, concealment is associated with their infection advancing faster than for those who do not conceal their homosexual identity.[45,46] Furthermore, gay men who are sensitive to rejection generally have a greater decrease in CD4 cell count and a longer time to AIDS diagnosis, in comparison to gay men who conceal their identities and are protected, hiding their identity from others and shielding themselves from possible rejection.[47] This is the dilemma that many LGBT people face: Being "out" reduces the amount of internal stress that hiding one's identity creates, but it may sever important social connections that people rely on for support and resources.[48,49]

Levels of alcohol, tobacco, and illicit substance use among gay men and lesbians are higher than those of the general population. One study found that young gay or bisexual men were twice as likely, and lesbian and bisexual women four times as likely, to have used marijuana in the previous year.[50] In the same study, gay and bisexual men were three times more likely, and lesbian and bisexual women four times more likely, to have used the street drug Ecstasy (MDMA) in the previous year. Lesbian and bisexual women were also three-and-a-half times more likely to have smoked in the previous month. Other studies have linked LGBT people's substance use to their experiences of discrimination.[33,49,51-53] While smoking in the general adult population is decreasing, gay men and lesbians are still more likely to smoke than the general adult population.[54-56] Preliminary comparisons between young gay men and lesbians have found that lesbians actually smoke more than their gay male counterparts.[57] However, it is difficult to assess rates of smoking or other forms of substance use in this population because few such studies include measures of sexuality and gender identity.

Cardiovascular Disease and Cancer

LGBT men and women are at increased risk for cardiovascular disease.[58–60] Lesbians smoke more and have, on average, a higher body mass index (BMI) than heterosexual women, which may place them at higher risk for cardiovascular disease.[61–63] Tobacco use of lesbian and bisexual women influences their cancer risks. Because lesbian and bisexual women tend to smoke more, use alcohol more, are less likely to undergo routine gynecological screenings, and have more sexual partners, they are at a greater risk of lung, cervical, and other forms of cancer.[64–70]

LGBT men and women experience many problems with access to health care.[34] For example, a transsexual man died of cervical cancer because he could not get a physician to treat him until it was too late.[71] A masculine lesbian discussed her experiences trying to get access to health care for a serious health condition; she was refused treatment, comments were made about her by staff members, and a physician claimed her ill health was a result of her immoral lifestyle.[72] In general, many LGBT people are afraid to disclose their lives for fear of being discriminated against. Moreover, health care providers are likely to fail to collect important information if they make certain assumptions about person's sex/gender or sexuality. For example, transsexual patients may need medical assistance for problems that members of their identified gender may not be expected to have, such as transsexual men needing gynecological examinations and transsexual women needing prostate examinations.

The Centers for Medicare & Medicaid Services (CMS) of the U.S. Department of Health and Human Services implemented new rules in 2010 preserving the rights of all patients to choose who may visit them within Medicare- and Medicaid-participating hospitals and critical access hospitals.[73] Even with this change, many partners of LGBT men and women experience problems when taking care of their sick or hurt loved ones that do not exist for heterosexual men and women. Some of the issues include:

- Inability to make legal decisions for incapacitated partners
- Lack of access to health insurance for one's partner and partner's children
- Lack of coverage for medical expenses by their health insurance
- Denial of the right to make funeral arrangements and to address other end-of-life issues, such as child custody
- Denial of many financial rights, such as those related to Social Security, property ownership, and tax benefits.[74]

These problems create an added burden for LGBT people in addition to the stress and worry related to having a sick or injured partner. Not only can LGBT persons lose the persons whom they have loved, but they can also lose their homes and custody of their children and have to pay huge health care bills that are not covered by insurance.

At a deeper level, class status may play a significant role in preventing access to health services through lack of adequate health coverage. In this respect, LGBT (as well as racial) stigmatization and discrimination in schools, universities, and employment may undermine the potential of LGBT people to secure the sort of incomes or jobs that would make health service more affordable. For example, the Los Angeles Transgender Health Study found that 69 percent of the participants did not have post-secondary education, 50 percent earned less than $12,000 annually, 50 percent reported that commercial sex work was a major source of income, and 64 percent reported lacking any health insurance coverage. These findings suggest that class, race, and LGBT disadvantages in education and employment act together in complex ways to prevent adequate access to health services.

▞ ROOT CAUSES AND UNDERLYING ISSUES

One needs to recognize not only the existence of stigmatizing views about LGBT people, but also the role of simplistic categorization in the promotion of social injustice. The diversity found among LGBT people affects research and access to health care resources. Failure to appreciate this complexity may promote social injustice.

The category "LGBT" contains considerable diversity within it, making it difficult to provide a unified account of the social injustice that confronts LGBT people. Unsophisticated or reductive accounts that attempt to address LGBT social injustice may fail to address all of the problems, and may even leave some individuals out of the solution by failing to address specific issues. For example, some transgender people may seek various body-altering medical technologies, such as hormones and surgeries; these technologies, when accessed through "black markets," raise specific health concerns that are easily ignored in a simplistic description of LGBT health, especially those that emphasize sexual orientation.

More generally, the tense relationship between gender-based and sexuality-based social injustice points to the complexity of LGBT issues.[75] For while it may be initially tempting to draw a clear distinction between gender-based and sexuality-based social injustice, the diversity within the category "LGBT" makes it difficult to draw this distinction. For example, "lesbian," "gay," and "bisexual" are categories of sexual orientation, but "transgender" and "transsexual" are categories of gender and gender identity. This diversity makes more difficult attempts to explain (a) LGBT discrimination and stigmatization in terms of the oppression of non-normative sexualities alone, and (b) social injustice only in terms of the enforcement of strict gender norms.[76]

More deeply, it is difficult to distinguish between being assaulted because of one's gender presentation and one's perceived sexual orientation.[77] Gay bashing in public space, for example, may be facilitated by non-normative gender cues. Stigma against gay men, lesbians, and bisexual people may often be gender-based; for example, gay men may be represented as "feminine"—"not real men."[76] Moreover, gender presentation and gender identity may be important in some gay and lesbian relationships, such as "butch" and "femme" identities. By contrast, transgender and transsexual individuals may find themselves subject to reductive representations—such as "really a gay man" or "really a lesbian"—and subject to violence on the basis of their perceived sexual orientation.[77] Hence, gender and gender identity may be implicated in social injustice against LGB individuals, and sexuality implicated in social injustice against transgender individuals.

The social injustice faced by LGBT people lies in the complex intersections of gender-based and sexuality-based oppressions, where deep cultural views about gender and sexually appropriate conduct are enmeshed. It is useful to distinguish between different forms of stigma and the background assumptions that ground them. For example, one might distinguish LGBT stigmas that are grounded in religious perspectives (LGBT individuals seen as "sinful") from those that flow from more "scientific" or "medical" discourses (LGBT sexualities and identities seen as "pathological"). One might also identify prevalent cultural views about gender, such as "the natural attitude about gender," and distinguish them from higher-order theoretical legal, medical, or other discourses that also promote stigmatizing views in different, albeit related, ways.[78-80]

In addition, such social injustice is often linked with other forms of injustice, making it difficult to separate LGBT injustice from other forms of injustice. For example, lesbians may face discrimination not only on the basis of sexuality, but also as women. The existence of hybrid forms of discrimination is especially important with respect to (a) the intersections between race- and class-based injustice and LGBT injustice, and (b) the possibility of complex, hybrid forms of social injustice. There are many LGBT people of color who also experience hybrid forms of discrimination.

LGBT discrimination and stigma may have distinctive forms in culturally specific contexts. For example, within some Latino cultural contexts, religion plays an important role in promoting negative views about LGBT people.[81] The very way in which "LGBT" identities are negotiated may vary considerably depending on cultural context. For example, homosexuality may be conceptualized differently in Latin America and North America, suggesting different sexual identifications of Latinos and Latinas who live in different places.[82] Moreover, it is not clear that language and culturally specific terms may be easily translated or assimilated into Anglo "LGBT" terms without significant distortion.[83] For example, the Chicano colloquial term *jota* may be roughly translated as "dyke" or "lesbian," but such translations cannot easily capture the roles that such terms play in the culturally specific ways of life within which such terms are actually deployed and negotiated.

Related to this, mainstream U.S. "LGBT" identifications can be seen from certain vantage points as distinctively "white Anglo," and consequently any identification with such terms may also take on connotations of cultural betrayal.[84]

It may be difficult to discuss the ways in which homosexuality has been viewed as "aberrant" without also discussing the ways in which racialized sexualities have been stereotyped and devalued. For example, African American sexuality has been historically represented in mainstream white American discourse as "degenerate" or "dirty."[85] Given this, it is unclear to what extent one may seriously discuss representations of homosexuality as "sick" or "degenerate" without also appreciating the possible connections with racial representations and the role that both sorts of stigma may have on African American homosexuals and lesbians.[86]

An analysis of the social injustice faced by LGBT people, therefore, should consider its race and class stratification as well as the specific gender and sexuality differences among LGBT people. For example, discrimination against LGBT people may be more likely in lower-paying jobs; therefore, race and class could interact with gender and sexuality to a create a context that is far more problematic for people than either would be separately. Internalized LGBT stigmatization and its impact on self-esteem may not always be easily separated from internalized racial stigmatization. And the ability of medical and social service organizations to provide services to LGBT people may be impaired by failures to accommodate culturally specific issues—indeed, by their ignorance of LGBT communities of color.

▓ WHAT NEEDS TO BE DONE

Legislative and Other Policies

Legislative and other policies that explicitly prohibit discrimination and violence against LGBT people may reduce the social injustice experienced by LGBT individuals and thereby improve their health. Such policies can also reduce their own internalized prejudice against LGBT people and straight people who do not follow traditional norms of gender and sexuality, thereby improving their mental health. This strategy may also decrease discrimination at school and work so that LGBT people can afford and access adequate medical care. Nevertheless, such policies need to be thoroughly examined for possible racist or classist assumptions and/or consequences that provide advantage to particular groups within LGBT communities while harming others.

Under the Barack Obama administration, many governmental agencies are addressing the health disparities experienced by LGBT people.[87] The Healthy People program, a federal program to identify objectives for improving the health of Americans, is giving more attention to LGBT health disparities. Federally sponsored health studies have increasingly included LGBT individuals. In 2011, the policy that barred the enlistment in U.S. military service by openly lesbian, gay, or bisexual men and women was rescinded, allowing LGB military personnel to serve without the fear of harassment or dismissal. While the change was seen as a "non-event" among those within the military, the rescinding of this policy has been socially significant concerning the role of LGB people in society. This change does not affect *transgender* service members, who are still subject to dismissal from military service.

Domestic partner legislation that gives partners of LGBT men and women many of the same benefits as married heterosexual couples has been a welcome development for many LGBT families. The legal recognition of same-gender relationships in a manner similar to heterosexual relationships will have major implications toward improving the lives of LGBT people. As of 2012, eight states allowed same-sex marriage, and an additional five states and the District of Columbia allowed civil unions. In a related development, a study found that LGBT individuals living within regions with greater concentrations of same-sex relationships reported lower prevalence of psychiatric disorders.[88]

Transgender/transsexual individuals also need legislation and policies that legitimize their lives and identities.[89-91] The ability of transgender/transsexual men and women to change important legal documents varies by document and locality. In some localities, little to no medical intervention is required to change one's legal sex or name, while in others, surgery is required. However, in many instances, even this may not be sufficient, as many places do not allow people to change their legal sex designations on documents, or to be able to live their lives fully. There have been recent court cases with mixed responses to opposite-gender marriages of transsexual individuals; all of these cases involved people who underwent some operative procedure as a requirement for changing their legal sex designation.

Transgender/transsexual men and women need affordable and more reliable access to medical care that will enable them to better embody their gender identity. As such, legislative and other policies must prevent denial of public and private insurance coverage for such procedures, because doing so restricts people's ability to interact in society in their identified gender. Many transgender men and women are considered to be one gender in some instances and another gender in others. The process of changing one's gender must be made easier so that people do not need to guess what to do next and whether they can afford access to medical services necessary to change legal gender. Some private companies and academic institutions have started to offer transgender-related health benefits to their employees and students. There is support from the medical community for employers offering health benefits to their transgender employees.[92,93]

Roles of Health Care Facilities and Organizations

Health care facilities and organizations need to have policies that protect the dignity of those accessing care and prohibit discrimination or harassment based on people's LGBT status. Organizations must allow domestic partners and all children being raised by same-gender couples to have the same rights as those in opposite-gender relationships. As such, they must respect the existence of domestic partners and treat them as they would any other partner in a committed relationship—including end-of-life activities.

In addition to policies and procedures that do not discriminate against LGBT men and women, personnel within these organizations need training about issues relating to LGBT health. This training needs to inform people about the diversity found among LGBT people and not focus on specific stereotypes or media images. Although HIV/AIDS is important, especially for gay men, it should not be seen as the only health risk faced by LGBT people. Diversity among LGBT people needs to be recognized and understood, especially the relevance of race, culture, and class. Health care workers need to know how to promote sensitivity and to provide culturally relevant care.

Educational Measures

Because access to educational resources affects employment opportunities, which, in turn, affects access to adequate health insurance and overall health and well-being, teachers and school administrators need to be trained to treat LGBT youth without discrimination and to educate students about LGBT issues. Such measures help provide LGBT students with a safe place to learn and promote supportive cultural attitudes. These educational approaches should be sensitive to race, class, and culture. In addition, programs are needed that enable disenfranchised LGBT people to access educational resources.

Research Issues

The Institute of Medicine's report entitled *The Health of Lesbian, Gay, Bisexual, and Transgender People*[94] identified a research agenda to advance knowledge and understanding of LGBT health. Its overall priorities for LGBT health research include:

- Demographic research to examine diversity among LGBT populations
- Research to examine the effect of social factors on health
- Research to examine the barriers that LGBT people face in accessing health care
- Research to develop interventions to reduce health disparities among LGBT populations
- Greater research on transgender health issues.

The report also identified the need to have data on the health of LGBT people collected in federally funded studies.

There is a need to ensure that measures are included to identify LGBT people within health care research. Most studies of LGBT people use relatively small convenience samples that greatly limit their generalizability to the larger population. To be inclusive, survey instruments should:

- Differentiate between "sexual orientation" and "gender" (transgender and bisexual individuals should not be assimilated into "lesbian" or "gay" categories).
- Allow people to self-identify as lesbian, gay, or bisexual, and allow transgender/transsexual individuals to self-report their gender identity and sexual orientation—rather than having interviewers or staff members decide. Instruments should also be sensitive to language- and culture-specific identifications.
- Allow people to identify unmarried domestic partners, rather than forcing categorization as "single" or "married."
- Be aware of, and allow for, the diversity of attitudes and behaviors found among LGBT people.
- Be cognizant of—and sufficiently sophisticated to investigate—other forms of social injustice and the impact that these might have on some LGBT people. For example, studies that examine possible correlations between LGBT stigma and health outcomes should be sufficiently sophisticated to measure the role of race and race stigma in promoting worse health outcomes among LGBT people of color.
- Recognize that some terminology—including "LGBT," "gay," "lesbian," "transgender," and "queer"—may have white/Anglo cultural connotations that can undermine the promotion of social justice.

■ CONCLUSION

There has been improvement in the status of LGBT people in the United States, as evidenced by the 2003 Supreme Court decision regarding laws criminalizing same-gender sexual relationships. But much remains to be done. Changes in legislation and social policies are needed to provide LGBT people with adequate resources and benefits. Health care providers need to be informed about LGBT issues in culturally sensitive ways to address inadequacies in health care. And researchers need to be sufficiently sophisticated to investigate the complexity of LGBT issues and their intersection with other forms of injustice.

Most of all, there needs to be a change in the social environment that creates social injustice against LGBT people—a change that can only be brought about through education and by addressing multiple forms of social injustice. To foster greater change, coalitions need to be developed and nurtured, not only among the diverse groups found within the LGBT population, but also with other groups that experience social injustice.

During the past 8 years, there has been much improvement in the provision of resources to reduce social and health disparities among LGBT men and women.

Much of this improvement can be attributed to political leaders who have supported LGBT causes. However, LGBT people are not in less danger from social injustice. The lives of LGBT people are still politicized, and the positive developments that occurred with the past few years could be reversed.

The United States continues to be divided on the treatment of LGBT people. Legislative issues, such as same-gender marriage and anti-discrimination legislation, continue to vary by jurisdiction. In 2012, North Carolina added an amendment to its state constitution banning same-gender marriage as well as civil unions and domestic partnerships, becoming the 30th state to have a constitutional amendment banning legal recognition of same-gender relationships.[95] Soon after, President Obama become the first sitting president to state his support for same-gender marriage.[96] These developments represent the dissonance that LGBT people experience in society: Opportunities and societal changes have developed for LGBT people, and, at the same time, societal stigma continues to adversely affect their health and well-being.

■ REFERENCES

1. *John Geddes Lawrence and Tyron Garner, Petitioners, v. Texas.* 539 U.S. 558, 2003.
2. Smith GA. Remembering our dead. 2012. Available at: http://www.rememberingour-dead.org. Accessed March 6, 2013.
3. Lombardi E. Understanding genderism and transphobia. Unpublished.
4. Lombardi EL, Wilchins RA, Priesing D, et al. Gender violence: Transgender experiences with violence and discrimination. *J Homosex* 2001;42:89–101.
5. Clements K. The Transgender Community Health Project: Descriptive results. San Francisco: San Francisco Department of Public Health, 1999.
6. Reback CJ, Simon PA, Bemis CC, Gaston B. The Los Angeles Transgender Health Study: Community report. Los Angeles: Van Ness Recovery House, Prevention Division, 2001.
7. Burke LK, Follingstad DR. Violence in lesbian and gay relationships: Theory, prevalence, and correlational factors. *Clin Psychol Rev* 1999;19:487–512.
8. Ristock JL. Exploring dynamics of abusive lesbian relationships: Preliminary analysis of a multisite, qualitative study. *Am J Commun Psychol* 2003;31:329–341.
9. Merrill GS, Wolfe VA. Battered gay men: An exploration of abuse, help seeking, and why they stay. *J Homosex* 2000;39:1–30.
10. Sacco DT, Silbaugh K, Corredor F, et al. An overview of state anti-bullying legislation and other related laws. Cambridge, MA: Berkman Center for Internet and Society at Harvard University, 2012.
11. Russell ST, Ryan C, Toomey RB, et al. Lesbian, gay, bisexual, and transgender adolescent school victimization: Implications for young adult health and adjustment. *J Sch Health* 2011;81:223–230.
12. Toomey RB, Ryan C, Diaz RM, et al. Gender-nonconforming lesbian, gay, bisexual, and transgender youth: School victimization and young adult psychosocial adjustment. *Dev Psychol* 2010;46:1580–1589.
13. Chesir-Teran D, Hughes D. Heterosexism in high school and victimization among lesbian, gay, bisexual, and questioning students. *J Youth Adolesc* 2009;38:963–975.

14. Malebranche DJ. Black men who have sex with men and the HIV epidemic: Next steps for public health. *Am J Public Health* 2003;93:862–865.
15. Clifton CE. A black gay man's call to action to the black community. *Positively Aware* 2003;14:7.
16. Leslie NS, Deiriggi P, Gross S, et al. Knowledge, attitudes, and practices surrounding breast cancer screening in educated Appalachian women. *Oncol Nursing Forum* 2003;30:659–667.
17. Gross M. When plagues don't end. *Am J Public Health* 2003;93:861–862.
18. Chen M, Rhodes PH, Hall IH, et al. Prevalence of undiagnosed HIV infection among persons aged >/=13 years—National HIV Surveillance System, United States, 2005–2008. *MMWR* 2012;61(Suppl):57–64.
19. Prejean J, Song R, Hernandez A, et al. Estimated HIV incidence in the United States, 2006–2009. *PLoS One* 2011;6:e17502.
20. Clements-Nolle K, Marx R, Guzman R, et al. HIV prevalence, risk behaviors, health care use, and mental health status of transgender persons: Implications for public health intervention. *Am J Public Health* 2001;91:915–921.
21. Simon PA, Reback CJ, Bemis CC. HIV prevalence and incidence among male-to-female transsexuals receiving HIV prevention services in Los Angeles County. *AIDS* 2000;14: 2953–2955.
22. Sykes DL. Transgendered people: An "invisible" population. *California HIV/AIDS Update* 1999;12:80–85.
23. Nemoto T, Luke D, Mamo L, et al. HIV risk behaviours among male-to-female transgenders in comparison with homosexual or bisexual males and heterosexual females. *AIDS Care* 1999;11:297–312.
24. Brennan J, Kuhns LM, Johnson AK, et al. Syndemic theory and HIV-related risk among young transgender women: The role of multiple, co-occurring health problems and social marginalization. *Am J Public Health* 2012;102:1751–1757.
25. Nuttbrock L, Bockting W, Rosenblum A, et al. Gender abuse, depressive symptoms, and HIV and other sexually transmitted infections among male-to-female transgender persons: A three-year prospective study. *Am J Public Health* 2012; 103: 300–307.
26. Reback CJ, Shoptaw S, Downing MJ. Prevention case management improves socioeconomic standing and reduces symptoms of psychological and emotional distress among transgender women. *AIDS Care* 2012;24:1136–1144.
27. Boehmer U. Twenty years of public health research: Inclusion of lesbian, gay, bisexual, and transgender populations. *Am J Public Health* 2002;92:1125–1130.
28. Dean L, Meyer IH, Robinston K, et al. Lesbian, gay, bisexual, and transgender health: findings and concerns. *J Gay Lesbian Med Assoc* 2000;4:102–151.
29. Strathdee SA, Hogg RS, Martindale SL, et al. Determinants of sexual risk-taking among young HIV-negative gay and bisexual men. *J Acquir Immune Defic Syndr Hum Retrovirol* 1998;19:61–66.
30. Greenwood GL, White EW, Page-Shafer K, et al. Correlates of heavy substance use among young gay and bisexual men: The San Francisco Young Men's Health Study. *Drug Alcohol Depend* 2001;61:105–112.
31. White House Office of National AIDS Policy. National HIV/AIDS strategy for the United States. Washington, DC: White House Office of National AIDS Policy, 2010.
32. Herek GM, Gillis JR, Cogan JC. Psychological sequelae of hate-crime victimization among lesbian, gay, and bisexual adults. *J Consult Clin Psychol* 1999;67:945–951.

33. Skinner WF. The prevalence and demographic predictors of illicit and licit drug use. *Am J Public Health* 1994;84:1307–1310.

34. Lee R. Health care problems of lesbian, gay, bisexual, and transgender patients. *West J Med* 2000;172:403–408.

35. Meyer IH. Minority stress and mental health in gay men. *J Health Soc Behav* 1995;36: 38–56.

36. Garnets L, Herek GM, Levy B. Violence and victimization of lesbians and gay men: Mental health consequences. In: Herek GM, Berrill KT, eds. Hate crimes: Confronting violence against lesbians and gay men. Newbury Park, CA: Sage, 1992:207–226.

37. Meyer IH. Prejudice, social stress, and mental health in lesbian, gay, and bisexual populations: Conceptual issues and research evidence. *Psychol Bull* 2003;129:674–697.

38. Williamson IR. Internalized homophobia and health issues affecting lesbians and gay men. *Health Educ Res* 2000;15:97–107.

39. Brotman S, Ryan B, Jalbert Y, et al. The impact of coming out on health and health care access: The experiences of gay, lesbian, bisexual and two-spirit people. *J Health Soc Policy* 2002;15:1–29.

40. Huebner DM, Davis MC, Nemeroff CJ, et al. The impact of internalized homophobia on HIV preventive interventions. *Am J Commun Psychol* 2002;30:327–348.

41. American Psychiatric Association. Diagnostic and Statistical Manual of Mental Disorders: DSM-IV-TR (Text Revision). 4th ed. Washington, DC: American Psychiatric Association, 2000.

42. Campo J, Nijman H, Merckelbach H, et al. Psychiatric comorbidity of gender identity disorders: A survey among Dutch psychiatrists. *Am J Psychiatry* 2003;160:1332–1336.

43. Habermeyer E, Kamps I, Kawohl W. A case of bipolar psychosis and transsexualism. *Psychopathology* 2003;36:168–170.

44. Haraldsen I, Dahl A. Symptom profiles of gender dysphoric patients of transsexual type compared to patients with personality disorders and healthy adults. *Acta Psychiatr Scand* 2000;102:276–281.

45. Cole SW, Kemeny ME, Taylor SE, et al. Accelerated course of human immunodeficiency virus infection in gay men who conceal their homosexual identity. *Psychosom Med* 1996;58:219–231.

46. Cole SW, Kemeny ME, Taylor SE, et al. Elevated physical health risk among gay men who conceal their homosexual identity. *Health Psychol* 1996;15:243–251.

47. Cole SW, Kemeny ME, Taylor SE. Social identity and physical health: Accelerated HIV progression in rejection-sensitive gay men. *J Personal Soc Psychol* 1997;72:320–335.

48. Meyer IH. Prejudice, social stress, and mental health in lesbian, gay, and bisexual populations: Conceptual issues and research evidence. *Psychol Bull* 2003;129:674–697.

49. Stall R, Wiley J. A comparison of alcohol and drug use patterns of homosexual and heterosexual men: The San Francisco Men's Health Study. *Drug Alcohol Depend* 1988;22:63–73.

50. McCabe SE, Boyd C, Hughes TL, et al. Sexual identity and substance use among undergraduate students. *Substance Abuse* 2003;24:77–91.

51. Stall R, Paul JP, Greenwood G, et al. Alcohol use, drug use and alcohol-related problems among men who have sex. *Addiction* 2001;96:1589–1601.

52. McKirnan DJ, Peterson PL. Psychosocial and cultural factors in alcohol and drug abuse: An analysis. *Addict Behav* 1989;14:555–563.

53. Hughes TL, Eliason M. Lesbian, gay, bisexual, and transgender issues in substance abuse. *J Prim Prev* 2002;22:263–298.

54. Emery S, Gilpin EA, Ake C, et al. Characterizing and identifying "hard-core" smokers: Implications for further reducing smoking prevalence. *Am J Public Health* 2000;90: 387–394.

55. Ryan H, Wortley PM, Easton A, et al. Smoking among lesbians, gays, and bisexuals: A review of the literature. *Am J Prev Med* 2001;21:142–149.

56. Stall RD, Greenwood GL, Acree M, et al. Cigarette smoking among gay and bisexual men. *Am J Public Health* 1999;89:1875–1878.

57. Skinner W, Otis MD. Drug and alcohol use among lesbian and gay people in a southern U.S. sample: Epidemiological, comparative, and methodological findings from the Trilogy Project. *J Homosex* 1996;30:59–92.

58. Roberts SA, Dibble SL, Nussey B, et al. Cardiovascular disease risk in lesbian women. *Women's Health Issues* 2003;13:167–174.

59. Ungvarski PJ, Grossman AH. Health problems of gay and bisexual men. *Nursing Clin North Am* 1999;34:313–331.

60. Valanis BG, Bowen DJ, Bassford T, et al. Sexual orientation and health: Comparisons in the Women's Health Initiative sample. *Arch Fam Med* 2000;9:843–853.

61. Bradford J, Ryan C, Honnold J, et al. Expanding the research infrastructure for lesbian health. *Am J Public Health* 2001;91:1029–1032.

62. Moran N. Lesbian health care needs. *Can Family Physician* 1996;42:879–884.

63. White J, Dull VT. Health risk factors and health-seeking behavior in lesbians. *J Women's Health* 1997;6:103–112.

64. Burnett CB, Steakley CS, Slack R, et al. Patterns of breast cancer screening among lesbians at increased risk for breast cancer. *Women Health* 1999;29:35–55.

65. Dibble SL, Roberts SA, Robertson PA, et al. Risk factors for ovarian cancer: Lesbian and heterosexual women. *Oncol Nursing Forum* 2002;29:E1–E47.

66. Matthews AK, Brandenburg DL, Johnson TP, et al. Correlates of underutilization of gynecological cancer screening among lesbian and heterosexual women. *Prev Med* 2004;38:105–113.

67. Rankow EJ, Tessaro I. Cervical cancer risk and Papanicolaou [Pap] screening in a sample of lesbian and bisexual women. *J Fam Pract* 1998;47:139–143.

68. Cochran SD. Emerging issues in research on lesbians' and gay men's mental health: Does sexual orientation really matter? *Am Psychol* 2001;56:931–941.

69. Horn-Ross PL, Canchola AJ, West DW, et al. Patterns of alcohol consumption and breast cancer risk in the California Teachers Study cohort. *Cancer Epidemiol Bio-markers Prevent* 2004;13:405–411.

70. Hamajima N, Hirose K, Tajima K, et al. Alcohol, tobacco and breast cancer— Collaborative reanalysis of individual data from 53 epidemiological studies, including 58,515 women with breast cancer and 95,067 women without the disease. *Br J Cancer* 2002;87:1234–1235.

71. Davis K. Southern comfort [documentary]. HBO Theatrical Documentary, 2001.

72. Feinberg L. Trans health crisis: For us it's life or death. *Am J Public Health* 2001;91: 897–900.

73. Centers for Medicare & Medicaid Services, U.S. Department of Health and Human Services. Medicare and Medicaid programs: Changes to the hospital and critical access

hospital conditions of participation to ensure visitation rights for all patients. *Federal Register* 2010;75:70831–70844.

74. Cahill S, Mitra E, Tobias S. Family policy: Issues affecting gay, lesbian, bisexual and transgender families. Washington, DC: National Gay and Lesbian Task Force, January 22, 2003.

75. Rubin G. Thinking sex: Notes towards a radical theory of the politics of sexuality. In: Vance C, ed. Pleasure and danger: Exploring female sexuality. Boston: Routledge and Kegan Paul, 1984:267–319.

76. Namaste VK. Genderbashing. In: Namaste VK, ed. Invisible lives: The erasure of transsexual and transgendered people. Chicago: University of Chicago Press, 2000.

77. Butler J. Against proper objects. In: Weed E, Schor N, eds. Feminism meets queer theory. Indianapolis: Indiana University Press, 1997:1–30.

78. Garfinkel H. Studies in ethnomethodology. Englewood Cliffs, NJ: Prentice-Hall, 1967.

79. Bornstein K. Gender outlaw: On men, women, and the rest of us. New York: Routledge, 1994.

80. Kessler SJ, McKenna W. Gender: An ethnomethodological approach. New York: John Wiley and Sons, 1978.

81. Trujillo C. Chicana lesbians: The girls our mothers warned us about. Berkeley, CA: Third Woman Press, 1991.

82. Almaguer T. Chicano men: A cartography of homosexual identity and behavior. *Differences: A Journal of Feminist Cultural Studies* 1991;3:75–100.

83. Lugones M. El pasar discontínuo de la cachapera/tortillera del barrio a la barra al movimiento [The discontinuous passing of the cachapera/tortillera from the barrio to the bar to the movement]. In: Lugones M, ed. Pilgrimages/peregrinajes: Theorizing coalition against multiple oppressions. New York: Rowman & Littlefield, 2003:167–180.

84. Moraga C. Loving in the war years: Lo que nunco pasó por sus labios. Boston: South End, 1983.

85. West C. Black sexuality: The taboo subject. In: West C, ed. Race matters. Boston: Beacon Press, 1994: 81–91.

86. Collins PH. The sexual politics of black womanhood. In: Collins PH, ed. Black feminist thought: Knowledge, consciousness, and the politics of empowerment. 2nd ed. New York: Routledge, 2000:123–148.

87. United States Department of Health and Human Services. Statement by Secretary Kathleen Sebelius on LGBT Health Awareness Week 2012. Washington, DC: United States Department of Health and Human Services, 2012. Available at http://www.hhs.gov/news/press/2012pres/03/20120326a.html. Accessed on June 19, 2012.

88. Hatzenbuehler ML, Keyes KM, McLaughlin KA. The protective effects of social/contextual factors on psychiatric morbidity in LGB populations. *Int J Epidemiol* 2011;40:1071–1080.

89. Swartz L. Updated look at legal responses to transsexualism: Especially three marriage cases in U.K., U.S. and New Zealand. *Int J Transgenderism* 1997;1. Available at http://www.wpath.org/journal/www.iiav.nl/ezines/web/IJT/97-03/numbers/symposion/ijtc0201.htm. Accessed on June 19, 2012.

90. Dasti JL. Advocating a broader understanding of the necessity of sex-reassignment surgery under Medicaid. *NY Univ Law Rev* 2002;77:1738–1775.

91. Frye PR. The International Bill of Gender Rights vs. The Cider House Rules: Transgenders struggle with the courts over what clothing they are allowed to wear on

the job, which restroom they are allowed to use on the job, their right to marry, and the very definition of their sex. *William Mary J Women Law* 2000;7:133.

92. American Medical Association. AMA Resolution 122: Removing financial barriers to care for transgender patients. Available at http://www.tgender.net/taw/ama_resolutions.pdf. Accessed on June 19, 2012.

93. Committee on Health Care for Underserved Women of The American College of Obstetricians and Gynecologists. Committee Opinion No. 512: Health care for transgender individuals. *Obstet Gynecol* 2011;118:1454.

94. Committee on Lesbian, Gay, Bisexual, and Transgender Health Issues and Research Gaps and Opportunities; Board on the Health of Select Populations; Institute of Medicine. The health of lesbian, gay, bisexual, and transgender people: Building a foundation for better understanding. Washington, DC: National Academies Press, 2011.

95. Robertson C. Ban on gay marriage passes in North Carolina. *New York Times*, May 8, 2012. Available at http://www.nytimes.com/2012/05/09/us/north-carolina-voters-pass-same-sex-marriage-ban.html. Accessed on June 19, 2012.

96. Calmes J, Baker P. Obama says same-sex marriage should be legal. *New York Times*, May 9, 2012. Available at http://www.nytimes.com/2012/05/10/us/politics/obama-says-same-sex-marriage-should-be-legal.html?pagewanted=all. Accessed on June 19, 2012.

8 People with Disabilities

■ NORA ELLEN GROCE

■ **INTRODUCTION**

The image of the little boy in the polio-prevention poster was arresting. Perhaps 4 or 5 years of age, he had obviously responded to the photographer's request by pulling himself up on his crutches, looking straight into the camera, and beaming his most winning smile. The caption, however, was what caught one's attention. "Let's make him the last," it told the reader, pleading for more active commitment to the local polio immunization campaign.

Preventing polio is an admirable public health goal, but it is not the only one.* What will become of the little boy in the poster? Certainly, his life should be worth more than simply encouraging public health professionals to redouble their efforts. Yet research clearly shows that, compared with his peers, this boy will be far less likely to receive adequate health care or education, or to participate in the social, economic, and religious life of his community.

According to the *World Report on Disability* (2011) by the World Health Organization (WHO) and the World Bank, more than 1 billion people (15 percent of the world's population) live with a physical, sensory, intellectual, or mental health impairment significant enough to make a difference in their daily lives.[1] Eighty percent of these people live in developing countries (Figure 8–1).[2] Social justice cannot be achieved unless these people with disabilities—among the poorest and the most marginalized—are fully included in all aspects of life. (See Box 8–1.)

Over the past decade, significant progress has been made in giving disability issues higher priority, most notably in the United Nations Convention on the Rights of Persons with Disabilities (CRPD), which guarantees full participation and equal access to resources to all persons with disabilities (Figure 8–2).[3] But there is still a long way to go. The Convention and much new legislation within countries that have ratified it, designed to ensure that national laws are in compliance with the overarching Convention, may mean little if these laws are not enforced at the individual and community levels.

---

* While many types of disability may be preventable, some individuals and families with certain hereditary disorders, such as deafness and dwarfism, have made a strong case for continuing to have children with these traits, who can share their family's genetic heritage and social legacy. The assumption that all types of disability should be prevented is not, therefore, as straightforward as it is sometimes presented.

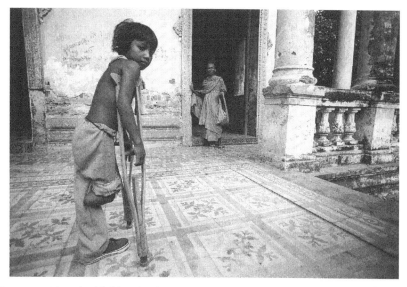

Figure 8-1 A boy disabled by a land mine stands in a courtyard of a UNICEF-assisted rehabilitation center in Cambodia. This boy is one of the fortunate few. Most people with disabilities in both developing and developed countries have inadequate access to necessary services, and reduced opportunities in education, employment, and other aspects of life. (Photograph: UNICEF/HQ92–0629/Roger Lemoyne.)

▪ DISABILITY AS A SOCIAL JUSTICE ISSUE

The primary issues faced by persons with disabilities are not their specific impairments, but social stigma, reduced access to resources, and poverty that can limit their full potential. For example, in many countries, children with disabilities often receive less nurturing and have less access to basic resources, such as food and health care, with resultant developmental delays.[4] Despite increasing levels of education, 90 percent of all children with disabilities are not in school,[5] and literacy rates for adults with disabilities may be less than 5 percent globally.[6] Few young people with disabilities are trained for jobs or given the opportunity to learn a skill that will allow them to support themselves as adults. Even when skilled, persons with disabilities are often simply not hired. Unemployment rates for people with disabilities are frequently 80 percent or higher.[7] Indeed, a common form of employment for disabled individuals outside of their households remains begging.[8] Compounding this, people with disabilities are denied the right to decide when, where, and with whom they will live. They often have no say over how they will support themselves and may be denied the right to have a relationship or marry and have a family.[9] Gender and ethnic or minority status can compound these inequities.[9] Hundreds of thousands continue to be institutionalized against their will, although community-based inclusionary models provide far better and more cost-effective services.[10]

BOX 8-1 ■ Terminology

Much attention has been devoted to getting away from pejorative terms and phrases. Older terms such as *cripple* have given way to more politically neutral terms. To say that someone is a "wheelchair user," rather than "confined to a wheelchair," shifts the emphasis to an individual who is making use of an appliance rather than being a victim imprisoned in an object.

Some issues of terminology are of more relevance in one language than are others. For example, the term *handicap* ("cap in hand" or "beggar") has a more pejorative connotation in English than in French, where it carries a more neutral connotation.

At its best, this debate over proper language fosters rethinking and reevaluation of basic assumptions by members of society and, as such, is analogous to the shifts in many languages brought about by women's rights movement. (This is particularly true in languages where general terms about those with a disability include concepts like "the unfortunates" and "the cursed.") At its worst, however, controversy over the proper language about disability has taken much time and energy, which could more fruitfully be directed at more substantive issues facing disabled populations. It has also led to the generation of a number of terms (usually by people who are not themselves disabled) that are "politically correct" but unlikely to enter common speech, such as *the differently abled*. A good rule of thumb is to ask members of the local disability community what terms they prefer be used. Another solution to this ongoing debate over terminology was offered by a mother at a meeting of parents of young children with severe intellectual disabilities in Canada. The mother turned to the audience, composed largely of human rights lawyers and physicians, and said, "Please promise me you will tell the professionals you work with that there is one term that applies to everyone with a disability, no matter what type of disability they have. Tell them the term is 'citizen.'"

Globally, one family in four has a member with a significant disability, and this proportion is increasing.[1,11] Disabilities due to violence and inadequate health services, which continue to disable millions of people, are preventable. Many other disabilities are not. Improved health care, especially for critically ill newborns and those who are seriously injured or chronically ill, enables them to survive, but often with disabilities.

Although there is extensive literature on disability, most of it addresses clinical, rehabilitative or vocational issues—not public health. Outside of specific data sets from developed countries, where social protection schemes and public health laws and policies have prompted officials to keep statistics for rehabilitative or educational services, few epidemiological and demographic data on disabled populations are available.[1,11] Little attention has been paid to how people with disabilities can and should be incorporated into broader public health initiatives or social justice campaigns.

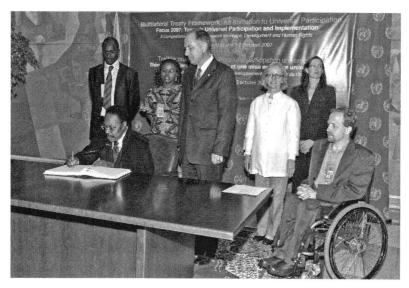

Figure 8–2 Omar Bongo Ondimba, President of Gabon, signs the Convention on the Rights of Persons with Disabilities in 2007 at United Nations Headquarters in New York. (UN Photo/Devra Berkowitz.)

Yet people with disabilities are often at increased risk for (a) many chronic conditions, such as Alzheimer's disease; (b) infectious diseases, such as HIV/AIDS; (c) social and behavioral problems, such as domestic violence and substance abuse; and (d) health concerns caused by deprivation of resources, such as malnutrition.[2,12,13] They are also more likely to be denied legal, social, and political rights, largely because, in many countries, they continue to face severe stigma and discrimination.[1,14]

Much of this stigma and discrimination is linked to negative traditional beliefs, although ignorance and lack of familiarity with persons with disabilities are also limiting factors. For example, disability is often assumed to be evidence of "bad blood" or incest, divine displeasure, or punishment for sins. Such social interpretation of disability is important because disability cannot be understood outside of a cultural context. Within every society, attitudes and inclusionary or exclusionary practices are, in part, shaped by beliefs about why a disability occurs and what the anticipated adult roles are for people with disabilities.[14] Differences in socioeconomic status, class, caste, and educational level also make a significant difference in the quality of life for people with disabilities.[15]

Where disability is stigmatized, a common corollary is that people with disabilities are deprived of the resources of that society. In such societies, people with disabilities often contend with a "charity model." This model gives them no inherent right to the resources of a community. In poorer societies, the unmet needs of people with disabilities are sought through individualized appeals for charity—begging on a street corner or the steps of a church, temple, or mosque. In developed countries, such unmet needs are often addressed by more organized appeals, such as telethons and other types of public fund-raisers. These kinds of charitable appeals, whether done by individuals or organizations, differ significantly from a social justice-driven "rights-based" model, in which all individuals are believed to be entitled to an equitable share of the community's resources.

▓ DISABILITY, POVERTY, AND INEQUALITY

While not all people who are born with or later develop a disability are poor, there is a strong feedback loop between disability and poverty. People who are poor are more likely to become disabled.[16,17] Those who are poor are more likely to live and work in physically dangerous environments, have less to eat, and receive poorer quality medical care or none at all. Similarly, those who are disabled are more likely to be poor because they receive less education, have fewer skills, and are much more likely to be unemployed. If employed, persons with disability are more likely to be underemployed or employed in positions that are marginal and poorly paid, and they are often the first to be fired if the economy declines. Thus, there is a heightened chance that once a disability occurs, those who lived above the poverty line will be driven into poverty, and those who were poor before the disability occurred are more likely to become destitute.[18,19]

This feedback loop between disability and poverty places people with disabilities at a marked disadvantage at every stage of their lives.[20] Disabled children, especially those with more visible disabilities, are frequently assumed to be in frail health and unlikely to survive into adulthood. Indeed, in many countries, a significantly disabled child is referred to as "an innocent" or a "little angel."[8] From this perspective, sending such children to school, including them in social interactions, or preparing them for participation in the adult world seems unnecessary. Families with disabled children have often anticipated their early death, but not their possible survival. (See Box 8–2.)

Disabled adolescents and young adults are rarely allowed to learn marketable skills or participate in the formal and informal "rites of passage"—such as learning to drive, playing sports, or dating—that prepare all other young people for their transition to adulthood. Where no services exist, such young people usually must either continue to live as "children" in their parents' households, face institutionalization, or find themselves on the street. One-third of all street children are disabled.[10]

As adults, people with disabilities are often denied the right to work outside the home. They are also often forbidden to marry, to have children, or to participate in the religious, social, and recreational activities that would mark their status as adult members of society. They often have no political voice and frequently are barred from taking oaths or giving testimony in court, which severely restricts their ability to call upon protection from the legal system or to question legal decisions made for them by their family or society.[21]

BOX 8-2 ■ Disability and Education

Sara had looked forward to school for years. Third in a family of five children, Sara, age 8, has waited an additional 2 years to start school because of her parent's reluctance to let her venture beyond their rural homestead. As Sara was born with a withered right arm, her parents feared that she would be the object of ridicule by local children and a sign to other parents that their family had been "cursed." But she was bright and inquisitive, and a full season of pestering on her part had finally led her parents to relent. As she took her seat in the classroom, the surrounding students looked at her uneasily. Many were playmates who already knew her from home. It was the teacher who would decide her fate, however, and the teacher's reaction was swift and uncompromising. "You would be a distraction to other children," the teacher told her. "And besides, I do not know how to teach crippled children. There is a special school for your kind in the city if you want to go." Sara dissolved into tears and returned home. Twelve years later, her eyes still fill with tears as she recounts the incident.

Sara's experience in her West African village school is hardly unique. UNESCO estimates that despite significant gains in primary school enrollment rates for children with disabilities over the past decade, more than 90 percent of all disabled children are not in primary school, and possibly one-third of all those currently still not in primary school are children with disabilities.[1] In 1994, the Salamanca Declaration and the ongoing UNESCO Education for All initiative[2] spurred strong interest in and commitment to ensuring attendance of children with disabilities in their local schools.

Attendance in mainstream schools by children with disabilities, known as *inclusive education*, is increasingly common, and in line with the UN Convention, which calls specifically for children to be provided with services in the "least restrictive" environments. Such inclusion, in some countries, has been going on for many years. For example, Dr. Michael Miles noted that up to 40 percent of disabled children in one area of rural northwest Pakistan were attending school in general classrooms.[3] But, historically, special schools have been the only option available for most children with disabilities who seek an education.

Unfortunately, in many countries there has been only a handful of such schools, often located in regional centers or capital cities, which tend to serve children from more affluent families. While such schools are helpful for those who attend or for teachers who can receive some training through them, the capacity of these schools is limited. They are usually under-funded and short of staff and facilities; and they can rarely educate more than a few hundred children at a time. In many countries, this means that there are potentially waiting lists for such schools of tens of thousands of children.

There is another concern. Special schools are operated as boarding schools for most of their students, especially those from distant rural areas. Disabled children as young as 5 years of age may be sent across the country to such institutions for years, rarely returning home. Ties to their families weaken, and their links to home communities dissolve, often leaving these children estranged from their families and support networks.

However, change has begun. The right of children with disabilities to receive an education and to receive this education while living at home with their own families and in their own communities has given rise to a strong movement towards inclusive education. For millions of children, their specific disability would not preclude them from being able to function easily within a general classroom. In other cases, only minor adaptations are necessary—allowing a child with poor eyesight to sit closer to the blackboard, or moving a class from the second floor to the ground floor of a building so a child who has mobility problems will not lose out on an education because she cannot climb a set of stairs. Special adaptations require more resources, such as sign-language interpretation or instruction for children who are deaf, or special adaptations for children with intellectual disabilities.

Regrettably, in many countries, education for disabled children is still a low priority. And, if disabled children are unable to attend school or drop out of school early, their ability to gain literacy and numeracy skills later in life is more limited. Persons with disabilities are rarely targeted by or included in general adult literacy campaigns.[4] Any attempt to bring them into the economic, social, and political mainstream or to reach them effectively in public health campaigns will not occur unless their educational needs are seriously considered.

Box References

1. UNESCO. Education for all. Available at http://www.unesco.org/new/en/education/themes/leading-the-international-agenda/education-for-all/. Accessed on June 25, 2012.
2. UNESCO. The Salamanca Statement and Framework for Action on Special Needs Education, 1994. Available at http://www.unesco.de/fileadmin/medien/Dokumente/Bildung/Salamanca_Declaration.pdf. Accessed on June 25, 2012.
3. Miles M. Children with disability in ordinary schools: An action study of non-designed educational integration in Pakistan. Peshawar: National Council of Social Welfare, 1986.
4. Groce N, Bahkshi P. Illiteracy among adults with disabilities in the developing world: A review of the literature and a call for action. *International Journal of Inclusive Education* 2011;15:1153–1168.

To be female and disabled is frequently referred to as being "doubly disabled." (See Chapter 4.) Survival itself is often at issue. For example, a poor family may delay buying medicine for a disabled daughter, hesitating to spend scarce resources on a female child, while hoping that the condition will clear on its own. An indication of the extent of this problem can be seen in the survival figures from a small-scale study of former polio patients from Nepal, where the polio survival rate for males was twice that for females.[22] The 2011 *World Report on Disability* found that the global incidence of disability is 11 percent higher for women than for men due to unequal access to basic resources, such as food, adequate health care, and freedom from violence and abuse.

Bishnu Dhungana, writing on the lives of disabled women in Nepal, cited a striking example of this gender imbalance in her interview with a disabled young woman who had a twin brother born with an identical disability.[23] The brother attained a university degree, with the strong support of his parents, who had carried him to school daily to ensure that he received a good education. The sister had never attended school and, despite the middle-class status of her family, was illiterate.

Women with disabilities often receive significantly less education, are less likely to marry, and have much more difficulty finding employment than do disabled males or non-disabled women.[9] With little ability to support themselves and few prospects for marriage, millions of women with disabilities live in abject poverty and at increased risk of physical and psychological abuse.[24]

People with disabilities who are members of ethnic and minority populations are also at increased risk. Coming from traditions that differ from that of the majority population, they are less likely to be included in available services and programs. Women with disabilities from ethnic or minority communities often find themselves contending with forces that exclude them on the basis of gender as well as disability and heritage.[25]

■ SOCIAL INJUSTICE AND ACCESS TO HEALTH CARE

Public health work is frequently framed in terms of disability prevention. However, public health workers often overlook the need to ensure that people with disabilities have the opportunity to maintain good health—this is not surprising, because few schools of public health or medicine integrate disability into their curricula. When addressed at all, information on disability is usually offered in electives taken only by students with an already established interest in the subject.

In health services and programs in the community, the question of whether people with disabilities are being reached and served is rarely raised—whether the focus is breast cancer screening, dental care, or reproductive health services. Research is rarely performed on the distribution of chronic and infectious diseases among disabled people and on their knowledge, attitudes, and practices concerning various health and social-welfare issues.

Access of disabled people to non–disability related medical care is also limited. Health care facilities are frequently inaccessible. Stairs block access for wheelchair users. Medical equipment that does not require patients to transfer from a wheelchair or to stand—such as examining tables, dental chairs, and x-ray machines—is difficult to locate. A lack of sign-language interpreters makes medical consultation difficult for many deaf people. Access to clinics, testing sites, and counseling programs may require more organization and planning than individuals with mental health problems or intellectual impairments are capable of providing. (See Box 8–3.) Yet, in many cases, people with disabilities can be included in health programs, and health facilities can be made accessible at little or no additional cost. For example, in many countries, ramps into clinics can be made of pounded sand, stone, or bamboo. Malaria-prevention campaigns or smoking-cessation messages for the general public can easily be designed to be simple and straightforward in order to enable individuals with intellectual impairments to understand them.

BOX 8-3 ■ **Similarities and Differences Among People with Disabilities**

People with different types of disability often face markedly different sets of problems. For example, an individual with a physical impairment who needs assistance with activities of daily living, such as dressing, toileting, and feeding, may benefit significantly from environmental adaptations, such as ramps, grab bars, and automated doors. An individual who is deaf may have no physical restrictions, but will need a sign-language interpreter in order to communicate effectively with the surrounding hearing world. An individual who is intellectually impaired may be physically fit and fully able to communicate, but may need help in organizing and performing daily responsibilities. An individual with a mental health problem may be fully able to meet both physical and intellectual challenges, but need support and appropriate medication in order to continue to function successfully in the community.

Historically, persons with disabilities have been divided into distinct constituencies on the basis of their specific disabilities. The concept of "disability" as a politically viable category developed in the 1960s and 1970s, when people with a broad range of disabilities started to join together in an emerging global disability rights movement. They argued that no matter what types of disabilities they had, they faced common challenges. Their lives were structured and their options determined by (a) complex medical, legal, and educational bureaucracies; (b) a Social Security system or social protection scheme that limited their options and denied the right of persons with disabilities independence and self-determination; and (c) a broader society wherein prejudice and stereotypes were still widespread.

Because resources for people with disabilities are extremely limited, disability advocacy and service organizations are frequently forced to compete with each other for these limited resources. Organizations working on behalf of those who are blind or physically disabled, for example, must often justify funding for their projects or programs by arguing that they will yield greater benefits, or why their constituents are more worthy of support than are individuals with other types of disabilities. The UN Convention on the Rights of Persons with Disabilities and a growing collaboration between groups representing people with different types of disabilities at the grassroots levels have begun to alter this landscape, with many disability advocacy groups placing increased emphasis on the similar concerns that all individuals share—no matter what type of disability they have. This common sense of purpose is important, but in many places groups representing the interests of people with different types of disabilities are still asked to justify why their particular constituency is more "in need" or "worthy of support" than others.

Problems go beyond accessibility. In both developed and developing countries, those who seek care for conditions not related to their disabilities report that clinicians seem fixated on their disabilities—no matter for what condition they are seeking care.[26] Clinicians often refuse to provide basic vaccinations, reproductive health information, or chemotherapy to people with disabilities because they assume that people with disabilities do not have a need for these services or do not have the right to use scarce resources.[27] During times of disaster and political upheaval, disabled people face additional challenges. (See Box 8–4.)

BOX 8-4 ■ Disability During Times of Disaster and Political Upheaval

During times of natural disasters and political upheaval, individuals with disabilities often face a complex set of problems. A study by the Center for Services and Information on Disability (CSID) examined the fate of individuals with physical mobility problems during times of natural disasters in 10 coastal districts in Bangladesh.[1] Only 17 percent of individuals with mobility impairments had been taken to cyclone shelters, 55 percent of them remained at home while their families went to shelters. The remaining 28 percent either sought safer shelter in a built structure nearby or were forced to cling to a tree or other permanent structures.

Following the disaster, individuals with mobility problems were much less likely to be able to access relief supplies—largely because, in order to get emergency food rations, building materials, or medicines, people were required to travel to central distribution sites and stand in line for long hours—difficult or impossible for many of those with mobility impairments. Only 2 percent of the families with a disabled individual in the study had received any special attention during the rehabilitation phase following the disaster.

Such problems are compounded when families are forced to flee their homes. Individuals with disabilities are often left behind in times of war and famine when families flee, especially when they are forced to flee on foot. Being left behind in times of emergency is not related solely to the physical inability of individuals with some types of disabilities to keep up. In many disaster situations, families who anticipate becoming refugees (seeking asylum in another country) may fear that all members of the family will be denied asylum if someone in the family is disabled. This is a realistic fear. Prior to the Convention on the Rights of Persons with Disabilities,[2] many countries, including the United States, routinely denied asylum because of disability status, arguing that the new immigrants would be unlikely to become self-supporting.

There are additional concerns. In times of crisis, social and political unrest often leads to the closure of health care institutions, schools, and other organizations that have been responsible for providing support and advocacy for disabled people. In such situations, individuals with disabilities are often abandoned unattended in facilities, sent home to families who do not have experience in providing care, or left behind with meager systems of social support systems—distant relatives or neighbors who promise to occasionally check in on them. Some relief organizations have responded to queries about serving individuals with disabilities by stating that they actually see few individuals with disabilities. So where are these people?

There has been increasing attention to the fate of people with disabilities during humanitarian crises and natural disasters. Since Hurricane Katrina in the United States[3] and the tsunamis in Thailand, Indonesia, and Japan, there is growing realization that many people with disabilities are at greatly increased risk because they are unable to receive or respond to warnings about imminent danger. For example, deaf individuals will be unable to hear warning sirens, and people with mobility impairments may be unable to flee and to be accommodated should they reach refugee camps or other places of refuge.[4]

Progress is being made, however. For example, *The Sphere Handbook,* one of the most widely used guidelines for humanitarian response in times of disaster and emergency has incorporated disability issues throughout its most recent updated version.[5] And the needs of persons with disabilities in times of emergency are specifically addressed in the Convention on the Rights of Persons with Disabilities,[6] which states that signatory countries shall ensure the protection and safety of persons with disabilities in situations of risk, including armed conflict, humanitarian emergencies, and natural disasters."[6]

Box References

1. Rahman N. Disasters and disability: Service delivery or rights? Dhaka, Bangladesh: National Forum of Organizations Working with Disability, 2004.
2. United Nations General Assembly. Convention on the Rights of Persons with Disabilities, Article 5. December 6, 2006. Available at http://www.un.org/esa/socdev/enable/rights/convtexte.htm#convtext. Accessed on June 25, 2012.
3. Prabu DP, Wingate M, Butler J, et al. 2006–2007 ASPH/CDC Vulnerable Populations Collaboration Group preparedness resource kit. Atlanta: Centers for Disease Control, 2008. Available at http://preparedness.asph.org/perlc/documents/VulnerablePopulations.pdf. Accessed on June 25, 2012.
4. Kett M, van Ommeren M. Disability, conflict and emergencies. *Lancet* 2009;374:1801–1803.
5. The Sphere Project: The Sphere handbook: Humanitarian charter and minimum standards in humanitarian response. Geneva: The Sphere Project, 2011. Available at http://www.sphereproject.org/handbook/. Accessed on June 25, 2012.
6. United Nations General Assembly. Convention on the Rights of Persons with Disabilities, Article 11. December 6, 2006. Available at http://www.un.org/esa/socdev/enable/rights/convtexte.htm#convtext. Accessed on June 25, 2012.

▓ DISABILITY-SPECIFIC RESOURCES

Issues of unmet rehabilitative needs for some also lessen their ability to fully participate in society. Not all people with disabilities need rehabilitative care; some never need it, and many more need it for limited amounts of time or intermittently during their lives.

However, the availability of rehabilitative care and assistive devices, such as artificial limbs, wheelchairs, hearing aids, and eyeglasses, must be specifically addressed because it is usually given a low priority by health professionals and policy-makers.[28] Lack of such assistive devices often restricts people with disabilities far more than do their specific impairments.

Globally, WHO estimates that only 17 to 37 percent of those who need rehabilitation services or assistive devices receive them, and men are more likely to receive them than women.[29] In addition, rehabilitative services tend to be concentrated in urban areas and can be prohibitively expensive. Programs that require long-term care are unavailable to many, especially women in societies where they are not allowed to travel or live away from home unescorted by a male relative. In developing countries, community-based rehabilitation (CBR), in which services and expertise is offered at the community level with a triage system to access greater expertise, offers great promise. WHO guidelines on CBR have helped clarify future prospects for this intervention.[30] However, CBR programs are chronically under-funded, have rarely been brought to scale, and often are the first to be cut when funding is reduced.

▓ HIV/AIDS AND DISABILITIES

The impact of HIV/AIDS on the global disability community helps illustrate the interlocking problems faced by people with disabilities. Although AIDS researchers have studied the disabling effects of HIV/AIDS on previously healthy people, little attention has been given to the risk of HIV/AIDS for people with existing disabilities. A review of the thousands of articles and information sites available on HIV/AIDS in both the published literature and the grey literature* yielded fewer than 100 articles on the HIV risk to people with pre-existing disabilities, with most attention focused on people affected by both mental illness and drug addiction.[31] (See Chapter 13.)

Why have people with disabilities not been included? It appears to be because it is commonly assumed that people with disabilities are not at risk of acquiring HIV infection. They are incorrectly thought to be sexually inactive, unlikely to use drugs, and at less risk for violence or rape than their non-disabled peers. Yet they actually have equal or increased risks for all known risk factors for HIV/AIDS compared to non-disabled people.

For example, extreme poverty and social sanctions against marrying an individual with a disability mean that people with disabilities, especially women with disabilities, are likely to become involved in a series of unstable relationships and have less ability to negotiate safer sex within these relationships.[9] Bisexuality and homosexuality have been reported within disabled populations at rates comparable to that of the general population. People with disabilities are at increased risk of substance abuse and less likely to have access to interventions. Disabled adolescents are rarely reached by safer-sex campaigns. Factors such as increased physical vulnerability, the need for attendant care, life in institutions, and the almost universal belief that persons with disabilities cannot be reliable witnesses on their own behalf place many disabled children and adults (both males and females) at an increased risk of being victims of sexual abuse and rape—at rates up to three times as high as that of their non-disabled peers.[32] In cultures in which it is believed that HIV-positive individuals can rid themselves of the virus by having sex with virgins, there has been a significant rise in the rape of disabled children and adults, who have been specifically targeted because they are assumed to be virgins.[33] Educating disabled populations about HIV/AIDS is also difficult. Lack of access to primary education has resulted in extremely low literacy rates, which makes communication of messages

---

* That which is produced by government, academia, business, and industry in print and electric formats, but not controlled by commercial publishers.

about HIV/AIDS even more difficult. These low literacy rates, compounded by lack of sex-education programs for persons with disabilities, is reflected in significantly lower rates of knowledge about HIV-prevention in disabled populations.[34-36] Few HIV/AIDS educational campaigns target or include disabled populations. Indeed, where HIV/AIDS educational campaigns are on radio or television, deaf and blind people are at a distinct disadvantage.

People with disabilities who become HIV-positive are equally disadvantaged, having far less access to health services than do non-disabled people. Indeed, care is often both physically inaccessible and too expensive for impoverished individuals with disabilities. A growing number of reports point to significant unreported rates of HIV-related infection, disease, and death globally among people with disabilities.[32]

Despite these risk factors, only a few HIV/AIDS pilot programs and interventions for disabled populations exist, and these projects continue to work on shoestring budgets and have difficulty in being brought to scale. Including people with disabilities in mainstream interventions intended for the all members of the general public is rarer still. There is a pressing need to understand the impact of HIV/AIDS on disabled populations and to design and implement programs and policies for them in a more coherent and comprehensive manner. And HIV is only one of many public health problems in which such exclusion has occurred.

■ SOCIAL JUSTICE AND THE CONVENTION ON THE RIGHTS OF PERSONS WITH DISABILITIES

In 2002, the first of a series of meetings was held at the United Nations in New York as the global disability community, began writing a UN convention to ensure the rights of persons with disabilities. The Convention, which was approved in 2006 and came into force in 2008, does not contain new rights, but rather brings together and affirms that all existing human rights guaranteed under other UN conventions pertain equally to persons with disabilities. The Convention also introduces mechanisms to monitor and evaluate progress in ensuring that these rights are enforced.

As of 2013, the Convention had been ratified by 130 countries. In ratifying the Convention, each country must rewrite its own national laws to ensure they are in accord with the Convention. The Convention guides the work of all UN agencies; as a result, UN agencies increasingly are addressing disability issues. For example, the UN Department of Economic and Social Affairs (DESA) published a report in 2011 specifically reviewing the integration of disability issues into the Millennium Development Goals (MDGs);[37] UNICEF has established a Disability Unit; and UNICEF's *State of the World's Children* report for 2013 focuses on children with disabilities.

WHO, in conjunction with the World Bank in 2011, published *The World Report on Disability*,[2] an evidence-based review of disability and health—a critically important new reference point for the collection and dissemination of data on this subject. WHO has also produced a series of guidelines and reports on disability-related topics, such as community-based rehabilitation, assistive devices, and child development, that are contributing to the evidence base on disability and health.[37]

■ WHAT NEEDS TO BE DONE

The global disability rights movement and the Convention on the Rights of Persons with Disabilities hold great promise. But such rights and the equitable access to resources guaranteed in the Convention are still far from being available to millions of persons with disabilities at the individual or community levels. And commitments at the international or national level mean little if they are not funded and enforced. A critical first step is building awareness that people with disabilities must be included in all work on development, social justice, and health, and building the commitment to do so (Figure 8–3).

The need for equity and inclusion must be understood and accepted as a legally established right by those working on ensuring social justice and promoting and protecting health. "I would very much like to help disabled children in my community," a colleague recently confided after I had given a talk on social injustice and disabled adolescents. "But I can't even get services to non-disabled children."

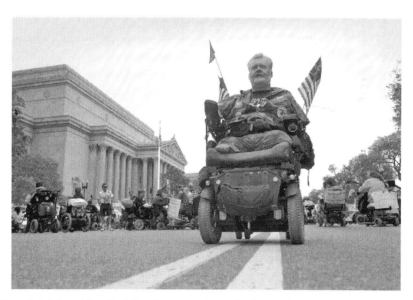

Figure 8–3 Man with a disability demonstrating at the Justice Department in Washington, DC, advocating for better Medicare and Medicaid benefits for long-term care for disabled people. (AP Photo/Susan Walsh.)

There is no reason why the needs of children or adults with disabilities should be addressed only after the needs of non-disabled people. Indeed, under the Convention on the Rights of Persons with Disabilities, deciding to have persons with disabilities wait until after the needs of non-disabled individuals are addressed is not a decision for individual care providers or administrators. Inclusion is a right—not a charitable gesture.

And it is important to emphasize that other global health and development problems will not be solved unless people with disabilities—who compose 15 percent of the world's population—are part of common solutions. As former World Bank president James Wolfensohn has noted: "Unless disabled people are brought into the development mainstream, it will be impossible to cut poverty in half by 2015 or to give every girl and boy the chance to achieve a primary education by the same date—goals agreed to by more than 180 world leaders at the United Nations Millennium Summit."[38]

There is a growing number of resources available to help public health workers address these issues. Over the past three decades, the global disability rights movement has achieved an impressive record. Disability advocates and organizations representing disabled people can serve as a major resource for public health workers and their organizations.

An increasing number of people with disabilities who are receiving education in public health, law, medicine, political science, and other fields now serve as both advocates and experts in helping identify and define the needs and concerns of disabled populations. Non-disabled experts in rehabilitation or medicine can provide information and guidance. But decisions on behalf of people with disabilities can no longer be made without their input at all stages of policy and program planning. To quote the slogan of the global disability rights movement: "Nothing about us without us."

▪ CONCLUSION

Advocates in public health and social justice must rethink many basic assumptions about disability. The issue is not disability prevention *or* disability services, but recognition that disability is—and will continue to be—an inevitable part of life. Although disability is inevitable, denial of human rights to people with disabilities, lack of equitable access to public health and social resources, and the disproportionate rates of poverty and social exclusion faced by persons with disabilities are not inevitable. These threats to social justice are socially determined and, as such, can be socially redefined.

The expectation that an individual with a disability will soon either recover or die does not fit reality. People with disabilities will now often live for decades after they are born with or acquire a disability—whether or not they receive an education, are provided medical and rehabilitative care, or are included in the social, religious, and economic activities of their communities. Their existence and our own, however, will be much richer if they are allowed to develop to their full potential.

The public health and social justice needs of people with disabilities are strikingly similar to those of their non-disabled peers. What distinguishes people with disabilities is not their common needs, but the fact that many of these needs continue to be unmet. Public health workers can play important roles in meeting this challenge, ensuring that disability issues are routinely included in all phases of public health practice, education, and research.

■ REFERENCES

1. World Health Organization and the World Bank. World report on disability. Geneva: WHO/World Bank, 2011. Available at http://whqlibdoc.who.int/publications/2011/9789240685215_eng.pdf. Accessed on June 25, 2012.
2. UNICEF. Monitoring child disability in developing countries: Results from the Multiple Indicator Cluster Surveys. New York: UNICEF Division of Policy and Practice, 2009. Available at http://www.childinfo.org/files/Monitoring_Child_Disability_in_Developing_Countries.pdf. Accessed on June 25, 2012.
3. United Nations Convention on the Rights of Persons with Disabilities, G.A. Res. 61/106, U.N. Doc. A/RES/61/106, December 13, 2006. Available at http://www.un.org/disabilities/default.asp?id=150. Accessed on June 25, 2012.
4. UNICEF. 2012. Child development: The child with disability. Available at www.unicef.org/disability. Accessed on July 12, 2012.
5. UNESCO. Education for all. Available at http://www.unesco.org/new/en/education/themes/leading-the-international-agenda/education-for-all/. Accessed on June 25, 2012.
6. Groce N, Bahkshi P. Illiteracy among adults with disabilities in the developing world: A review of the literature and a call for action. *International Journal of Inclusive Education* 2011;15:1153–1168.
7. International Labour Organization. ILO/Japan technical consultation meeting on vocational training and employment of people with disabilities in Asia and the Pacific. Information note. Available at http://www.ilo.org/public/english/region/asro/bangkok/ability/background.htm. Accessed on June 25, 2012.
8. Groce N, Murray B, Loeb M, et al. Disabled beggars in Addis Ababa, Ethiopia: Employment Sector (Employment Working Paper No. 142). Geneva: International Labour Office, 2013.
9. UNFPA/WHO. Promoting sexual and reproductive health for persons with disabilities: WHO/UNFPA guidance note. Geneva: WHO, 2009. Available at http://whqlibdoc.who.int/publications/2009/9789241598682_eng.pdf. Accessed on June 25, 2012.
10. UNICEF. Violence against children with disabilities: UN Secretary General's report on violence against children. Thematic Group on Violence against Children with Disabilities. July 28, 2005. Available at http://www.unicef.org/videoaudio/PDFs/UNICEF_Violence_Against_Disabled_Children_Report_Distributed_Version.pdf. Accessed on June 25, 2012.
11. United Nations Department of Economic and Social Affairs (DESA). United Nations Enable: Development and human rights for all. Available at http://www.un.org/disabilities/default.asp?id=17. Accessed on March 5, 2013.

12. Officer A, Groce N. Key concepts in disability. *Lancet* 2009;374:1795–1796.

13. UNICEF. Disability prevention efforts and disability rights: Finding common ground on immunization efforts. Available at www.unicef.org/disability. Accessed on July 12, 2012

14. Ingstad B, Whyte S, eds. Disability and culture. Berkeley, CA: University of California Press, 1995.

15. Groce N, Zola I. Disability in ethnic and minority populations. *Pediatrics* 1993;91;5:1048–1055.

16. Braithwaite J, Mont D. Disability and poverty: A survey of World Bank poverty assessments and implications. SP Discussion Paper No. 0805. Washington, DC: The World Bank, 2008.

17. Mehta AK, Shah A. Chronic poverty in India: Incidence, causes and policies. *World Development* 2003;31:491–511.

18. Filmer, D. Disability, poverty, and schooling in developing countries: Results from 14 household surveys. *World Bank Economic Review* 2008:22:141–163.

19. Yeo R, Moore K. Including disabled people in poverty reduction work: Nothing about us without us. *World Development* 2003;31:571–590.

20. UN Department of Economic and Social Affairs (DESA). Disability and the Millennium Development Goals: A review of the MDG process and strategies for inclusion of disability issues in Millennium Development Goal efforts. New York: United Nations, 2011. Available at http://www.un.org/disabilities/documents/review_of_disability_and_the_mdgs.pdf. Accessed on June 25, 2012.

21. Groce N, London J, Stein M. Intergenerational poverty and disability: The implications of inheritance policy and practice on persons with disabilities in the developing world. Available at http://www.ucl.ac.uk/lc-ccr/centrepublications/workingpapers/WP17_Disability_and_Inheritance.pdf. Accessed on June 25, 2012.

22. Helander E. Prejudice and dignity: An introduction to community-based rehabilitation. New York: United Nations Development Program, 1998.

23. Dhungana B. The lives of disabled women in Nepal: Vulnerability without support. *Disability & Society* 2006;21:133–146.

24. Nosek M, Howland C, Hughes R. The investigation of abuse and women with disabilities: going beyond assumptions. *Violence Against Women* 2001;7:477–499.

25. Maxwell J, Belser W, David D. Women and disability—A health handbook for women with disabilities. Palo Alto, CA: Hesperian Foundation, 2007. Available at http://hesperian.org/wp-content/uploads/pdf/en_wwd_2008/en_WWD_2008_full%20book.pdf. Accessed on June 25, 2012.

26. Shakespeare T, Iezzoni L, Groce N. The art of medicine: Disability and the training of health professionals. *Lancet* 2009;374:1815–1816.

27. UNICEF. Disability prevention efforts and disability rights: Finding common ground on immunization efforts. 2012. Available at www.unicef.org/disability. Accessed on July 12, 2012.

28. World Health Organization. Assistive Devices/Technologies. Geneva: WHO, 2010. Available at www.who.int/disabilities/technology/en/. Accessed on June 25, 2012.

29. WHO/USAID. Joint position paper on the provision of mobility devices in less resourced settings. Geneva: WHO, 2011. Available at http://www.who.int/disabilities/publications/technology/jpp_final.pdf. Accessed on June 25, 2012.

30. WHO. Community based rehabilitation. Geneva: WHO, 2010. Available at http://www.who.int/disabilities/cbr/guidelines/en/index.html. Accessed on June 26, 2012.

31. Groce N, Rohleder P, Eide A, et al. HIV issues and people with disabilities: A review and agenda for research. *Social Science and Medicine* 2013;77:31–40.

32. The World Bank. HIV/AIDS and disability: Capturing hidden voices. Washington, DC: The World Bank, 2004. Available at http://siteresources.worldbank.org/DISABILITY/Resources/Health-and-Wellness/HIVAIDS.pdf. Accessed on June 26, 2012.

33. Groce N, Trasi R. Rape of individuals with disability: AIDS and the folk belief of virgin cleansing. *Lancet* 2004;363:1663–1664.

34. Gaskins S. Special population: HIV/AIDS among the deaf and hard of hearing. *J Assoc Nurses AIDS Care* 1999;35:75–78.

35. Collins P, Geller P, Miller S, et al. Ourselves, our bodies, our realities: An HIV prevention intervention for women with severe mental illness. *J Urban Health* 2001;78:162–175.

36. McGillivray J. Level of knowledge and risk of contracting HIV/AIDS amongst young adults with mild/moderate intellectual disability. *Journal of Applied Research on Intellectual Disabilities* 1999;12:113–126.

37. UN Department of Social and Economic Affairs (DESA). Disability and the Millennium Development Goals: A review of the MDG process and strategies for inclusion of disability issues in Millennium Development Goal efforts. Available at http://www.un.org/disabilities/default.asp?id=1470. Accessed on June 26, 2012.

38. Wolfensohn J. Poor, disabled and shutout. *The Washington Post*, December 3, 2002, A25.

9 Prisoners

■ ERNEST DRUCKER

▓ INTRODUCTION

Over the past four decades, mass incarceration has become a driving force of social injustice in the United States. Overuse of imprisonment in the United States derails the lives of millions of people by damaging their opportunities for work, education, housing, and stable family life—undermining many of the foundations of personal health and well-being as well as community cohesion, which are the principal safeguards against crime in any society.[1] When incarceration occurs at a very high rate and with great disparities—such as between African Americans and Caucasians in the United States—the criminal justice system worsens public health and perpetuates social injustice.[2]

Understanding the role of mass incarceration enables us to understand the roots of many persistent health and social problems in the United States. Incarceration policies and practices in the United States derive from a long history of state laws and socioeconomic mechanisms that create and perpetuate social injustice. Over the course of more than two centuries of U.S. history, these laws and socioeconomic mechanisms have accounted for slavery, state laws that perpetuated racial segregation of public facilities in Southern states until 1965, discriminatory immigration policies, official hostility to trade unions, and social welfare policies that isolated, stigmatized, and marginalized economically disadvantaged people—a pattern that is perpetuated by mass incarceration.[3]

The contrast of U.S. incarceration policies to those of other developed societies is profound. While the United States has only 5 percent of the world's population, it has 25 percent of all prisoners.[1] At any given time, over 7 million Americans—almost *5 percent* of the adult population—are under the control of the criminal justice system (Table 9–1). In January 2012, over 2.2 million Americans were in federal, state, and local prisons and jails, and another 5 million were on probation and parole.[4] Since 1975, over 25 million Americans have been incarcerated, more than the total number imprisoned in the previous 100 years. The number of people incarcerated peaked in 2009; 2010 was the first year in three decades with a decrease in the prison population (by less than 1 percent)—although the rates of arrests and other police interventions are still increasing.[3]

The U.S. imprisonment rate is the highest of any nation—more than 700 per 100,000 people[5] (Figure 9–1). European countries average less than one-fifth this rate, and many other countries average only one-tenth of it.[4] (However, as described in Box 9–1, in many other countries people have been incarcerated as a result of their political beliefs or actions.)

TABLE 9–1 *Estimated Prison Rates in State and Federal Prisons per 100,000 U.S. Residents, Total and Age 18–29, by Sex, Race, Hispanic Origin, and Age, United States, December 31, 2010*

	Male			Female		
Age Group	White	Black	Hispanic	White	Black	Hispanic
18–19	149	1,555	563	11	40	31
20–24	638	4,618	1,908	72	182	122
25–29	980	6,349	2,707	125	299	202
Total (all ages)	459	3,074	1,258	47	133	77

(*Source:* U.S. Department of Justice, Bureau of Justice Statistics. Prisoners in 2010. December 2011, NCJ 236096, p. 27. Available at: http://bjs.ojp.usdoj.gov/content/pub/pdf/p10.pdf. Accessed March 1, 2013.)

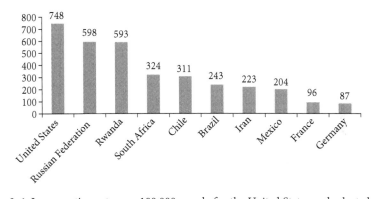

Figure 9–1 Incarceration rates per 100,000 people for the United States and selected other countries. Most data are for the years from 2006 to 2009. The total global incarceration rate was 168 per 100,000. (*Source:* ChartsBin. World prison population rates per 100,000 people. Available at http://chartsbin.com/view/eqq. Accessed January 9, 2013.)

Prison budgets in the United States also reached their highest level in this period, averaging over $30,000 per inmate, or about $80 billion annually. Most of this money comes from state governments—money which, during economic downturns, is needed for health, education, and social services. Spending $100 billion to build new prisons since 1980, the United States has created a "prison industrial complex"[6]—a system of over 5,000 federal, state, and local prisons and jails that have millions of inmates and employ about the same number of law-enforcement and correctional workers. The corrections "industry" is huge, including the operation of prisons, prison construction, subcontracts for inmate services (such as health care), food services, and the provision and maintenance of equipment.

The operation of private "for-profit" prisons has become a significant feature of the U.S. correctional system. More than half of states in the United States are contracting with private corporations to operate prisons or to staff them with guards and other workers. In 2010, these companies were operating over 6 percent of the entire system (25 percent of the beds in the 25 states that contract with private correctional services) and 12 percent of the 140,000-bed federal system. Two

BOX 9-1　■　Political Prisoners

William F. Schulz

Political prisoners are at least as old as the days of Greek mythology. Anyone who challenged the authority of the gods of Olympus was cast into the pit of Tarturus. The term *political prisoner* refers to those who have been incarcerated largely, if not entirely, as a result of their political beliefs or actions.

Usually rulers will claim that such prisoners broke laws. Some of these laws are legitimate. For example, it is not inappropriate for a government to outlaw violence. Other laws have been created in order to enforce discrimination or stifle dissent. The "Pass Laws" that enforced apartheid in South Africa were clearly discriminatory, and those imprisoned for violating them were considered "political prisoners."

In addition, repressive governments often interpret even legitimate laws in ways that are designed to control their political opponents. The hundreds of political prisoners released in Myanmar (Burma) in the spring of 2012 were charged with crimes up to and including treason. It is appropriate for a government to make treason illegal, but it is not appropriate to consider nonviolent protest treasonous.

A subcategory of political prisoners is called *prisoners of conscience* (POCs)—a phrase coined in the early 1960s by the global human rights organization Amnesty International (AI) to refer to those who pursue their goals nonviolently. Even some of the most famous political prisoners were not considered POCs by AI; Nelson Mandela, for example, was not regarded as a POC because he and his African National Congress favored the violent overthrow of South Africa's apartheid government.

Many Americans would claim that the United States, with its commitment to democracy, free speech, and freedom of association, has never had political prisoners. That would be a surprise to Eugene V. Debs, the great socialist leader, who was sentenced in 1918 to 10 years in prison simply for giving a speech in opposition to the World War I military draft. At his sentencing, he uttered the famous words, "While there is a lower class, I am in it, while there is a criminal element, I am of it, and while there is a soul in prison, I am not free." When Martin Luther King, Jr., was imprisoned in 1963 in Birmingham, Alabama, for nonviolently protesting laws that promulgated racial segregation, he became a political prisoner of the state. More recently, some human rights organizations have suspected that political factors played a role in the prosecution of Leonard Peltier, the American Indian Movement (AIM) leader who was convicted of killing two Federal Bureau of Investigation agents.[1]

Whole classes of people have been considered political prisoners—especially in countries where freedom is limited. For example, belonging to the Muslim Brotherhood in Hosni Mubarak's Egypt was considered a crime, even in the absence of overt illegal action. Falun Gong practitioners in China are regularly arrested and imprisoned for their beliefs.

It is impossible to tell how many political prisoners are being held in jail cells globally because the definition of "political prisoner" is somewhat elastic, and because no organization keeps a careful count. After all, most governments do not brag about the number of prisoners they have locked up simply because they do not like their views. But it is fair to say that significant numbers of such prisoners remain in China, Belarus, Zimbabwe, and elsewhere. Amnesty International lists

POCs in at least 24 countries—although some POCs may be in prison for reasons other than political reasons.

There are now more organizations working to free political prisoners than ever before. The Internet has made it increasingly difficult for governments to hide the persecution of their opponents from public view. The growth in democracy globally means that it is less acceptable in the eyes of the international community to imprison and mistreat dissenters than it once was. And the reach of international courts, including the International Criminal Court, signals a newfound commitment to holding governments accountable for human rights abuses.

As long as there are political voices arrayed against powerful governments that are indifferent to human rights protections, there will be political prisoners. And as long as there are individuals who are devoted to liberty, there will be movements dedicated to setting these prisoners free.

Box Reference

1. Amnesty International. USA: Appeal for the release of Leonard Pelletier, July 14, 1999. Available at http://amnesty.org/en/library/info/AMR51/160/1999/en. Accessed on June 27, 2012.

publicly traded international security firms accounted for three-fourths of these operations.[6-8]

■ MASS INCARCERATION AND RACE

Mass incarceration in the United States is characterized by significant economic, ethnic, and racial disparities that perpetuate institutionalized racism. While they constitute about 12 percent of the U.S. population, African Americans account for nearly 50 percent of the prison population—and African American males represent more than 10 percent of all prisoners globally.[2,3]

In the late 1800s in New York State, about four African Americans were imprisoned for every Caucasian; in 2000, that ratio was 12:1 (Figure 9–2).[3] For nonviolent drug offenses—about 30 percent of all crimes in the state—that ratio is 40:1. (The Hispanic–Caucasian ratio is 30:1.)[1,9]

Drug-related incarcerations are the main factor driving the increase in racial and ethnic disparities in U.S. prisons, although there is no evidence of any major difference in the rates of illicit drug use among African Americans, Hispanics, and Caucasians.[10] Incarceration for drug-related offenses compounds the adverse effects of welfare policies, unemployment, and broken families. It also predicts future criminal involvement: Drug-related offenses often lead subsequently to more serious ones.[11]

Incarceration has become the norm for many African American men. Over one-third of them in the 20- to 29-year-old age group are in prison or jail, or on parole and probation. More African American males go to jail than to college.[2] In Washington, DC, more than 90 percent of all African American men can expect to be incarcerated at some point in their lives.[4] A random telephone survey in

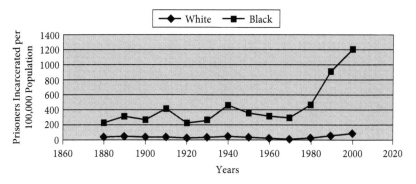

Figure 9–2 Incarceration rates by race for 1880–2000 in New York State. (*Source*: U.S. Census; and Hupart JH, unpublished report on New York State historical data on prison rates. Based on New York State Department of Prisons [1880–1960], New York State Department of Correctional Services[1961–2000].)

Central Harlem in New York City in 2002 found that 9 percent of all respondents had been in jail in the previous year, and between 35 and 40 percent knew of someone who had been released from prison in the previous year.[11,12] Among men born between 1965 and 1969, 3 percent of whites and 20 percent of blacks had served time in prison by their early 30s. The risks of incarceration are highly stratified by education: 30 percent of those without college education and almost 60 percent of high school dropouts had been imprisoned by 1999. Some consider incarceration as a new stage in the life course of young, low-skill African American men.[12]

This pattern of racial and ethnic disparities is not new, and its magnitude is not unprecedented in U.S. history. Major racial disparities in prison rates have always existed. They existed in the post–Civil War era of Reconstruction, when freed slaves were converted to prisoners and brought back to plantations in chains under vagrancy laws.[13] Among women, there has been some recent reduction in racial disparity, with an increased percentage of immigrants and poor white women among those recently incarcerated.[14] However, the 4.5 million African Americans in prison or jail, or on parole or probation, is still more than the number of slaves in 1860.[3]

■ **COLLATERAL DAMAGES OF INCARCERATION**

The impact of incarceration extends well beyond those in prison, with profound consequences for families and communities. African American and Hispanic prisoners generally are poor and come from specific urban communities that account for more than 80 percent of all inmates in the United States. Over 600,000 people re-enter these communities each year following their release from prison, and many more do so after arrests and brief detention in local jails. This influx of former prisoners adversely affects these communities, in part because of their having become socially, politically, and economically dis-enfranchised in prison.[1,3] More than 2.5 million school-age children have an incarcerated parent, which accounts for mental health problems in these children, even after their parents are released.

How Social Injustice Affects the Health of Those Incarcerated and Their Families

Mass incarceration has long-term consequences for prisoners and their families and communities during their imprisonment and after their release. Most recently released prisoners, including those who have completed their sentences, continue to be under supervision (on parole) and subject to a wide range of restrictions on their movement and behavior. Failure to comply with these restrictions often results in re-incarceration.

The Health of Prisoners

Many serious physical and mental health problems affect prisoners.[1] In general, the same health problems that are present in these communities are more prevalent among prisoners. Most of the health problems are associated with poverty: elevated rates of chronic disease (such as hypertension, diabetes, and cardiovascular disease) and infectious diseases. And all of the problems are exacerbated by drug addiction and alcoholism, mental illness, and inadequate access to medical care. Prison conditions amplify these problems, such as the transmission of hepatitis B and C viruses and HIV by the sharing of contraband drug-injecting equipment, and the spread of sexually transmitted infections by rape.

Inadequate health services for inmates persist in many prisons in the United States. Despite the constitutional entitlement to "decent medical care" (under the Eighth Amendment barring "cruel and unusual punishment") and frequent court mandates to provide it, persistent failures to fulfill this obligation are common.[1]

Incarcerated people are drawn overwhelmingly from poor and minority communities. The health risks and the disparities in health care that are present in prisons mirror those in these communities. In addition, many specific health risks and patterns of social injustice faced by incarcerated people persist after their release. Multiple periods of incarceration, frequently experienced by poor African American and Hispanic men, are socially disabling, leading, for example, to loss of eligibility for many jobs—and, for drug offenders, loss of many federal health entitlements. Multiple periods of incarceration are a major determinant of ill health.

While in some circumstances, such as in court-ordered care for HIV/AIDS, prisoners may receive better medical care in prison than they receive outside of prison, usually they receive inadequate care. Since prisoners often have serious health issues when they enter prison, in the aggregate, they have a pattern of complex health problems unlike that of any other institutionalized population in the United States. More than 80 percent of U.S. inmates enter prison with problems of drug abuse or dependency, and drug use often continues throughout prison stays—sometimes with injection of drugs in even more dangerous circumstances. And after release, they face increased risks of acquiring bloodborne diseases or sexually transmitted infections, or dying from an overdose.[15]

The violence and stress of prison life and the poor quality of diet and medical care there increase the risks of complications of diabetes, hypertension, and other chronic diseases, which are prevalent among prisoners—especially African American and Hispanic inmates and those with histories of tobacco and/or alcohol abuse.

The Affordable Care Act, beginning in 2014, will extend the right of prisoners to health care while in prison to the period after they are released—thereby integrating prison and community health care services. This extension of services will be most helpful for those with chronic diseases and older former inmates.

Mental health problems are prevalent among prisoners. After many psychiatric hospitals in the United States closed from the 1950s through 1970s, the criminal justice system became responsible for providing care for many people—especially poor people—who had both mental health and drug abuse problems. Aggressive criminal prosecution of these people led to many of them being imprisoned. About half a million inmates in the United States have a major psychiatric disorder, which has a high likelihood of persisting or recurring. Over 40 percent of those in solitary confinement—which is widely used to discipline prisoners—have major psychiatric disorders.[1,16]

Those inmates in solitary represent 5 percent of the prison population, but they account for almost half of suicides among prisoners. Homelessness before and after incarceration is widespread; almost 25 percent of those released from prison will be in a shelter or on the street within 6 months of release.[17]

Abuse by U.S. military prison guards during the wars in Iraq and Afghanistan and at Guantanamo may be understood in the context of the harsh conditions and racial disparities in prisons in the United States and the portrayals of these prisons in the news media in ways that desensitize the public to their true nature. Although incarceration in the United States has become so widespread, the damaging effects of incarceration on individuals and their families are generally not recognized—and the blame is often shifted to the prisoners, their families, and their communities.

Collateral Damage: Effects on Prisoners' Families and Communities

Mass incarceration causes many adverse effects on prisoners' families and communities. More than half of male prisoners and 80 percent of female prisoners have children under age 18. And more than half of these men and 80 percent of these women were living with their children when they were sent to prison.

In New York State, where there were 70,000 prisoners in 2001, there were more than 23,000 children who had a parent in prison on drug charges and about 125,000 children who had at least one parent imprisoned as a result of the state's street-drug laws.[11] In the United States, there are more than two million children who have a parent in prison, and, since the early 1970s, more than 20 million children have had a parent in prison.[1]

Incarceration of a parent disrupts children's social environments and the financial stability of their families, weakens parental bonds, and places severe stress on caregivers. As a result, children are often not disciplined. They often develop shame and anger that become manifest in behavioral problems at school and elsewhere. Poor school performance, unsupervised free time, financial strain, decreased contact with adults, and suppressed anger often lead to delinquency. Despite widespread awareness of these problems, and the burdens of disadvantage that they place on the families of incarcerated parents, there has been no systematic effort by the criminal justice system to minimize the impact of parental incarceration on children.

Parental imprisonment alters the social experience of so many African American children, affecting vital statistics of the entire black population of the United States.[18] By age 14, over half of all African American children born in 1990 to a father who was a high school dropout had a parent imprisoned.

Imprisonment harms children in ways previously unrecognized, including an increased likelihood of being in a gang and a shortened life expectancy. Parental incarceration is associated with increased infant mortality. African American infants are known to have 2.3 times the mortality rate of non-Hispanic whites and are four times as likely to die due to complications of low birthweight. In addition, in 2005, African Americans had 1.8 times the mortality rate for sudden infant death syndrome (SIDS) as non-Hispanic whites. And African American mothers were 2.5 times more likely than non-Hispanic white mothers to begin prenatal care in the third trimester or to not receive any prenatal care.[19]

Recent parental incarceration increases the risk of infant death by 30 percent. If the imprisonment rate in the United States had remained at its 1973 level (about 120 per 100,000), the U.S. infant mortality rate would be 5.1 percent lower today, and, in 2003, the black–white inequality in infant mortality rates would have been 23 percent less.

An estimated 10 to 15 million children have been directly exposed to parental incarceration. In some families and communities, there are three generations of children who have had parents in prison—a profound consequence, more damaging than illegal drugs or nonviolent drug-related crimes.

Drug-enforcement policies account for most racial disparities in incarceration rates. More people are incarcerated in the United States for drug offenses than all the people incarcerated for all offenses in the European Union. Beginning in 1973, the "Rockefeller drug laws" in New York State (initiated by Governor Nelson Rockefeller) mandated long prison sentences for nonviolent drug offenders. They have became a model for other states and the federal government. Between 1975 and 2000, the rate of drug-related incarcerations in New York State increased from 8 percent of the prison population to more than 30 percent.[1,19-21]

Since 1974, more than 150,000 people have been incarcerated in New York State, where over 110,000 person-years of life have been lost to imprisonment for drug offenses between 1974 and 2002.[22] About 90 percent of them have been male. In 2000, their median age was 35. Seventy-eight percent have been New York City residents—70 percent from just six neighborhoods. Ninety-four percent have been black or Hispanic.

In the United States, there are currently more than 450,000 people incarcerated for nonviolent drug offenses, and almost two million drug offenders on parole or probation. Given the chronic inadequacies of drug-addiction treatment in the United States, drug offenders often violate the terms of their probation and parole; positive drug tests frequently lead to re-incarceration.

Economic Disenfranchisement

Felony conviction usually means a greatly reduced chance of gainful employment. In most states, 75 to 95 percent of jobs requiring a state license are barred to those with felony records. Felons lose their driver's licenses and the many job opportunities that require one, they lose eligibility for military service, and they are disqualified for many professional licenses, such as those for beauticians, barbers, and taxi drivers, and for work in the U.S. Postal Service. Felons with drug offenses are also temporarily or permanently prohibited from visiting their families in public housing, and barred from federal benefits, such as home and school loans, that might help them avoid committing crimes. As one inmate said, "My sentence really began the day I was released."[23] These extensions of felons' incarceration into their post-sentence life also adversely affect their families and communities.

Civic Death: Felony Disenfranchisement

Felony convictions also mean the loss of the right to vote—in prison, while on parole, and, in some states, while on probation. In 15 states, convicted felons are barred from voting for life. Approximately 4 million Americans—about half of them African American—are prohibited from voting even after they have "paid their debt" to society.[24]

■ ROOT CAUSES AND UNDERLYING ISSUES

With "the war on drugs," the arrest and incarceration of nonviolent drug offenders has increased the prison population tenfold over the past three decades. Although the prevalence of illicit drug use differs only slightly by race and ethnicity, a highly disproportionate percentage of African Americans is imprisoned for drug-related offenses. This disparity is largely due to (a) the huge illegal drug industry that operates openly in most minority communities, and (b) the vulnerability of low-level user-dealers in these communities to "buy and bust" operations by police—low-risk methods that increase arrest rates of police officers and conviction rates of prosecutors—with 95 percent of cases ending in plea bargains and not going to trial. In New York City, despite huge drops in crime over the past decade, more-aggressive police activities for marijuana possession and "stop-and-frisk" encounters continue to target young minority males.[25-27]

Drug laws and prosecution practices are deeply embedded in our criminal justice system. Their restrictions of judicial discretion, by mandatory sentencing policies, represent the ascendancy of right-wing political power during the past few decades and the acquiescence by liberal politicians fearful of being labeled as "soft on crime." New York governor Nelson Rockefeller, perceived as a moderate Republican by many people, promoted these laws to distinguish himself from the liberal wing of his own party. In appearing to aggressively address the burgeoning heroin epidemic of the 1970s, he succeeded in undermining the newly successful methadone programs, which were just beginning to demonstrate their efficacy.[22]

The unprecedented use of incarceration in the United States has created an imbalance of power in the judicial system. It has moved the country away from rehabilitation toward a punitive approach of retribution, increasing the power of prosecutors, weakening the capacity of defense attorneys, and decreasing judicial discretion and power—especially in drug-related cases where harsh mandatory sentences account for much of the national increase in incarceration since 1975. Incarceration is the default position of the criminal justice system—instead of alternatives that leave offenders in the community and provide drug abuse treatment, job and housing programs, and restorative justice to compensate and heal victims' families. Mass incarceration undermines the family and community life of African Americans on a scale not seen since slavery. It does this by destroying the very social capital needed to prevent crime[1,28,29]—adversely affecting the already disparate physical and mental health of three generations of African Americans.[30,31]

When any state system of punishment grows substantially and targets racial or ethnic minorities, it is more the sum of punishment of individuals for individual crimes. The unprecedented scale of imprisonment of African Americans in the past four decades and its profound impact on health clearly makes mass incarceration a public health issue. The rate of incarceration can be seen as a parameter of the health of the nation, like rates of infant and child mortality, HIV/AIDS, obesity, and gun-related deaths.

■ WHAT NEEDS TO BE DONE

Incarceration should be used sparingly, especially for nonviolent offenders who are parents of young children. The following measures can help reduce incarceration and its adverse effects on families and communities.

Improve Community Services

Involvement in drug use—and, for poor people, involvement in the local drug trade—can be addressed by improving the quality of education, providing after-school and other activities for youth, and supporting families in poor communities. Non-judgmental, accessible, and high-quality health care in these communities, especially for mental health problems, drug abuse, and sexually transmitted infections and HIV/AIDS, would significantly improve personal and community health.

Improve Prison Health Services

The need for improving health services in prisons has become a greater challenge as states cut budgets and privatize prison health services. There is also a need to improve health and social services for people recently released from prison and/or on probation or parole.

Reform Drug Laws

Marijuana laws in the United States account for more than 300,000 people in prison and over 800,000 arrests annually. New policies concerning marijuana, many of which have significant public support, offer opportunities for reform. Medical use of marijuana (now approved in 16 states in the United States) should be legalized, and the possession of small amounts of marijuana for personal use should be decriminalized, as has been done in the United Kingdom and Australia and is now being considered in Canada. In 2012, voters in Colorado and Washington State approved the full legalization of marijuana. (The author sees this as beginning a new era in U.S. drug policy and law reform.)

Modify or Repeal Mandatory Sentencing Laws

Mandatory sentencing laws should be repealed, especially those for nonviolent drug-related offenses. Some progress is being made with the use of "drug courts," which order treatment of nonviolent drug offenders, rather than incarceration. New drug laws are needed that allow judges to make distinctions between dangerous criminals and the vast number of defendants with drug-dependency problems. New York State, the original source of mandatory sentencing laws for drug offenders, has, over the past decade, weakened or eliminated many laws that had increased the number of inmates in its state prison system from 12,000 to 73,000 over the previous 30 years. These changes have led to a 30 percent decline in the state's prison population—to 53,000 in 2012—and have become a model for reforms in other states.

Assist Family Members

Policies and programs should be implemented to help children, families, and communities when their loved ones are imprisoned—and when they are discharged. For example, in New York City, the Family Justice Program of the Vera Institute of Justice provides intensive support to drug offenders' families when they are released from prison, to reduce the likelihood that they will again commit crimes. To reduce the harm to children when a parent is incarcerated, several programs of the Osborne Association and the Fortune Society in New York City support families of inmates and now offer children counseling, educational tutoring, and assistance with writing letters to their incarcerated parents. Since more than 80 percent of children with parents in prison never get to visit them, these programs organize visits to often-remote prisons where their parents are incarcerated. Some programs are using video technology to enable "tele-visiting" between inmates and their family members at home.

Enable Former Prisoners to Vote

In many states, former inmates are being re-registered to vote. Having their voting rights restored is a way of re-involving them in civic society in positive ways. More of this work needs to be done. In addition, the Legal Defense Fund of the National Association for the Advancement of Colored People (NAACP) and the Brennan Center for Constitutional Rights at New York University School of Law are bringing legal action against policies that disenfranchise former felons, basing this action on racial disparities in criminal penalties. This approach needs to be expanded and more widely supported.

▨ CONCLUSION

The principal reforms needed to address mass incarceration are (a) changing drug policies to decriminalize drug use, and (b) applying a public-health model to address drug problems, replacing prosecution with treatment, education, and prevention. Laws that are unjust and counterproductive should be reformed—especially the antiquated and discredited drug laws that have made imprisonment the norm for so many Americans. The huge expenditures for the criminal justice system in the United States—more than $100 billion annually—should be redirected to housing, health care, education, and social support in the communities heavily impacted by mass incarceration.

Incarceration—especially in response to youthful drug use—should be replaced with residential care. Other means should be found to enforce laws. The rate of incarceration should be reduced to levels of other democratic countries where there are less punitive models of responding to crime. Restorative justice models should be used to reintegrate offenders into their communities and rehabilitate them.

▓ ACKNOWLEDGMENTS

The author's work has been supported by the Jeht Foundation and the Soros Justice Fellowship program of the Open Society Institute. He acknowledges the seminal work and encouragement of Nils Christie, and the research and helpful conversations about these issues with Ricardo Barreras, Marc Mauer, Jacob Hupart, Bob Gangi, Jamie Fellner, Diane Wachtell, Tara Grove, Joanne Page, and Elizabeth Gaines.

▓ REFERENCES

1. Drucker E. A plague of prisons. New York: The New Press, 2011.
2. Mauer M. Race to incarcerate. 2nd ed. New York: The New Press, 2000.
3. Alexander M. The New Jim Crow. New York: The New Press, 2010.
4. Walmsley R. World prison population list. 8th ed. 2009. Available at http://www.apcca. org/stats/8th%20Edition%20(2009).pdf. Accessed November 25, 2012.
5. Christie N. Crime control as industry. 3rd ed. London: Routledge, 2002.
6. U.S. Department of Justice, Bureau of Justice Statistics. Private adult correctional facility census, 2010. Washington, DC: Bureau of Justice Statistics, 2012. Available at http://bjs.ojp.usdoj.gov/index.cfm?ty=dcdetail&iid=255. Accessed November 25, 2012.
7. Greene J. Bailing out private jails. The American Prospect, September 2001. Available at: http://prospect.org/article/bailing-out-private-jails. Accessed March 1, 2013.
8. Greene J. Entrepreneurial corrections: Incarceration as a business opportunity. In: Mauer M, Chesney-Lind M, eds. Invisible punishment: The collateral consequences of mass imprisonment. New York: The New Press, 2002.
9. New York State Department of Prisons (1880–1960), New York State Department of Corrections (1961–2000).
10. Braman D. Families and incarceration. In Maurer M, Chesney-Lind M, eds. Invisible punishment: The collateral consequences of mass imprisonment. New York: The New Press, 2002.
11. Western B. Punishment and inequality in America. New York: Russell Sage Foundation, 2006.
12. Pettit B, Western B. Mass imprisonment and the life course: Race and class inequality in U.S. incarceration. *American Sociological Review* 2004;69:151–169.
13. Oshinsky DM. Worse than slavery: Parchman Farm and the ordeal of Jim Crow justice. Glencoe, IL: Free Press, 1997.
14. Mauer M. The Sentencing Project: The changing racial dynamics of women's incarceration. February 2013. Available at: http://www.sentencingproject.org/doc/publications/rd_Changing%20Racial%20Dynamics%202013.pdf. Accessed March 19, 2013.
15. Binswanger IA, Stern MF, Deyo RA, et al. Release from prison—A high risk of death for former inmates. *N Engl J Med* 2007;356:157–165.
16. Fellner J. Collateral damage: Children of inmates incarcerated in New York State under Rockefeller drug laws. New York: Human Rights Watch, June 2002.

17. Metraux S, Culhane D. Homeless shelter use and reincarceration following prison release: Assessing the risk. *Criminology & Public Policy* 2004;3:139–160.
18. Pettit B. Invisible men: Mass incarceration and the myth of black progress. New York: Russell Sage Foundation, 2012.
19. Wildeman C. Parental imprisonment, the prison boom, and the concentration of childhood disadvantage. *Demography* 2009;46:265–280.
20. Gabel K, Johnstone E, eds. Children of incarcerated parents. Lanham, MD: Lexington Books, 1995.
21. Drucker E. Drug prohibition and public health: 25 years of evidence. *Public Health Rep* 1999;114:14–29.
22. Drucker E. Population impact of mass incarceration under New York's Rockefeller drug laws: An analysis of years of life lost. *J Urban Health Bull NY Acad Med* 2002;79: 434–435.
23. Gonnerman J. Life on the outside: The prison odyssey of Elaine Bartlett. New York: Picador, 2004.
24. The Sentencing Project and Human Rights Watch. Losing the vote: The impact of felony disenfranchisement laws in the United States. New York; Washington, DC: Human Rights Watch and The Sentencing Project, October 1998.
25. Mauer M, Chesney-Lind M, eds. Invisible punishment: The collateral consequences of mass imprisonment. New York: The New Press, 2002.
26. Dwyer J. Whites smoke pot, but blacks are arrested. *The New York Times*, December 22, 2009. Available at http://www.nytimes.com/2009/12/23/nyregion/23about.html?_r=0. Accessed November 30, 2012.
27. New York Civil Liberties Union. Report: NYPD stop-and-frisk activity in 2011 (2012). Available at http://www.nyclu.org/publications/report-nypd-stop-and-frisk-activity-2011–2012. Accessed November 30, 2012.
28. Rose DR, Clear TR. Incarceration, social capital, and crime: Examining the unintended consequences of incarceration. *Criminology* 1998;36:441–479.
29. Putnam DR. Bowling alone. Carmichael, CA: Touchstone Books, 2001.
30. Geiger HJ. Racial and ethnic disparities in diagnosis and treatment: A review of the evidence and a consideration of causes. Washington, DC: Institute of Medicine, 2002.
31. Byrd MW, Clayton LA. Report of the Secretary's Task Force on Black and Minority Health. Washington, DC: National Center for Health Statistics, 1994.

10 Homeless People

■ LISA ARANGUA AND LILLIAN GELBERG

▓ INTRODUCTION

Homelessness is a focus of increasing social and public health concern globally, even in countries with superior safety nets. The United Nations Committee on Human Rights (UNCHR) defines *absolute homelessness* as the condition of those without any physical shelter who sleep outdoors, in vehicles, or in abandoned buildings or other places not intended for human habitation, as well as people staying in temporary forms of shelter, such as emergency shelters or in transition houses.[1] An estimated 100 million people globally, by this definition, suffer from absolute homelessness.[2] In the United States, at any given point in time, there are approximately 250,000 people living on the streets (unsheltered)—representing a decrease over the past two decades—but, during a 1-year period, approximately 1.6 million use homeless shelters.[3-5] In contrast, in England and in France, there are at least 500,000 homeless people,[6-8] and in Canada, there are tens of thousands of homeless people.[9]

The demographic characteristics of homeless people vary among countries. In high-income countries, 60 to 95 percent of homeless people are male (Figure 10–1). Single men account for most chronically homeless people (those with a current homeless episode of 1 year or longer). Homeless families are frequent in the United States, but are rare in other countries. The median age of homeless people in the United States is 32 years; in most European countries, it is 40. Minority and indigenous persons are over-represented in the homeless population.

Mortality and disease severity of homeless people, which far exceed those of the general population and the housed poor population, are due to factors such as extreme poverty, delays in seeking care, non-adherence to therapy, substance-use disorders, and psychological impairment. Homeless people in their 30s and 40s develop severe disabilities and seek hospital care at rates comparable to those of people decades older. Lack of shelter is a powerful contributor to adverse health outcomes; as evidence, street-dwelling homeless people have significantly worse health outcomes than do homeless-shelter residents.

The many social and health problems that homeless people endure reflect a variety of social injustice issues. Homelessness represents the convergence of multiple factors, including poverty, high housing costs, and a shortage of subsidized public housing units. The exposure to substandard environmental conditions that affects the health of homeless people is related to failures of urban development.

The complex health, social, and psychological problems commonly experienced by homeless people as a result of these factors present therapeutic challenges.

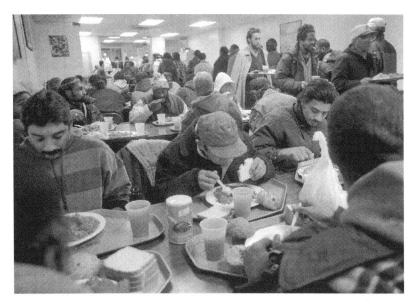

Figure 10-1 Homeless people eating dinner at the Bowery Mission in New York, which serves 500 to 600 meals a day. (AP Photo/Bebeto Matthews.)

Many health care providers lack the time or necessary training to treat homeless persons. Even in countries with socialized medicine, primary care physicians often fail to fully register homeless people who seek care at a medical practice because of associated social problems, complex health problems, substance abuse, and lack of medical records.

■ HOW SOCIAL INJUSTICE AFFECTS THE HEALTH OF HOMELESS PEOPLE

Homeless people, as a group, are exposed to very high levels of almost all the social and environmental risk factors for adverse health effects. They therefore pose serious public health challenges. The impact of homelessness on health can be profound for the newly homeless, long-term homeless, formerly homeless, or episodically homeless. Even relatively short bouts of homelessness expose individuals to deprivations, such as hunger and poor hygiene, and to victimization through robbery, physical assault, or rape.[10] Homeless persons have a very high prevalence of untreated acute and chronic physical, mental, and substance-abuse problems. Many health problems, such as infections due to crowded living conditions in shelters, hypothermia from exposure to extreme cold, and malnutrition due to limited access to food and cooking facilities, are a direct result of homelessness.[11] Homeless persons who have a substance-abuse or mental disorder or a physical disability are at increased risk of remaining homeless.[12] Poor health among homeless people is due to many factors, including extreme poverty, inadequate family and other social supports, the pressing demands of day-to-day survival, delays in seeking care and reduced access to care, non-adherence to therapy, and cognitive impairment.

■ HEALTH STATUS

Approximately 35 percent of homeless people in high-income countries report having fair or poor health,[13-16] compared with 18 percent of housed persons of lower socioeconomic status (SES) and 3 percent of housed persons of higher SES.[15-17] Even newly homeless persons report experiencing significant physical and mental problems before becoming homeless.[18] Factors such as the length of time people are homeless or the condition of living on the streets, significantly increase the probability of perceived poor or fair health status.[16,19]

Contagious diseases and infections, such as tuberculosis (TB),[20] HIV infection,[21] hepatitis B virus (HBV) infection,[22] and hepatitis C virus (HCV) infection,[23] are more common among the homeless than among housed people. In most high-income countries, TB prevalence rates among homeless people are 3 to 20 times greater than in the general population.[24,25] Prevalence of HIV infection among homeless people in high-income countries ranges from 2 to 9 percent—3 to 10 times greater than that of the general population.[26,27] Among homeless adults in the United States, 23 to 47 percent have had previous exposure to HBV, compared with 5 to 8 percent in the general population; and 12 to 16 percent are currently infected with HBV, compared with 0.1 to 0.5 percent in the general population.[28,29] In high-income countries, between 22 and 44 percent of homeless adults and between 5 and 17 percent of homeless adolescents have tested positive for HCV infection[30-34]—rates that are 10 to 12 times greater than adults and adolescents in the general population.

■ SUBSTANCE USE

Between 69 and 82 percent of homeless people in high-income countries smoke—more than double the rate of lower SES groups and more than three times the rate in the general population.[35] Homeless persons describe high rates of alcohol and drug use. The prevalence of alcohol dependence among homeless people ranges from about 25 percent in England, France, and Spain, to 60 percent in the United States, to 73 percent in Germany[36-39]—three to five times greater than rates in the general population in these countries. The very high rates in the United States and Germany may result from high per-capita use, easy accessibility, and the relatively low cost of alcohol.

Rates of illicit drug dependence are also high among homeless people. More research needs to be done on the direct and indirect effects of illicit drug use as a cause of homelessness. Some evidence, albeit slight, suggests that early homeless experiences are predictive of drug dependence.[40] In Germany, England, Spain, and

France, the prevalence of drug dependence among homeless people ranges from 9 to 16 percent.[36,37,39,41] Drug dependence is more prevalent among homeless people in the United States (30 to 49 percent), Canada (40 percent), and the Netherlands (60 percent).[42-44] Rates of drug dependence among homeless people are four to six times greater than those in the general population in these countries. Drugs of choice among homeless people in Canada and the United States are commonly cocaine and marijuana, whereas in Spain and the Netherlands they are opioids and heroin. The prevalence of both alcohol and drug abuse is higher among homeless men than among homeless women.

■ OBESITY AND A SEDENTARY LIFESTYLE

The prevalence of obesity in homeless people ranges from 23 percent in Germany to 39 percent in the United States—almost three times the rate in the general population.[45,46] In contrast, homeless people in Japan do not appear to have any significant problems with obesity.[47] Limited physical activity is significantly more common among homeless persons (47 percent), compared with the general population (15 percent). Heart disease, diabetes, and hypertension are higher among homeless people, largely because of their sedentary lifestyles.[48]

■ MENTAL HEALTH

Since the 1960s, mental health services have gone through major transitions in high-income countries, leaving an increasing number of mentally ill people living on the streets or in shelters or hostels.[49] Over the course of their lives, 34 to 45 percent of homeless people in England and almost 60 percent of homeless people in the United States and France experience a serious mental disorder—rates that are two to four times those in the general population.[41,50,51] Lifetime major depression (20 percent) and recent major depression (15 percent) are their most prevalent mental disorders. More than half of homeless people suffering from a chronic mental health disorder also experience comorbid substance abuse/substance dependence problems.[42] Rates of schizophrenia among homeless people range from 4 to 9 percent in Germany, Canada, the United States, Spain, and England, to 15 percent in France.[36,39,52,53] Rates of mental disorders among homeless people are higher for men than they are for women, except for rates of lifetime depression and serious mental disorder without associated substance abuse. (See Chapter 16.)

■ MORTALITY

Homelessness is strongly associated with an increased risk of death in several countries.[54-56] For homeless people in high-income countries, the average age at death is between 45 and 50 years.[54-56] The age-adjusted number of years of potential life lost (YPLL) before age 75 is three to four times higher for home-less people than for the general population.[57,58] Even among sheltered homeless families, who tend to acquire homes quicker than single homeless adults, both homeless adults and children in these families experience higher rates of mor-tality than the general population and the low-income housed population.[59]

Causes of death among homeless people differ substantially among countries. For example, in the United States, homicide, accidents, substance abuse, liver dis-ease, heart disease, HIV infection, pneumonia, and influenza are the leading causes of death among homeless people.[54,57,59] In some other countries, leading causes of death are substance abuse, cardiovascular disease, alcoholic liver disease, and suicide.[55,58,60] Homeless people in other high-income countries have much lower mortality rates than those in the United States[56-58]; access to social and health ser-vices as well as cultural factors may explain this difference.

■ HEALTH CARE ACCESS AND UTILIZATION

Among homeless people in Canada and the United States, 75 percent report receiving some form of health care in the past year.[61] However, 73 percent of homeless persons report at least one past-year unmet need for health care, and 49 percent report two or more past-year unmet needs.[62] For the preceding year, 32 percent of homeless people report an unmet need for medical or surgical care, 36 percent report an unmet need for prescription medications, 21 percent report an unmet need for mental health care or counseling, 41 percent report an unmet need for eyeglasses, and 41 percent report an unmet need for dental care.[62]

In addition, most homeless people seek care at places that do not provide the continuous, quality care that can address their complex health problems. Of those homeless people in the United States who sought care in the past year, 32 per-cent received care at a hospital emergency department, 27 percent at a hospital outpatient clinic, 21 percent at a community health clinic, 20 percent at a hos-pital as an inpatient, and 19 percent at a private physician's office.[3] High rates of emergency-department use among homeless persons represent the substitution of emergency department care for conditions more suitable for outpatient primary care. Even newly homeless people heavily use the medical care system—especially emergency departments—while homeless and after finding housing.[18] Having a regular source of care, which is strongly associated with access to health services and the use of preventive health services, is very rare among homeless people, with more than half lacking a regular source of care.

In the United States and Canada, about 24 percent of homeless people are hos-pitalized each year.[61,63] About 75 percent of hospitalized homeless people are hos-pitalized for conditions that are often preventable, such as substance abuse, mental disorders, trauma, respiratory disorders, skin disorders, and infectious diseases (except AIDS)—a rate 15 times that of the general population.[64] Following hospital discharge, 40 percent of homeless people are readmitted to the hospital within 14 months, usually with the same diagnosis. The finding that most homeless inpatients could have been treated less expensively in an outpatient setting highlights the difficulty in sustaining treatment intensity for homeless persons outside the hospital. Despite higher rates of medical hospitalization and higher rates of disease, homeless people are less likely to use medical ambulatory services than others. Homeless people often delay seeking medical attention at an early stage when illness or complications of illness could be prevented. Homeless adults, given their increased need for care, may benefit from improvement in and increased availability of primary and preventive care.

■ DISPARITIES IN HEALTH STATUS AMONG HOMELESS PEOPLE

The degree of homelessness—as measured by number of homeless episodes, length of time homeless, and living in unsheltered conditions—has profound effects on a homeless person's health status and use of health services. Unsheltered homeless people are more likely to use illegal drugs, have acute skin injuries, report daily alcohol use, be victimized, experience accidents and injuries, and be exposed to TB than are sheltered homeless people.[65] Unsheltered homeless women are more likely than sheltered women to report fair or poor health status, be engaged in risky sex, have poor pregnancy outcomes, have more gynecological conditions, be forcibly raped, have poor mental health, and use drugs and alcohol.[66-69]

Despite their overwhelming health needs, unsheltered and long-term homeless people are significantly less likely to use health services. Sheltered homeless people are more likely to report use of health services than are unsheltered homeless people.[63,70] Unsheltered and long-term homeless people are (a) less likely to use non-urgent ambulatory care services or be hospitalized, and (b) more likely to have unmet needs for care and use emergency departments than more stably housed homeless people.[66,71,72] Long-term homeless people are also less likely to have a regular source of care and to receive substance-abuse treatment. Homeless people with extended homelessness have twice the mortality rates of others, even after controlling for all other factors.[73]

■ ROOT CAUSES AND UNDERLYING ISSUES

Historically, two competing political and economic models—the social democratic model and the individual rational-choice model—have profoundly influenced health and social policies regarding homeless people. The social democratic model, which stresses the social rights of citizens in society, emphasizes that everyone is entitled to the resources that provide good health. Therefore, society should seek to maximize the aggregate health of all people. Under this model, the better health enjoyed by upper-class people is evidence that poor and homeless people could enjoy better health. As a result, poor and homeless people are less healthy than they could be, and, with the right policies in place, society could achieve better aggregate health for all. The social democratic model is the foundation of the Canadian and European health care systems and their superior safety nets, which emphasize the social ethic of the principle of solidarity. This model also found its way into the U.S. health care system during the "Great Society" initiative of the Lyndon B. Johnson administration in the 1960s, and strains of it have persisted through the public health insurance systems of Medicaid, Medicare, and Social Security Insurance (SSI).

The individual rational-choice model, which advocates individual effort and the freedom to exercise individual choice, stresses that people bear some responsibility for their individual risks for illness and death. Differences in health status reflect choices—in lifestyles, social conditions, and health habits—that have a greater influence on health status than medical care. Because individuals bear responsibility for their health, this model calls into question whether differences in health can be construed as "injustices." The model incorporates a justification for curbing political excesses, controlling administrative costs, and preventing overutilization of resources. Therefore, the market becomes the framework through which many rights can be achieved. This model facilitates a distinction between the "deserving poor" and the "undeserving poor." Advocates of this model harness public fear that undeserving, able-bodied malingerers will get a "free ride" on other people who contribute compulsorily to the provision of public health benefits. "Deserving homeless" groups, in this model, include veterans, people with disabilities, people who are mentally ill, older people, and families with children.

However, neither of these models has clearly addressed a population-health perspective that focuses on the social determinants of health in society. (See Chapter 2.) The social democratic model has created a system that increases access to medical care. The persistence in disparities in health among homeless people in countries with universal health care demonstrates that access alone will not eliminate health disparities. Many who support this model and its emphasis on medical care assert that a health care system that focuses on subspecialty care, which requires more health care resources and is used largely by people who are better off socioeconomically,[74-76] perpetuates health disparities. They advocate for a strong network of primary care providers for improving health status. However, emphasizing the role of medical care to explain why high-SES people are healthier than, for example, homeless people, overlooks the fact that social and cultural environments and other factors profoundly influence morbidity and mortality.

The individual rational-choice model relies heavily on economic growth to improve population health. It is true that the Industrial Revolution (from about

1760 to about 1830) improved sanitation, food safety, housing conditions, and life expectancy. However, there is no guarantee that economic advance will improve population health status. In the early modern period (from about 1500 to about 1800), economically advanced towns had the highest mortality rates among the lower classes.[77] A recent study found that chronically ill homeless people who were offered stable housing and case management had fewer hospital days and fewer emergency department visits, but not a lower mortality rate or better health outcomes.[78]

Population health can also serve as an index for economic strength. Historically in societies, long-term economic strength ensues when economic growth is combined with a carefully regulated and managed political response to population health. In 19th-century Great Britain, the absence of a significant political response to population health during a period of increased economic growth resulted in devastation to population health that lasted half a century and significantly affected the economy.[79] Japan and Sweden, in anticipation of economic growth, passed comprehensive public health laws and adopted preventive health policies that were mainly implemented by government and funded by taxes. These countries used economic growth to improve health for most people, resulting in very long life expectancy and, in turn, further economic growth.

Recently, there has been an overzealous application of the individual rational-choice model, even in countries that have espoused the social democratic model. In the past 30 years, international policy priorities have been marked by suspicion of central government and by heavy promotion of free trade and rapid economic growth—with decreased government investment in welfare and health services. Leading economists, including finance ministers, have not supported the consideration of social determinants of health in all major government initiatives. The United Kingdom, Canada, and the United States have implemented fiscal policies over the past three decades that have restricted public spending and increased income inequality by giving generous tax benefits to those with higher incomes.[80] Homeless people and other disadvantaged persons may be suffering from poorer health status because of policies that support the growth of the global market economy. Increasing population health problems—such as obesity, mental health disorders, and the comorbidity of chronic diseases—have provoked some governments, such as those of Canada and England, to seriously examine the merits of the "social determinants" movement.[81,82]

Canada developed a new model of population health, shifting its focus beyond health care to social and economic determinants. As part of this new focus, it established the Canadian Institutes for Health Research, which funds research on the social determinants of health. In 1997, the Labour government in England focused its health agenda on reducing health inequalities and issued related policy documents and targets. The current coalition government in England (Conservative, Liberal Democratic) has expressed a commitment to reducing health inequalities by transferring responsibility for addressing social determinants and population health to local authorities and by creating incentives for positive outcomes. (See Chapter 2.)

■ WHAT NEEDS TO BE DONE

Public health agencies should assure the conditions in which homeless people can be healthy. This means assuring that homeless people have access to public health and social services, quality medical care, adequate and safe food, and secure shelter.

Homeless people, even in countries with superior safety nets, do not receive adequate health care because of the stigma of being homeless and the prejudice of health care providers. Even at equivalent levels of access to care, low-income people have unmet health care needs, receive a lower quality of health care, and are less likely to receive even routine medical procedures than higher-income people. A study of the universal health care system in Canada found that 32 percent of homeless people did not have a primary care provider, and about 17 percent reported unmet health care needs—significantly more than the general population.[83] Being a victim of physical assault and having worse physical and mental health status were significantly associated with unmet health care needs.[62,83] In addition, homeless young adults and homeless people who are recent victims of violence face important non-financial barriers to health care, such as distrust of health care providers.[83,84] Providers of health care for homeless people should carefully consider how their diagnostic and treatment procedures and their advice will be experienced by these people. Appropriate models of care should be developed, taught to clinicians, and replicated in communities. These models of care should include up-to-date protocols for disease management, comprehensive health screening, and preventive health interventions that target behavioral change. Medical education should include developing attitudes and behaviors that are sensitive to the needs of homeless people. Because most care provided to homeless people is in emergency departments—rather than in special clinics for homeless people—all medical students and physicians in training should develop cultural competence in caring for poor and homeless people.

Globally, clinics that treat homeless people have difficulty in recruiting physicians. Reforms of medical education and health care could increase physician recruitment by these clinics by improving their working conditions and salaries, reducing physician bias against homeless patients, and increasing respect for this work by the medical profession.

Inadequate health care, however, is only one of the complex factors that account for poor health among homeless people. Social and environmental factors also play important roles. Unhealthful health behaviors, such as cigarette use, consumption of a poor diet, and behaviors that increase the risks of infectious diseases are also shaped by the social and physical environments where homeless people live— dominated by stores that heavily market cigarettes, alcohol, and unhealthful food. In addition, substandard and crowded shelters as well as social influences increase their risk of socially and environmentally induced health problems—such as asthma due to mold and other factors, tuberculosis associated with crowded shelters, and infections with HIV, HBV, and HCV due to intravenous drug abuse and unsafe sex.

Redeveloping low-income neighborhoods can improve the health of poor and homeless people. Countries that equally distribute resources for sanitation, air quality, food and water safety, housing, nutrition, and physical exercise have significantly narrowed health disparities among socioeconomic groups.[85-87] Countries that have not equally distributed these resources need to redirect these resources, with their governments making significant investments and promoting collective efficacy—the capacity of community members to improve social and structural development based on collective principles and desires.

The *institutional rational-choice model*, in which the social and environmental context facilitates and perpetuates patterns of behavior,[88] could help develop a guiding social ethic in health. This model, which broadens the focus from individuals to institutions (or context), challenges the individual rational-choice model. Therefore, factors such as the sensitivity of health care providers, the general quality of health care, and the social and physical environments in which homeless people live are seen as influencing individual behavior and health. This includes many of the complex institutional, environmental, and social structures that profoundly influence the health of homeless people.

The widening gap in health disparities between homeless people and high-income people is largely the result of society's acceptance of health improvement approaches that focus exclusively on altering individual behavior. The institutional rational-choice model recognizes how prevailing economic structures, cultural norms, and health care institutions shape policies that undermine self-determination and equality for homeless and poor people. Therefore, use of this model can help influence social, economic, and health policies to promote health among vulnerable people, facilitate development of a new social ethic in health care, and achieve social justice.

■ CONCLUSION

Consideration of the health of homeless people globally should not be limited to addressing their physical health, mental health, and substance abuse problems. It should also address attitudes toward and treatment of poor people, as well as welfare and housing policies. Globally, we have become ever more intimately interdependent on each other and on the consequences of our collective actions. Social justice for homeless people must reflect the collective work of local and global political leaders and cross-class alliances. This collective approach requires complete mobilization and participation of the population in a social ethic that focuses on the institutional, social, and physical elements that profoundly influence the health of homeless people.

■ **REFERENCES**

1. Springer S. Homelessness: A proposal for a global definition and classification. *Habitat International* 2000;24:475–484.
2. United Nations Centre for Human Settlements (Habitat). Strategies to combat homelessness. Nairobi, 2000. Available at http://ww2.unhabitat.org/programmes/housingpolicy/documents/HS-599x.pdf. Accessed November 15, 2012.
3. Burt MR, Aron LY, Lee E, Valente J, eds. How many homeless people are there? In: Helping America's homeless: Emergency shelter or affordable housing? Washington, DC: Urban Institute, 2001:23–54.
4. U.S. Interagency Council on Homelessness. Opening doors: Federal strategic plan to prevent and end homelessness. Washington, DC: US Interagency Council on Homelessness, 2010. Available at http://www.ich.gov/PDF/OpeningDoors_2010_FSPPreventEndHomeless.pdf. Accessed November 15, 2012.
5. U.S. Department of Housing and Urban Development. The 2010 Annual Homeless Assessment Report to Congress. Washington, DC: HUD, 2011. Available at <http://www.hudhre.info/documents/2010HomelessAssessmentReport.pdf>. Accessed January 22, 2013.
6. Leff J. All the homeless people: Where do they all come from? *BMJ* 1993;306:669–670.
7. Connelly J, Crown J, eds. Homelessness and ill health: Report of a working party of the Royal College of Physicians. London: Royal College of Physicians, 1994.
8. Chauvin P, Mortier E, Carrat F, et al. A new out-patient care facility for HIV-infected destitute populations in Paris, France. *AIDS Care* 1997;9:451–459.
9. Hwang S. Homelessness and health. *Can Med Assoc J* 2001;164:229–233.
10. Link B, Susser E, Stueve A, et al. Lifetime and five year prevalence of homelessness in the United States. *Am J Public Health* 1994;84:1907–1912.
11. Fischer P, Breakey W. Homelessness and mental health: An overview. *Int J Mental Health* 1986;14:6–41.
12. Culhane D, Kuhn R. Patterns and determinants of public shelter utilization among homeless adults in New York City and Philadelphia. *J Policy Analysis Manag* 1998;17:23–43.
13. A report on the qualitative exploration for the entrants of winter season's temporary accommodation. Tokyo: Society of Welfare Office Director of Tokyo's 23 Wards;, 1995.
14. Usherwood T, Jones N, Hanover Project Team. Self-perceived health status of hostel residents: Use of the SF-36D health survey questionnaire. *J Public Health Med* 1993;15:311–314.
15. Gallagher T, Andersen R, Koegel P, et al. Determinants of regular source of care among homeless adults in Los Angeles. *Med Care* 1997;35:814–830.
16. Nyamathi A, Leake B, Gelberg L. Sheltered vs. non-sheltered homeless women: Differences in health, behavior, victimization and utilization of care. *J Gen Intern Med* 2000;15:565–572.
17. Adams PF, Martinez ME, Vickerie JL, Kirzinger WK. Summary health statistics for the U.S. population: National Health Interview Survey, 2010. National Center for Health Statistics. *Vital Health Stat* 10(251), 2011. Available at http://www.cdc.gov/nchs/data/series/sr_10/sr10_251.pdf. Accessed January 17, 2013.
18. Schanzer B, Dominguez B, Shrout PE, Caton CL. Homelessness, health status, and health care use. *Am J Public Health* 2007;97:464–469.

19. White MC, Tulsky JP, Dawson C, et al. Association between time homeless and perceived health status among the homeless in San Francisco. *J Commun Health* 1997;22: 271–282.

20. Barnes P, Yang Z, Preston-Martin S, et al. Patterns of tuberculosis transmission in central Los Angeles. *JAMA* 1997;278:1159–1163.

21. Zolopa A, Hahn J, Gorter R, et al. HIV and tuberculosis infection in San Francisco's homeless adults. *JAMA* 1994;272:455–461.

22. Gelberg L, Robertson M, Leake B, et al. Hepatitis B among homeless and other impoverished U.S. military veterans in residential care in Los Angeles. *Public Health* 2001;115:286–291.

23. Beech BM, Myers L, Beech DJ, et al. Human immunodeficiency syndrome and hepatitis B and C infections among homeless adolescents. *Semin Pediatr Infect Dis* 2003;14:12–19.

24. Yamanaka K, Akashi T, Miyao M, et al. Tuberculosis statistics among the homeless population in Nagoya City from 1991 to 1995. *Kekkaku* 1998;73:387–394.

25. Gelberg L, Panarites C, Morgenstern H, et al. Tuberculosis skin testing among homeless adults. *J Gen Intern Med* 1997;12:25–33.

26. Robertson MJ, Clark RA, Charlebois ED, et al. HIV seroprevalence among homeless and marginally housed adults in San Francisco. *Am J Public Health* 2004;94:1207–1217.

27. Manzon L, Rosario M, Rekart ML. HIV seroprevalence among street involved Canadians in Vancouver. *AIDS Educ Prevent* 1992;Fall:86–89.

28. Gelberg L, Stein J, Andersen RM, Robertson M. impact of hepatitis on homeless persons' health services utilization: A test of the Gelberg-Andersen Behavioral Model for Vulnerable Populations. 38th NAPCRG [North American Primary Care Research Group] 2010 Annual Meeting, Seattle, WA, November 14, 2010.

29. McQuillan G, Coleman P, Kruszon-Moran D, et al. Prevalence of hepatitis B virus infection in the United States: The National Health and Nutrition Examination surveys, 1976 through 1994. *Am J Public Health* 1999;89:14–18.

30. Desai R, Rosenheck R, Agnello V. Prevalence and risk factors for hepatitis C virus infection in a sample of homeless veterans. *Soc Psychiatry Psychiatric Epidemiol* 2003;38: 396–401.

31. Nyamathi A, Dixon E, Robbins W, et al. Risk factors for hepatitis C virus infection among homeless adults. *J Gen Intern Med* 2002;17:134–144.

32. Gelberg L, Robertson MJ, Arangua L, et al. Prevalence, distribution, and correlates of hepatitis C virus infection among homeless adults in Los Angeles. *Public Health Rep* 2012;127:407–421.

33. Strehlow AJ, Robertson MJ, Zerger S, et al. Hepatitis C among clients of health care for the homeless primary care clinics. *J Health Care Poor Underserved* 2012;23:811–833.

34. Stein JA, Andersen RM, Robertson M, Gelberg L. Impact of hepatitis B and C infection on health services utilization in homeless adults: A test of the Gelberg-Andersen Behavioral Model for Vulnerable Populations. *Health Psychol* 2012;31:20–30.

35. Kermode M, Crofts N, Miller P, et al. Health indicators and risks among people experiencing homelessness in Melbourne [Australia], 1995–1996. *Aust NZ J Public Health* 1998; 22:464–470.

36. Kovess V, Magin-Lazarus C. The prevalence of psychiatric disorders and use of care by homeless people in Paris. *Soc Psychiatry Psychiatric Epidemiol* 1999;34:580–587.

37. Munoz M, Koegel P, Vazquez C, et al. An empirical comparison of substance and alcohol dependence patterns in the homeless in Madrid (Spain) and Los Angeles (CA, USA). *Soc Psychiatry Psychiatric Epidemiol* 2002;37:289–298.

38. Vazquez C, Munoz M, Sanz J. Lifetime and 12-month prevalence of *DSM-III-R* mental disorders among the homeless in Madrid: A European study using CIDI [Composite International Diagnostic Interview]. *Acta Psychiatr Scand* 1997;95: 523–530.

39. Fichter M, Quadflieg N. Prevalence of mental illness in homeless men in Munich, Germany: Results from a representative sample. *Acta Psychiatr Scand* 2001;103: 94–104.

40. Johnson TP, Fendrich M. Homelessness and drug use: Evidence from a community sample. *Am J Prev Med* 2007;32:S211–S218.

41. Shanks N, George S, Westlake L, et al. Who are the homeless? *Public Health* 1994;108: 11–19.

42. Koegel P, Sullivan G, Burnam A, et al. Utilization of mental health and substance abuse services among homeless adults in Los Angeles. *Med Care* 1999;37:306–317.

43. Sleegers J. Similarities and differences in homelessness in Amsterdam and New York City. *Psychiatric Serv* 2000;51:100–104.

44. Grinman MN, Chiu S, Redelmeier DA, et al. Drug problems among homeless individuals in Toronto, Canada: Prevalence, drugs of choice, and relation to health status. *BMC Public Health* 2010;10:94.

45. Luder E, Ceysens-Okada E, Koren-Roth A, Martinez-Weber C. Health and nutrition survey in a group of urban homeless adults. *J Am Diet Assoc* 1990;90:1387–1392.

46. Langnase K, Muller MJ. Nutrition and health in an adult urban homeless population in Germany. *Public Health Nutrition* 2001;4:805–811.

47. Takano T, Nakamura K, Takeuchi S, et al. Disease patterns of the homeless in Tokyo. *J Urban Health* 1999;76:73–84.

48. Gelberg L, Linn L. Assessing the physical health of homeless adults. *JAMA* 1989;262:1973–1979.

49. Koegel P, Burnam A, Farr R. The prevalence of specific psychiatric disorders among homeless individuals in the inner city of Los Angeles. *Arch Gen Psychiatry* 1988;45: 1085–1092.

50. Victor C. Health status of the temporarily homeless population and residents of North West Thames region. *BMJ* 1992;15:6850.

51. Tompkins CN, Wright NM, Sheard L, et al. Associations between migrancy, health and homelessness: A cross-sectional study. *Health Soc Care Commun* 2003;11:446–452.

52. Munoz M, Vazquez C, Koegel P, et al. Differential patterns of mental disorders among the homeless in Madrid (Spain) and Los Angeles (USA). *Soc Psychiatry Psychiatric Epidemiol* 1998;33:514–520.

53. Geddes J, Newton R, Young G, et al. Comparison of prevalence of schizophrenia among residents of hostels for homeless people in 1966 and 1992. *BMJ* 1994; 308: 816–819.

54. Hwang S, Orav E, O'Connell J, et al. Causes of death in homeless adults in Boston. *Ann Intern Med* 1997;126:625–628.

55. Ishorst-Witte F, Heinemann A, Puschel J. Morbidity and cause of death in homeless persons. *Arch fur Kriminol* 2001;208:129–138.

56. Babidge N, Buhrich N, Butler T. Mortality among homeless people with schizophrenia in Sydney, Australia: A 10-year follow-up. *Acta Psychiatr Scand* 2001;103:105–110.

57. Hibbs J, Benner L, Klugman L, et al. Mortality in a cohort of homeless adults in Philadelphia. *N Engl J Med* 1994;331:304–309.

58. Hwang S. Mortality among men using homeless shelters in Toronto, Ontario. *JAMA* 2000;283:2152–2157.

59. Kerker BD, Bainbridge J, Kennedy J, et al. A population-based assessment of the health of homeless families in New York City, 2001–2003. *Am J Public Health* 2011;101:546–553.

60. Nordentoft M, Wandall-Holm N. 10-year follow-up study of mortality among users of hostels for homeless people in Copenhagen. *BMJ* 2003;327:81.

61. Hwang S, Gottlieb J. Drug access among homeless men in Toronto. *Can Med Assoc J* 1999;160:1021.

62. Baggett TP, O'Connell JJ, Singer DE, Rigotti NA. The unmet health care needs of homeless adults: A national study. *Am J Public Health* 2010;100:1326–1333.

63. Kushel M, Vittinghoff E, Haas J. Factors associated with the health care utilization of homeless persons. *JAMA* 2001;285:200–206.

64. Salit S, Kuhn E, Hartz A, et al. Hospitalization costs associated with homelessness in New York City (special article). *N Engl J Med* 1998;338:1734–1740.

65. Gelberg L, Andersen R, Leake B. The behavioral model for vulnerable populations: application to medical care use and outcomes. *Health Serv Res* 2000;34:1273–1302.

66. Lim Y, Andersen R, Leake B, et al. How accessible is medical care for homeless women? *Med Care* 2002;40:510–520.

67. Wenzel S, Leake B, Gelberg L. Health of homeless women with recent experience of rape. *J Gen Intern Med* 2000;15:265–268.

68. Stein J, Lu M, Gelberg L. Severity of homelessness and adverse birth outcomes. *Health Psychol* 2000;19:524–534.

69. Wenzel S, Andersen R, Gifford D, et al. Homeless women's gynecological symptoms and use of medical care. *J Health Care Poor Underserved* 2001;12:323–341.

70. O'Toole T, Gibbon J, Hanusa B, et al. Utilization of health care services among subgroups of urban homeless and housed poor. *J Health Politics Policy Law* 1999;24:91–114.

71. Lewis J, Andersen R, Gelberg L. Health care for homeless women: Unmet needs and barriers to care. *J Gen Intern Med* 2003;18:921–928.

72. Kushel M, Perry S, Bangsberg D, et al. Emergency department use among homeless and marginally housed: Results from a community-based study. *Am J Public Health* 2002;29:778–784.

73. Barrow S, Herman D, Cordova P, et al. Mortality among homeless shelter residents in New York City. *Am J Public Health* 1999;89:529–534.

74. Alter D, Iron K, Austin PC, Naylor D. Socioeconomic status, service patterns, and perceptions of care among survivors of acute myocardial infarction in Canada. *JAMA* 2004;291:1100–1107.

75. Goddard M, Smith P. Equity of access to health care services: Theory and evidence from the U.K. *Soc Sci Med* 2001;53:1149–1162.

76. Van Doorslaer E, Wagstaff A, van der Burg H, et al. Equity in the delivery of health care in Europe and the U.S. *J Health Econ* 2000;19:553–583.

77. Wrigley EA. A simple model of London's importance in the changing British society and economy, 1650–1750. *Past Present* 1967;37:44–70.

78. Sadowski LS, Kee RA, VanderWeele TJ, Buchanan D. Effect of a housing and case management program on emergency department visits and hospitalizations among chronically ill homeless adults: A randomized trial. *JAMA* 2009;301:1771–1778.

79. Hamlin C. Public health and social justice in the age of Chadwick: Britain 1800–1854. Cambridge, England: Cambridge University Press, 1998.

80. Carter M. Transient people, transient policies: A study of recent policy initiatives towards single homeless people. London: London School of Economics Homeless Group, 1992.
81. Acheson D. Report of independent inquiry into inequalities in health. London: Stationery Office, 1998.
82. Robertson A. Shifting discourses on health in Canada: From health promotion to population health. *Health Promotion International* 1998;13:155–166.
83. Hwang SW, Ueng JJ, Chiu S, et al. Universal health insurance and health care access for homeless persons. *Am J Public Health* 2010;100:1454–1461.
84. Barkin SL, Balkrishnan R, Manuel J, et al. Health care utilization among homeless adolescents and young adults. *J Adolesc Health* 2003;32:253–256.
85. Wagstaff A, Van Doorslaer E. Equity in the finance and delivery of health care: Concepts and definitions. In Van Doorslaer E, Wagstaff A, Rutten F, eds. Equity in the finance and delivery of health care: An international perspective. Oxford, England: Oxford University Press, 1993:7–19.
86. Wilkinson RG. Unhealthy societies: The afflictions of inequality. London: Routledge, 1996.
87. Wilkinson RG. Socioeconomic determinants of health. Health inequalities: Relative or absolute material standards? *SMJ* 1997;314:591–595.
88. Marlis E, Kannan M, eds. Preferences, institutions and rational choice. Oxford, England: Oxford University Press, 1995.

11 Forced Migrants: Refugees and Internally Displaced Persons

■ MICHAEL J. TOOLE

■ INTRODUCTION

One of the starkest examples of the relationship among social injustice, inequality, and poor health outcomes occurs among populations that are forcibly displaced. The major forced population movements in the past 50 years have been a result of (a) systematic persecution of certain population groups, such as religious or ethnic minorities; (b) widespread human rights abuses, such as torture, imprisonment, deprival of legal rights, and inadequate access to food, health care, education, and other social services; and (c) exposure to systematic violence intended to terrorize communities. Most of these situations have evolved in the context of economic uncertainty, political transition, and the emergence of predatory social formations.

During the Cold War period from 1947 to 1991, civil war, persecution, and forced displacement of civilian populations were often masked by the ideological nature of the parties involved in armed conflict. In the 1970s and early 1980s, millions of refugees fled civil wars, which were mainly between pro- and anti-Communist forces in Central America (Guatemala, El Salvador, and Nicaragua), Asia (such as in Vietnam and Afghanistan), and Africa (such as in Ethiopia and Angola). Even during this period, however, movements that were apparently politically motivated sometimes disguised the underlying oppression of minorities by powerful elites. For example, the right-wing Guatemalan government directed military action against indigenous Mayan communities; the new communist Pathet Lao government in Laos targeted members of the Hmong ethnic minority; and the socialist government in Ethiopia (dominated by the Amhara ethnic group) oppressed other ethnic groups (such as the Tigrayans). In each situation, many oppressed ethnic minorities fled, as refugees, into neighboring countries.

After the Cold War ended, most of the factions in armed conflicts ceased to masquerade as being ideologically motivated, and civilians were increasingly targeted by violence—simply because they belonged to ethnic or religious minority groups. Many of these post–Cold War conflicts arose during periods of economic uncertainty and political transition. For example, as newly established nations that had been part of Yugoslavia abandoned communism, a small nationalist elite emerged in Serbia. It violently resisted independence movements in these new nations and implemented a massive campaign of "ethnic cleansing." In Africa, armed conflicts

187

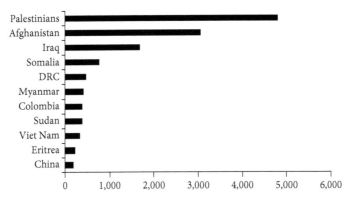

Figure 11–1 Sources of the world's largest refugee populations in 2010 (in thousands). (*Source:* UNHCR: The UN Refugee Agency. UNHCR Global Trends 2011. Geneva: UNHCR, 2011.)

known as *resource wars* were fueled by desires to control natural resources, such as the "blood diamonds" in countries such as Sierra Leone and Liberia.[1]

In late 2011, there were approximately 10.5 million refugees and approximately 26.4 million internally displaced persons.[2] These refugees had crossed international borders, fleeing war or persecution because of their race, ethnic or tribal group, religion, nationality, or membership in a specific social or political group. Most had come from countries in Asia, the Middle East, and Africa (Figure 11–1). The five countries hosting the largest numbers of refugees in 2011 were Pakistan, Iran, Jordan, Syria, and Kenya. "Refugees" are clearly defined by international conventions and, therefore, entitled to protection and assistance by UNHCR: The UN Refugee Agency.

In contrast, internally displaced persons, who have fled their homes for the same reasons as refugees, but who have remained inside their own countries, do not have this protection and assistance.[3] They are therefore generally more vulnerable to threats to their health, safety, and well-being; have less access to safe food and water, medical care, and other basic needs; and enjoy less assurance of their human rights. They have often been beyond the reach of international agencies, which rely on the cooperation of national governments to deliver relief assistance. In 2011, the country with the most internally displaced persons was Colombia, where 3.9 million people were displaced. The other four countries with more than a million internally displaced persons were Iraq, Sudan, the Democratic Republic of the Congo (the DRC), and Somalia.[3]

■ IMPACT OF SOCIAL INJUSTICE

Social injustice experienced by civilians who are forced to flee their homes and become refugees or internally displaced persons—or victims of a siege, such as the residents of Sarajevo, in the former Yugoslavia—often suffer direct consequences on their physical and mental health. More recent conflicts, such as the conflict in West Darfur, Sudan, which began in 2004, highlight the social injustice of civil (internal) wars. These wars have been characterized by (a) use of repressive techniques to evict people from their homes and to undermine their sense of security and safety, and (b) targeted use of force to destroy social, political, and economic structures. An especially insidious development has been the targeting of violence toward individuals and groups because of their religion or ethnicity—known as *ethnic cleansing*. Opportunistic politicians have often inflamed perceived differences between groups, especially during times of economic and political uncertainty, resulting in armed conflict.

The story of Kosovo illustrates this type of situation. Starting in 1989, when Serbian nationalism was being inflamed by the ruling elite in Belgrade, Kosovar Albanians experienced gradually escalating discrimination: They could not easily obtain land titles, could not access professional employment, and could not enter universities. By 1998, Serbian police imposed severe restrictions on their physical movement, and frequently intimidated and harassed them.[4] Eventually they could not access health care. Their travel to hospitals was restricted by random detention at checkpoints and lengthy identification checks, and, because of the general climate of fear, they could not travel to hospitals after dark. Albanians were arbitrarily charged for their medical treatment, while Serbs did not have to pay. By early 1999, heavily armed police patrolled the main hospital in Pristina, rooftop snipers terrorized patients, Albanians injured by violence were increasingly denied treatment, and all Albanian hospital employees had been fired.[4]

This spiral of human rights abuses included arbitrary arrest and detention, rape and other forms of sexual violence, forced expulsion, and arbitrary killing, culminating in massacres of Albanian civilians in their villages—all of which led to intervention by the North American Treaty Organization (NATO) in March 1999. By the end of May, about 1.4 million Kosovars had been uprooted, including 442,000 to Albania, 250,000 to Macedonia, more than 600,000 to Kosovo, and over 67,000 to Montenegro.[5]

The international community's assistance to Kosovar refugees was generous and effective in preventing disease outbreaks and excess mortality.[6] However, the impact of the forced migration on mental health was significant. A study by the Centers for Disease Control and Prevention in late 1999 found that 17 percent of adult Kosovar Albanians had psychiatric disorders, and, not surprisingly, 90 percent expressed strong feelings of hatred toward Serbs. And half of these Kosovar Albanians reported strong desires for revenge.[7]

■ IMPACT OF VIOLENCE

In other situations that have led to mass population displacement, the extent to which basic human rights have been denied has varied, but it has included the worst possible types of violations. The systematic discrimination experienced by Kosovar Albanians was also experienced by Muslims in Bosnia, Serbs in Croatia, and Muslims in Chechnya—leading in all three cases to open armed conflict, many civilian deaths—for example, between 25,000 and 60,000 in Bosnia, and millions of people being displaced.

The most dramatic manifestation of these human rights violations has been genocide. Indisputably, genocide has occurred at least twice since World War II: in Cambodia from 1975 to 1979 when a fanatical elite (the Khmer Rouge) declared war on its educated urban population, and in Rwanda in 1994, when Hutu extremist leaders exploited long-standing ethnic animosity to slaughter approximately one million ethnic Tutsis.

A more recent conflict in Sudan has also led to charges of genocide. In 2003, systematic human rights abuses began to be perpetrated by the *janjaweed* militia against the Zaghawa, Masaalit, and Fur peoples in the Darfur region. The Sudan government was accused of supporting the militia. Consequently, in 2010, the International Criminal Court issued an arrest warrant for President Omar Al-Bashir, the head of state of Sudan, for crimes against humanity. By the end of 2011, more than 300,000 civilians had been killed, 2.7 million had been internally displaced, and 264,000 were living in refugee camps in neighboring Chad.[8] It was not until 2007 that the United Nations Security Council authorized the deployment of a joint United Nations–African Union Force, which is now the largest UN peacekeeping mission in the world. In early 2012, it had more than 19,500 military personnel and a robust mandate to protect civilians. (See Box 17–4 in Chapter 17.)

■ INDIRECT EFFECTS ON HEALTH

Refugees and internally displaced persons have often been exposed to long periods of deprivation and denied access to food and basic services. This deprivation has in many cases been linked directly to membership in a specific ethnic, religious, or social group, such as South Sudanese Christians, Bosnian Muslims, Kosovo Albanians, non-Arab Muslims in Western Sudan, and East Timorese people who support independence.

Political disturbances, as they evolve in a country, generally have substantial adverse consequences for the national and local economy. In some cases where there have been underlying tensions among political factions, ethnic or religious groups, or people in disadvantaged geographic areas, such as in Indonesia in 1998, an economic crisis may initiate political turmoil. In such situations, especially in low-income countries, one of the first health effects is under-nutrition in vulnerable populations caused by food insecurity. Two-thirds of the 18 countries with the highest rates of undernourishment in the world have recently experienced armed conflict (Table 11–1).[9]

During political disturbances, local farmers may not plant crops as extensively as usual, or they may decrease the crop diversity due to uncertainty created by the

TABLE 11-1 *Countries with Prevalence (Rates) of Undernourishment (Defined by FAO as Inadequate Dietary Intake) Greater Than 30 Percent of Their Population, 2012*

Afghanistan 58%	Kenya* 30%
Angola 44%	Liberia 32%
Burundi 73%	Mozambique* 37%
Chad 33%	North Korea* 32%
Central African Republic 41%	Rwanda 40%
Democratic Republic of Congo 75%	Sierra Leone 46%
Eritrea 66%	Somalia 65%
Ethiopia 40%	Tanzania*39%
Haiti* 44%	Zambia* 47%

*Not recently affected by armed conflict. (*Source*: Food and Agriculture Organization. The state of food insecurity in the world 2012. Rome: FAO, 2012.)

economic and/or political situation. The cost of seeds and fertilizer may increase, and government agricultural extension services may be disrupted, resulting in lower yields. Distribution and marketing systems may be adversely affected. Currency devaluation may drive down the price paid for agricultural produce, and the collapse of the local food-processing industry may further reduce demand for agricultural products.

If full-scale armed conflict occurs, fighting may damage irrigation systems, crops may be intentionally destroyed or looted by armed soldiers, distribution systems may completely collapse, and there may be widespread theft and looting of food stores. In countries that do not normally produce agricultural surpluses or that have large pastoral or nomadic communities, especially in sub-Saharan Africa, the impact of food deficits on the nutritional status of civilians may be severe. If drought occurs—as it often has during the past 30 years in Sudan, Somalia, Chad, Ethiopia, and other countries—the outcome may be catastrophic famine. A study that compared actual mean food production per capita with "peace-adjusted" values for 14 countries found that, in 13 of these countries, food production was lower in wartime—a mean decrease of 12.3 percent, with declines ranging from 3.4 percent in Kenya to over 44 percent in Angola.[10]

When food aid programs are established, there may be inequitable distribution due to political and gender factors, damage to or destruction of food stores, theft of food, diversion of food to military forces, and obstruction of food distribution.[11] Resultant food shortages may cause prolonged hunger and eventually drive families from their homes in search of food. Diversion of food aid has occurred often, such as in Mozambique and Ethiopia in the 1980s and in southern Sudan, and the former Yugoslavia in the 1990s. In the Central African Republic, 40 to 50 percent of the cattle owned by members of the pastoralist federation were killed during fighting between pro-government and anti-government forces between October 2002 and March 2003.

People who are uprooted from their homes have high mortality rates—as high as 25 times the baseline mortality rate in their country of origin. The

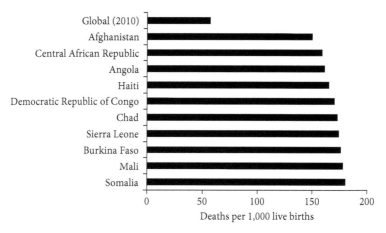

Figure 11-2 The 10 countries with the highest child mortality rates in 2010. Eight of them have experienced recent conflict. (Based on data in Inter-agency Group for Child Mortality Estimation, Levels & Trends in Child Mortality. New York: UNICEF, 2011.)

highest mortality rate recorded among refugees during the past 30 years was among Rwandans who fled to eastern Zaire in 1994. During the first month after this exodus, this population's mortality rate averaged 25 deaths per 10,000 per day, or approximately 50 times higher than the usual death rate in Rwanda.[12]

For refugees in low- and middle-income countries, the major causes of death have consistently been measles, diarrhea (including outbreaks of cholera and dysentery), malaria, acute respiratory infections, hepatitis, and meningitis—reflecting the crowding, contaminated water, and poor sanitation in many refugee camps.[13] Severe malnutrition has affected many refugee populations, concomitant with increased mortality due to infectious diseases. Children affected by armed conflicts have often had extremely high mortality rates (Figure 11–2). Armed conflict has also adversely affected the global campaign to eradicate polio. Of the six countries where wild polio virus was still circulating in 2012, five had experienced recent armed conflict (Pakistan, Afghanistan, Nigeria, the DRC, and Chad); the sixth country (Angola) is recovering from decades of civil war. (See Figures 11–3 and 11–4.)

▪ ROOT CAUSES AND UNDERLYING ISSUES

The definition of *refugees* in the Convention and Protocol Relating to the Status of Refugees (1951)[14]—people who have crossed international borders "fleeing war or persecution for reasons of race, religion, nationality, or membership in particular social and political groups"—implies that they have experienced systematic injustice. However, this definition was developed immediately after World War II in response to massive movements of refugees within Europe. It suggests a political context in which one government is the oppressor and

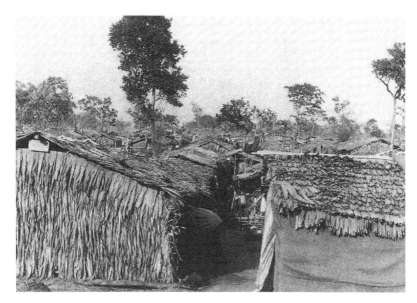

Figure 11-3 Huts made of thatch and burlap at Khao-I-Dang camp for Cambodians in Thailand in 1980. (Photograph by Barry S. Levy.)

another government is offering asylum and protection for refugees. The situation today is far more complex than in 1951, when the Convention was adopted.

Article 25 of the Universal Declaration of Human Rights, proclaimed by the United Nations General Assembly in 1948, states that "everyone has the right to a

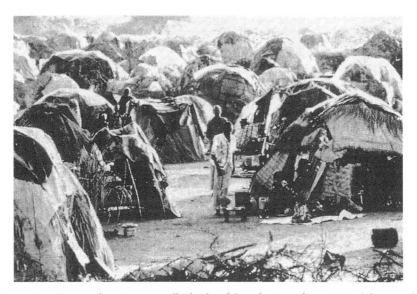

Figure 11-4 Tent city housing internally displaced Somalis in Baidoa in 1992. (Photograph by Michael J. Toole.)

standard of living adequate for the health and well-being of himself and of his family, including food, clothing, housing and medical care....." In times of war, this declaration and other declarations, laws, covenants, and treaties that constitute the body of human rights law are complemented by international humanitarian law. The latter is "a set of rules aimed at limiting violence and protecting the fundamental rights of the individual in times of armed conflict."[15] (See Chapters 22 and 27.)

These legal instruments relate to the obligations of nation-states and their governments. However, recent studies have suggested that many millions of people live in situations where "traditional distinctions between people, army, and government have been blurred, and new ways of projecting power have emerged."[16] Many people can no longer rely on their governments—or even organized resistance groups, once called *liberation movements*—to protect their basic human rights. They live in areas governed by warlords, international criminals, and opportunists who have developed and have sustained "shadow" economies that link, for example, diamond dealers in the conflict zones of Sierra Leone with members of the Russian Mafia, jade mine owners in northern Burma with government and secessionist army generals and international drug traffickers, leaders of ethnic separatist movements in the Balkans with leaders of prostitution rings in Western Europe, and warlords in the DRC with international money launderers and diamond smugglers. These "parallel economies" or black markets within an increasingly unregulated global economic system have created wealthy and powerful elites who live outside the boundaries of international law and national law of sovereign states. They remain wealthy and powerful by exploiting poor and powerless people, often sustaining their influence by exploiting fears generated by perceived differences among various ethnic and religious groups. For example, the Serbian power elite in Belgrade exploited such fears in the early 1990s, provoking widespread ethnic violence, while enriching themselves by controlling illegal trade operations that avoided economic sanctions. Another example, exploitation of the mineral coltan, used in the manufacture of mobile phones, has made several Congolese warlords, such as General Laurent Nkunda, multimillionaires.[17] Likewise, Somali warlords exploited traditional differences among familial clans, eventually eroding the authority of the central government and leading to the total collapse of governance. These alternative economies have thrived, in part, because the liberalized international economic system has increasingly marginalized the poorest countries of Africa.

In this lawless environment, social injustice has greatly increased. Not only are people subject to discrimination and terror, but they also have minimal access to basic social services. The DRC is an extreme example of this situation. This country is "ground zero" of what has been called an "African world war."[17] Nearly 20 armed groups—Congolese and foreign—have been vying for political advantage or economic gain. Attempts to curb the war, through peace accords signed in Zambia, have been desperately inadequate, as has the United Nations force meant to keep the peace—the second largest United Nations peacekeeping force anywhere in the world. The intractable war has occurred after decades of misrule and misappropriation of the country's vast natural wealth. The DRC's infrastructure and health system are in ruins. Of the 300 health districts in the country, 79 are more than 62 miles (100 km) from their referral hospitals. The lack of government funds and foreign aid means that 100 districts are left without any external funding. Human resources fare no better: The country's 70 million people have only 7000 Congolese physicians to serve them. Life expectancy in 2011 was 48 years. Twenty percent of children die before 5 years of age. Only 2 percent of roads are paved; therefore, large parts of the country are inaccessible to humanitarian assistance. A national mortality survey of 19,500 households performed in 2004 found that the crude mortality rate of 2 deaths per 1000 per month was 67 percent higher than before the war (which began in 1998), and that 3.8 million people had died due to the conflict, almost all as a result of damage to the health-supporting infrastructure.[18]

The custodian of international humanitarian law is the International Committee of the Red Cross (ICRC). For several decades after World War II, the ICRC was able to negotiate adherence to the Geneva Conventions by its signatory parties involved in internal conflicts. However, since 1990, ICRC and other neutral humanitarian non-governmental organizations (NGOs) have had increasing difficulty in ensuring the protection of civilians affected by civil wars. Its staff members have often been targets of violence, despite the sanctity of the Red Cross symbol. ICRC's chief delegate in Bosnia was killed in a vehicle clearly marked with the symbol. Delegates have been killed in Pakistan, Chechnya, Sudan, and Central Africa. Five Médecins Sans Frontières (MSF, or Doctors Without Borders) aid workers were murdered in Afghanistan in 2004, and three others were killed in Somalia in 2008.

In addition to these incidents, humanitarian agencies have increasingly been forced to compromise their neutrality by negotiating with warlords to ensure safe passage—and even paying to have armed guards to protect their staff members, as was the norm in Somalia in 1992 and 1993. This practice has often bestowed legitimacy on armed groups that are little more than criminal gangs, contributing, in turn, to these groups' intimidating people in local communities.

■ POOR HEALTH AS A RISK FACTOR FOR CONFLICT

Poor national health indicators may be associated with an elevated risk of conflict within a country. Population Action International studied the relationship between civil conflict in the 1970s, 1980s, and 1990s and demographic and social indicators, using data from 180 countries. It found that countries in the early stage of the demographic transition (from high to low birth rates and infant mortality rates) were at higher risk of armed conflict. It also found that a decline in the annual birth rate of 10 per 1000 corresponded with a reduction by about 10 percent in risk of civil conflict during the following decade (Table 11–2).[19]

TABLE 11-2 *Birth Rate, Infant Mortality Rate, and Risk of Civil Conflict*

Birth Rate 1985–1990 (births per 1,000 people)	Average Infant Mortality Rate, 1985–1990 (infant deaths per 1,000 live births)	Risk of Outbreak of Civil Conflict, 1990–2000 (Percent)
>45	125	53
35–44	78	34
25–34	42	24
15–24	20	16
<15	10	5

(*Source*: Cincotta R, Engelman R, Anastasion D, The security demographic. Washington, DC: Population Action International, 2003.)

■ INTERNATIONAL RESPONSES

The vulnerability of populations subjected to extreme conditions of injustice has often been compounded by the inconsistency of the international community's response to their plight. Inequity has characterized the global response to their needs. Although the impact of these conflicts on populations has varied greatly, the response by the "international community"—itself a relatively new concept since 1990—has generally not been based solely on humanitarian needs.

The scale of the response has often been determined by (a) media interest, such as the *New York Times*'s coverage in July 1992 of the Somalia famine (five stories in 8 days); (b) geopolitical concerns, such as in Kuwait, Iraq, Kosovo, and Afghanistan; (c) the domestic agendas of donor nations, such as President George H. W. Bush's support for United Nations intervention in Somalia during the next to the last month of his presidency in December 1992; and (d) the strength of international advocacy groups, such as those in Australia that provided extensive public support for intervention in Timor L'Este (East Timor). In 1999, President Bill Clinton exhorted the world community to take action in Kosovo ("a moral imperative"), citing Serb atrocities against Kosovar Albanians. This concept of a "moral imperative" has been selectively used to mobilize support for similarly oppressed populations in Africa. It was not applied in Rwanda, Sierra Leone, Western Sudan, Liberia, or, as of late 2012, even Syria. It was, however, employed to intervene in Libya in 2011.

A dramatic shift in geopolitical priorities has occurred as a result of the terrorist attacks in the United States in 2001. Among high-income countries that have the resources to intervene militarily, the pressing concerns of ensuring national security overshadow humanitarian motives that were prominent in the 1990s. NATO and U.S. interventions have been largely confined to countries whose governments were perceived as supporting terrorists who were targeting Western countries. Afghanistan is an example of the blurring of humanitarian and military objectives. Humanitarian action depends on (a) concern for humanity, (b) impartiality of assistance, (c) independence of the organization delivering aid, and (d) neutrality in the relevant conflict. These principles are only adhered to if there is unhindered access to people in danger, independent evaluation of their needs, independent and impartial distribution of aid according to the level of need, and independent monitoring of the impact of aid. NGOs are concerned that humanitarian action has been severely compromised in recent humanitarian programs taking place in military environments, such as in Kosovo, Afghanistan, Timor L'Este, and Iraq, where military objectives have subsumed humanitarian goals. In addition, grave humanitarian needs of large populations in Liberia, Sierra Leone, Angola, and the DRC have largely been ignored by major government donor agencies.

■ WHAT NEEDS TO BE DONE

Social injustice and inequality are most pronounced in politically unstable and impoverished countries where armed conflict has occurred and where the line between political struggle and organized crime is blurred. These conditions are not confined to countries where civil wars are widely recognized, such as in Africa (including the long civil war in the DRC, which has involved troops from seven African countries), Central Asia, the Middle East, or Central and Eastern Europe. These conditions also exist in Colombia, where right-wing and left-wing guerrilla movements spread terror; in Sri Lanka, where government forces coerced hundreds of thousands of ethnic Tamils into camps at the end of the civil war in 2009; and in Pakistan, where Islamic extremists terrorize local communities.

During the 1990s, these situations were referred to as "complex political emergencies." The response to them often consisted of complex humanitarian operations that focused on the delivery of food and medicine but neglected the underlying causes of conflict. This approach was evident in Bosnia between 1993 and 1995, when United Nations "peacekeepers" averted their eyes from the most widespread abuses of human rights in Europe since World War II. More recently, the focus on short-term humanitarian responses has broadened to the relationship among economic and social development, national and international security (and the prevention of terrorism), and humanitarian emergencies.

Under-development and resultant exclusion and destabilization in developing countries are threats to global security. The threats can be decreased by a "pro-poor system of global liberal governance,"[16] in which poverty is reduced by a commitment to equity and substantial investment in access to basic education and health services. Poverty alleviation, good health, and education promote economic growth, political stability, and national security. Improved quality of life of poor people can help prevent the emergence of extremist movements and reduce international terrorism and the need for counter-terrorist military interventions.

Armed conflicts rarely occur in economically prosperous countries. Therefore, economic development helps prevent complex emergencies. So do the Millennium Development Goals (MDGs), three of which relate directly to public health. (See Table 21–7 in Chapter 21 and Chapter 29.)

From 2000 to 2009, high-income countries stepped up their commitments to addressing global health inequities. Generous pledges were made at the Millennium Summit. The Global Fund to Fight AIDS, Tuberculosis and Malaria was established and strongly supported by donor governments. The U.S. President's Emergency Plan for AIDS Relief (PEPFAR) and the President's Malaria Initiative were launched. And private-sector initiatives, such as the Global Alliance on Vaccines and Immunization and programs of the Bill and Melinda Gates Foundation, were established. The G8 (Group of Eight) meeting in 2005 led to the Gleneagles Communiqué, which included a "renewed commitment to Africa" to help achieve the MDGs.

These commitments, however, have lessened since the onset of the global financial crisis in 2007. For example, in the Gleneagles Communiqué, G8 nations were to increase total official development assistance from $58 billion in 2004 to $106 billion in 2010; but, by 2010, this aid had only reached $89 billion. In many donor countries, the proportion of gross domestic product (GDP) spent on official development assistance has been steadily declining; in others, such as Ireland, Spain, Portugal, and Greece, GDP has declined, leading to reduced development aid. Only Denmark, Norway, the Netherlands, Luxembourg, and Sweden exceed the United Nations official development assistance target of 0.7 percent of GDP; the United States spends only 0.2 percent of its GDP on official development assistance, the fifth-lowest among the 34 Organization for Economic Co-operation and Development countries. (See Figure 21–1 in Chapter 21.)

A consistent international response to conflict-related emergencies must be based on humanitarian need, rather than political expediency. More work is needed to resolve conflicts with diplomacy, supported, when necessary, by a proportionate use of force—a contentious and highly emotional issue. There is still no consensus on what should bring about a forceful international response to massive human rights abuses. The public demands intervention to prevent widespread human rights abuses, but also demands withdrawal if that intervention goes sour (as in Somalia) or leads to excessive "collateral damage" (as in Kosovo). The conviction of Charles Taylor in the International Criminal Court for war crimes in Sierra Leone is a positive sign that international law may play a positive role in the prevention of armed conflicts. (See Chapter 27.)

■ CONCLUSION

In 2011, approximately 37 million people were refugees or internally displaced people because of threats of persecution and violence. Many people have experienced much social injustice, which has limited their freedom of movement and employment and has restricted their access to food, water, health services, education, and other human needs. Many of these people can no longer rely on their governments to protect their human rights or to provide basic services. In many cases, they are being exploited by quasi-criminal groups that masquerade as legitimate political movements. These groups wield increasing power and influence and amass significant wealth by exploiting the people under their control. Many of these groups collude with governments and non-state actors to sustain a parallel unregulated economy. Poor and powerless people are eventually faced with no option other than to flee their homes—and sometimes their country—to survive. The toll on their health is profound. The plight of these people can be addressed only if the international community is serious about addressing the root causes of poverty, poor governance, exploitation, and inequities between rich and poor countries.

▪ REFERENCES

1. Bieri F. From blood diamonds to the Kimberley process: How NGOs cleaned up the global diamond industry. London: Ashgate, 2010.
2. UNHCR: The UN Refugee Agency. UNHCR Global Trends 2011. Geneva: UNHCR, 2011. Available at http://www.unhcr.org/pages/4fd9a0676.html. Accessed on December 21, 2012.
3. Internal Displacement Monitoring Centre. Global Overview 2011. People internally displaced by conflict and violence. Geneva: Norwegian Refugee Council, 2012. Available at http://www.internal-displacement.org/publications/global-overview-2011. Accessed on November 1, 2012.
4. Organization for Security and Cooperation in Europe. Kosovo/Kosova: As seen, as told. An analysis of the human rights findings of the OSCE Kosovo Verification Mission, October 1998 to June 1999. Warsaw: OSCE, 1999. Available at http://www.osce.org/odihr/17774. Accessed on November 1, 2012.
5. Winter R, ed. World refugee survey 2000. Washington, DC: United States Committee for Refugees, 2001.
6. United Nations Subcommittee on Nutrition. Refugee nutrition information system. Geneva: United Nations, 1999.
7. Lopes CB, Vergara A, Agani F, et al. Mental health, social functioning, and attitudes of Kosovar Albanians following the war in Kosovo. JAMA 2000;284:567–577.
8. Degomme O, Guha-Sapir D. Patterns of mortality rates in Darfur conflict. Lancet 2010;375:294–300.
9. Food and Agriculture Organization. The state of food insecurity in the world. Rome: FAO, 2011.
10. Messer E, Cohen M, Marchione T. Conflict: A cause and effect of hunger. In: Environmental change and security project report No. 7. Washington, DC: Woodrow Wilson International Center for Scholars, Smithsonian Institution, 2001.
11. Macrae J, Zwi A, eds. War and hunger: Rethinking international responses to complex emergencies. London: Zed Books, 1994.
12. Toole MJ, Waldman RJ. Complex emergencies. In: Merson M, Black R, Mills A, eds. Global health: Diseases, programs, systems, and policies. Burlington, MA: Jones and Bartlett Learning, 2012.
13. Toole MJ, Waldman RJ. Refugees and displaced persons: War, hunger, and public health. JAMA 1993;270:600–605.

14. UNHCR: The UN Refugee Agency. Convention and protocol relating to the status of refugees. Geneva, Switzerland: UNHCR, 2010. Available at http://www.unhcr.org/3b66c2aa10.html. Accessed on November 1, 2012.

15. Perrin P. Handbook on war and public health. Geneva: International Committee of the Red Cross, 1996:381.

16. Duffield M. Introduction. In: Global governance and the new wars: The merging of development and security. London: Zed Books, 2001.

17. Prunier G. Africa's world war: Congo, the Rwandan genocide, and the making of a continental catastrophe. New York: Oxford University Press, 2008.

18. Coghlan B, Brennan R, Ngoy P, et al. Mortality in the Democratic Republic of Congo: Results from a nationwide survey. *Lancet* 2006;367:44–51.

19. Cincotta R, Engelman R, Anastasion D. The security demographic. Washington, DC: Population Action International, 2003.

PART III

How Social Injustice Affects Aspects of Public Health

12 Medical Care

■ OLIVER FEIN AND H. JACK GEIGER

▓ INTRODUCTION

In the United States, medical care—access to personal medical services, both curative and preventive—is ironically an area of grave social injustice. Deep dysfunctions in the organization, financing, and distribution of medical care have profound consequences for individuals in avoidable suffering and preventable death, cumulatively damaging the health status and life prospects of whole populations and incurring staggering costs to society.

These costs and damages are not the inevitable result of fundamental economic laws or the nature of health care—as the much-better experience of all other industrialized democracies attests. They are instead the consequence of a deliberate ideological and political choice to treat medical care as a market commodity to be rationed by one's ability to pay—rather than as (a) a social good to be distributed in response to medical need, (b) a responsibility of government, and (c) a fundamental right embodied in a social contract. As a consequence, the opportunities in the United States to maintain a healthy and long life and to fulfill one's human potential are skewed by income, education, primary language, race, ethnicity, and area of residence. This injustice is not due to random chance in the distribution of disease; it is injustice by design.

The roots of this injustice lie in U.S. political culture and history. Neither government nor the shared beliefs of the public have ever fully recognized a human right to health care, as they have done—albeit after a slow political evolution—for other social goods, such as education. The health status of the U.S. population is now clearly seen as a matter of essential national interest. But massive inequalities in the health status of variously disadvantaged or marginalized population groups—by race, ethnicity, social class, and gender—are officially viewed, at best, as problems requiring intervention, not as issues of social justice. Indeed, these inequalities have often been viewed as the *fault* of these groups due to their alleged biological inferiority or lifestyle choices.

While nominal fairness is seen as an important criterion for many policy choices, health care in the United States is not widely considered a part of what John Rawls defined as *primary social goods*: rights and liberties, power and opportunity, income and wealth, and a social basis of self-respect.[1] Views on health care in the United States are therefore reflective of society's willingness to tolerate very large inequalities in income, wealth, and economic and political power. The more unequal a society is in economic parameters, the more unequal it is likely to be in health outcomes.[2] Yet many ethicists, following John Rawls, have asserted that health care is special, and that, in this domain, inequality is injustice because poor health care and poor health so profoundly limit opportunities for the full realization of one's potential for employment, relationships, and social and political participation. From this perspective, justice in health care is good for the public's health, and the public's good health, in turn, broadens opportunities and facilitates a more just society.[3]

■ THE IMPACT OF SOCIAL INJUSTICE IN MEDICAL CARE

The consequences for public health of social injustice in medical care are complex. Personal medical services contribute only modestly to the health status of a population—in morbidity, mortality, life expectancy, or health-related quality of life. Health is not merely a function of one's access to medical care; to a much greater extent, health is a function of the cumulative experience of social conditions throughout one's lifetime.[4]

The most powerful influences on the public's health are social determinants, including:

- Income level
- Employment
- Quality and affordability of housing
- Educational opportunities
- Workplace safety
- Quality of air, water, and food
- Sanitation
- Less tangible, but pervasive, factors, such as racism, class bias, and political inequality

Medical care, however, does make a difference to both personal and population health—a difference that is revealed when care is absent or denied. For example, lack of prenatal care is associated with higher rates of infant and maternal mortality among minority groups and uninsured people. As another example, low-income adults removed from programs that fund access to care, such as Medicaid, have more uncontrolled illnesses and preventable deaths within a year of removal.[5] It is estimated that approximately 45,000 deaths associated with lack of health insurance occur annually among Americans age 18 to 64.[6]

Inaccessible health care causes unjust assumption of risks, as when untreated hypertension leads to a disabling stroke or a lethal heart attack. Low-income adults who are uninsured consistently assume these risks, even though most of them are full-time workers. Low-income retirees also assume these risks when they are denied coverage or suddenly abandoned by their private-sector, for-profit Medicare "Advantage" plans—which have frequently cancelled coverage and withdrawn from the health care marketplace when they found it insufficiently profitable.[7] Whole communities may be affected: Neighborhoods with high rates of uninsured people attract few physicians and health care facilities, making access more difficult for all people—even those who *do* have coverage. Consequences ripple through the health care system. For example, hospitals that are burdened with the huge expenses of un-reimbursed emergency department visits and inpatient care for uninsured people shift these costs by increasing charges for insured patients, thereby driving up the cost of health insurance premiums.

Members of minority groups and poor people who do access medical care receive less-comprehensive and lower-quality diagnostic and therapeutic services compared with others—even when their insurance status, severity of disease, and other characteristics are comparable.[8] These people bear a triple burden: (a) they generally reside in the most dangerous biological and physical environments and are exposed to the worst social determinants of health; (b) they have the least access to care; and (c) even when they receive care, it tends to be of poor quality.

These are longstanding patterns. At no time in the history of the United States has the health status of African Americans, Hispanic Americans, Native Americans, and several Asian American subgroups equaled or even approximated that of Caucasians. It is largely because of such systemic defects that the United States, while paying the highest per-capita expenditures for medical care among all nations, ranks 51st in life expectancy at birth—far behind other countries, even much poorer ones like Bosnia.[9]

After prolonged political struggle and during a period of broader social change in the United States, a significant advance toward the assumption of social responsibility for medical care was made in the 1960s with the passage of both Medicare (to insure elderly people) and Medicaid (to insure many low-income people). However, U.S. policy has remained ambivalent. Medical care has continued to be treated as a consumer good, subject to the rules of the marketplace and alleged competition, even as Medicare and Medicaid represented a partial recognition of the principle that justice is embodied in a shared social responsibility.

The degree of this recognition has fluctuated over time. With no effective control over total health care costs (including the costs of health insurance and prescription drugs) in a system that has depended on employers providing health insurance as a benefit, more employers and more patients over time have been priced out of the health insurance market. Societal pressure has led to incremental increases in publicly funded coverage, especially for children, further increasing total health expenditures. By the early 2000s, the medical care system in the United States—the only industrialized democracy without universal health insurance—was accelerating into crisis.

■ THE U.S. HEALTH CARE CRISIS AND SOCIAL JUSTICE

This crisis has three dimensions: access, cost, and quality—each with implications for social justice.

Access

In a system in which citizens have no legal right to health care (beyond emergency treatment) and no guarantee of access to adequate care unless they have the means to pay for it, 48.6 million Americans in 2011 lacked private or public health insurance of any kind.[10] In 2011, the total number of uninsured people included at least 37 million workers and almost 8 million children.

The distribution of uninsured people follows patterns of racial and ethnic discrimination. Among all working adults, 13 percent of whites, 21 percent of African Americans, and 32 percent of Hispanics are uninsured.[11] Substantially higher percentages of these groups are uninsured for part of any given year.

Lack of health insurance has profoundly reduced access to care. For example, in 2012, 26 percent of uninsured adults went without needed medical care in the previous year, compared with about 7 percent of insured adults.[12] And 53 percent of uninsured adults did not have a personal physician or usual source of care compared with 10 percent of insured adults.[12] Uninsured adults, compared to insured adults, are far less likely to have their blood pressure or serum cholesterol checked or be screened for cancer.[12] As a consequence, uninsured people are diagnosed later in the course of disease, and they die earlier than those with insurance. Therefore, lack of insurance—mainly due to inability to pay for it despite full-time employment—is associated with poorer health and the reduced opportunities that accompany poorer health. Gaining health insurance restores access to health care and diminishes the adverse effects of having been uninsured.[13] (Lack of insurance does not mean total absence of health care for sick people. Some care is delivered to uninsured patients during emergency department visits and unavoidable—but uncompensated—hospitalizations.)

Even among those who have insurance, an estimated 36 million people (including those covered by Medicare and Medicaid) are unable to access care because there are too few physicians in their communities—or no physicians who will accept Medicare or Medicaid patients. And there are millions more people who are underinsured, either because of the unaffordable cost of adequate coverage or because of insurance policies that exclude coverage of those with preexisting disease. These people and those without any insurance—totaling about 27 percent of the U.S. population—are medically underserved.

In sum, the health care system arbitrarily—but selectively—increases inequality in ways that have little to do with individual merit. Except for the passage of Medicare in 1965, U.S. policy has abandoned the concept of shared social responsibility—a general obligation to protect all people against disease, disability, and premature death.[3]

Cost

In 2010, health care spending in the United States totaled $2.6 trillion—nearly 18 percent of the gross domestic product (GDP), with an average expenditure of $8,402 per person, the highest of any country.[14] Total medical costs for uninsured people range from about $56 to $73 billion per year.[15] Health care spending is projected to grow to 21 percent of GDP by 2019 if the system does not change.

From 1999 to 2012, the premiums that employers paid to provide health insurance for their employees increased 172 percent. In response, many employers reduced benefits, increased deductibles and co-payments, and required their workers to pay a steeply rising share of the premiums—employee contributions to premiums increased 180 percent during this 13-year period. Since worker's earnings only increased 47 percent and inflation was 38 percent during this period,[16] some employees could not afford to pay these costs and either became uninsured, or dropped coverage for other family members. Some employers eliminated insurance benefits for retirees or discontinued all health insurance for employees. And the health insurance coverage many employers did continue was almost always incomplete. In 2012, the average premium for employer-provided health insurance was $5615 for individuals and $15,745 for families. Employee contributions, on average, toward those premiums was $925 for individuals and $4215 for families.[16,17]

Problems with costs were compounded by fragmentation of care, the consequence of an employer-based system that relies primarily on thousands of (mostly for-profit) private-sector insurers, with widely varying benefit packages, frequent limitations on patient choice of physicians and hospitals, and complex regulations. The costs of administering this system—to employers, insurance companies, hospital administrators, and health care providers—is high: Administrative costs add $2685, on average, to the cost of health care for every insured person in the United States, compared with only $809 in Canada's government-operated, single-payer system.[18]

Quality

Vast expenditures, however, do not ensure quality of care. There are wide variations in the appropriateness and comprehensiveness of the medical care that patients receive. The Institute of Medicine has called the gap between what is done and what should be done a "quality chasm."[19] Many patients experience poor-quality care, receiving only 50 to 60 percent of recommended treatments for common acute and chronic conditions, such as diabetes, asthma, hypertension, and heart disease, as well as reduced preventive care.[20] Lower-quality, less-comprehensive care for African Americans, Hispanics, and other minorities is pervasive and systemwide, resulting in substantial personal and social costs.[21] (See also Chapter 3.) The United States—despite massive health care expenditures and its international leadership in biomedical research and technological innovation in health care, as well as repeated claims that its market-based health care system is the best in the world—has neither ensured quality of care nor produced equitable improvements in health status.

■ MEDICARE "REFORM" IN 2003: THE TRIUMPH OF INJUSTICE

Since the establishment of Medicare and Medicaid, incremental expansions of coverage, such as the Children's Health Insurance Program (CHIP), have lent support to the view that ensuring access to health care is the government's responsibility. (However, reliance on employment-based health insurance has meant that the proportion of the population covered has varied with changes in the economy.) In 2003, this pattern of incremental improvement was reversed with Medicare changes enacted by the U.S. Congress and signed into law by President George W. Bush. We believe that there remains a need to ensure health care for all. The focus of the 2003 legislation, the Medicare Prescription Drug, Improvement and Modernization Act (MMA), was primarily characterized by its proponents as helping elderly patients pay for the staggering costs of prescription medications. This goal was only partially achieved by the drug provisions of the MMA. However, the Act's other, less-emphasized, provisions reveal a much broader intent: to abandon Medicare as a social insurance system in which risks and costs are shared by all older people—healthy and ill, rich and poor alike—with free choice of physicians and hospitals, under a government guarantee to pay for their medical care as an entitlement—a right. This intent has been demonstrated in the MMA's creation of multiple strategies to (a) fragment the common-risk pool; (b) move most older people into a spuriously competitive, private-sector, profit-driven marketplace of managed care plans with limited choices; and (c) transform an entitlement into a voucher for the purchase of care as a commodity. The intent of the MMA was to use government funds to subsidize the for-profit, private sector in its attempt to establish exclusive control over the provision of care.

The strategy to fragment the common-risk pool was based on a subsidy. Under the Act, the U.S. government makes huge preferential payments to private-sector, for-profit health insurance companies and health maintenance organizations (HMOs)—up to 14 to 16 percent more than the traditional Medicare program. These payments enable those companies to lower (and in some cases to eliminate) their monthly premium charges to patients, offer more-generous prescription drug coverage, and "compete" on a favorably tilted playing field with traditional, public fee-for-service Medicare. The playing field is favorably tilted further by provisions allowing these companies to negotiate with pharmaceutical companies for lower drug prices, but prohibiting traditional Medicare, despite its massive potential for bulk purchasing power, from doing the same—a startling deviation from free-market philosophy by the conservative advocates who supported the Act.

In addition, the MMA allows Medicare patients to withdraw almost entirely from traditional Medicare—if they are wealthy enough to make this choice. It created this option by establishing large, tax-free *health savings accounts*, which are tax shelters in which people can use their own money to pay for medical expenses—rather than paying monthly premiums for Medicare coverage—while remaining in the common-risk pool of all older people. As a result, the healthiest and wealthiest older people can enroll in private-sector plans (Medicare Medical Savings Accounts) and effectively withdraw from traditional Medicare, while the sickest and poorest older people remain in the system. The increased medical needs and costs of the sickest and poorest people inevitably increase the expenses of traditional Medicare, requiring its premiums to rise sharply and thereby escalating Medicare's drain on general governmental revenues. (Since everyone can use health savings accounts—not just older people, the withdrawal of healthy and wealthy people from other insurance plan pools similarly increases the cost of employment-based health insurance.) To ensure that these outcomes appear to be a triumph of the private marketplace and that the principle of social insurance is demeaned, the MMA arbitrarily states that, when more than 45 percent of traditional Medicare costs come from general tax revenues, Medicare will be declared—by fiat, rather than fact—to be in "crisis" and Medicare will have to be restructured.

Well-established evidence does not support the strategies that underlie the MMA. Privatized Medicare managed-care ("Advantage") plans cost more than public fee-for-service Medicare, incur higher out-of-pocket costs for subscribers, frequently deny services (sometimes with disastrous medical results), and often require limitation or elimination of patients' free choice of health care providers. Some plans abandoned their subscribers entirely when they began to lose money. For example, between 1999 and 2003 (before the MMA), private Medicare health maintenance organizations (HMOs) dropped 2.2 million of their elderly patients.[22] The administrative costs of commercial health insurers and private-sector, managed-care plans are approximately 20 percent, compared to 3 percent for traditional Medicare. Health economists have long demonstrated that health care— unlike commodities—cannot be efficiently managed by the marketplace.[23]

The real goal of the MMA was to abandon the principle of shared social responsibility—government action to embody a right—in favor of an intrinsically unjust allocation of resources, favoring the most affluent people and those least in need. In effect, the MMA created an Orwellian system in which some people are more equal than others in receiving health care.

This system is more clearly understood if one examines it in relation to another system that is widely recognized as a government responsibility to serve the whole population: police protection for the security of individuals and property. Suppose the government enacted legislation to (a) use public funds to subsidize private guards and commercial security companies to lower their fees and expand their services; (b) create tax-sheltered *security savings accounts* so that citizens could use their own money to hire bodyguards and private patrols; and (c) reduce the local property taxes of these people by one-third because they no longer depended primarily on the public police system. Inevitably, those people with the highest incomes, the most property to protect, and the most to gain from tax shelters would be those most likely to enter this subsidized marketplace for private guards and commercial security companies. Just as inevitably, local governments' revenues from property taxes would fall, forcing them to either raise taxes on everyone else or close police stations and fire police officers, making life more dangerous for middle-class and poor people. Either way, the principle of collective security would be abandoned. That is precisely what is threatened by the planned "de-socialization" and "de-universalization" of health insurance. In both cases, what is denied is a general social obligation to provide systems of protection for individuals and families. In the case of health care, this social obligation involves the willingness of healthy and wealthy people to share in the cost of care for people who are sicker and poorer—a matter of distributive justice.

■ HEALTH CARE "REFORM" IN 2010

Although many advisors counseled President Barack Obama not to address health care reform during his first term, he decided to do so. In early 2009, he convened the White House Health Care Summit,[24] bringing together stakeholders, advocates, and leaders of relevant congressional committees to declare his intent and begin the process. Not wanting to repeat the errors of the Clinton administration's health care reform attempt in the 1990s, he announced that the process would be transparent (no secret White House task force) and highly dependent on Congress. He said that he did not want "to start from scratch." It was clear that he had decided to build on private health insurance, rather than expand Medicare to people under age 65. Despite the widespread popularity of Medicare (76 percent of all adults and even 62 percent of Tea Party supporters have said that Medicare was worth its cost to taxpayers),[25] "Medicare for All" was never considered by the relevant congressional committees at any time in the process. Even though eight activists were arrested in Congress, trying to provide testimony favoring an expansion of the public Medicare program to all people, proposed options were limited to those with mandates to buy private health insurance.

There was, however, consideration of a public option, which, in its most robust form, would have made Medicare available to everyone who wanted it—even those with private, employment-based health insurance. A study, financed by the private health insurance industry, estimated that 131 million Americans would enroll in the public option, 81 million of whom had private health insurance.[26] But neither the public option nor the proposal to expand Medicare to all Americans was enacted into law after lobbyists representing business groups, private health insurance companies, and pharmaceutical corporations spent $1.2 billion in 2009 to lobby Congress.[27]

The Patient Protection and Affordable Care Act (ACA)—labeled "Obamacare" by right-wing opponents—was passed by Congress and signed into law in March 2010. It contained no public option and reduced spending on Medicare. Based on a "mandate model" for expanding health insurance coverage, the ACA mandates that all people buy private health insurance or annually pay a penalty ($695 for an individual and $2085 for a family). Employers of 50 employees or more who do not offer health insurance to their employees must also pay an annual penalty ($2000 per employee). The ACA mandates that states expand eligibility for their Medicaid programs to 133 percent of the federal poverty level (which, in 2012, equaled an income of $14,856 for an individual, and an income of $25,390 for a family of three). However, the Supreme Court weakened this mandate, by giving states the ability to opt out of this requirement. The ACA also makes subsidies to purchase private health insurance available to individuals and families earning between 133 percent and 400 percent of the federal poverty level.

The ACA mandates were essential for the survival of the private health insurance industry, which had lost close to 30 million enrollees in the previous 30 years. Private health insurance had increasingly become a defective product, with high premiums ($5615 for an individual and $15,745 for a family), escalating deductibles (ranging from $1000 to $15,000 a year) and significant co-payments.[28] It is estimated that over 80 million Americans are *underinsured*, which means that they spend over 10 percent of their income "out-of-pocket" on health care in a calendar year; most of them have health insurance! It is therefore not surprising that 62 percent of all personal bankruptcies in the United States are due to medical expenditures, and that more than 75 percent of people who claim bankruptcy due to medical expenditures had health insurance at the start of their bankrupting illness.[29]

The ACA also includes some regulatory features, such as permitting coverage of young adults (up to age 26) on their parents' insurance policies, prohibiting denial of health insurance coverage because of preexisting conditions, and eliminating annual and lifetime limits on health insurance coverage. The individual and small group markets for private health insurance may benefit by the creation of the state-based *health insurance exchanges*, which will create a more transparent marketplace in which one can compare health insurance products. Private health insurance will also have to demonstrate a *medical loss ratio* (defined as total health benefits divided by total premiums) of 80 to 85 percent. This term embodies the perspective of stockholders in a private health insurance company, for whom every dollar spent by the company for a physician, a hospital, or a medication is perceived as a loss. As a result, the company has a strong incentive to deny coverage and delay payment.

There are many other features included in the ACA: enhanced funding for community health centers, support for comparative effectiveness research, encouragement of quality by imposing hospital-readmission penalties and by denying payment for treatment of hospital-acquired infections, funding for the public health infrastructure, patient-centered medical homes (PCMHs), and accountable care organizations (ACOs).

When it comes to addressing the three primary challenges facing the U.S. health care system—access, cost, and quality—ACA, however, leaves much to be desired. An estimated 29 million people, by 2019, will remain uninsured. The ACA is extremely weak on controlling costs, heavily relying on the "market"—if many uninsured people are young, mandating that they buy health insurance will expand the risk pool with generally healthy people and therefore premiums for everyone should decrease. But there is considerable concern that, with high premiums ($5615 for an individual and $15,745 for a family), the ACA's annual penalties for not buying insurance ($695 for an individual and $2085 for a family, and, for employers, $2000 per employee) may not be high enough. Many people and employers might pay the penalty rather than buy insurance. In addition, the ACA may lead to more people being under-insured, as private insurance companies, in order to keep premiums low, create policies with high deductibles and high co-payments. An additional shortcoming of the ACA is that it does not explicitly address disparities in the quality of health care.

Conservative legislators had threatened, from 2010 to 2012, to repeal the ACA. But, with the Supreme Court upholding the constitutionality of the ACA and President Obama being re-elected, repeal became unlikely. But the ACA does not change the provisions in the MMA that created Medicare Medical Savings Accounts, which have the potential to undermine the social insurance principles in the traditional Medicare program. In fact, those in Congress opposed to the ACA may not only obstruct its implementation, but they may also attempt to privatize Medicare (through *premium support*),[30] by converting Medicare from a *defined-benefit* program (in which it pays for a list of benefits irrespective of their cost) to a *defined-contribution* program (in which it gives each enrollee a fixed amount of money—a "voucher"—to buy private insurance). If this were achieved, private insurance premiums would likely rise far above the value of the voucher, thereby transferring medical costs to enrollees.

Is the ACA a step forward or backward for the U.S. health care system? Many defenders of the ACA point to its expansion of coverage, its potential to increase Medicaid enrollment, its provision of preventive care without co-payments, and its support for community health centers, primary care, and public health. Many critics of the ACA point out that it strengthens the forces that want to privatize Medicare by taking public tax money and pouring it into the private, for-profit health insurance industry. A third point of view is that the ACA is a great leap sideways: It does not guarantee universal coverage. It will not control costs. And it will not lead to major improvements in quality of care. But it is the first time that the U.S. Congress has implicitly stated that the government is responsible for providing health care to all Americans.

We believe that there remains a need for health care reform beyond the ACA—best achieved by implementing an improved, single-payer, public, "Medicare for All" health care program.[31] (See Box 12–1.)

BOX 12-1 ■ Single-Payer Health Care

Steffie Woolhandler and David U. Himmelstein

In a single-payer health care system, virtually all health care funds flow through a single public (or quasi-public) agency that pays for care for an entire population.

Single-payer systems vary somewhat. In some countries, such as Canada or Taiwan, the government operates the single-payer insurance plan, but most physicians are in private practice and most hospitals and clinics are operated by private, nonprofit organizations. Such insurance-based, single-payer systems are generally called *national health insurance*—or sometimes *Medicare for All*. However, unlike U.S. Medicare, a true "single payer" is not one among many insurance plans, but one that covers the entire population—and, in a single-payer system, private insurance that duplicates public insurance is prohibited.

In some countries with single-payer systems, such as Great Britain and Spain, the government not only pays for care, but also owns most hospitals and employs most medical workers—a model known as a *national health service*. This model resembles the Veterans Health Administration in the United States, but it covers the entire population—not just veterans.

Both of the single-payer models described above facilitate greater equity in care because everyone is covered, and hospitals and physicians are paid the same amount to care for patients irrespective of their income or wealth. Therefore, in Canada, poor people get slightly more care than wealthy people—although, given their high rates of illness due to greater exposure to hazardous physical and social environments, poor people should probably get an even greater share of care. While class gradients in infant mortality (and other health outcomes) remain, even the poorest 20 percent of Canadians have a lower infant mortality rate than the overall infant mortality rate for the United States. Indeed, health outcomes in almost every nation with a single-payer system surpass those in the United States.

A single-payer system facilitates cost containment through several mechanisms. First, having virtually all funds flow through a single "spigot" enables setting and enforcing an overall health care budget. In contrast, in multi-payer systems like that in the United States, hospitals, clinics, and physicians collect fees from hundreds of insurance plans and tens of millions of individual patients, making it almost impossible to track and control the flow of money.

A multiplicity of payers also generates mountains of needless paperwork. Providers must maintain elaborate internal cost-accounting systems to keep track of whom to bill for each bandage and aspirin tablet. And insurance firms—which profit when they avoid paying for care—demand extensive documentation to justify each bill. Therefore, both insurers and providers employ legions of workers to joust over payment and documentation.

In contrast, the government in Canada pays each hospital a global budget that covers all of the care that hospital delivers—similar to the way local governments in the United States pay their fire departments. Hospitals in Canada do not bill for individual patients or need to get an approval from an insurer for each diagnostic procedure or treatment. As a result, Canadian hospitals spend about 13 percent of their revenues on administration—compared to about 24 percent spent by U.S. hospitals. And billing by Canadian physicians is also far simpler; every patient has the same insurance plan, with the same simple set of rules. Canadian physicians have billing costs that are two-thirds lower than those of U.S. physicians.

A single-payer system also saves on insurance overhead, which consumes about 14 percent of premiums in the United States, compared to 1 percent in Canada. Overall, a properly structured single-payer system in the United States could decrease insurance overhead and physicians' paperwork costs by about $400 billion annually.

A single-payer system in the United States could realize additional savings through improved health planning to assure that hospitals and other "high-tech" facilities are available where they are needed and not duplicated where they are wasteful—or even harmful. An excessive number of hospital beds and excessive medical technology induce over-treatment—a phenomenon first noted by Milton Roemer, who articulated "Roemer's Law": "A built (hospital) bed is a filled bed."

In order to minimize incentives for gaming the payment system and to match investment to need, control of new capital expenditures is essential, by forbidding hospitals and clinics from retaining any surplus funds (or profit) left over from their operating budgets. If hospitals and clinics could use these leftover funds to buy new buildings and high-tech equipment, they could avoid unprofitable patients and services and seek out profitable ones in order to expand. Conversely, in this scenario, hospitals and clinics that provide needed—but unprofitable—care could be starved for new investment. Therefore, effective health planning requires that funds for new capital be allocated through a transparent and democratic process.

In the United States, legislation to implement a single-payer system has been introduced in Congress and several state legislatures. Such a system would automatically enroll all residents and fully cover them for all medically necessary care. Patients would have free choice of physicians and hospitals. Hospitals and clinics would be freed of insurers' burdensome micromanagement, but would have to adhere to their budgets.

Polls show substantial support for such reform, both among the general public and among health professionals. In contrast, pharmaceutical and insurance firms, which would lose huge amounts of money under a single-payer system, continue to spend enormous sums to influence politicians to keep a single-payer system off the political agenda. In the United States, groups such as Physicians for a National Health Program (www.pnhp.org), Healthcare-NOW! (www.healthcare-now.org), the National Nurses Organizing Committee (www.NationalNursesUnited.org), and Public Citizen (www.citizen.org) are working to educate the public about single-payer health care and to build the popular movement that can lead to its being established.

Futher Reading

Woolhandler S, Campbell T, Himmelstein DU. Health care administration costs in the U.S. and Canada. *N Engl J Med* 2003;349:768–775.

Woolhandler S, Himmelstein DU, Angell M, Young QD. Proposal of the Physicians' Working Group for single-payer national health insurance. *JAMA* 2003;290:798–805.

Himmelstein DU, Woolhandler S. Competition in a publicly funded health care system: The U.S. experience. *BMJ* 2007;335:1126–1129.

▧ ROOT CAUSES OF PARADOX AND FAILURE

Most Americans, dissatisfied with incremental expansions in health care, favor universal health care coverage—as do substantial numbers of physicians and other health care providers.[32] There is deep public concern about increasing costs and shrinking and uncertain coverage, access, and quality. Yet, attempts to establish universal coverage and universal access to care in the United States have failed. Political analysts attribute this failure to the power of two basic American cultural beliefs: a persistent mistrust of government, and an ideological commitment to individual autonomy and entrepreneurship. Other factors are structural:

- The long-term political absence in the United States of a labor party—a key supporter of universal health coverage in other industrialized democracies
- A federalist political system designed to resist populist pressures and constrain large-scale changes, even when they have widespread public support (In this context, the passage of Medicare was an aberrant event, due to a rare period in which one political party controlled the White House and, by wide margins, both the Senate and the House of Representatives.)
- The organized power and money of corporate interests to influence the political process at the federal and state level through campaign contributions, lobbying, and advertising

The ACA will result in multibillion-dollar profits for the health insurance and pharmaceutical industries.[33] The Supreme Court's ruling in the *Citizens United* case in 2010 has markedly increased corporate influence on the political process, by enabling corporations and labor unions to spend unlimited funds to influence voters. Against this power, progressive change is difficult. Uninsured people have no organized constituency or voting bloc.

▧ WHAT NEEDS TO BE DONE

Almost 50 years of incremental remedies have reduced, but not fundamentally changed, the inequities and inefficiencies in the U.S. health care system. The movement to establish access to health care as a right has faced significant challenges, and is likely to continue to face these challenges unless basic changes are made.

There remains unresolved in the political and social thinking of the American public an ideological conflict between (a) those who see government as an instrument of shared social responsibility, and (b) those who view government as a threat to individual freedom and autonomy. The latter group, despite contrary evidence, believes that, in health care and other areas, the marketplace and entrepreneurship are key to effective outcomes. This conflict, however, may be resolved when increasing costs, deteriorating access to care, and uncertain quality threaten the viability of the U.S. health care system. At that point, the American public may embrace fundamental change and adopt a single-payer system with universal access. Such a change will require real campaign finance reform to support the public interest and block corporate power.

State-level reforms in health care may provide an intermediate step toward a federal system for universal health care. Legislatures in Vermont, Hawaii, and several other states have embarked on a pathway toward single-payer, universal coverage.[34] While a patchwork of varied state programs is no substitute for a uniform and efficient national program, success at the state level may spur support for federal initiatives.

Fundamental change will also require that health care providers and patients recognize that they have common interests and that the present system is not merely unsatisfying, but also profoundly unjust. Health care providers and patients share concerns about the loss of autonomy, uncontrollable costs, exhausting burdens of administration and paperwork, and difficulties in providing and receiving appropriate and high-quality care. The egalitarian and ethical commitments of health care providers and the self-interest of patients are in alignment.

■ CONCLUSION

Social injustice is built into the fabric of the health care system of the United States—the only industrialized democracy that does not define access to health care as a right and a government responsibility, and therefore does not provide universal health care coverage. Instead, access to health care is treated as a commodity to be purchased by those who are able to pay or as a partially subsidized benefit of employment—in a system that is increasingly dominated by for-profit insurance companies, pharmaceutical manufacturers, and corporate medical providers. As a consequence, almost 50 million people, including members of many working families, lack any ensured access to health care; millions more are inadequately insured; and overall expenditures—the highest per person of any country—have increased to the point of crisis. Untreated illness as well as preventable disability and mortality limit personal opportunities for social, political, and economic participation and violate fundamental principles of distributive justice.

The burdens of this unjust system fall most heavily on low-income people and racial and ethnic minorities—the populations at greatest risk and in greatest need—and contribute significantly to their poorer health status, already impaired by exposure to hazardous chemical, physical, biological, and social environments and other social determinants of poor health. Since 1965, Medicare as well as other means-tested programs and safety-net systems have improved access to medical care for poor people. Since the early 2000s, however, even these programs have been politically attacked, by laws and regulations that encourage healthy and wealthy people to withdraw from systems of shared risk and shared cost, providing them with incentives to purchase tax-sheltered private health insurance.

At the root of these injustices are ideological and political philosophies that: (a) rely on the marketplace, which is ill suited to health care; (b) invoke suspicions of government; and (c) permit health-sector corporations to spend enormous amounts of money to influence legislation and regulation. The present system, at the point of crisis, leaves the United States far behind other industrialized democracies in population health status. A health care system that ensures universal access to care through public-sector social insurance can restore the social contract and the primacy of the interests of patients and health care providers in a just and equitable system.

▓ REFERENCES

1. Rawls J. A theory of justice. Cambridge, MA: Harvard University Press, 1971.
2. Kawachi I, Kennedy BP, Wilkinson RG, eds. Income inequality and health. New York: W.W. Norton and Company, 1999: xvi.
3. Daniels N. Justice, health and health care. In: Rhodes R, Battin MP, Silvers A, eds. Medicine and social justice. New York: Oxford University Press, 2002.
4. Berkman LF, Kawachi I, eds. Social epidemiology. New York: Oxford University Press, 2000.
5. Institute of Medicine Committee on the Consequences of Uninsurance. Insuring health: Hidden costs, value lost. Washington, DC: National Academies Press, 2003.
6. Wilper AP, Woolhandler S, Lasser K, et al. Health insurance and mortality in U.S. adults. *Am J Public Health* 2009;99:2289–2295.
7. AHIP Coverage. FLASHBACK: Previous Medicare advantage cuts caused seniors to lose coverage. Available at: http://www.ahipcoverage.com/2013/02/25/flashback-previous-medicare-advantage-cuts-caused-seniors-to-lose-coverage/. Accessed February 25, 2013.
8. Institute of Medicine Committee on Understanding and Eliminating Racial and Ethnic Disparities in Health Care. Unequal treatment: Confronting racial and ethnic disparities in healthcare. Washington, DC: National Academies Press, 2001.
9. U.S. Central Intelligence Agency. The world fact book – 2012. Available at: https://www.cia.gov/library/publications/the-world-factbook/rankorder/2102rank.html. Accessed November 4, 2012.
10. U.S. Census Bureau. Health insurance: Highlights 2011. Available at: http://www.census.gov/hhes/www/hlthins/data/incpovhlth/2011/highlights.html. Accessed March 18, 2013.
11. Kaiser Commission on Medicaid and the Uninsured. Key facts about Americans without health insurance. October 2012. Available at http://www.kff.org/uninsured/upload/7451-08.pdf. Accessed November 29, 2012.
12. Institute of Medicine Committee on the Consequences of Uninsurance. Insuring health: Hidden costs, value lost. Washington, DC: National Academies Press, 2003.
13. Sommers BD, Baicker K, Epstein AM. Mortality and access to care among adults after state Medicaid expansions. *N Engl J Med* 2012;367:1025–1034.
14. Martin AB, Lassman D, Washington B, Catlin A. Growth in U.S. health spending. *Health Affairs* 2012;31:208–219.

15. Office of the Assistant Secretary for Planning and Evaluation, U.S. Department of Health and Human Services. The value of health insurance: Few of the uninsured have adequate resources to pay potential hospital bills. Available at: aspe.hhs.gov/health/reports/2011/ValueofInsurance/rb.shtml. Accessed November 17, 2012.

16. Kaiser/HRET Survey of Employer-Sponsored Health Benefits, 1999–2012. Bureau of Labor Statistics, Consumer price index, U.S. city average of annual inflation (April to April), 1999–2012. Bureau of Labor Statistics, Seasonally adjusted data from the Current Employment Statistics Survey, 1999–2012 (April to April). Available at http://facts.kff.org/chart.aspx?ch=2834,2836,2837. Accessed November 29, 2012.

17. Gabel JR, McDevitt R, Lore R, et al. Trends in underinsurance and affordability of employer coverage, 2004–2007. *Health Affairs* 2009;28:w595–w606.

18. Personal communication with S Woolhandler and DU Himmelstein concerning their estimates for 2011, based on their methodology in: Woolhandler S, Campbell T, Himmelstein DU. Costs of health care administration in the United States and Canada. *N Engl J Med* 2003;349:768–775.

19. Institute of Medicine Committee on the Quality of Health Care in America. Crossing the quality chasm: A new health system for the 21st century. Washington, DC: National Academies Press, 2001.

20. Kerr EA, McGlynn EA, Adams J, et al. Profiling the quality of care in twelve communities: Results from the CQI [Community Quality Index] study. *Health Affairs* 2004;23:247–256.

21. Agency for Healthcare Research and Quality. National Healthcare Quality and Disparities Report, 2011. Available at:http://www.ahrq.gov/research/findings/nhqrdr/nhqrdr11/qrdr11.html. Accessed November 17, 2012.

22. Davis K, Schoen C, Doty M, et al. Medicare versus private insurance: Rhetoric and reality. *Health Affairs* 2002(*Suppl web exclusives*):W311–W324.

23. Savedoff WD. Kenneth Arrow and the birth of health economics. *Bull World Health Organ* 2004;82:139–140.

24. Fein O. A report from the White House Health Care Summit. March 5, 2009. Available at http://www.pnhp.org/archives.

25. Spotlight on Poverty and Opportunity. *New York Times*/CBS News poll, April 5–12, 2010. Available at: http://www.spotlightonpoverty.org/AgingAndPovertyPolling.aspx?id=fe3387e1-f1dd-4ac4-96a1-156e53d8d334. Accessed March 18, 2013.

26. Shiels J, Haught R. The cost and coverage impact of a public plan: Alternative design options. Available at http://www.lewin.com/~/media/lewin/site_sections/publications/lewin%20cost%20and%20coverage%20impacts%20of%20public%20plan%20alternative%20design%20options%20final.pdf. Accessed November 18, 2012.

27. Eaton J, Pell MB, Mehta A. Washington lobbying giants cash in on health overhaul. March 26, 2010. Available at http://www.scpr.org/news/2010/03/26/13457/lobbying-giants-cash-in-on-health-overhaul/. Accessed November 29, 2012.

28. Kaiser Family Foundation and Health Research & Educational Trust. Employer health benefits: 2012 annual survey. Available at http://ehbs.kff.org/pdf/2012/8345.pdf. Accessed November 29, 2012.

29. Himmelstein DU, Thorne D, Warren E, Woolhandler S. Medical bankruptcy in the United States, 2007: Results of a national study. *Am J Med* 2009;122:742–746.

30. Brookings Institution. Premium support: A primer. December 16, 2011. Available at http://www.brookings.edu/research/papers/2011/12/16-premium-support-primer. Accessed November 29, 2012.

31. Physicians for a National Health Program. Proposal of the Physicians' Working Group for single-payer national health insurance. Available at http://www.pnhp.org/publications/proposal-of-the-physicians-working-group-for-single-payer-national-health-ins urance. Accessed November 25, 2012.

32. Carroll AE, Ackerman RT. Support for national health insurance among U.S. physicians: Five years later. *Ann Intern Med* 2008;148:566–567.

33. Brown S, Doyle S. Op-Chart: The Medicare Index. *New York Times*, January 28, 2004:A25.

34. Wallack AR. Single payer ahead—Cost control and the evolving Vermont model. *N Engl J Med* 2011:365;584–585.

13 Infectious Disease

■ JOIA S. MUKHERJEE AND
PAUL E. FARMER

▓ INTRODUCTION

"The Black Death"—the bubonic plague—is the epitome of a devastating infectious disease epidemic. In 1348, Europe was ravaged by its first attack of *Yersinia pestis*. In just the first 5 years of the outbreak, 24 million people perished in Europe—over one-third of the European population.[1] Plague-stricken communities lacked strategies to deal with the rapidly spreading disease and resorted to measures such as burning masses of people alive—a method considered to be a rational public health strategy at the time. Other defensive measures included banishing members of society who followed lifestyles seen as offensive to God, partaking in public processions to appease angry deities, or simply awaiting a realignment of the planets.

The plague claimed the lives of up to half of urban dwellers throughout Europe, disproportionately impacting the poor. Wealthy people could avoid the plague by physically running from it: "by fleeing early, fleeing far, and returning late."[2] Indeed, many physicians, having greater means themselves, moved to safer, less plague-ridden areas.[3]

Today, despite many advances in prevention and treatment, infectious diseases continue to plague people unequally (Figure 13–1). Although the establishment of the Global Fund to Fight AIDS, Tuberculosis and Malaria (the Global Fund) in 2002 realigned the global community's focus on increasing prevention and treatment of the major fatal infectious diseases in low-income countries, many challenges remain.[4] In 2010, there were 8.8 million new cases of tuberculosis (TB) globally and more than 1 million deaths from TB.[5] Despite a decade of impressive gains in its control and treatment, malaria claimed an estimated 655,000 lives in 2010—91 percent in Africa and nearly 90 percent in children under 5 years of age.[6] Globally, approximately 33 million people are infected with HIV, and approximately 1.5 million die of AIDS-related diseases each year.[7]

While the H5N1 virus ("avian flu") caused an epidemic concentrated in megacities in Asia, it claimed relatively few lives. In the 8 years since the initial recognition of H5N1, there have been 566 confirmed human cases and 332 deaths.[8] In contrast, rotavirus, a common pathogen, receives little attention by the media or public health officials, but is responsible for at least 527,000 deaths per year in children under 5 years of age–with more than 85 percent of those deaths occurring in low-income countries.[9]

There are several reasons for the differential attention focused on a new epidemic like H5N1 rather than on a much more serious killer like rotavirus; however,

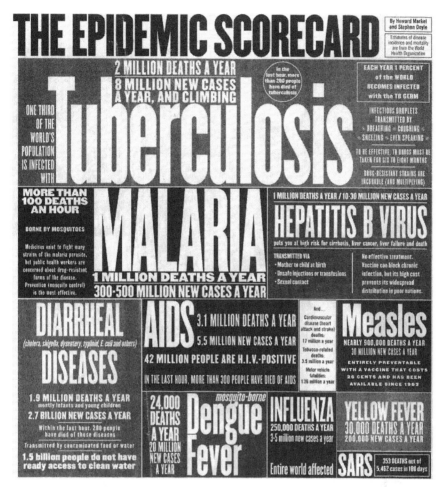

Figure 13-1 The epidemic scorecard (in 2003): "The sudden appearance of an epidemic typically inspires rapt attention, panic and action. Once the initial crisis subsides, public attention wanes although the threat of contagion continues, especially among the poor. Compare our response to severe acute respiratory syndrome (SARS), with the more familiar germs that plague us daily. When facts are few, it is easy for fear to fill the vacuum." (*Source*: Markel H, Doyle S. The epidemic scorecard. *New York Times*, April 30, 2003: A31.)

the impact of an infection on a richer, more mobile population and its resultant effects on the economy play a central role.[10] Long before the development of the germ theory of disease, it was recognized that overcrowding, lack of sanitation, and poverty exacerbate the spread of epidemic diseases. For centuries, people with control over the basic aspects of their lives—such as where to live and work and what to eat and drink—have experienced a significantly lower risk of developing infectious diseases than those without such control. Structural risks and lack of control, borne largely by poor people, have been major causes of most infectious disease epidemics.[11] Therefore, disease-prevention programs that do not address the social determinants of health are inevitably limited in their effectiveness.

This chapter focuses on (a) the causative relationship between social injustice and infectious diseases, and (b) the processes by which the disproportionate burden of infectious diseases furthers a vicious cycle of poverty and injustice. The remediation of social injustice must be at the root of global work to successfully prevent, treat, and control infectious diseases. Therefore, current public health paradigms for the prevention and treatment of infectious diseases must be altered to incorporate an ethos of social justice and human rights.

▪ THE IMPACT OF SOCIAL INJUSTICE ON INFECTIOUS DISEASES

The burden of infectious disease cases and deaths falls most heavily on people in low-income countries, as illustrated in Table 13–1 for malaria and respiratory infections. Structural inequities—from insecurity concerning housing, food, and water, to discrimination in employment and education—account for much of the disproportionate burden of infectious diseases on poor people. These marked disparities are also reflected in Table 13–2, which demonstrates a much higher prevalence of HIV infection and a much higher incidence of TB among people living in low-income countries.

Transmissible infectious diseases respect few boundaries and can freely cross both national borders (which are often permeable) and also socioeconomic boundaries (which are generally less porous). For example, a man may travel to a neighboring country to seek work in a mine. While isolated and away from home for many months, he may acquire HIV from a commercial sex worker who became infected at age 15, when she was raped by an older man in her village for whom she had worked as a domestic servant. Both she and the newly infected man may then spread the virus in their home villages and elsewhere.

TABLE 13–1 *Estimated Burden of Disease and Deaths, for Selected Diseases, by Areas of the World*

WHO Region	Burden of disease (in thousands of DALYs*), by cause, 2004		Deaths (in thousands), by cause, 2008	
	Malaria	Respiratory infections	Malaria	Respiratory infections
Africa	30,928	43,058	756	1,151
The Americas	89	3,877	1	245
Eastern Mediterranean	1,412	12,421	15	407
Europe	4	2,907	0	220
Southeast Asia	1,341	29,078	51	1,080
Western Pacific	169	6,363	4	431

*DALYs: Disability-adjusted life years.
Adapted from: World Health Organization. Disease and injury regional estimates. Cause-specific mortality: regional estimates for 2008. Available at http://www.who.int/healthinfo/global_burden_disease/estimates_regional/en/index.html. Accessed on August 22, 2012.

TABLE 13-2 *Prevalence of HIV Infection and Incidence of Tuberculosis in Selected Developing Countries and the United States*

Country	Prevalence of HIV (in percent), 2009		Incidence of tuberculosis (per 100,000 people), 2010
	Males, Age 15–24	Females, Age 15–24	
Afghanistan	NA	NA	189
Guatemala	0.5	0.3	62
Haiti	0.6	1.3	230
Iraq	NA	NA	64
Kenya	1.8	4.1	298
Pakistan	0.1	<0.1	231
Peru	0.2	0.1	106
Sierra Leone	0.6	1.5	682
South Africa	4.5	13.6	981
Vietnam	0.1	0.1	199
United States	0.3	0.2	4

Source: World Bank, 2012 World Development Indicators. Washington, DC: World Bank, 2012. Available at http://data.worldbank.org/data-catalog/world-development-indicators/wdi-2012. Accessed on August 22, 2012.

However, it is unlikely that either of them will spread HIV to a wealthy banker in Durban or a research scientist in the United States. Why? The same structures that create a disproportionate burden of infectious diseases among the poor—lack of housing, employment, land ownership, and education—also physically and socially separate poor people from wealthy people. Such structural divisions effectively concentrate and magnify the impact of infectious diseases to epidemic proportions in the most impoverished and vulnerable communities. Because these forces are embedded in ubiquitous social structures and occur wherever people are disadvantaged by political, legal, economic, or cultural factors, prevention programs must address these fundamental and widespread inequities in order to significantly decrease the transmission of infectious disease to—and within—the most vulnerable populations.

Thanks to modern medicine and public health measures, life expectancy for women in high-income countries continues to rise, now reaching 83 years. Yet over the past two decades—largely due to the AIDS pandemic—life expectancy for men in sub-Saharan Africa has decreased to 53 years.[12] The vast difference in life-expectancy trends in rich and poor nations can largely be explained by disparities in infectious disease prevalence and mortality. For example, 60 percent of all adult deaths in Africa are caused by infectious diseases, compared with only 10 percent in high-income countries.

The health data for children are also grim. Both child and infant mortality rates were greatly reduced in the 1970s and 1980s, due largely to the widespread implementation of oral rehydration therapy and infant vaccination. But these gains have been slowed—or reversed—over the past decade in the poorest countries, where diarrheal diseases, pneumonia, and malaria are now the leading causes of child and infant mortality. In 2010, the average under-5 mortality rate in low-income countries was 108 deaths per 1000 live births; in lower-middle-income countries, 69; in upper-middle-income countries, 20; and in upper-income countries, 6. On the surface, this 18-fold difference in under-5 mortality rates between low- and upper-income countries can largely be explained by the high rate of infectious gastrointestinal disease in low-income countries.[12–15] Yet even in upper-income countries, poor children suffer disproportionate morbidity from diarrheal disease, largely related to structural factors, including inadequate maternal education, substandard and transient housing, and lack of access to sanitation and clean water.[16,17] A study in Latin America and the Caribbean found the following five structural factors to be inversely related to under-5 mortality rates: use of oral rehydration therapy, access to safe water, vaccination levels, female literacy, and per-capita gross national product.[18]

▪ ROOT CAUSES AND UNDERLYING ISSUES

Preventive interventions, such as the use of DDT to control malaria north of the Panama Canal[19] and vaccinations to decrease child mortality,[20] have been great victories in public health. Social injustice, however, accounts for the enormous differences in the distribution of diseases. When unequal access to food, water, housing, and employment promote the transmission of infectious diseases, the most impoverished and vulnerable communities have neither the resources nor the capabilities at governmental, community, or personal levels to prevent these diseases.

Inadequate Support for Public Works and Infrastructure

Risk factors for the transmission of infectious diseases are often directly related to existing infrastructure. This relationship was first recognized in 1854, when John Snow traced a cholera epidemic in London to unclean water originating from one communal pump.[21] By removing the handle of that pump, he stopped the epidemic. While this intervention was simple, the structural inequalities affecting access to clean water are usually far more complex. As of 2010, at least 780 million people lacked access to clean drinking water, and 2.5 billion lacked improved sanitation.[22] The ability to construct adequate wells and sanitation systems lies beyond the economic means of many lower-income countries. In addition, under the guise of development programs and loans, international financial institutions have often imposed structural adjustment policies that further constrain the ability of poor countries to provide basic services to their citizens.[23] (See Chapter 21.)

For example, South Africa, although not as poor as many of its neighbors, still struggles to overcome inequalities stemming from decades of oppression and injustice under apartheid. Only after its transition to democracy in 1994 did South Africa begin to provide clean water to residents of the former homelands.

However, bowing under pressure from international financial institutions, programs that provided clean water were subsequently privatized and user fees were imposed. Not surprisingly, a cholera epidemic in KwaZulu Natal in 2000 was directly linked to stopping free provision of clean water to an informal settlement, whose residents were then unable to pay the new user fees.[24]

All too often, prevention strategies fail to address the structural inequities that perpetuate disease at the most basic level. For example, decentralizing and privatizing health care—another tenet of structural adjustment and neo-liberal economic reform—has severely weakened the public health infrastructure in many poor countries.[25,26]

The function of the public sector is to provide health, education, and other services to all citizens, including, and often especially, to poor people. Privatization of the health sector and the imposition of user fees in the public sector reduces the utilization of services, especially by poor people.[27–29] Such cost-recovery measures, although widely considered to be regressive, are still being implemented to force poor countries to spend less in the public sector and move toward market economies. As countries faced, and continue to face, the reality of HIV/AIDS, such policies were called into question. For example, in 2003, Uganda was awarded a grant from the Global Fund to implement an HIV-treatment program. Pursuant to preexisting stipulations of international financial institutions, however, the grant would have exceeded health care spending limits. Afraid of repercussions from the international financial institutions, the Ugandan government recommended that the money be put into the financial sector.[30] Even a physician without formal economic training wonders if the neo-liberal agenda of many international financial institutions might be increasing the risk of infectious diseases by "slapping the hands" of those who attempt to treat sick people who are poor.

Social and Economic Rights

The spread of infectious diseases is strongly linked to lack of access to services and to substandard living conditions. However, fulfilling basic social and economic rights, such as the right to adequate housing, education, and food, is not often linked to strategies for preventing infectious diseases. Disparities in housing, level of education, and nutritional status are causally linked to the disproportionate burden of infectious disease in impoverished communities. This relationship is demonstrated in the spread of airborne diseases among the poor, most notably TB. Conditions of urban poverty, including overcrowding, poor housing, and poor nutrition, continue to promote the spread of TB globally. While TB treatment is highly effective, it was not treatment that first reduced TB incidence in higher-income countries, but rather improvement of living conditions.

In the 1940s, before the advent of effective TB treatment, the incidence rate of active TB sharply decreased in New York City, mainly due to the post–World War II economic boom and the migration of people from tenements in cities to single-family homes in the suburbs. TB then strikingly increased in the United States in the 1990s,[31] fueled by HIV co-infection and structurally associated with overcrowding in prisons, increased homelessness, and cuts in government funding that led to deterioration of the public health infrastructure.[32] Similarly, the incidence of childhood acute respiratory infections in lower-income countries has been directly linked to conditions in the home environment, including inadequate food, concomitant diarrheal illness, little maternal education, and indoor cooking fires.[33,34] As is true with all infectious diseases, eradication of respiratory infections will require remediating the conditions of poverty that place people at risk and impede effective treatment.

Economic Freedom

The spread of sexually transmitted infections brings the concept of *structural violence* to an individual level. HIV/AIDS, the worst pandemic disease of our time, spreads with a strikingly unequal distribution among populations, both locally and globally.

Methods promoted by global health experts to prevent the sexual transmission of HIV/AIDS include delaying the onset of sexual intercourse, decreasing one's number of sexual partners, and using condoms. "Knowledge, attitudes, and practices" surveys and prevention strategies based on their results have been used for more than two decades to try to limit the spread of HIV/AIDS. The risk of acquiring HIV depends less on knowledge of how the virus is transmitted, however, and more on having the freedom to apply this knowledge.

Poverty is a major factor limiting such freedom. Many people who acquire HIV infection do so despite having more than enough information to protect themselves. Migration for work, domestic servitude, and exchange of sex for food, money, and survival are among the main risk factors fueling the epidemic.[35–37]

While sub-Saharan Africa is wracked by violence, not enough has been written about the increase in HIV infection after political conflict, war, or genocide.[38,39] Yet rape as a war crime is front-page news when it occurs in Europe.[40] People at high risk of HIV infection today include those who live lives of constrained choices— such as child servants who are raped by their masters, men who work in mines far from their homes, and married women who remain faithful to men who have multiple partners. Often their acute survival is contingent on maintaining or enduring the situations that put them at risk for HIV infection in the first place.

Access to Treatment

Improved treatment of infectious diseases has been a hallmark of modern medicine. The discovery of penicillin in the 1940s was quickly followed by discovery of other antimicrobials in the 1950s, including cures for previously fatal bacterial diseases such as pneumonia, endocarditis, and TB. HIV/AIDS, when it arose, presented one of the first widespread incurable infections. Highly active antiretroviral therapy (HAART), which was developed in 1996 (15 years after the first reported cases of AIDS), has dramatically prolonged and enhanced the lives of people infected with HIV.[41]

Drug Development and Market Forces

The treatment of TB illustrates how market forces, rather than disease burden, drive the development of new drugs. Globally, over 2 billion people (nearly one-third of the world's population) are infected with the TB bacillus, and TB accounts for nearly 4000 deaths every day.[42] Although resistance to anti-TB drugs has been growing, there has not been a new drug developed for TB since the 1970s. Drugs are not developed if there is no market able to pay—even for the most devastating diseases. Pharmaceutical companies often assert that it takes years to recoup the research and development costs of a new drug, but many companies spend twice as much money on advertising and marketing as they do on research and development.[43]

In higher-income countries, determined constituents are sometimes able to circumvent market-based research and development agendas, even when no obvious market exists. For example, in 1983, the U.S. Congress passed the Orphan Drug Act to encourage the development of drugs for *orphan diseases*: 6000 rare diseases and conditions that together affect approximately 25 million Americans.[44] Brought about through lobbying by those affected by these rare diseases, the Act enabled the federal government to use tax incentives to safeguard pharmaceutical companies against the financial losses they might incur in the research and development of therapies that were expected to generate relatively small sales.[45,46] In contrast, the hundreds of millions of TB patients globally, whose ability to pay for life-saving drugs is limited, have no such lobbying power.

The Use of Substandard Therapies

Utilitarian public health strategies have promoted a nihilistic approach to the treatment of some diseases. For example, the standard treatment for diarrheal disease in low-income countries is oral rehydration therapy (ORT). Although ORT is a life-saving intervention, invasive bacterial gastrointestinal infections, such as typhoid, often require antibiotics and occasionally surgical management. Case-fatality rates of untreated typhoid range from 10 to 50 percent, and children 1 to 5 years of age are at the highest risk of death. However, antibiotics are not included in the standard of care for diarrheal diseases, even when dysentery is present. Constrained choices are cited as the reason for focusing solely on ORT.[47–49]

A similar choice has historically been made in the treatment of drug-resistant TB. While multidrug-resistant tuberculosis (MDR TB) is treatable, duration of treatment is 18 months or longer with second-line anti-TB drugs, which cost significantly more than first-line drugs.[50] The cost of second-line treatment and constrained choices, in addition to policies within the international public health community that promote the use of standard anti-TB drugs to treat patients known to have MDR TB,[51] have left many of those infected with MDR TB without adequate or appropriate treatment.

Patents and Access to Pharmaceuticals

Many years after the development of HAART,[41] this life-saving treatment remained largely unused in sub-Saharan Africa, the epicenter of the epidemic; in 2002, fewer than 50,000 of the 20 million people infected with HIV were receiving treatment, largely due to cost.[52] African countries and activist groups attempted to address this problem through legal channels under the 1994 Agreement on Trade-Related Aspects of Intellectual Property Rights (TRIPS) of the World Trade Organization. Under Articles 8 and 31 of that treaty, a country facing a national emergency and needing to provide a product otherwise pro-tected by intellectual property protections and prohibitively priced may either issue a compulsory license to develop a product locally, or import, in parallel with the brand-name product, a generic version.[53] Brazil and Thailand, both with strong public health programs, began producing, during the early years of the AIDS epidemic, antiretroviral therapy for public, noncommercial use to meet the needs of their populations.[54] For invoking the flexibilities in TRIPS to manufacture AIDS drugs for public use, both countries faced sanctions from the United States.[55,56] Yet both Brazil and Thailand, by aggressively providing early HIV treatment as a public good, helped limit the epidemic.[57] In Brazil, the annual incidence of HIV infection decreased from 24,816 cases in 1998 to 7361 in 2001.[58]

Unfortunately, similar swift responses were neither seen nor supported in sub-Saharan Africa, where the HIV epidemic was far more widespread. In 2001, fully 5 years after the dramatic success of HAART was documented in the United States and Europe, several African countries began legal processes to procure generic drugs.[59,60] In 1998, several pharmaceutical companies brought suit against the government of South Africa to prevent its implementing the flexibility of complusory-licensing and parallel-importing provisions of TRIPS as they applied to HAART. Activists and people living with HIV who were still without access to therapy were able to draw significant attention to this issue, and, in 2001, the suit was dropped.[61]

Ironically, in the same year in the United States, President George W. Bush invoked TRIPS, also in response to a national emergency related to an infectious disease. In October 2001, envelopes containing spores of *Bacillus anthracis* were mailed to two U.S. senators and several news media offices. While only 23 cases (five of which were fatal) resulted from these attacks, thousands of people were thought to have been exposed. Fortunately, anthrax can be successfully treated with ciprofloxacin, a drug patented by Bayer Pharmaceuticals. The U.S. government, perceiving a national emergency, claimed that the price of the drug was too high and that it would be forced to parallel-import the generic form in order to have a sufficient stockpile. Eventually, in part due to political pressure, Bayer lowered the price from $1.80 to $1.00 per tablet, reducing the cost of a 6-week course of therapy from about $150 to about $80.[62]

Also in 2001, HIV activists from civil society organizations met in Doha, Qatar, and advocated for more specificity in implementing the flexibility of compulsory-licensing and parallel-importing provisions of TRIPS for public health purposes. This pressure led to a declaration that gave governments protections to manufacture patented drugs or import generic equivalents for public use, and opened the possibility for large-scale use of generic HAART in resource-poor settings.[63]

To address the social injustice demonstrated by the differential prevalence of infectious diseases, a holistic approach that acknowledges the social determinants of health and promotes prevention and treatment of disease is needed. This approach should be embedded in a rights-based framework (Chapter 22). The experiences of addressing social injustice related to TB and HIV demonstrate that advocacy by civil society organizations can lead to the creation of laws and funding mechanisms that improve access to health care. Indeed, in 2011, the number of people receiving antiretroviral treatment in resource-poor settings increased to 8 million, with 54 percent of eligible patients receiving treatment.[64]

▪ WHAT NEEDS TO BE DONE

The World Health Organization's Declaration of Alma-Ata (1978), with its goal of "health care for all by the year 2000,"[65] was the last such ambitious rights-based call for improved access to health care. The rights-based goals of the Declaration were straightforward: (a) 90 percent of children should have a weight-for-age that corresponds to reference values; (b) every family should be within a 15-minute walk of potable water; and (c) women should have access to medically trained attendants for childbirth. In addition, it was widely agreed that these goals could not be achieved without increased international aid. However, the right to universal basic health care proposed in the Declaration of Alma-Ata was attacked by some international health experts as naïve and too expensive. Since 1978, distribution of limited resources for health has been determined more by markets than by rights.[66] With foreign debt mounting, international financial institutions have required low-income countries, as they moved toward market-based economies, to decrease the proportion of their gross national product spent on health. Reforms in the health sector have emphasized user fees, privatization, and other cost-recovery measures. The effects of these so-called reforms have been devastating in most countries where they have been implemented.

Revitalizing the public health infrastructure and improving the delivery of essential services, such as immunization, sanitation, and the provision of clean water, are critical to addressing the social injustices that underlie and perpetuate infectious disease. Governments need to assume responsibility for the health of their people by setting rational, stable, and rights-based policies that guarantee health care for all—especially for their poorest and most vulnerable citizens. Health-sector reforms in low-income countries have often resulted in (a) chaotic implementation of services; (b) unclear lines of authority for specific tasks, such as drug purchasing; and (c) a lack of institutional memory. For example, inadequate planning and health system changes have adversely affected TB control in many countries.[67,68]

Governments of the poorest countries cannot begin to address the right to health without substantial financial assistance. Advocacy to address social injustice and the health of the poor must recognize that international financial institutions, by requiring restrictions on health spending, promote inequity in health care and perpetuate social injustice. Recent calls for debt relief are rooted in the belief that governments that spend less money paying off debt can invest more money in health and education. In addition, novel strategies to allocate more money to the health sector have been implemented, such as the Global Fund (the largest multilateral public health fund) and the U.S. President's Emergency Plan for AIDS Relief (PEPFAR—the largest single-disease funding mechanism). Since its inception in 2002, the Global Fund has disbursed $22.9 billion to more than 1000 programs in 151 countries.[4]

In order to remediate inequalities in access to health care, treatments must reach those who need them most. The World Health Organization's (WHO) Model List of Essential Medicines serves as a guide to the medications that have the greatest benefit for health. But all too often poor people have severely limited access to these essential drugs. The Millennium Development Goals (Table 21–7 in Chapter 21) were established to improve factors that most affect health and development, one of which is access to essential medicines. Without external assistance, however, these goals are out of the reach of most low-income countries.[69] The Global Drug Facility was established by the Stop TB Partnership in 2001 to coordinate bulk procurement of low-priced, quality-assured anti-TB drugs. Governments of low-income, heavily-indebted countries can apply to the Facility to obtain these drugs free of charge. Price reductions and tiered pricing systems are additional methods of decreasing inequities in treatment.[70]

In addition to strengthening the public sector, assuring the right to health requires the engagement of civil society. Encouragingly, even among vulnerable people, there are powerful examples of such engagement. The civil society movement of people living with disabilities demanded governmental changes to make buildings accessible and to end discrimination in hiring and education (Chapter 8). In countries such as India and Brazil, civil society movements have used instances of exclusion and poor health care to bring about legal action for fulfilling the right to health—even enshrining the right to health in their national constitutions. With

increasing globalization, civil society must engage with the international community as well as governments in order to assure the right to health.

■ THE AIDS MOVEMENT

Unlike any other disease in history, AIDS has spurred an effective social movement characterized by solidarity between the global North and South and by grassroots engagement in accelerating and distributing the benefits of scientific progress.
Activists argued that an approach based on human rights—as opposed to markets—was the only realistic strategy for tackling AIDS, an epidemic concentrated in
poor and marginalized communities without access to health care or the ability to
pay for treatment. The global campaign to improve access to AIDS treatment has
resulted in remarkable gains in establishing the concept of health as a right.

The global AIDS movement began as a fight against discrimination, and
quickly took up equitable access to treatment as its clarion call. As the HIV epidemic reached unprecedented infection rates in the mid-1990s, groups such as the
AIDS Coalition to Unleash Power (ACT-UP) and the Treatment Action Group
(TAG) began advocating for the U.S. Food and Drug Administration (FDA) to
speed up development of, and access to, new therapies. The pressure to develop
a treatment began to subside when new antiretroviral drugs were introduced in
the mid-1990s, and advocacy began to focus on gaining access to this treatment
for HIV-infected people in low-income countries. In response, people living with
AIDS and civil rights activists began pressuring pharmaceutical companies, health
care organizations, research institutes, and public health and other government
agencies to deliver treatment and care to the millions of HIV-positive people in
low-income countries. The AIDS movement was fueled by the stories of people
like Ryan White, an American boy who suffered profound discrimination after he
was infected with HIV, and Zackie Achmat, a South African man who refused to
take HAART until his nation's government committed to providing HAART to all
people who needed it, regardless of their ability to pay. Enlisting more than 16,000
members, the South Africa-based Treatment Action Campaign, which Achmat
founded, uses strategies of treatment literacy and community health advocacy to
provide grassroots education on HIV treatment to patients and their allies.

Transnational momentum for treatment access grew, resulting in the formation
of many civil society groups, including the Health Global Access Project (Health
GAP). Today, the successes of TAG, Health GAP, and ACT-UP are lauded for helping to remove barriers to care and improving access to, and quality of, HIV treatment. A multifaceted success, this movement brought together the international
community and the private sector, and linked the creation of a new global funding
mechanism for AIDS treatment to rights-based arguments over patents and the
fruits of scientific progress. In addition, much of the money provided for AIDS
treatment went to governments for programs that were delivered free of charge in
the public sector—which in some cases far exceeded the public-sector spending

caps imposed by international financial institutions. Although challenges remain in maintaining and expanding funding for health as a right (Chapter 22), the movement for access to AIDS treatment has enabled at least 6.6 million people in low- and middle-income countries to receive treatment.[71] The AIDS movement vividly illustrates how deep and lasting transnational solidarity in civil society can use rights-based arguments to apply strategic pressure on international duty-bearers, governments, and private-sector organizations to expand access to treatment for a pandemic infectious disease.

The AIDS movement also successfully challenged neo-liberal economic policy, which imposed restrictions on spending international aid funds in the public sector. A major policy achievement of the AIDS movement was the exemption of AIDS expenditures from fiscal constraints, using the argument that countries heavily affected by HIV must invest in treatment if they were to become "self-sufficient." Once the structural barriers to AIDS financing were overcome, a strategy was needed to provide equitable access and delivery. Activists lobbied governments of high-income countries to share responsibility for the health of all people living with HIV. Partly in response to such pressure, donor governments pledged unprecedented support to the global AIDS campaign, culminating in the creation of the Global Fund and PEPFAR. The international community's commitment to fund governments that sought to deliver treatment on a large scale marked a new human-rights paradigm of shared responsibility.

Grants from the Global Fund harness the impact and potential of partnerships between governments and non-governmental organizations (NGOs). In 2007, the Global Fund's board of directors endorsed *dual-track financing*, which requires two equal principal recipients—one a governmental implementer and the other an NGO—to submit a collaborative proposal for funding. The intentional pairing of recipients promotes (a) faster use of grant funds to provide care; (b) increased sustainability through capacity-building of weaker sectors; and (c) improved reach of service delivery to all people, especially those who are most vulnerable. By establishing dual-track financing, the Global Fund affirmed the value of coordination between governments and NGOs in strengthening health systems by complementing each other's advantages. Governments provide the standardization of national protocols and the capacity to bring programs to scale, while NGOs can ensure that target populations include marginalized patients and communities frequently neglected by government initiatives. Dual-track financing better assures implementation of health measures that are equitable, effective, and accountable to both individual patients and the general public.

■ CONCLUSION

Human suffering due to infectious disease can be alleviated if social injustice is comprehensively addressed by governments of all countries and by the international business and financial communities. Governments have a responsibility to ensure basic social and economic rights, including the right to health care, education, and access to food, water, and shelter. Large debt burdens and their associated economic stress prevent the governments of deeply impoverished countries from ensuring these rights. If the donor community were to abolish punitive structural-adjustment policies and provide debt relief, low-income countries could spend more money addressing the social injustices that are the underlying causes of disease. In addition, novel approaches are needed to ensure that the advances of science are shared equitably by all.

Risk mitigation, prevention, and care for those suffering from infectious diseases must be seen as a public good. The justifications for such ambitious initiatives include the needs of those already sick, the prevention of ongoing transmission of disease, the rectification of previous clinical and policy errors, and—perhaps most importantly—the ethical unacceptability of tolerating a lower standard of care for poor people. To substantially improve global health, we must make social justice a central component of public health.

Focusing solely on prevention fails to address the needs of those already infected or sick. Prevention is considered cheap when compared to treatment, and yet real preventive measures—the provision of safe water sources, adequate housing, and gainful employment—have not traditionally been promoted as integral components of public health strategies. Rather, these factors are relegated to the "development" sphere and most often linked with market reforms that exclude poor and vulnerable people.

Improving the lives of sick people, especially those who are poor, requires large-scale, novel, multilateral, and innovative funding strategies as well as implementation of policy reforms, such as debt relief and reinterpretation of intellectual property rights laws and trade agreements. Despite the unprecedented outpourings of funding, the global community must still do more to address the inequalities that promote the occurrence of infectious diseases. Social justice in global public health requires commitments to eliminating the structural violence caused by inequity and to treating all populations. Without a social justice approach, public health will be relegated to the historical ledger as having offered, in the face of global cataclysm, cheap and inadequate palliation rather than sustainable remediation.

■ REFERENCES

1. Haensch S, Bianucci R, Signoli M, et al. Distinct clones of *Yersinia pestis* caused the Black Death. *PLOS Pathog* 2010;6e1001134. doi:10.1371/journal.ppat.1001134.
2. Watts S, ed. Epidemics and history. New Haven, CT: Yale University Press, 1997.
3. Kiple K, ed. The Cambridge world history of human disease. Cambridge, UK: Cambridge University Press, 1993.
4. The Global Fund To Fight AIDS, Tuberculosis and Malaria. Who we are. 2012. Available at http://www.theglobalfund.org/en/about/whoweare/. Accessed on July 24, 2012.

5. World Health Organization. WHO report 2011: Global tuberculosis control. Geneva: World Health Organization, 2011.

6. World Health Organization. World malaria report: 2011. Geneva: World Health Organization, 2011.

7. UNAIDS. Report on the global AIDS epidemic 2010: Global report, 2010. Available at http://www.unaids.org/globalreport/global_report.htm. Accessed on August 15, 2012.

8. World Health Organization. Cumulative number of confirmed cases for avian influenza A/(H5N1) reported to WHO, 2003–2011. Available at http://www.who.int/influenza/human_animal_interface/EN_GIP_Latest CumulativeNumberH5N1cases.pdf. Accessed July 25, 2012.

9. Parashar UD, Burton A, Lanata C, et. al. Global mortality associated with rotavirus disease among children in 2004. *J Infect Dis* 2009;200(Suppl 1):S9–S15.

10. Marmot M. Social determinants of health inequalities. *Lancet* 2005;365:1099–1104.

11. Burris S. Law as a structural factor in the spread of communicable disease. *Houston Law Rev* 1999;36:1755–1786.

12. World Bank. World development indicators 2010. Available at http://data.worldbank.org/sites/default/files/wdi-final.pdf. Accessed on June 22, 2012.

13. Porignon D, Noterman JP, Hennart P, et al. The role of the Zaïrian Health Services in the Rwandan refugee crisis. *Disasters* 1995;19:356–360.

14. Bern C, Ortega Y, Checkley W, et al. Epidemiologic differences between cyclosporiasis and cryptosporidiosis in Peruvian children. *Emerg Infect Dis* 2002;8:581–585.

15. Akram DS, Agboatwalla M. A model for health intervention. *J Trop Pediatr* 1992;38:85–87.

16. Baker D, Taylor H, Henderson J. Inequality in infant morbidity: Causes and consequences in England in the 1990s. ALSPAC Study Team: Avon Longitudinal Study of Pregnancy and Childhood. *J Epidemiol Commun Health* 1998;52:451–458.

17. Abate G, Kogi-Makau W, Muroki NM. Health seeking and hygiene behaviours predict nutritional status of pre-school children in a slum area of Addis Ababa, Ethiopia. *Ethiopia Med J* 2000;38:253–265.

18. Moore D, Castillo E, Richardson C, et al. Determinants of health status and the influence of primary health care services in Latin America, 1990–1998. *Int J Health Plann Manage* 2003;18:279–292.

19. Najera JA. Malaria control: Achievements, problems and strategies. *Parassitologia* 2001;43:1–89.

20. Morley D. Saving children's lives by vaccination. *BMJ* 1989;299:1544–1545.

21. Vinten-Johansen P, Brody H, Paneth N, et al, eds. Cholera, chloroform, and the science of medicine: A life of John Snow. New York: Oxford University Press, 2003:115–116.

22. WHO/UNICEF Joint Monitoring Programme for Water Supply and Sanitation. Progress on drinking water and sanitation: 2012 update. New York: UNICEF and World Health Organization, 2012.

23. Kim JY, Millen J, Irwin A, eds. Dying for growth: Global inequality and the health of the poor. Monroe, ME: Common Courage Press, 1999.

24. Pauw J. The politics of underdevelopment: Metered to death—How a water experiment caused riots and a cholera epidemic. *Int J Health Serv* 2003;33:819–830.

25. Hanson S. Health sector reform and STD/AIDS control in resource poor settings—The case of Tanzania. *Int J Health Plann Manage* 2000;15:341–360.

26. Yoder RA. Are people willing and able to pay for health services? *Soc Sci Med* 1989;29:35–42.

27. Benson JS. The impact of privatization on access in Tanzania. *Soc Sci Med* 2001;52:1903–1915.

28. Ching P. User fees, demand for children's health care and access across income groups: The Philippine case. *Soc Sci Med* 1995;41:37–46.

29. Mbugua JK, Bloom GH, Segall MM. Impact of user charges on vulnerable groups: The case of Kibwezi in rural Kenya. *Soc Sci Med* 1995;41:829–835.

30. Wendo C. Uganda and the Global Fund sign grant agreement. *Lancet* 2003;361:942.

31. Frieden TR, Sherman LF, Maw KL, et al. A multi-institutional outbreak of highly drug-resistant tuberculosis: Epidemiology and clinical outcomes. *JAMA* 1996;276:1229–1235.

32. Brudney K, Dobkin J. Resurgent tuberculosis in New York City: Human immunodeficiency virus, homelessness and the decline of tuberculosis control programs. *Am Rev Respir Dis* 1991;144:745–749.

33. Hortal M, Contera M, Mogdasy C, et al. Acute respiratory infections in children from a deprived urban population from Uruguay. *Rev Inst Med Trop Sao Paulo* 1994;36:51–57.

34. Denny FW, Loda FA. Acute respiratory infections are the leading cause of death in children in developing countries. *Am J Trop Med Hygiene* 1986;35:1–2.

35. Quinn TC. Population migration and the spread of HIV types 1 and 2 human immunodeficiency viruses. *Proc Natl Acad Sci USA* 1994;91:2407–2414.

36. International Organization for Migration and Joint United Nations Programme on HIV/AIDS. Mobile populations and HIV/AIDS in the Southern African Region. Geneva: IOM and UNAIDS, 2003.

37. Chen L, Prabhat J, Stirling B, et al. Sexual risk factors for HIV infection in early and advanced HIV epidemics in sub-Saharan Africa: Systematic overview of 68 epidemiological studies. *PLoS One* 2007;3:1–14.

38. Donovan P. Rape and HIV/AIDS in Rwanda. *Lancet* 2002;360(Suppl):S17–S18.

39. Smallman-Raynor MR, Cliff AD. Civil war and the spread of AIDS in Central Africa. *Epidemiol Infect* 1991;107:69–80.

40. Acheson D. Health, humanitarian relief, and survival in former Yugoslavia. *BMJ* 1993;307:44–48.

41. Hammer SM, Squires KE, Hughes MD, et al. A controlled trial of two nucleoside analogues plus indinavir in persons with human immunodeficiency virus infection and CD4 cell counts of 200 per cubic millimeter or less. AIDS Clinical Trials Group 320 Study Team. *N Engl J Med* 1997;337:725–733.

42. World Health Organization. Tuberculosis fact sheet no. 104, March 2012. Available at http://www.who.int/mediacentre/factsheets/fs104/en/. Accessed on June 24, 2012.

43. Families USA. Off the charts: Pay, profits and spending by drug companies. Washington, DC: Families USA Foundation, 2001:3.

44. United States Congress. Public Law 107–280, Rare Diseases Act of 2002, November 6, 2002. Available at http://history.nih.gov/research/downloads/PL107-280.pdf. Accessed on August 15, 2012.

45. van Woert MH. Orphan drugs: Proposed legislative help. *N Engl J Med* 981;304:235.

46. Asbury CH, Stolley PD. Orphan drugs: creating a policy. *Ann Intern Med* 981;95:221–224.

47. Bhandari N, Bahl R, Taneja S, et al. Pathways to infant mortality in urban slums of Delhi, India: Implications for improving the quality of community- and hospital-based programmes. *J Health Popul Nutr* 2002;20:148–155.

48. Goldman N, Pebley AR, Beckett M. Diffusion of ideas about personal hygiene and contamination in poor countries: Evidence from Guatemala. *Soc Sci Med* 2001;52:53–69.

49. Goldman N, Pebley AR, Gragnolati M. Choices about treatment for ARI and diarrhea in rural Guatemala. *Soc Sci Med* 2002;55:1693–1712.

50. Mukherjee J, Rich M, Socci A, et al. Programmes and principles in treatment of multi-drug-resistant tuberculosis. *Lancet* 2004;363:474–481.

51. World Health Organization. Prevention and control of multi-drug-resistant tuberculosis and extensively drug-resistant tuberculosis, May 22, 2009. Available at http://apps. who.int/gb/ebwha/pdf_files/A62/A62_20-en.pdf. Accessed on August 15, 2012.

52. Mukherjee JS, Farmer PE, Niyizonkiza D, et al. Tackling HIV in resource poor countries. *BMJ* 2003;327:1104–1106.

53. The Joint United Nations Programme on HIV/AIDS, World Health Organization, and United Nations Development Programme. Using TRIPS flexibilities to improve access to HIV therapy: UNAIDS, WHO and UNDP policy brief, 2011. Available at http://www. undp.org/content/dam/undp/library/hivaids/Using%20TRIPS%20Flexibility%20 to%20improve%20access%20to%20HIV%20treatment.pdf. Accessed on August 15, 2012.

54. Ford N, Wilson D, Costa Chaves G, et al. Sustaining access to anti-retroviral therapy in the less developed world: Lessons from Brazil and Thailand. *AIDS* 2007;21(Suppl 14):S21–S29.

55. Sweeney R. The U.S. push for worldwide patent protection meets the AIDS crisis in Thailand: A devastating collision. Pacific Rim & Policy Journal, 2000. Available at https://digital.lib.washington.edu/dspace-law/bitstream/handle/1773.1/814/9PacRim LPolyJ445.pdf?sequence=1. Accessed on August 15, 2012.

56. Teixeira PR, Vitória MA, Barcarlo J. Anti-retroviral treatment in resource-poor settings: The Brazilian experience. *AIDS* 2004;18(Suppl 3):S5–S7.

57. Marins JRP, Jamal LF, Chen SY, et al. Dramatic improvement in survival among adult Brazilian AIDS patients. *AIDS* 2003;17:1675–1682.

58. Dados Epidemiológicos do Brasil. Boletin Epidemiológico—AIDS, 27ª a 40ª Semanas Epidemiológicas Julho a Setembro de 2001. 2002:15.

59. Siringi S. Genetic drug battle moves from South Africa to Kenya. *Lancet* 2001;357:1600.

60. Nattrass NJ. The (political) economy of anti-retroviral treatment in developing countries. *Trends Microbiol* 2008;16:574–579.

61. Barnard D. In the high court of South Africa, case no 4138/98: The global politics of access to low-cost AIDS drugs in poor countries. *Kennedy Inst Ethics J.* 2002;12:159–174.

62. Resnik DB, DeVille KA. Bioterrorism and patent rights: "Compulsory licensure" and the case of Cipro. *Am J Bioeth* 2002;2:29–39.

63. World Trade Organization. Declaration on the TRIPS agreement and public health. Ministerial Conference, 4th Session, November 14, 2001. Available at https://www.wto. org/english/thewto_e/minist…/mindecl_trips_e.doc. Accessed on August 15, 2012.

64. Kaiser Family Foundation. U.S. global health policy fact sheet: The global HIV/AIDS epidemic. November 2012. Available at http://www.kff.org/hivaids/upload/3030-17. pdf. Accessed on December 12, 2012.

65. Declaration of Alma-Ata. International Conference on Primary Health Care, Alma-Ata, USSR, September 6–12, 1978. Available at http://www2.paho.org/hq/

dmdocuments/2010/PHC_Alma_Ata-Declaration-1978.pdf. Accessed on November 26, 2012.

66. Hall JJ, Taylor R. Health for all beyond 2000: The demise of the Alma-Ata Declaration and primary health care in developing countries. *Med J Aust* 2003;178:17–20.

67. Kritski AL, Ruffino-Netto A. Health sector reform in Brazil: Impact on tuberculosis control. *Int J Tuberc Lung Dis* 2000;4:622–626.

68. Bosman MC. Health sector reform and tuberculosis control: The case of Zambia. *Int J Tuberc Lung Dis* 2000;4:606–614.

69. World Health Organization. Health-related Millennium Development Goals out of reach for many countries. *Bull WHO* 2004;82:156–157.

70. Berman D. AIDS, essential medicines, and compulsory licensing. *J Int Assoc Physicians AIDS Care* 1999;5:24–25.

71. Joint United Nations Programme on HIV/AIDS (UNAIDS). UNAIDS data tables 2011. Available at http://www.unaids.org/en/media/unaids/contentassets/documents/unaidspublication/2011/JC2225_UNAIDS_datatables_en.pdf. Accessed on August 15, 2012.

14 Nutrition

■ J. LARRY BROWN

■ INTRODUCTION

Poor nutritional status leads to adverse health outcomes. In both developing and developed countries, there is a strong association between poor nutrition in vulnerable populations and poverty, inequality, and other manifestations of social injustice (Figure 14–1). (See Box 21–2 in Chapter 21.)

■ INADEQUATE NUTRITION: THE U.S. CONTEXT

In 1966, a team of physicians commissioned by the Field Foundation studied areas of endemic poverty in the United States: migrant labor camps, Indian reservations, urban slums, and small towns in the Mississippi Delta. In their report to the U.S. Congress the following year, they underscored the desperate circumstances they had found: "If you go look, you will find America a shocking place. No other Western country permits such a large population of its people to endure the lives we press on our poor. To make four-fifths of a nation more affluent than any other people in history, we have degraded one-fifth mercilessly."[1,2] It was common, the team reported, for poor infants and young children to have no milk to drink because their parents did not have the money to purchase it. Hunger was widespread. Many households had little, or sometimes nothing, to eat for several days each month. Kwashiorkor, a form of severe malnutrition usually associated with Third World conditions of starvation, was not uncommon. It was seen in African American children whose black hair had turned yellow, in Native American children with sunken eyes and rotted teeth, and in the protruding abdomens and thin limbs of children in migrant camps and city slums. (See Box 14–1 for definitions of *hunger, malnutrition*, and related terms.)

These shocking findings provoked enough public outrage to galvanize President Richard Nixon, a Republican, and the U.S. Congress, then controlled by the Democratic Party, into action.[3] The Food Stamp Program was expanded from a pilot effort reaching only 2 million poor households to a national program covering 10 times that number.[4] The federal school lunch program was augmented with a parallel school breakfast program; feeding programs for older people were begun; and the Special Supplemental Food Program for Women, Infants, and Children (WIC) was established.[5] This collective policy response, viewed by political leaders as a wise investment in the nation's future,[6] produced remarkable results. A decade later, the team of physicians returned to the same areas and reported to

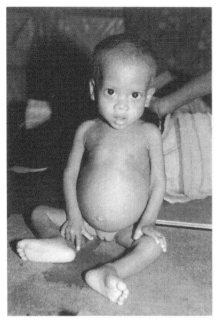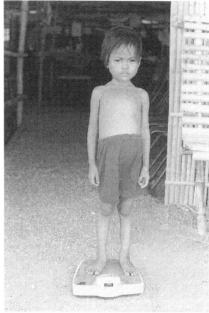

Figure 14-1 Malnutrition among children in a Cambodian refugee camp in 1980. *Left*: Young child with kwashiorkor, a severe form of malnutrition. *Right*: Seven-year-old girl with severe malnutrition who weighed only 27 pounds. Much hunger and malnutrition occurred among Cambodians during the genocidal regime of Pol Pot in the late 1970s. (Photographs by Barry S. Levy.)

BOX 14-1 ■ Definitions of Key Terms

Food deprivation
Involuntary lack of access to an adequate diet, typically associated with poverty and low income status.

Food insecurity
The condition of not knowing where one's next meal will come from, going without enough to eat, cutting back on adequate nutritional intake, and/or reliance on charitable handouts.

Hunger
Defined by the federal government as a "painful sensation" associated with inadequate food intake. The scholarly community considers hunger to be the chronic under-consumption of adequate food and nutrients associated with inadequate income. (Pain is not the only, or even a necessary, outcome.)

Malnutrition
A general term referring to severe impairment of health and/or mental function that results from chronic failure to receive adequate nutrients in the diet.

Congress that, while poverty remained a significant problem, hunger was no longer widespread.[5] This conclusion was later borne out by university-based scholars and national nutrition surveys.[7,8]

The success, however, would be short-lived. The first official recognition that hunger had reappeared came in 1982 from the U.S. Conference of Mayors.[9] From 1980, the news media had been reporting locally and regionally on what would become a national phenomenon: increasing bread lines and soup kitchens in the United States.[10] The mayors termed hunger "a most serious emergency," and some, like the mayors of Detroit and Salt Lake City, called the situation "a national tragedy and a national disgrace."[11] In 1983, a study commissioned by the U.S. Department of Agriculture (USDA) found that hunger was growing across the nation "at a frenetic pace"[12]; however, the Ronald Reagan administration ordered that these findings not be released. They became known only because low-level civil servants, angered by the suppression of the study, gave copies to the media.[13]

The first authoritative calculation of the extent of hunger in the United States was published in the 1985 report of the Harvard-based Physician Task Force on Hunger in America, entitled "Hunger in America: The Growing Epidemic." This group estimated the number of people affected by hunger to be 20 million[11] (9 percent of the U.S. population)—a number challenged by the Reagan administration, for which the problem had political overtones.[14]

There was then no universally accepted definition of hunger. The Harvard-based physician group defined *hunger* as "chronically inadequate nutritional intake due to low income status."[11] Whether chronic or episodic in nature, hunger was the lack of sufficient calories and nutrients for physical growth or the maintenance of good health. Frequently extending over longer periods, hunger can lead to serious chronic health conditions in both children and adults.

Since 1995, the U.S. government has used its own measure of nutritional deprivation, based on an annual survey conducted by the U.S. Census Bureau as part of its Current Population Survey. Known as the "Federal Hunger and Food Security Module"[15] and annually released by the USDA, this survey consistently supported estimates that the number of Americans living in households with serious food problems was more than 30 million. The latest report, published in 2010, placed this number at nearly 49 million U.S. residents (14.5 percent of the population).[16]

The federal standard designates any person having food-access problems as *food insecure*, including (a) people experiencing the pangs of hunger, (b) those who do not eat what they know they need because they cannot buy it, and (c) those who have no idea where their next meal will come from. However, the federal standard also has a subcomponent: households that it terms "hungry." Oddly, its official definition of hunger is far more conservative than its own survey justifies. *Hunger* is defined as a "painful sensation," meaning that its victims must experience abdominal pain before they are considered hungry.[15] Not only is this definition not reflective of its survey questions, but it also has little basis in science. Abdominal pain is neither the first nor the only consequence of being hungry.

Moreover, many people who experience hunger report no pain at all; others who experience pain report that it passes with time.[17,18] In other words, "pain" is neither a necessary—nor a sufficient—definition of hunger. Whether or not people experience pain, their nutrient intake may be inadequate for optimal health and productivity.

It is with this backdrop—a nation carrying the burden of nearly 49 million people without adequate nutrition—that we can examine what hunger does to its victims and why it occurs amid extravagant wealth.

■ THE IMPACT OF SOCIAL INJUSTICE ON NUTRITION

While debate about the causes and remedies of hunger is conducted in the political arena, hunger itself is a public health issue. The adverse consequences of chronic under-nutrition, as well as the social sequelae, make hunger a critical problem for the nation. Moreover, an increasing body of knowledge points to the problem of obesity as a health consequence frequently associated with inadequate income and even hunger.[19] (See Box 14–2.)

In the United States, hunger presents quite differently than it does in developing nations. (See Box 21–2 in Chapter 21.) Protein-calorie malnutrition, or marasmas, and kwashiorkor, characterized by adequate calories but extreme protein deficiency, now occur in the United States only rarely.[20] Instead, hunger in this country typically takes the form of what the World Health Organization calls "silent undernutrition."[21] It is reflected in young children who are several pounds beneath the low end of the pediatric growth chart. They may simply look like thin children, but a trained health professional will recognize that they are experiencing growth failure. Although their symptoms are different from those of malnourished children in developing countries, they are, from a health perspective, in difficulty. (See Box 5–1 in Chapter 5 for a comparison between the United States and other developed countries.)

Because children grow and their height and weight gains are plotted on internationally used pediatric growth charts, they are perhaps the easiest population group in which to detect the consequences of inadequate nutrition. Typically, youngsters who fall below the 5th percentile in weight-for-height or height-for-age on growth charts are candidates for further investigation. Normally, 5 percent of any population is expected to fall in this low end of the range; but, in studies of low-income children, 10 to 15 percent do so. This indicates that what is being observed is not normal genetic variation but rather a "human-made" outcome. Moreover, this analysis is confirmed in the work of child development clinics in urban teaching hospitals throughout the United States, where children experiencing growth failure due to poverty are nursed back to health with appropriate nutrition.

While the relationship between inadequate nutritional intake and health status reflected in the height and weight of children is well established, scientific research

---

BOX 14-2 ■ Obesity

Research has shed light on the paradox of obesity among low-income households that experience food insecurity and hunger. Obesity itself is now at epidemic proportions in the United States, as an increasing proportion of people are affected by the social causes of high energy consumption and/or inadequate expenditure of energy through exercise. Ironically, this problem also affects poor people. It is reasonable to wonder how people who do not get enough to eat can become obese.

Hunger exists when people lack access to an adequate diet because they do not have enough money to purchase what they need to eat. Their dietary purchases are limited to cheaper, more-filling foods that produce the sensation of being full. Healthier foods, such as vegetables and fruit, especially those with necessary micronutrients, cannot be purchased.[1] Instead, many poor families rely on diets of macaroni and cheese, biscuits and gravy, and hamburgers and French fries at fast-food restaurants—a "good buy" from a caloric perspective, filling the body with cheap calories to stave off hunger. In the short term, the stomach is not an intelligent organ; it knows when it is full, not whether it has had an adequate meal.

Researchers are now studying several aspects of the hunger–obesity relationship.[2,3] One aspect is the need of people with limited money to buy food to maximize caloric intake in order to stave off hunger. The greater their economic constraints, the harder it is for families to achieve the nutritional quality they need in their diets.[2,4] This *economic roulette*, in turn, produces a tradeoff between quantity and quality of food. Households go through a succession of coping strategies to try to get by. They first reduce overall food expenditures, they then change the quality and variety of their food intake, and ultimately, if forced, they also reduce the quantity of their food intake. Parents consistently reduce their own intake first to protect that of their children, but often both children and parents reduce their food intake. Overall, the primary goal of households faced with not enough money to eat right is to consume enough to not feel hungry. Theirs is a tradeoff of quantity over quality, with resulting obesity.

Obesity also can be an adaptive response when food availability is unreliable. Chronic food shortages related to low income lead people to overeat when food is available. This cycle often results in weight gain. The body then experiences physiological changes designed to help conserve energy when it is available. It compensates for periodic shortages by becoming more efficient at storing more calories as fat.

In the future, researchers will learn still more about how the social injustice that produces hunger in America also produces obesity among many of its victims.

Box References

1. Basiotis PP. Validity of the self-reported food sufficiency status item in the U.S. Department of Agriculture's food consumption surveys. In: Haldeman VA, ed. American Council on Consumer Interests 38th Annual Conference: the proceedings. Columbia, MO: American Council on Consumer Interests 38th Annual Conference, 1992.
2. Darmon N, Ferguson EL, Briend A. A cost constraint alone has adverse effects on food selection and nutrient density: An analysis of human diets by linear programming. *J Nutr* 2002;132:3764–3771.

3. Radimer KL, Olson CM, Greene JC, et al. Understanding hunger and developing indicators to assess it in women and children. *J Nutr Educ* 1992;24:36S–45S.
4. Townsend MS, Peerson J, Love B, et al. Food insecurity is positively related to overweight in women. *J Nutr* 2001;131:1738–1745.

in recent years has broadened our understanding of other insidious effects. Direct links exist between inadequate food intake and a variety of poor developmental outcomes in children. The health status of children from impoverished homes experiencing hunger and food insecurity is much worse than that of other children. They get sick more often, have much higher rates of both iron deficiency anemia and serious ear infections, and are hospitalized more frequently.[22]

As a result, low-income children miss more days of school and are less prepared to learn when they do attend, making the relationship among food intake, health status, and learning far more poignant than previously understood. Further exacerbating this interactive impairment of young bodies and minds are behavioral and emotional outcomes that accompany food deprivation. Poorly nourished children have significantly higher rates of emotional problems, mental disorders, and withdrawn or disruptive behavior.

Household food insufficiency is associated with overall declines in general health.[23,24] In one U.S. national study, food-insufficient preschool and school-aged children had elevated rates of stomachaches, headaches, and colds.[23,24]

Other studies have corroborated these results and reported additional ones. In a multi-state study of low-income families, hungry children under the age of 12 had twice the rate of anemia of non-hungry children in low-income households.[25] Hungry children also have higher rates of visits to emergency departments and physicians.[25]

Food deprivation is associated with considerable psychological and emotional distress in children. In controlled studies, low-income children from households with inadequate food were more likely to exhibit impaired psychosocial functioning, including higher levels of anxiety, irritability, hyperactivity, and aggression.[26,27] In a U.S. national sample, children from food-deprived households manifest significantly higher levels of aggressive, destructive, and withdrawn behavior.[28] Related outcomes apparently also extend into the teenage years. Two studies have shown that food-insufficient teenagers are more likely to have no friends and to exhibit both depressive disorders and suicidal behaviors.[29] Such effects, not surprisingly, seem to also be expressed in the educational environment. Hungry children are much more likely to have had mental health counseling and to require special education services.[27,28]

Nutritional status and cognitive function in children are strongly linked. Children from food-insufficient households do not perform as well on academic achievement tests as those from food-sufficient households. In some studies, hungry children not only have higher rates of tardiness and absence, but also are more likely to have to repeat a grade in school. For example, in two U.S. national studies of elementary school children, household food hardships were negatively correlated with school test results and achievement test results.[28–30] In another national study of kindergartners, children from food-deprived households not only entered school less prepared to learn mathematics, but also learned less over the course of the year.[31]

Food deprivation impairs cognitive function.[32] In a nutrient-deprived state, the body allocates energy first to critical organ function, then to height and weight gain, and then to the role of the nervous system in one's interaction with the environment, including listening to parents, dealing with peers, and learning. If there is insufficient energy to enable a child to carry out the latter activities, cognitive dysfunction results. Children from hungry and food-insecure homes are more likely to repeat grades,[26,27,29,30] be absent or late,[25,33] and be suspended from school.[29,30] The public health and economic implications of all this evidence are significant. (See also Chapter 5.)

In general, low-income families know what constitutes a nutritious diet as well as other families.[34] Because limited income constrains their purchasing choices— for example, fresh fruits and vegetables typically are too expensive for them—their intake of required nutrients is significantly lower than both the recommended dietary allowances (RDAs) of the Institute of Medicine and that of the general population.[35]

Pregnancy is a period of significant risk from dietary inadequacy because a woman needs nutrient energy not only for herself, but also for the developing fetus. Stores of maternal nutrients may be depleted, and maternal anemia can be one consequence. The primary risk is borne by the fetus, including prematurity (birth at less than 37 weeks of gestation) and low birthweight (less than 2500 grams, or approximately 5.5 pounds). Infants born too early or too small, or both, are not well equipped for extrauterine life. Sequelae include respiratory distress syndrome, weakening of the immune system, and long-term developmental problems. The most paramount threat, however, is death, because low–birthweight infants account for 75 percent of deaths to infants in the first month of life (neonatal deaths).[36]

Older people are another highly vulnerable population for food deprivation. In old age, the risk factors associated with not having enough to eat are heightened by the circumstances associated with aging. Chief among these are chronic conditions, such as hypertension, coronary artery disease, and diabetes, at least one of which affects 85 percent of people over age 65.[13] Other factors impairing health status in older people that are associated with food intake are deficiency diseases, such as osteoporosis, and conditions that impair digestion.[37] In addition, older people have a heightened vulnerability to infection, and their risk of infection is increased significantly when their diet is constrained by limited income for purchase of appropriate foods. (See also Chapter 6.)

■ ROOT CAUSES AND UNDERLYING ISSUES

Why do so many people in the wealthiest nation have an inadequate food supply? Several factors are commonly cited. I will critique the first two, which are
myths, and then address the actual cause.

There Is Not Enough Food to Go Around (Myth 1)

In fact, not only does the United States produce enough food for all its people,
but some experts estimate that it has the capacity to also feed most of the hungry people in the world.

The Poor Make Bad Purchasing Choices (Myth 2)

President Ronald Reagan once suggested that the poor simply are "too
ignorant."[38] Scholarly analysis sheds a different light on the situation. All population groups could learn more about getting better nutritional value for each
dollar spent on food. Too many non-nutritious purchases are made, and too few
healthy diets are the norm. But no evidence suggests that low-income households make poorer food-purchasing choices than other households do. Indeed,
the Continuing Survey of Food Consumption suggests that poor households do
as well as non-poor households in knowing what they should purchase. They
simply do not have the money to do it. Furthermore, hunger in the United
States increases or decreases from year to year. Were we seeing hunger resulting
from ignorance, it is not likely that it would vary over time.

The Underlying Cause: Social Injustice

How, then, are we to understand why there are about 49 million people in the
United States without enough to eat? We need to consider some of the components of social injustice: the economy, wages, poverty, and related public
policies. Virtually all food deprivation and its adverse health consequences are
the direct or indirect outcome of social injustice—human actions that include
policy decisions.

To see how human actions can create food deprivation in the United States, consider that hunger in this country seemed largely under control during the 1970s,
but it returned with a vengeance in the early 1980s. Within a few years, bread lines
and soup kitchens markedly increased in each major city.[11] Clearly, something had
abruptly changed the situation: At that time, a national recession led to a high
unemployment rate and unusually high interest rates. Millions of people lost their
jobs, thousands of farmers lost their livelihood, and many people once secure in
their middle-class existence were laid off from their jobs due to downsizing and
then reentered the labor market with much lower incomes. While the recession

was significant, it was not unprecedented; the United States had experienced some tough economic circumstances not too many years earlier, but that period did not have a proliferation of bread lines and soup kitchens. The phenomenon in the 1980s had not been seen since the Great Depression of the 1930s. Something else was occurring.

The return of hunger was not due to the economic recession, but rather to new public policy that was adopted as more households were becoming vulnerable. Starting in 1982, the Reagan administration submitted its first 4-year budget (for the 1982–1985 period)—the Omnibus Budget and Reconciliation Act. It was passed by a Democratic Congress, largely as submitted. This budget cut more than $12 billion from the federal food program safety net that had been created during the late 1960s and early 1970s. Nearly $8 billion was cut from the Food Stamp Program, largely through reducing the allotment or value of the stamps to an average of $0.72 per person per meal. An additional $4 billion was cut from child nutrition programs, such as the school breakfast program.

In sum, more people jobless during a recession, together with the intentional weakening of federal programs to feed people during tough times, led to more bread lines and soup kitchens. Hunger was the inevitable product of political choices made at the time. Although we cannot always predict or control the national economy or the well-being of individual households, we can protect families from the occasional vicissitudes of the economy.

For more than a decade, the number of those experiencing food deprivation in the United States has remained relatively stable, at about 30 million people. But, the combination of the recession that began in 2008, the slow economic recovery in the years since, and changes that Congress made in nutrition programs increased food deprivation to more than 49 million people—a dramatic increase.

At the end of 1999—the peak of the boom—the average hourly wage was $11.87, lower than it had been in 1979: $12.05 (adjusted for inflation). For salaried workers, the median weekly income was $567 in 1999, about the same as in the 1970s, when it was $558. In 1999, the per-capita annual income of the poorest quintile of the labor market earned $13,320, compared with $13,540 in 1979 (in constant dollars). In contrast, in this 20-year period, the richest quintile increased its per-capita annual income to $45,000.

In terms of wealth, inequality is even more striking. The bottom four quintiles own 4 percent of the nation's wealth, compared with the richest 1 percent who own 48 percent. Hunger and food deprivation exist in the United States because we are tolerating such great inequality. When our nation's nutrition-policy safety net is so threadbare, such economic disparities are destined to have a profound impact.

■ WHAT NEEDS TO BE DONE

Two avenues exist to remedy hunger and other forms of nutritional deprivation in the United States: to treat the symptom and to address the root cause of the problem—the growing inequality in both income and wealth that affects an increasing number of people.

It is possible to end hunger without addressing poverty and inequality—the quicker, easier, and less costly approach for now. Hunger in the United States could be ended by the President and Congress within 6 months by fully funding and utilizing existing programs for people in need. For an estimated $12 to $15 billion a year over current spending,[39] we could:

- Better fund the Food Stamp Program and extend it to the 45 percent of eligible people that it now fails to reach
- Mandate that all schools offer the federal school breakfast program and that all communities with low-income children participate in the federally funded summer food program
- Expand the provision of after-school snacks
- Increase the coverage of feeding programs for older people

Implementation of these measures and some fine-tuning of a handful of other federal programs, such as WIC and Head Start, would mean that no one in the United States would go hungry or need to demean themselves by taking their children to eat at a soup kitchen.

We can also work to address the structural injustices that cause hunger. This will require a reconstruction of the social contract—the nature of the relationship between government and households. The social contract that had been the hallmark of social policy since the New Deal has eroded dramatically over the past three decades due to regressive social policies that have removed much protection for those most vulnerable.

The most likely policy construct through which a new social contract might be built is referred to as *asset development policy*.[40] To reach middle-class living standards, households need (a) income; (b) financial wealth, in the form of a home, a savings account, investments, and a retirement plan; and (c) human capital assets, such as a good education and skill-based training.

This new policy construct is based on long-standing U.S. government policies. The Homestead Act of another era, or, more recently, the GI Bill, was a federal policy that invested in asset-building through the promotion of property ownership, home ownership, and higher education. Millions of military personnel, for example, entered the middle class through this form of governmental largesse. Currently, many people benefit through other governmental investments, such as pretax retirement accounts, home mortgage deductions, and college loan funds—all of which help household members accrue the assets they need for economic security and well-being.

What has been good government policy for the many, however, has not been extended to the downtrodden. Social policy has seen most Americans as targets of governmental investments, but poor people as a drain on the economy. The new vision of asset-based social policy, however, is to treat all households as targets of government investment so that people in low-income households, like other Americans, can acquire the assets they need for greater independence and security.

This transformation can be achieved in numerous ways,[41] as the following examples illustrate:

- By indexing the minimum wage to inflation, and restoring it to at least its purchasing power of, for example, the 1970s, we can ensure that no working people bring home paychecks insufficient to feed the family.
- Similarly, the Earned Income Tax Credit (EITC) can be expanded, along with its state tax corollary, to ensure adequate household incomes.
- Individual development savings accounts (IDAs) can be provided to help low-income people accrue wealth.
- Home ownership can be expanded through set-aside savings plans, whereby part of the rents paid by public housing tenants are placed into dedicated accounts so they can save for down payments on homes.
- Children's savings accounts (CSAs) can be created whereby, for example, each child born in the United States would receive a $10,000 investment in a dedicated account. The investment could be matched in subsequent years by other federal investments and/or be augmented by family contributions. The original investment could grow to $50,000 or more by the time a child reached college age, and $500,000, if left to accrue until retirement. Moreover, CSAs could be earmarked for specific purposes, such as a college education, a first home, the establishment of a business, or retirement income.

The beauty of asset development policy is that it is universal, treating rich and poor people alike. It is built on the widely shared values of work, responsibility, meaningful opportunity, and reward.

■ CONCLUSION

Social injustice in the United States has many adverse effects. Few are as troubling as hunger. Seven thousand years after the first cities were established to ensure food security, the wealthiest country in the history of the world is incapable of doing the same. But hunger, as we have seen, stems not from a shortage in the food supply or from lack of capacity and know-how, but rather from structural inequalities built into the U.S. economy and social system.

While it is possible to end hunger in the United States within a year by better using the federal programs designed to feed those at risk, it is also possible to address the root cause of food insecurity by reframing the nation's social contract. Government policy that invests in all households—rather than some—and narrows disparities in income and wealth—rather than widening them—will end hunger and also the many other adverse health outcomes that result from social injustice.

■ REFERENCES

1. Citizens' Board of Inquiry into Hunger and Malnutrition in America. Hunger USA. Boston: Beacon Press, 1968:4.
2. Subcommittee on Employment, Manpower and Poverty, Committee on Labor and Public Welfare, U.S. Senate. Poverty: Hunger and federal food programs background information. Washington, DC: U.S. Government Printing Office, 1967.
3. Brown JL. Hunger USA: The public pushes Congress. *J Health Soc Behav* 1970;11:4.
4. Select Committee on Nutrition and Human Needs, U.S. Senate. Hunger 1973 and press reaction. Washington, DC: Government Printing Office, 1973:1–74.
5. Citizens' Board of Inquiry into Hunger and Malnutrition in America. Hunger USA revisited. New York: Field Foundation, 1977.
6. McGovern G. Testimony before the U.S. House of Representatives, Select Committee on Hunger. Washington, DC: USGPO, 1984.
7. Allen JE, Gadson KE. Nutritional consumption patterns of low-income households. In: Elimination of the purchase requirement in the Food Stamp Program. Washington, DC: USDA Economic Research Service, 1979.
8. Radzikowski J. National evaluation of school nutrition programs: Final report executive summary. Washington, DC: USDA Office of Analysis and Evaluation, 1983.
9. U.S. Conference of Mayors. Human services in FY82. Washington, DC: U.S. Conference of Mayors, 1982.
10. Brown JL, Pizer H. Living hungry in America. New York: Mentor, 1987.
11. Physician Task Force on Hunger in America. Hunger in America: The growing epidemic. Middletown, CT: Wesleyan University Press, 1985:12–14.
12. Social and Scientific Systems. Report on nine case studies of emergency food assistance programs. Washington, DC: USDA, 1983.
13. Brown JL, Allen D. Hunger in America. *Annu Rev Public Health* 1988;9:503–526.
14. Bode JW, Bauer GL, Brown JL. Letters. *Scientific American* 1987;255.
15. Abt Associates, Center on Hunger and Poverty, Cornell University Division of Nutritional Sciences, CAW Associates. Household food security in the United States in 1995. Alexandria, VA: USDA Food and Nutrition Service, 1996.
16. Coleman-Jensen A, Nord M, Andrews M, Carlson S. Household food security in the U.S. 2010, Economic Research Report No. (ERR-125). U.S. Department of Agriculture, September 2011. Available at http://www.ers.usda.gov/publications/err125/. Accessed on June 22, 2012.
17. DeCastro J, Elmore DK. Subjective hunger relationships with meal patterns in the spontaneous feeding behaviors of humans. *Physiol Behav* 1987;43:159–165.
18. Ogden J, Wardle J. Cognitive restraint and sensitivity to cues for hunger and satiety. *J Physiol Behav* 1990;47:477–481.
19. Center on Hunger and Poverty, Food Research and Action Center (CHPFRAC). The paradox of hunger and obesity in America. Boston, MA, and Washington, DC: CHPFRAC, September, 2003.
20. Listernack R, Christoffel K, Pace J, et al. Severe primary undernutrition in U.S. children. *Am J Dis Child* 1985;139:1157–1160.
21. World Health Organization. Toward a better future: Maternal and child health. Geneva: WHO, 1980.
22. Center on Hunger and Poverty. The consequences of hunger and food insecurity for children: Evidence from recent scientific studies. Waltham, MA: Brandeis University, 2002.

23. Alaimo K, Olson CM, Frongillo EA, et al. Food insufficiency, family income and health in preschool and school-aged children. *Am J Public Health* 2001;91:781–786.

24. Casey PH, Szeto K, Lensing S, et al. Children in food insufficient low-income families: Prevalence, health and nutrition status. *Arch Pediatr Adolesc Med* 2001;155:508–514.

25. Wehler CA, Scott RI, Anderson JJ. Community Childhood Hunger Identification Project. Washington, DC: Food Research and Action Center, 1995.

26. Kleinman, RE, Murphy JM, Little M, et al. Hunger in children in the United States: Potential behavioral and emotional correlates. *Pediatrics* 1998;101:E3.

27. Murphy JM, Pagano ME, Nachmani J, et al. The relationship of school breakfast to psychosocial and academic functioning. *Arch Pediatr Adolesc Med* 1998;152: 899–907.

28. Reid LL. The consequences of food insecurity for child well-being: An analysis of children's school achievement, psychological well-being and health. Joint Center for Poverty Research Working Paper 137. Chicago: JCPR, Northwestern University, 2000.

29. Alaimo K, Olson CM, Frongillo EA. Family food insufficiency, but not low family income, is positively associated with dysthymia and suicide symptoms in adolescents. *J Nutr* 2002;132:719–725.

30. Alaimo K, Olson CA, Frongillo EA. Food insufficiency and American school-aged children's cognitive, academic and psychosocial development. *Pediatrics* 2001;108:44–53.

31. Winicki J, Jemison K. Food insecurity and hunger in the kindergarten classroom: Its effects on learning and growth (mimeograph). Washington, DC: USDA Economic Research Service, 2001.

32. Brown JL, Pollitt E. Malnutrition, poverty and intellectual development. *Scientific American* 1996;274:38–43.

33. Murphy JM, Wehler CA, Pagano ME, et al. Relationship between hunger and psychosocial functioning in low-income American children. *J Am Acad Child Adolesc Psychiatry* 1998;37:163–170.

34. Science and Education Administration, Department of Agriculture. Food consumption and dietary levels of low-income households, nationwide food consumption survey, preliminary report, No. 8. Washington, DC: USDA, 1991.

35. Martin KS, Cook J. Differences in nutrient adequacy among poor and non-poor children. Waltham, MA: Center on Hunger and Poverty, Brandeis University, 1995.

36. Child Health Outcomes Project. Monitoring the health of America's children: Ten key indicators. Chapel Hill, NC: University of North Carolina, 1984.

37. Franz M. Nutritional requirements of the elderly. *J Nutr Elderly* 1981;1:39–56.

38. Reagan R. President's news conference on foreign and domestic issues. *New York Times,* July 24, 1984.

39. Brown JL. Letter to members of Congress. Waltham, MA: Center on Hunger and Poverty, Brandeis University, April 2001.

40. Brown JL, Beeferman L. From New Deal to new opportunity. *American Prospect* February 12, 2001.

41. Beeferman LW, Venner SH. Promising state asset development practices: A resource guide for policymakers and the public. Waltham, MA: Asset Development Institute, Center on Hunger and Poverty, Brandeis University; April 2001.

15 Chronic Non-Communicable Disease

■ KAREN R. SIEGEL,
K.M. VENKAT NARAYAN, AND
DEREK YACH

▓ INTRODUCTION

When considering global health disparities, public health workers tend to focus on infectious diseases, hunger, and poor access to medical care. This focus has become entrenched in the priorities and spending patterns of international donors and health agencies. (See Box 15–1.) As a result, major chronic diseases—or non-communicable diseases (NCDs)—that kill many people and cause considerable suffering have been neglected.

Approximately 57 million deaths occurred globally in 2008. Four NCDs accounted for 36 million (63 percent) of these deaths:

- Cardiovascular disease (CVD), especially coronary heart disease (CHD) and stroke, which caused 17 million deaths
- Cancer, which caused 7.6 million deaths
- Chronic respiratory disease, which caused 4.2 million deaths
- Diabetes mellitus, which caused 1.3 million deaths

Almost 80 percent of deaths due to NCDs occurred in low- and middle-income countries, where they tend to occur at younger ages. Globally, one-fourth of NCD deaths occur before the age of 60. In low- and middle-income countries, 29 percent of NCD deaths occur prematurely, compared to 13 percent in high-income countries.[1] Figure 15–1 shows the probability of dying prematurely from a chronic disease in various regions.[2] Mental health problems are leading contributors to the burden of disease in many countries.[3] (See Chapter 16.) They contribute significantly to the incidence and severity of many chronic diseases, including CVD and cancer. Overall, NCD deaths are projected to increase by 15 percent between 2010 and 2020, with the greatest increases in Africa, the Eastern Mediterranean, and Southeast Asia.[1]

Given the profound burden of NCDs, their disproportionate impact on poor people, and the availability of cost-effective treatment and prevention measures,[4] the neglect of NCDs is a major social injustice. Differences in morbidity and mortality rates of NCDs and their risk factors—by gender, race and ethnicity, and socioeconomic status—account for a significant proportion of the disparities in survival and quality of life within a population. However, appropriate policies and programs can reduce these inequalities. This chapter addresses mainly the socioeconomic dimensions of social injustice and NCD risks. Gender aspects have been reviewed elsewhere.[5]

BOX 15-1 ■ Who Neglects the Global Burden of Chronic Diseases?

Here are some of the "actors" who have neglected chronic diseases.

Heads of State

Heads of state of the eight major industrial democracies (which form the G8), in 2000, recognized health as a global challenge, acknowledging that health is the "key to prosperity" and "poor health drives poverty." They mobilized resources to address infectious diseases, which led to establishment of the Global Fund for HIV/AIDS, Tuberculosis, and Malaria. Years passed without their similarly addressing non-communicable chronic diseases (NCDs). But, in 2011, heads of state, convening at the United Nations in New York, adopted the Political Declaration of the High-Level Meeting of the General Assembly, calling on WHO to recommend voluntary global targets for the prevention and control of NCDs and a framework for monitoring progress toward these goals. These global targets (including a 25 percent reduction in deaths from NCDs by 2025) have been drafted by the WHO, but more work is needed to ensure their implementation.

The World Health Organization (WHO)

Except for tobacco control, WHO's financial resources for prevention and control of NCDs are meager. WHO budget allocations are heavily skewed toward addressing infectious diseases—87 percent in 2006–2007. The skew toward infectious diseases is even greater for the WHO "extra-budget," which is allocated by donor organizations.[1]

Research Institutions

The exponential growth of funding for international research in recent decades has not been proportionally allocated to the growing burden of NCDs. Major international research institutes continue to focus their research programs almost entirely on infectious diseases. A notable exception is the Fogarty International Center of the National Institutes of Health, which has allocated one-third of its resources to NCD research and training programs in low-income countries.

Donor Organizations

NCDs in low-income countries have received substantially less attention than other health problems. Bilateral aid agencies rarely prioritize NCDs or related risk factors. The Bill & Melinda Gates Foundation does not yet include NCDs in its portfolio, with the sole exception of tobacco control. Many foundations in the United States support innovative domestic NCD research and training programs, but not in other countries. A recent analysis found that less than 3 percent of all spending by donor organizations is used to address NCDs.[2]

The World Bank and Regional Development Banks

The Health, Nutrition, and Population Sector Strategy of the World Bank recognizes the increasing burden of NCDs on poor people.[3] But this is not reflected by its limited investment in prevention and control of NCDs. It is also not reflected in its Poverty Strategy Reduction Papers, which are intended to guide investment priorities to reduce poverty in the poorest countries.

Public-Private Partnerships

There are now about 50 public-private partnerships that internationally address diseases related to poverty, but all of their focus has been on infectious diseases. There is much potential, for example, for new partnerships between government agencies and food-related industries to address diet and physical activity.

United Nations Agencies

United Nations health and development reports help set priorities for global health. Despite their impact in low- and middle-income countries, NCDs are infrequently recognized as a health or development issue. For example, the United Nations Population Fund (UNFPA) does not mention chronic illnesses in its strategy on population and development, and A World Fit for Children, a program of the United Nations Children's Fund (UNICEF), does not include chronic disease risk factors in its action plan for promoting healthy lives, despite strong evidence that tobacco use and obesity are major risk factors for children in low-income countries.

The NCD Alliance was founded by four international federations of non-governmental organizations (NGOs), representing the four main NCDs—cardiovascular disease, diabetes, cancer, and chronic respiratory disease. Together with other major international NGO partners, the NCD Alliance unites a network of over 2000 civil society organizations in more than 170 countries. The mission of the NCD Alliance is to combat the NCD epidemic by putting health at the center of all policies.[4]

Box References

1. Stuckler D, King L, Robinson H, McKee M. WHO's budgetary allocations and burden of disease: A comparative analysis. *Lancet* 2008;372:1563–1569.
2. Nugent RA, Feigl AB. Where have all the donors gone? Scarce donor funding for non-communicable diseases, 2010 (Working Paper 228). Available at http://www.cgdev.org/files/1424546_file_Nugent_Feigl_NCD_FINAL.pdf. Accessed on January 3, 2013.
3. Olusoji A, Smith O, Robles S. Public policy and the challenge of chronic noncommunicable diseases. Washington, DC: The World Bank, 2007. Available at https://openknowledge.worldbank.org/handle/10986/6761. Accessed January 3, 2013.
4. The NCD Alliance. Who we are. Available at http://www.ncdalliance.org/who-we-are. Accessed July 26, 2012.

Cardiovascular Disease

CVD is the leading cause of death globally. Over 80 percent of CVD deaths occur in low- and middle-income countries.[1] For example, in 2005, CVD accounted for 2.8 million deaths in China, dwarfing the combined totals of all deaths from infectious diseases in the country.[6,7] In low-income countries, the age at which people die of CVD is significantly younger than in high-income countries, leading to economic and family hardship on a large scale. In India and South Africa, for example, CVD death rates in working-age women are higher today than they were in U.S. women in the 1950s.[8] Asian Indians are

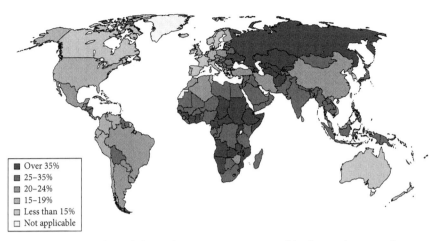

Figure 15–1 Probability of dying from a non-communicable disease between the ages of 30 and 70, in 2008. (*Source*: Daily chart: Death—where are you most likely to die from non-communicable disease? *The Economist*, June 1, 2012: http://www.economist.com/blogs/graphicdetail/2012/06/daily-chart. Accessed July 16, 2012.)

projected to account for 40 to 60 percent of the CVD burden globally over the next decade.

In Tanzania, stroke mortality rates are three times higher than in the United Kingdom. CVD rates for 30- and 40-year-olds in many low-income countries are now the same as for 40- and 50-year-olds in high-income countries.[9] While CVD deaths have declined by 50 percent since the 1960s in the United States, the United Kingdom, and many other high-income countries, they continue to increase rapidly in most low-income countries.[8]

Diabetes Mellitus

In 2010, approximately 285 million (6.6 percent) of people age 20 to 79 were estimated to have diabetes, 70 percent of whom were living in low- and middle-income countries.[10] By 2030, that number is expected to be 439 million (7.8 percent of all) people, an 18 percent increase from 2010 and a 54 percent increase from 2003.

Although diabetes affects both genders equally, working-age populations (40–59 years old) are disproportionately affected. Diabetes prevalence is higher in urban areas than in rural areas, although, in many low-income countries, this urban-rural gap is narrowing. The number of people with diabetes is projected to rise the fastest in three of the six developing regions: Africa

(98 percent increase), the Middle East and North Africa (94 percent increase), and Southeast Asia (72 percent increase). These increases are expected to be largest among children and adults of working age.

Diabetes prevalence globally is rising much faster than expected. In many countries, diabetes prevalence in 2010 already surpasses estimates for 2020. This is especially alarming in rural areas in low- and middle-income countries, where diabetes prevalence has quintupled over the past 25 years.[11]

The global diabetes burden may be higher than previously thought. In the United States, 40 percent of people with diabetes remained undiagnosed in 2009.[12] In regions of the world with less developed systems for diabetes detection and management, the proportion of people with undiagnosed diabetes may be 50 percent or higher. For example, in China, 92 million adults 20 years of age and older have diabetes, 61 percent of whom are undiagnosed.[13] There are also high percentages of undiagnosed diabetes cases in sub-Saharan Africa.[14] Assuming that similar proportions of undiagnosed diabetes are present in other countries, the actual number of people with diabetes may be closer to 651 million (509 million in low-income countries and 142 million in high-income countries).

Also increasing is the prevalence and number of people with "pre-diabetes"— who are at higher risk for developing diabetes. The global prevalence of impaired glucose tolerance (IGT) was 7.9 percent among adults (age 20 to 79) in 2010; this is projected to increase to 8.4 percent by 2030.[10] The annual rate of progression from pre-diabetes to diabetes, if no lifestyle modification occurs, is 5 to 10 percent.[15]

Cancer

Approximately 12.7 million people were diagnosed with cancer in 2008; global cancer incidence is projected to rise to 21.4 million by 2030. More than two-thirds of cancer diagnoses occur in low- and middle-income countries.

The major causes of cancer are (a) tobacco use, (b) chronic infections (especially in low-income countries), and (c) dietary, environmental, and other factors. Lung cancer, the most frequently occurring cancer globally that is primarily due to tobacco use, accounts for 1.2 million deaths annually—about 17 percent of all cancer deaths. Cancers caused by tobacco are increasing in most low-income countries—and among women in almost all countries. In a few high-income countries, the incidence of tobacco-related cancers is declining as men smoke less. In low-income countries, cancers caused by chronic infections and by food contaminants and food-preparation methods are declining. There has been little change in the incidence of breast cancer and cervical cancer over the past few decades. Survival rates remain very low for lung, liver, and stomach cancers, although they have increased for many other cancers, due mainly to early detection and increasingly effective treatment.[16]

Chronic Respiratory Diseases

Two major groups of chronic respiratory diseases are chronic obstructive pulmonary disease (COPD), which comprises chronic bronchitis and emphysema, and asthma. Globally, COPD causes approximately 7 percent of all deaths annually (4.2 million). Almost 90 percent of deaths from COPD occur in low- and middle-income countries. Major risk factors for COPD include tobacco use, occupational exposures, indoor air pollution from burning biomass fuel, and childhood respiratory infections. These risk factors are higher among people living in low-income countries and in poor communities in high-income countries. For example, more than half of COPD deaths among women in sub-Saharan Africa are due to indoor smoke from biomass fuel.[17]

▪ MAJOR RISK FACTORS

Major risk factors account for most cases of NCDs. Tobacco use, physical inactivity, unhealthy diet, and the harmful use of alcohol are responsible for more than half of the NCD burden.[6] In terms of attributable risk, the leading NCD risk factors are increased blood pressure (13 percent of deaths globally), physical inactivity (6 percent), and overweight and obesity (5 percent).[17] Nine of the ten leading mortality risk factors are related to NCDs (Figure 15–2).[18] Most of these risk factors cam be modified by policy and/or clinical interventions.[6]

The current burden of NCDs reflects cumulative lifetime risks. The future burden will be determined by the current presence of major NCD risk factors. Population growth and improved longevity, due mainly to a decline in fertility rates and a higher proportion of children living into adulthood, are important determinants of the NCD burden.[19] High-income countries are already under pressure to address the pensions and social insurance demands of aging populations; low-income countries will soon have to do so, although they have fewer resources.

Social Class and NCD Risks and Outcomes

For policy decisions, the rates and potential risks of NCDs can be conceptualized by use of a "chronic disease consumption curve" (Figure 15–3). In high-income and some middle-income countries, where risk factors for NCDs have been established for decades, NCDs caused by these risk factors are a major reason for health disparities by social class, ethnicity, and gender.[19-22] (See Chapters 2, 3, and 4.)

Socioeconomic disparities in the occurrence of CVD and cancer (and their major risks factors) are present from age 2, even in egalitarian countries with homogeneous populations, such as Iceland.[23] Studies of risk factors for NCDs in

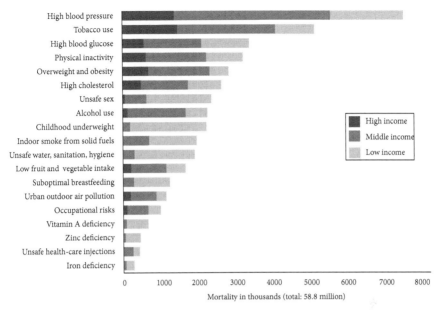

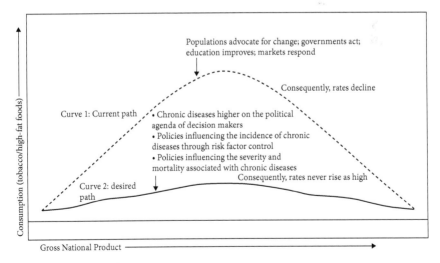

Figure 15-2 Deaths attributable to 19 leading risk factors, by country income level, 2004 WHO estimates. *Notes:* Data are from WHO Burden of Disease 2009. Key NCD risk factors include high blood pressure, tobacco use, high blood glucose, physical inactivity, overweight and obesity, high cholesterol, alcohol use, indoor smoke from solid fuels, low fruit and vegetable intake, and urban outdoor air pollution. (*Source:* World Health Organization. Global health risks: Mortality and burden of disease attributable to selected major risks. Available at: http://www.who.int/healthinfo/global_burden_disease/GlobalHealthRisks_report_full.pdf. Accessed March 19, 2013.)

Figure 15-3 Chronic disease consumption curve.

high-income countries—such as smoking, obesity, hypertension, and physical inactivity—have demonstrated that almost all risk factors are higher among people from the lowest social classes, mirroring trends in morbidity and mortality.[24] It has been estimated that 14 risk factors—smoking being the most important—explain about three-fourths of the socioeconomic disparities in the incidence and mortality for coronary heart disease.[25] (See Chapter 2.)

In the United States, a study investigated the influence of a small number of factors on life expectancy.[26] It identified "eight Americas," with substantial differences in life expectancy on the basis of race, county, population density, income, and homicide rate: Asians, northland low-income rural whites, Middle America, low-income whites in Appalachia and the Mississippi Valley, western Native Americans, black Middle America, low-income southern rural blacks, and high-risk urban blacks. For example, in 2001, the life expectancy gap between high-risk urban black males and Asian females was nearly 21 years. Within gender, the life expectancy gap was widest between Asian males and high-risk urban black males (15.4 years) and between Asian females and low-income rural black females in the South (12.8 years). The causes of death that were primarily responsible for these gaps were various chronic diseases and injuries.

In low-income countries, risks such as tobacco use, physical inactivity, and obesity are initially higher among those with the highest levels of disposable income. A "social-class drift" occurs as commodities and consumption patterns become available and affordable to poor people before health education and other preventive measures are implemented. For example, a study found an inverse relationship between socioeconomic status and the lifestyle index in the United States, but a direct relationship in China, explained by China's being on the ascending limb of Figure 15–3, and the United States on the descending limb.[27,28] Therefore, policymakers in low- and middle-income countries should not wait for the appearance of a social class gradient in the occurrence of chronic disease (or chronic disease risk factors) before implementing health-promotion and disease-prevention measures. Governments of low-income countries made this point during negotiations for the Framework Convention on Tobacco Control in 2003[29] and the United Nations High-Level Meeting on NCDs in 2011.[30]

Cumulative Exposure to Risks Increases Inequalities

A downward spiral occurs with NCDs. As Gunnar Myrdal, a recipient of the Nobel Prize for Economics, told the World Health Assembly, people are sick because they are poor, and become poorer because they are sick.[31]

Major risks for CVD, COPD, cancer, and diabetes begin in childhood with early termination of breastfeeding, suboptimal diets, exposure to tobacco and alcohol, indoor exposure to biomass fuel, and recurrent respiratory infections—all of which contribute to the development of NCDs in adulthood. Cumulative exposure to these risk factors as well as social and economic risk factors leads to disparities in the occurrence of NCDs. The risk of developing CVD or diabetes is influenced by biological and social factors starting during fetal development. About 85 percent of patients who develop clinically significant CHD and more than 95 percent of patients who have died of CHD have had at least one major cardiac risk factor—a history of smoking, diabetes, hypertension, and/or hypercholesterolemia.[32]

COPD and lung function decrement in adults result from cumulative exposures that start early in life. Studies in South Africa have shown that differences in lung size are probably due to (a) early childhood respiratory infections, occurring in crowded homes where biomass fuel is used; (b) tobacco use; and (c) hazardous occupational exposures.

Children are increasingly exposed to NCD risk factors and developing NCDs at earlier ages. For example, surveys in 2008 of 13- to 15-year-olds in South Africa and Mexico demonstrated that (a) one-fourth currently smoke cigarettes, and (b) almost as many girls as boys smoke. Overweight and obesity have become problems in low-income countries. For example, in 2004, 27 percent of children under age 15 in China were obese, 9 percent of 5- to 11-year-olds in Mexico were obese, and 22 percent of schoolchildren in South Africa were overweight or obese.[33] About 10 percent of children have been found to have elevated blood pressure in the Seychelles, Ghana, and Pakistan.[34-36] An estimated one-third of children born in the United States in 2000—perhaps one-half of minority children—will develop diabetes.[37] In most low-income countries, NCD risk factors have increased over time, and increases in obesity and tobacco use among children, especially in cities, portend a future increase in NCDs.

Asymmetrical Access to Healthy Messages

In countries and communities with low health-literacy, commercial "messages" have a strong influence on behavior. Low health literacy, prevalent in low-income countries and poor communities in other countries, undermines many public health measures to control NCDs. Low levels of health literacy are associated with reduced comprehension about causes of disease, the value of prevention and health promotion, how and when to seek care, and adherence to therapy—especially long-term therapy. Well-designed marketing campaigns by public health workers can promote health, but few have been designed to reach those with poor health literacy.

In contrast, global marketing of tobacco, alcohol, and salty, sugary, and fatty foods and beverages now reaches most parts of most countries—much of it targeting vulnerable populations, such as young people, minorities, and low-income people. Marketers use sophisticated methods to ensure that their messages "slip below the radar of critical thinking" and take advantage of inadequate regulations—while sometimes using false, misleading, or deceptive advertising to reach their targets.[38] Meanwhile, messages about healthy lifestyle choices do not reach poor people in most countries.

In low-income countries, companies perceive emerging markets, and they perform market research and strategize to reach specific populations. For example, in China, a brewery from Africa successfully targeted the mass market with locally brewed beer. In China and other Asian countries, international tobacco companies have used glamorous images to advertise "light" and "mild" cigarettes specifically to women. In many low-income countries, transnational food companies have used techniques specifically designed to attract children to eat at fast-food restaurants and consume high-sugar drinks and snacks. In Brazil, despite a relatively strong regulatory framework, technological advances in food manufacturing and distribution through larger multinational food companies may be displacing healthier, traditional diets and thereby increasing NCDs.[39]

Increased Comorbidity and Need for Long-term Care

Poor communities and countries suffer from the consequences of increased numbers of people with multiple chronic diseases—such as HIV/AIDS, tuberculosis (TB), CVD, cancer, and diabetes. (See also Chapter 13.) This situation has serious consequences for the provision of health care, especially long-term care. WHO estimates that low-income countries in sub-Saharan Africa, Latin America, and the Eastern Mediterranean area will experience three- to four-fold increases over the next several decades in people requiring long-term care (which is rudimentary in most of these countries).[40]

The role of certain infectious agents in causing cancer is increasingly recognized. For example, hepatitis B virus can cause liver cancer; human papilloma virus, cervical cancer; *Helicobacter pylori*, stomach cancer; HIV infection, Kaposi's sarcoma, non-Hodgkin lymphoma, and other malignancies; and *Schistosoma haematobium*, bladder cancer.[16] All of these cancers are common in low-income countries, where treatment resources are extremely inadequate. Availability of vaccines to prevent these infections and drugs to treat them can reduce the cancer burden.

There are interactions among TB, tobacco use, and diabetes. For example, people with diabetes are at higher risk of acquiring TB,[41,42] and tobacco increases the case-fatality rate of TB. In India, smokers are 4.5 times more likely to die of TB than are nonsmokers.[43] Although an estimated 80 percent of TB patients smoke, little progress has been made in helping them to quit. As a result, tobacco is probably the major cause of death in TB patients who have been treated.

Comorbidity of mental and physical disorders is common. About one-third of patients with depression also have common NCDs, such as CVD, diabetes, and cancer.[44] People with one or more chronic diseases have an increased risk of major depression.[45] The burden of comorbidity is borne disproportionately by poor people. (See also Chapter 16.)

Inadequate Access to Quality Medical Care

Poor people generally do not have access to tests for early detection of NCDs, such as diabetes, hypertension, and cervical cancer, leading to many cases presenting at an advanced stage. For example, in the United States, people in high-poverty areas are almost 2.5 times more likely to have an advanced stage of malignant melanoma and almost twice as likely to have an advanced stage of prostate cancer and breast cancer when they finally seek medical care for these diseases.

Patients in low social classes have consistently poorer survival for cancers of the bladder, colon, breast, and uterus.[21] In addition, chemotherapeutic agents most effective against the 10 leading cancers are not readily available in many low-income countries.[16] Neither is beclomethasone, an inhalable medication used to treat COPD and asthma.

Participation in breast cancer screening depends on income and education, health insurance, and the type of health service. Women of low social classes tend to have lower screening rates than those in higher social classes.[46] Women of low socioeconomic status have increased risk of cervical cancer, but they participate less in screening for cervical cancer. The major goals in screening programs for chronic diseases are to reduce barriers to early access and to ensure public resources for long-term sustainability of programs. Differences among socioeconomic groups in screening participation decrease when participation is promoted, cultural and economic barriers are removed, and social support is offered.

■ ROOT CAUSES AND UNDERLYING ISSUES

Macroeconomic Influences

The direct and indirect ways by which global and regional forces influence NCDs are complex. Economic status, reflected in household income, government expenditure, exchange rates, and prices, plays an important role. National income profoundly affects public-sector resources available for health, health-related behaviors (especially in low-income households), and the costs of health care.[7]

Economic development can increase national and personal income and subsequently improve all aspects of health. A global approach to economic development indeed has led to some positive consequences for health in low-income countries. The presence of supermarkets has rapidly expanded in low-income countries, increasing access to fresh foods and, in some cases, also increasing their affordability—possibly promoting consumption of more healthful foods. But there can also be negative health consequences.

Trade and investment drive economic development and may not encourage healthy behaviors. Open conditions for trade and investment can bring economic benefits, but also health risks. Expanded global trade of and foreign direct investment in tobacco have promoted demand. Among the top 100 non-financial transnational corporations (ranked by foreign assets in 2000) were several associated with NCD risks, including tobacco, food, and alcohol companies. These powerful companies often seek to prevent the public perception that health conditionalities (such as obesity) are linked to their investments, thereby weakening or preventing the implementation of regulations like those that have helped to reduce chronic disease risks in high-income countries.

Economic investment in the unregulated marketing of unhealthful products encourages development of risk factors for chronic diseases. Global tobacco, alcohol, food, and automobile companies all invest heavily in marketing their products, creating an environment where healthy choices by individuals are more difficult. Low-income countries experience many risks associated with globally interconnected economic development, without necessarily the investments made in many high-income countries required to protect against these risks.

Several studies have quantified the relationships between societal-level risk factors and chronic disease burdens.[47-50] One study found significant associations between diabetes prevalence and population-level availability of total calories, sugar, animal fat, and fruits and vegetables (as measured by agricultural production, imports, and exports).[50] It found that (a) a 10 percent higher availability of calories from fruits and vegetables is associated with 31 percent lower diabetes prevalence, (b) a 10 percent lower availability of calories from sugar is associated with 62 percent lower diabetes prevalence, and (c) a 10 percent lower availability of calories from animal fat is associated with 29 percent lower diabetes prevalence. It also found that availability of 500 fewer calories per person daily is associated with 5 percent lower diabetes prevalence.

Transnational corporations have attempted to avoid regulations and to suppress advocacy by governments and WHO for healthful consumption behaviors. For example, the tobacco industry has asserted that WHO should not focus on the "lifestyle issues" of affluent Western countries, such as tobacco. It has also attempted to redirect the tobacco-control resources of WHO, alleging that WHO was misspending its budget "at the expense of more urgent public health needs," especially in low-income countries, such as prevention of malaria and other communicable diseases.[51] Lobbyists for multinational companies in the tobacco, sugar, and other food industries have attempted to divert attention from the need to address consumption patterns that cause chronic diseases. Their views have been accepted by many national and international policymakers.[52]

Consumption patterns become increasingly unhealthy in countries and communities where (a) incomes are rising, (b) public health and regulatory capacities are weak, and (c) commercial pressures—often hidden from the public—are stronger than government's influence.

Over time, economic development often brings greater political awareness of the benefits of prevention, and often opposition to strong commercial interests in order to implement preventive measures. Therefore, countries with the highest levels of both income and education—and a high degree of openness in policy development—seem to have public health policies that encourage healthy consumption (Figure 15–3). In countries where government is democratic and the news media are not restricted, the intensity and quality of public discourse on addressing chronic disease is far better than elsewhere.

Some international policies, such as the WHO Framework Convention on Tobacco Control (FCTC), generally reduce risk factors for NCDs. However, even the FCTC has limited impact in low-income countries that may have a weaker regulatory framework. For example, although India is a signatory to the FCTC, the most common tobacco product there—the *bidi*, a hand-rolled cigarette—is not covered by the Convention. Even if it were, India could not easily tax it since it is often made by local people, who sell it in carts and stalls on the streets.[53,54]

Urban and Rural Factors

Urbanization exacerbates chronic disease risks, which increase with rising levels of disposable income, marketing of and better access to certain products, and cultural changes in taste and behavior. With urbanization, people often become less physically active and have increased availability of foods that are high in calories, fats, and sugars.

Rural populations are also at increasing risk for NCDs. From 1985 to 2010, diabetes prevalence quintupled in rural areas in low- and middle-income countries.[11] In some countries, obesity and diabetes rates are higher in rural areas than in urban areas. In Pakistan and South Africa, obesity rates, especially among rural women, exceed 35 percent.[55] Rates of all major chronic disease risk factors, except smoking, are higher in urban than in rural areas of Thailand,[56] but the number of people with risk factors is higher in rural areas. And rural populations often have limited availability of health care, which leads to worse health outcomes.

Generally Weak NCD Policies and Programs in Low-income Countries

Many countries give inadequate—or no—attention to NCDs.[57] In 2001, only about 40 percent of countries specifically budgeted for NCDs, and fewer than 50 percent of countries had a policy or plan for NCDs. In addition, essential medicines to treat NCDs were often not available in primary care facilities. By 2010, many countries had improved their policies and programs for NCDs. For example, more than 80 percent of countries reported NCD morbidity and mortality as part of their national disease reporting systems. However, 16 percent of countries had no morbidity or mortality surveillance at all.[1]

Implementing Comprehensive Policies That Reach the Poorest People

Gunnar Myrdal, a Swedish economist, sociologist, and politician, and a Nobel Laureate, cautioned over 50 years ago against quick fixes for complex public health problems. He said that work to achieve optimal health would need to be integrated within a broad economic and social reform policy.[31] Progress in addressing NCDs is being made in such a broader context. For example, in 2011, many heads of state at the UN High-Level Meeting on NCDs agreed that NCDs are a health, economic, and development priority. The UN General Assembly requested that WHO develop a comprehensive global monitoring framework for NCDs and voluntary global targets for their prevention and control.[58] It also set a global target of a 25 percent reduction in premature mortality from NCDs by 2025.

Low- and middle-income countries could better address NCDs with surveillance systems that could provide a reliable and timely data infrastructure to evaluate the effectiveness of interventions for NCDs. They will need to implement comprehensive, multisectoral approaches over the long term. They will need a combination of education, health services, and intersectoral action to reduce disparities in chronic disease outcomes. Education, in general, reduces health risks, improves health and well-being, and leads to more effective use of health services. Investment in health literacy in low-income countries could lead to more emphasis on prevention and primary care, and slow the demand for tertiary treatment, which distorts the relatively small health budgets of low-income countries.[59]

Placing Greater Emphasis on Prevention and Health Promotion

Application of existing knowledge can help prevent and control NCDs in a cost-effective manner. However, national governments and international organizations continue to focus on acute infectious diseases and do not give appropriate attention to NCDs. Only a few countries have developed and implemented comprehensive policies to prevent and control NCDs. And the tobacco industry and companies that produce and promote unhealthy food and beverage products[52,60,61] have advocated against the development and implementation of such policies. For example, in 2003 the sugar industry lobbied against WHO's Global Strategy on Diet and Physical Activity, threatening to sue; similarly, the tobacco industry worked hard to prevent the Framework Convention on Tobacco Control from being passed and implemented.

Globally, advocacy for prevention and control of NCDs generally is fragmented and specific to certain risk factors or diseases. However, the World Heart Federation, the International Diabetes Federation, the Union for International

Cancer Control, and the International Union Against Tuberculosis and Lung Disease have established the NCD Alliance. The Alliance is a network of more than 2000 civil-society organizations in more than 170 countries that is advocating for prevention and control of CVD, diabetes, cancer, and chronic respiratory disease—and, in doing so, is substantially increasing the attention being given to NCDs.

Increasingly, CVD, diabetes, and cancer are viewed as diseases of both development and poverty. In response, academic institutions, health professional organizations, consumer groups, and business organizations have supported policies and funding for prevention and control of NCDs. Initially, they have focused on single issues, such as tobacco control. Increasingly, there is a need for these organizations and their members to form broad alliances to advocate for the prevention and control of all NCDs, especially in low-income countries.

Strengthening Capacity and Mobilize Resources

Within most of these countries, human and financial resources for NCD prevention and control are inadequate. Governments of these countries and international aid organizations have been reluctant to invest in national institutions and infrastructure. In recent years, new private foundations have appropriately invested billions of dollars for HIV/AIDS, malaria, tuberculosis, and immunizable diseases. And international donor organizations have increased support for tobacco control. But there has not been any significant increase in funding for prevention and control of NCDs.

Developing Global Norms That Benefit Low-Income Countries

Many low-income countries lack the human resources to develop and implement laws and regulations as well as tax policies to support NCD control. For them, funding from international aid organizations can catalyze national action, and global norms can provide a needed "umbrella of legitimacy" for their developing, passing, and implementing national laws. Global norms on restricting the adverse influences of transnational corporations on NCDs can help to balance the otherwise unrestrained influences of powerful interests and can assist countries that have limited public health capacity, such as in national regulation of food and tobacco products and participation in such international regulatory bodies as the World Trade Organization.

For example, the Framework Convention on Tobacco Control (FCTC) is a global norm that can protect low-income countries from pressure by the tobacco industry as they introduce tobacco control policies and other measures. The FCTC, which was adopted by all 192 WHO member states in 2003 and came into force in 2005, represents the first time that WHO used its treaty-making right to advance public health goals. The FCTC facilitates bans on the advertising of tobacco products and promotes larger health-warning labels on these products, measures to protect against secondhand smoke, increases in prices and taxes on tobacco products, and the elimination of illicit trade in tobacco products. The FCTC provides a template for policy development for control of food-related chronic diseases. Other norms that support NCD control include:

1. The International Code of Marketing of Breast-milk Substitutes, which limits advertising for breast milk substitutes in order to encourage healthier breastfeeding
2. The Codex Alimentarius Commission, which was established by WHO and the Food and Agriculture Organization in 1963 to harmonize international food standards—with its likely increased focus on food labeling and health claims
3. Agricultural policy, which tends to focus on commodities such as grains that are converted into processed and packaged foods or fed to livestock—rather than healthy fruits and vegetables

International conventions alone cannot address the complex issues related to poor nutrition and physical inactivity and their relationship with NCDs. Codes and regulations that incorporate multiple stakeholder perspectives are better options to pursue, especially in relation to restricting the marketing of alcohol and food items to young children. Such approaches are already being implemented in low-income countries to improve labor conditions, environmental quality, and protection of human rights. These approaches are less expensive and faster to implement than legislative approaches that only take a single stakeholder perspective into account, but they require strong independent oversight to ensure they have the desired impact.

Reorienting Health Services to Address NCDs

Although well-established low-cost regimens exist for treating most of the major chronic diseases, many people die prematurely because of inadequate or low-quality treatment of these diseases,[62] especially in low-income countries and poor communities in high-income countries. Treatment of diabetes is an illustrative example.

There are many opportunities for prevention of NCDs, such as providing smoking-cessation programs and advising people on healthful diets and physical activity. For example, in the United Kingdom, smoking-cessation programs have reached many poor people who smoke. But relatively few initiatives have been undertaken elsewhere to target poor people with such interventions.

Non-governmental organizations, international organizations, pharmaceutical companies, and other entities have considerably improved access to antiretroviral drugs for HIV/AIDS, TB drugs, and several vaccines by substantially reducing prices. But similar progress has not been made for drugs for treating cancer, diabetes, and CVD. A patient with heart disease in a low-income country has the same right to effective treatment as a patient with malaria, TB, or HIV/AIDS.[63]

Promoting Broader Societal Changes

Legislative, financial, and engineering measures are needed to support prevention and control of NCDs. These measures, which can especially benefit poor people, include:

- Infrastructural changes that promote public transport and physical activity
- Laws that ban tobacco advertising and smoking in public places
- Tax policies that raise excise taxes on tobacco
- Government subsidies that provide schools and poor communities with improved access to fruits, vegetables, and other healthful foods

Building on Prevention and Control of Infectious Diseases

Strengthening some aspects of the prevention and control of infectious disease, especially related to chronic infectious diseases such as TB and HIV/AIDS, will benefit the prevention and control of CVD, diabetes, and cancer. Transformation of health care systems, such as is occurring in some sub-Saharan African countries, can improve prevention and treatment for both infectious diseases and non-infectious chronic diseases.[62] As countries, international organizations, and aid organizations are increasing their investments in the prevention and control of infectious diseases, the increased additional investment to prevent and control chronic diseases would yield substantial benefits to improve health, especially among people in low-income countries.

▓ CONCLUSION: AN AGENDA FOR ACTION

Social injustice concerning chronic diseases is neither inevitable nor acceptable. The following recommendations represent an agenda for action towards achieving social justice concerning chronic diseases:

- Promote reviews of government spending, by treasury or finance ministries, to identify ways in which national governments can reduce health disparities
- Develop partnerships among non-governmental and professional organizations, business groups, and community-based organizations
- Invest in programs that reduce risk factors for NCDs among children and young people
- Target prevention and control measures to population groups and diseases where they will have the greatest positive impact
- Provide better access and financial support to poor people for early detection and long-term treatment of chronic diseases

■ **REFERENCES**

1. World Health Organization. Global status report on noncommunicable diseases 2010: Description of the global burden of NCDs, their risk factors and determinants. Geneva: WHO, 2011. Available at http://www.who.int/nmh/publications/ncd_report2010/en/. Accessed January 3, 2013.

2. The Economist. Daily chart: Death—where are you most likely to die from non-communicable disease? *The Economist*, June 1, 2012. Available at http://www.economist.com/blogs/graphicdetail/2012/06/daily-chart. Accessed July 16, 2012.

3. Hyman S, Chisolm D, Kessler RC, et al. Mental disorders in disease control priorities related to mental, neurological, developmental and substance abuse disorders. Geneva: World Health Organization and The Disease Control Priorities Project, 2006:1–20. Available at http://www.dcp2.org/file/64/WHO_DCPP%20mental%20health%20book_final.pdf. Accessed January 3, 2013.

4. World Health Organization. Scaling up action against noncommunicable disease: How much will it cost? Geneva: WHO, 2011. Available at http://whqlibdoc.who.int/publications/2011/9789241502313_eng.pdf. Accessed January 3, 2013.

5. Brands A, Yach D. Noncommunicable diseases and gender. Geneva: World Health Organization, 2001.

6. World Health Organization. Chronic diseases: A vital investment. Geneva: WHO, 2005. Available at http://www.who.int/chp/chronic_disease_report/contents/en/index.html. Accessed January 3, 2013.

7. Beaglehole R, Yach D. Globalisation and the prevention and control of non-communicable disease: The neglected chronic diseases of adults. *Lancet* 2003;362:903–908.

8. Leeder S, Raymond S, Greenberg H. A race against time: The challenge of cardio-vascular disease in developing economies. New York: Center for Global Health and Economic Development, The Earth Institute, Mailman School of Public Health, Columbia University, 2004. Available at http://www.earth.columbia.edu/news/2004/images/raceagainsttime_FINAL_051104.pdf. Accessed January 3, 2013.

9. World Health Organization. World Health Report 2003: Shaping the future. Geneva: WHO, 2003. Available at http://www.who.int/whr/2003/en/index.html. Accessed January 3, 2013.

10. International Diabetes Federation. Diabetes atlas. 4th ed. Brussels: IDF, 2009.

11. Hwang CK, Han PV, Zabetian A, et al. Rural diabetes prevalence quintuples over twenty-five years in low- and middle-income countries: A systematic review and meta-analysis. *Diabetes Res Clin Pract* 2012;96:271–285.

12. Cowie CC, Rust KF, Ford ES, et al. Full accounting of diabetes and pre-diabetes in the U.S. population in 1988–1994 and 2005–2006. *Diabetes Care* 2009;32:287–294.

13. Yang SH, Dou KF, Song WJ. Prevalence of diabetes among men and women in China. *N Engl J Med* 2010;362:2425–2426; author reply, 2426.

14. Echouffo-Tcheugui JB, Dzudie A, Epacka ME, et al. Prevalence and determinants of undiagnosed diabetes in an urban sub-Saharan African population. *Prim Care Diabetes* 2012;6:229–234.

15. Gerstein HC, Santaguida P, Raina P, et al. Annual incidence and relative risk of diabetes in people with various categories of dysglycemia: A systematic overview and meta-analysis of prospective studies. *Diabetes Res Clin Pract* 2007;78:305–312.

16. Stewart B, Kleihaus P. World cancer report. Lyon, France: International Agency for Research on Cancer, 2003.

17. World Health Organization. Global health risks: Mortality and burden of disease attributable to selected major risks. Geneva: WHO, 2009. Available at http://www.who.int/healthinfo/global_burden_disease/GlobalHealthRisks_report_full.pdf. Accessed January 3, 2013.

18. World Health Organization. Mortality and burden of disease estimates for WHO member states in 2004. Geneva: WHO, 2009.

19. Aboderin I, Kalache A, Ben-Shlomo Y. Life course perspectives on coronary heart disease, stroke and diabetes: Key issues and implications for policy and research. Geneva: World Health Organization, 2001. Available at http://whqlibdoc.who.int/hq/2001/WHO_NMH_NPH_01.4.pdf. Accessed January 3, 2013.

20. Batty GD, Leon DA. Socio-economic position and coronary heart disease risk factors in children and young people. Evidence from U.K. epidemiological studies. *Eur J Public Health* 2002;12:263–272.

21. Reynolds T. Report examines association between cancer and socioeconomic status. *J Natl Cancer Inst* 2003;95:1431–1433.

22. Mackenbach JP, Cavelaars AE, Kunst AE, Groenhof F. Socioeconomic inequalities in cardiovascular disease mortality: An international study. *Eur Heart J* 2000;21:1141–1151.

23. Halldorsson M, Cavelaars AE, Kunst AE, Mackenbach JP. Socioeconomic differences in health and well-being of children and adolescents in Iceland. *Scand J Public Health* 1999;27:43–47.

24. Galobardes B, Costanza MC, Bernstein MS, et al. Trends in risk factors for lifestyle-related diseases by socioeconomic position in Geneva, Switzerland, 1993–2000: Health inequalities persist. *Am J Public Health* 2003;93:1302–1309.

25. Woodward M, Oliphant J, Lowe G, Tunstall-Pedoe H. Contribution of contemporaneous risk factors to social inequality in coronary heart disease and all causes mortality. *Prev Med* 2003;36:561–568.

26. Murray CJ, Kulkarni SC, Michaud C, et al. Eight Americas: Investigating mortality disparities across races, counties, and race-counties in the United States. *PLoS Med* 2006;3:e260.

27. Kim S, Symons M, Popkin BM. Contrasting socioeconomic profiles related to healthier lifestyles in China and the United States. *Am J Epidemiol* 2004;159:184–191.

28. Popkin BM. Will China's nutrition transition overwhelm its health care system and slow economic growth? *Health Aff (Millwood)* 2008;27:1064–1076.

29. World Health Organization. The WHO Framework Convention on Tobacco Control. Geneva: WHO, 2003. Available at http://www.who.int/fctc/text_download/en/index.html. Accessed January 3, 2013.

30. United Nations. 2011 High-Level Meeting on the prevention and control of non-communicable diseases. Available at http://www.un.org/en/ga/ncdmeeting2011/. Accessed July 16th, 2012.

31. Myrdal G. Economic aspects of health: Address to the World Health Assembly. Paper presented at the World Health Assembly, 1952, Geneva, Switzerland.

32. Canto JG, Iskandrian AE. Major risk factors for cardiovascular disease: Debunking the "only 50%" myth. *JAMA* 2003;290:947–949.

33. Yach D, Stuckler D, Brownell KD. Epidemiologic and economic consequences of the global epidemics of obesity and diabetes. *Nature Med* 2006;12:62–66.

34. Chiolero A, Madeleine G, Gabriel A, et al. Prevalence of elevated blood pressure and association with overweight in children of a rapidly developing country. *J Hum Hypertens* 2007;21:120–127.

35. Jafar TH, Islam M, Poulter N, et al. Children in South Asia have higher body mass–adjusted blood pressure levels than white children in the United States: A comparative study. *Circulation* 2005;111:1291–1297.

36. Agyemang C, Redekop WK, Owusu-Dabo E, Bruijnzeels MA. Blood pressure patterns in rural, semi-urban and urban children in the Ashanti region of Ghana, West Africa. *BMC Public Health* 2005;5:114.

37. Narayan KM, Boyle JP, Thompson TJ, et al. Lifetime risk for diabetes mellitus in the United States. *JAMA* 2003;290:1884–1890.

38. Walsh D, Gentile DA. Slipping under the radar: Advertising and the mind. Paper presented at the WHO Symposium on Marketing to Young People, 2002, Treviso, Italy. Available at http://www.fma.ie/Walsh_Gentile_WHO_-_Slipping_Under_the_Radar_-_Advertising_and_the_Mind.pdf. Accessed January 3, 2013.

39. Monteiro CA, Cannon G. The impact of transnational "big food" companies on the South: A view from Brazil. *PLoS Medicine* 2012;9:e1001252.

40. World Health Organization. A long-term care futures tool-kit. Geneva, Switzerland, and Washington, DC: World Health Organization and The Institute for Alternative Futures, 2002. Available at http://www.who.int/chp/knowledge/publications/ltctoolkit/en/index.html. Accessed January 3, 2013.

41. Dooley KE, Chaisson RE. Tuberculosis and diabetes mellitus: Convergence of two epidemics. *Lancet Infect Dis* 2009;9:737–746.

42. Dooley KE, Tang T, Golub JE, et al. Impact of diabetes mellitus on treatment outcomes of patients with active tuberculosis. *Am J Trop Med Hyg* 2009;80:634–639.

43. Gajalakshmi V, Peto R, Kanaka TS, Jha P. Smoking and mortality from tuberculosis and other diseases in India: Retrospective study of 43,000 adult male deaths and 35,000 controls. *Lancet* 2003;362:507–515.

44. Saraceno B, Gatti A. Personal communication with D. Yach, 2003.

45. Moussavi S, Chatterji S, Verdes E, et al. Depression, chronic diseases, and decrements in health: Results from the World Health Surveys. *Lancet* 2007;370:851–858.

46. Morgan MA, Behbakht K, Benjamin I, et al. Racial differences in survival from gynecologic cancer. *Obstet Gynecol* 1996;88:914–918.

47. Rabin BA, Boehmer TK, Brownson RC. Cross-national comparison of environmental and policy correlates of obesity in Europe. *Eur J Public Health* 2007;17:53–61.

48. Basu S, Stuckler D, McKee M, Galea G. Nutritional determinants of worldwide diabetes: An econometric study of food markets and diabetes prevalence in 173 countries. *Public Health Nutr* 2013;16:179–186.

49. Stuckler D. Population causes and consequences of leading chronic diseases: A comparative analysis of prevailing explanations. *Milbank Q* 2008;86:273–326.

50. Siegel KR, Echouffo-Tcheugui JB, Ali MK, et al. Societal correlates of diabetes prevalence: An analysis across 94 countries. *Diabetes Res Clin Pract* 2012;96:76–83.

51. World Health Organization. Tobacco company strategies to undermine tobacco control activities at WHO: Report of the Committee of Experts on Tobacco Industry Documents. Geneva: WHO, 2000. Available at http://www.who.int/tobacco/en/who_inquiry.pdf. Accessed January 3, 2013.

52. Brownell KD, Warner KE. The perils of ignoring history: Big Tobacco played dirty and millions died. How similar is Big Food? *Milbank Q* 2009;87:259–294.

53. Siegel K, Stuckler D. Comparative case studies from Brazil, China, India, Mexico, and South Africa. In: Stuckler D, Siegel K, eds. Sick societies: Responding to the global challenge of chronic disease. Oxford, England: Oxford University Press, 2011.

54. Steyn K, Bradshaw D, Levitt N, et al. Comparative case studies from Brazil, China, India, Mexico, and South Africa: Part 5, Chronic diseases in South Africa. In: Stuckler D, Siegel K, eds. Sick societies: Responding to the global challenge of chronic disease. Oxford, England: Oxford University Press, 2011.

55. Nanan DJ. The obesity pandemic—Implications for Pakistan. *J Pak Med Assoc* 2002;52:342–346.

56. The International Collaborative Study of Cardiovascular Disease in Asia (InterASIA). Cardiovascular risk factor levels in urban and rural Thailand. *Eur J Cardiovasc Prev Rehabil* 2003;10:249–257.

57. Alwan A, MacLean D, Mandil A. Assessment of national capacity for non-communicable disease prevention and control: The report of a global survey. Geneva: World Health Organization, 2001. Available at http://whqlibdoc.who.int/hq/2001/WHO_MNC_01.2.pdf. Accessed January 3, 2013.

58. World Health Organization. A comprehensive global monitoring framework, including indicators, and a set of voluntary global targets for the prevention and control of noncommunicable diseases: Revised WHO discussion paper. Geneva: World Health Organization, 2012. Available at http://www.who.int/nmh/events/2012/ncd_discussion_paper/en/index.html. Accessed January 3, 2013.

59. World Health Organization. Report of the WHO Commission on Macroeconomics and Health. Macroeconomics and health: Investing in health for economic development. Geneva: World Health Organization, 2001. Available at http://whqlibdoc.who.int/publications/2001/924154550x.pdf. Accessed January 3, 2013.

60. Yach D, Bettcher D. Globalisation of tobacco industry influence and new global responses. *Tob Control* 2000;9:206–216.

61. Nestle M. Food politics: How the food industry influences nutrition and health. Berkeley, CA: University of California Press, 2002.

62. Epping-Jordan JE, Bengoa R, Yach D. Chronic conditions—The new health challenge. *S Afr Med J* 2003;93:585–590.

63. The Lancet. WTO takes a first step. *Lancet* 2003;362:753.

16 Mental Health

■ CARLES MUNTANER, EDWIN NG,
HAEJOO CHUNG, AND
WILLIAM W. EATON

■ INTRODUCTION

Social epidemiologists were among the first scientists to ask the simple, yet critically important, question: "What is the relationship between social injustice and mental health?" They found an inverse association between socioeconomic position (SEP) and mental illness, demonstrating that the poor not only suffer from higher rates of mental disorders, but also receive inferior forms of treatment compared to more affluent people.[1] Many other studies have replicated this finding.[2,3]

Social injustice in mental health is not simply due to the varying attributes and behaviors of individuals. Rather, it reflects how societies produce and distribute valued resources between relatively more powerful and less powerful groups. It follows that mental health inequalities are generated and replicated through social processes that reflect societal forms of social injustice—political, economic, and cultural.

A social justice perspective on why deprived groups disproportionately bear the burden of mental disorders incorporates principles of equality, fairness, and solidarity. It also considers causal processes that directly or indirectly allocate rights, opportunities, resources, and capabilities.[4-6] Social systems of allocation confer more economic, political, and cultural opportunities and resources to some people than to others.[6] These processes systematically lead to unequal—and avoidable—mental health outcomes.

This chapter applies a social justice perspective and addresses the needs for (a) "preventive measures" to improve the unfair—and avoidable—living and working conditions that produce increased rates of mental disorders among poor workers, women, immigrants, and racial/ethnic and minorities[7-10]; and (b) "treatment options" to narrow persistent mental health inequalities by providing high-quality mental health services and psychiatric care.[7] Five major subjects are discussed:

1. Mental illness in a social-justice context, reviewing both individual and structural approaches to understanding the causes of mental health inequalities
2. The association between social stratification and mental health, focusing on how categories of people are ranked along social hierarchies
3. Specific dimensions of social injustice, implicating unequal power relations as a determinant of mental health inequalities and reviewing potential pathways that link social injustice and mental health

4. Mental health services as a source of social injustice, demonstrating that psychiatric care tends to favor those who are privileged at the expense of those who are marginalized

5. What needs to be done to achieve a more equal society, highlighting interventions to reduce inequalities mental health inequalities

▪ MENTAL ILLNESS IN A SOCIAL-JUSTICE CONTEXT

Social factors are closely associated with mental disorders, which contribute to the occurrence of many cases of disease and injury and much disability.[11–15] By 2020, mental and behavioral disorders are projected to be the most important cause of years lost to disability.[11,16] Adverse mental health consequences occur most often among those affected by social injustice. For example, the most common mental disorders, depression and anxiety, are significantly more prevalent among women than men.[17–19] Experiencing social discrimination, such as homophobia and racism, is associated with symptoms of psychological distress.[20]

There are two major opposing views of social justice in relation to mental health. Some assert that social behavior is a matter of individual agency, or volitional control, and this explains why workers, women, and some ethnic minorities experience a disproportionate burden of mental illnesses. From this individualist perspective, marginalized people are primarily responsible for their own social standing and their own mental illness. Outcomes such as poverty, low education, and mental illness are seen as the result of personal autonomous choices, and society as a whole has little or no obligation to prevent mental disorders or to provide treatment services.

In contrast, the structural view focuses on the social relations of class, race, ethnicity, and gender inequality as determinants of individual outcomes, including mental disorders. Instead of blaming victims for their own suffering, this view implicates social injustice—such as exploitation, domination, racism, and gender discrimination—as a major cause of mental health inequalities.[21] The structural view implies (a) a collective societal responsibility to empower people whose mental health is adversely affected by class, gender, and racial/ethnic inequalities; and (b) societal measures have the potential to significantly reduce mental health inequalities by increasing access to economic, political, and cultural resources.

Each of these views has gained support from academics, policymakers, and the general public.[22–24] Overall, however, more evidence supports the view that social class, gender, and racial/ethnic inequalities in mental health arise from social structures rather than from personal choices.

A society's unequal distribution of economic, political, and cultural resources will generate worse mental health among the relatively poor, powerless, and less educated. Economic inequalities in property generate an intergenerational transmission of poverty, which has disproportionately affected African Americans in the United States.[25] Political inequalities preclude immigrants from obtaining equal rights, while confining them to subordinate positions in society. Cultural factors, such as racism, patriarchy, or classism,[26] can lead to labor market discrimination and residential segregation, with adverse consequences for poor people, minorities, women, older people, ill or disabled people, and lesbian, gay, bisexual, and transgender/transsexual individuals. Public health workers share in the responsibility to improve the mental health of populations that arise from economic, political, or cultural inequalities.[27-29]

◾ SOCIAL STRATIFICATION AND MENTAL HEALTH

There is a strong, consistent, and inverse association between mental disorders and social stratification, measured in terms of SEP, race, ethnicity, nationality, gender, age, or sexual orientation.[30] The evidence is especially strong to support an association between (a) income, education, and higher occupational social class; and (b) frequent forms of psychiatric illness, such as depression, anxiety, and substance-use disorders.[3,30,31]

Low-income people have higher rates of depression than do people with higher incomes.[32,33] Factors such as financial strain and level of debt are associated with high rates of depression.[34,35] In the United States, people with annual household incomes of less than $20,000 have twice the prevalence of major depression of people with annual household incomes of $70,000 or more.[9] Some studies in U.S. metropolitan areas have found 11- to 16-fold higher rates of depression among low-income respondents.[7] One study found that financial dependence—indicating extreme deprivation—increased by 2.5-fold the risk of depression.[34]

Education is also associated with mental health.[36] Although high-income countries generally encourage education as means of social mobility, opportunities for educational attainment and mental health outcomes in these countries are unequally distributed. For example, a meta-analysis found that people with less education are at higher risk of depression.[37] Another study found that less education among working-age adults was associated with a high frequency of anxiety disorders.[38] Yet another study found that people with less education were 1.4 times more likely to have poor mental health.[39]

Occupational social class, a major determinant of income, wealth, and power, is strongly associated with mental illness. The prevalence of depression in the past 6 months among people employed in household services was found in one study to be 7 percent, compared to 2.5 percent among executive professionals.[40] Blue-collar workers are 1.5 to 2.0 times as likely to be depressed as white-collar workers.[1] Being born to parents who are manual laborers confers almost twice the risk of depression for women and almost four times the risk of depression for men, compared with those born to at least one parent not in the working class.[1] There is a 50 percent increase in depressive symptoms among workers engaged in temporary work compared to permanent employees.[41]

The association between low SEP and mental health is firmly established. People in the United States with low SEP have two to three times the prevalence of substance-use disorders, alcohol abuse or dependence, antisocial personality disorders, anxiety disorders, and all psychiatric disorders combined.[7,8] Internationally, even larger differences have been found.[8] However, the relationship between low SEP and poor mental health is infrequently considered, in that this link often relies on simply ranking individuals along different indicators of SEP. This represents a gradational approach, and it follows that some individuals earn more money, obtain more education, exercise more power at work, and enjoy better mental health outcomes. To gain a more complete understanding of how mental health inequalities are generated, gradational approaches should be augmented with relational mechanisms.

■ DIMENSIONS OF SOCIAL INJUSTICE AND MENTAL HEALTH INEQUALITIES

Relational mechanisms generate and reproduce mental health inequalities between relatively powerful and relatively powerless groups. Some groups benefit at the expense of others, thereby enjoying better mental health. Relationships between advantaged and disadvantaged groups are systematic and interdependent, and societies differ in what they deem to be fair and unfair. Structured forms of inequality in many societies lead to poverty, income inequalities, exploitation of employees, and gender, racial, and ethnic forms of discrimination.

Absolute poverty—deprivation of resources that is life-threatening—is a risk factor for depression, anxiety disorders, antisocial personality, substance use, and other mental disorders.[7,30,37] People experiencing absolute poverty often cannot afford basic housing and often become homeless. About one-fourth of all sheltered homeless persons have severe mental illness.[42] Cross-sectional and longitudinal studies have found consistent associations between poverty and mental disorders. The presence of a household member with a severe psychiatric disorder predicts a 52 percent increase in depth of poverty and more than a threefold increased risk of being poor.[43] In terms of relative poverty, greater levels of income inequality are usually associated with higher rates of mental disorders and drug abuse. Mental disorders may occur three times more frequently in societies that have more income inequality, compared with those that have less.[44,45]

Social class inequality, independent of SEP differences, is also associated with mental illness.[3,46-52] For example, low-level supervisors, who do not make policy—but can hire and fire workers, have higher rates of depression and anxiety than both upper-level managers, who have organizational control over policy and personnel, and front-line employees, who have neither. Low-level supervisors, while having little influence over company policy, are subjected to "double exposure": the demands of upper-level managers to discipline workers and the antagonism of subordinate workers—often placing them at greater risk of depression and anxiety disorders.

Studies of the influence of both gender and social class on mental health provide additional insights. Whereas the association between social class and poor mental health among men is partially explained by psychosocial and physical working conditions and job insecurity, this association among women is explained not only by working conditions, but also by material well-being at home and amount of household labor.[53]

Gender and racial discrimination also contribute to mental health inequalities. Women are at least twice as likely as men to have depression and anxiety disorders, partly because of their lower socioeconomic status and higher exposure to stressors.[54] Within the United States, women residing in states with the highest levels of income inequality, such as Louisiana, have substantially higher rates of depression than do women living in states with the lowest levels of income inequality, such as New Hampshire.[55] New mothers of low SEP have higher rates of postpartum depression symptoms than do new mothers of high SEP.[56]

Perceptions of racial and ethnic discrimination are associated with worse mental health.[57] Black women in the United States have a higher rate of anxiety disorders. Ageism and discrimination based on sexual orientation have also been found to adversely affect mental health.[58,59]

There is debate over the relative influence of neo-material determinants, such as owning a car or a house, and psychosocial determinants, such as perceptions of relative standing in income distribution, on mental health in high-income countries.[60-62] For example, a household survey in the United Kingdom found an association between (a) housing tenure and access to a car, and (b) "neurotic" disorders and depression.[63,64] It also found an association between a low material standard of living and depression and anxiety disorders.[63] Some studies have provided evidence of an association between (a) psychosocial factors, such as perceived job demands and perceived financial hardship, and (b) depression and anxiety disorders.[34,63] Psychosocial exposures may cause psychiatric disorders.[65] For example, job insecurity or remaining in a downsized company may cause anxiety and depression.

▓ MENTAL HEALTH SERVICES AS A SOURCE OF SOCIAL INJUSTICE

The quantity and quality of mental health services vary across geographic areas. There are systematic differences in the availability, accessibility, and appropriateness of treatment options for racial/ethnic minorities, homeless and incarcerated people, children in foster care, traumatized persons, refugees, and people with substance-use disorders or alternative sexual preferences. Inequalities in access to and quality of care often cause marginalized groups, who already have limited political power and economic resources, to suffer disproportionately from unmet mental health needs.[66] Since rates of mental illness are similar among people of different racial and ethnic backgrounds, inequalities in outcomes reflect: (a) varying abilities of mental health care providers to accurately diagnose and appropriately treat people from different backgrounds or with different characteristics; and (b) the willingness of people to receive treatment from mental health clinicians whom they mistrust or fear.[67]

The causes of racial/ethnic inequalities in mental health are due to patient, provider, and institutional factors—and the interaction among these factors.[68,69] Patient factors include cultural beliefs about health and medical care by members of a minority group, mistrust of the health care system based on past discrimination, language barriers and other difficulties in communication, and patient "preference." For example, members of minority groups may wish to find a mental health care provider of the same racial/ethnic background. Provider factors, which may influence diagnosis and treatment of minority patients, include inadequate cultural competence, ineffective provider-patient interactions, atypical symptom presentation, and negative stereotypes and other biases. Institutional factors include a lack of experience with certain patients and their problems, and policies to not treat patients who do not have health insurance. Recent measures to address racial inequalities in mental health services and outcomes of these services have included the incorporation of anti-racism and anti-oppression frameworks of practice. These frameworks refer to theories and practices that embrace a social justice perspective; seek to reduce, undermine, or eliminate racial discrimination; and include the use of empowerment, education, alliance building, language, alternative healing strategies, advocacy, activism, and reflexivity.[70]

The availability of mental health services depends on both (a) a sufficient number of competent providers to meet the complex mental health care needs of a population, and (b) the available care being culturally relevant. In the United States, most mental health patients who are members of minority groups are unable to find a provider of the same racial/ethnic background.[71,72] For example, only about 3 percent of mental health care providers are African American.[71] In addition, many African Americans live in areas where culturally competent mental health treatment is not available.[71] African Americans are incarcerated, homeless, in foster care, and uninsured at disproportionately high rates, and mental health services are far less available to people in these categories.[73-77] The situation is even worse for American Indians and Alaska Natives.[78-79] People who are not fluent in English often have limited access to services because of the absence—or inadequate numbers—of translators in mental health services.

Affordable health care and generous insurance coverage facilitate access to mental health services. Members of minority groups are less likely to have health insurance or the money to pay for mental health care.[80] Even with insurance, coverage for mental health problems seldom is equal to coverage for somatic disorders, even in states where parity is legislatively mandated. Children with mental disorders, even with coverage through the Children's Health Insurance Program (CHIP), are often inadequately insured for mental and substance-use disorders.[81]

Insurance coverage is often tied to employment; many blue-collar workers are unemployed and therefore unable to pay for mental health care.

Feelings of mistrust deter some minority patients from receiving mental health services.[82] Mistrust may derive from a historical legacy of discrimination and maltreatment or from experiences with culturally insensitive clinicians. One study found that 12 percent of African Americans and 15 percent of Latinos perceived that physicians treated them with disrespect or unfairly, compared with 1 percent of whites.[83] Immigrants to the United States from other countries whose governments persecuted their citizens—and American Indians—are also unlikely to trust authorities, including mental health care providers.[84]

Stigma about mental disorders and discrimination prevent marginalized groups from seeking necessary mental health care.[85] Stigma operates at the individual, family, community, and societal level. At the individual level, mentally ill persons who fear rejection due to their illnesses are often socially isolated and are less likely to seek, or adhere to, therapies. At the family and community levels, stigma against those with a mental illness disproportionately affects members of some minority groups. In some Asian cultures, for example, the shame of having a mentally ill family member adversely influences the potential of other immediate family members to marry or to work. Stigma by association is also present in other cultures. Contact of mentally ill patients with others improves their ability to integrate into the community.[86]

Implementation of the Americans with Disabilities Act (ADA) has reduced discrimination against mentally ill people in the United States. However, the stigma of mental illness can still prevent mentally ill people from acquiring housing and getting jobs—with accommodations, as required under the ADA—because they must disclose the nature of their disability to prospective employers, which they may be reluctant to do.[87,88] Patients with mental disorders often have multiple needs that extend beyond psychiatric care. As a result, they must negotiate their way through complex mental health care systems in order to receive adequate care. They often require income support, assistance in obtaining supported housing and employment, and legal aid. In theory, mental health services are designed to support people and provide a continuum of care; however, in practice, these services are often fragmented by sources of funding, geographic area, and diagnoses.[89] In response to these systemic barriers, case-management and community treatment models have been developed and implemented.[90,91]

Use of mental health services by minorities has been studied. African American patients do not underuse mental health services, compared to white patients, but they are more likely to receive care in a primary-care or general health-care setting, rather than in a mental-health specialty setting.[72,92] This may be due to African Americans' holding unfavorable attitudes toward mental health treatment or their perception of being forced to be "guinea pigs."[93] Among adolescents, African American males receive one-third the treatment of African American females and one-half that of white males, suggesting a referral bias based on racial discrimination.[94] Other plausible reasons for racial differences in treatment include African Americans' (a) having a higher threshold for tolerating symptoms before seeking help, (b) having lower expectations that treatment will be beneficial, and (c) possibly being shunted into the juvenile justice system. African American children, ages 5 to 14, on Medicaid are less than half as likely to be prescribed psychotropic medication as are white children.[95] In poor inner-city neighborhoods, there are fewer behavioral pediatricians and fewer options for children to receive psychiatric care. In addition, there are significant cultural differences in the interpretation of symptoms of attention deficit-hyperactivity disorder (ADHD) symptoms, which influence a family's decision to seek, or not to seek, psychiatric care.

There are racial differences in the amount and type of treatment for mental disorders. For example, compared to white patients, African Americans treated in an inpatient facility may have shorter lengths of stay and be more likely to have a urine drug screen.[96]

There may be an unconscious bias about the "treatability" of African Americans, especially when comorbid substance-use disorders are present.[96] African Americans may receive less close observation because they are reluctant to disclose suicidal thoughts and because they mistrust mental health care providers who are not minorities.[96] One study found African Americans had fewer sessions with a psychotherapist, compared with Asians and Latinos. Patients of low SEP are more likely to have fewer psychotherapy sessions, more sessions with an untrained mental health therapist, less medication, and less overall treatment.[97] Another study found that Mexican American ethnicity status interacts with low SEP to decrease social and institutional support, increase depression rates, and inhibit "treatment readiness."[98] Low SEP may inhibit participation in the mental health system, but may also create more distress from stressful life events.

Once a person receives mental health treatment, the outcome of care depends on the clinician's making a correct diagnosis and giving appropriate treatment. Treatment guidelines based on scientific evidence have been published by several professional organizations. Although these guidelines are supported and endorsed by various government agencies, their use in clinical practice is deficient for patients of all races, and especially deficient for minorities. For example, compared with whites, African Americans are less likely to receive guideline-based treatments for anxiety or depression,[99,100] less likely to receive an antidepressant, and more likely to be over-medicated with antipsychotic medications.[101,102] Minority patients are under-represented in clinical trials where interventions for major mental disorders are tested; therefore, the efficacy of many mental health treatments for minority patients has not been determined.[103] (See also Chapter 3.)

Social injustice against other groups adversely affects their mental health. For example, lesbian, gay, bisexual, and transgender/transsexual (LGBT) persons are exposed to various forms of homophobia and heterosexualism in the broader society.[104] (See Chapter 7.) They experience psychological distress as they cope with overt discrimination and internalization of hate messages. For LGBT males, rates of depression and panic attacks are higher than those for heterosexual men.[105] LGBT individuals who seek psychotherapy are generally satisfied with their experience,[106] although some are reluctant to disclose their sexual orientation to therapists.

Mental disorders and comorbid substance use are common among prisoners.[107-110] (See Chapter 9.) For young people entering the criminal justice system, these disorders are often unrecognized and undiagnosed. Prisoners have often experienced trauma and family disruption during childhood. Treatment of mental disorders during incarceration is often inadequate, and mental health care upon release is generally poor compared with treatment for somatic disorders. The experience of incarceration is traumatizing because inmates are daily exposed to stressful events, while correctional staff members can adversely affect the mental health of vulnerable inmates. "Supermax" prisons have been described as "incubators for psychosis"; sensory deprivation is severe, and electroshock instruments are often used to force compliant behavior.[111] The period of incarceration could present opportunities for focused treatment; however, this does not often occur, although some suggest that it would reduce recidivism. Collaboration between the mental health and criminal justice systems would better serve prisoners. So would re-conceptualizing the role of prisons to be restorative, rather than punitive.

Refugees are susceptible to mental disorders related to traumas they have experienced in their native countries.[112] (See Chapter 11.) Many have fled war, famine, or repressive regimes that use torture and intimidation to control their populations. Post-traumatic stress disorder is common among those who have been subjected to torture or rape or have witnessed murder. Often refugees are leaving behind relatives with no way to be assured of their safety or ability to contact them. Having arrived in host countries, refugees often experience difficulties with language, cultural assimilation, social isolation, and poverty. They are often at the bottom of the social strata. When mental health problems are recognized, refugees continue to face problems in treatment. Those from cultures in which emotional distress is somaticized may be misdiagnosed with somatic illnesses. Because of the extended period between traumatic event and treatment, outcomes of therapies are less than optimal. In some cultures, psychotherapy is not culturally acceptable, so different models of treatment must be used to assist refugees; trust is sometimes difficult when medical care providers in countries of origin participated in torture. Somatic and mental health care must be coordinated with services to assist with housing, language, employment, and income supports.

Children in foster care have high risks of mental disorders and developmental delays.[113] Many have been abused or neglected during the period of early brain development. Once they are in foster care, their behavioral problems often worsen because of attachment difficulties to foster caregivers, separation from siblings, and uncertainty about future relationships with biological parents. In the worst-case scenario, the foster care setting or the social service system increases stress on the child and can lead to mental disorders. Child welfare workers are a vital link to appropriate pediatric and mental health care services—if their caseloads are manageable—enabling foster children to be screened for behavioral symptoms. Older children who have failed to "catch up" emotionally are aged out of the system at age 18 and can have difficulties living independently. Child welfare workers face the challenge of coordinating care among social, health, and judicial systems, while advocating for the best interests of the child. (See Chapter 5.)

Homelessness and mental health problems are closely associated. About 30 percent of chronically homeless people experience mental disorders, and about 50 percent suffer from comorbid substance-use problems.[114-116] Treatment has been shown to be more effective when services for comorbid disorders are provided and when providers of community mental health care and shelter care systems are coordinated.[117] Independent housing and vocational rehabilitation programs have been developed that are assisting homeless people. (See Chapter 10.)

■ WHAT NEEDS TO BE DONE

Reversing the adverse mental health effects of social injustice will require more than addressing the immediate social determinants of mental illness, such as stigma, lack of access to treatment, and homelessness. Unless the United States comprehensively addresses broad social policies that affect mental health, such as poverty and racism, it will not adequately redress the mental health effects of social injustice.

Stigma profoundly affects the quality of life for patients with mental disorders. The only antidote to such discrimination is providing systematic, sustained, culturally appropriate public education that provides a realistic picture of mental illness. Media portrayals of individuals with mental disorders stress dangerousness, deviant behavior, and unpredictability. Accurate portrayals, such as those that include the biological basis for mental disorders, describe issues of discrimination, and demonstrate positive outcomes for those who receive optimal treatment, would challenge discriminatory beliefs and would expose the general public to real people with mental disorders.

Achieving social justice for people with mental illness will benefit if advocates use a "bottom-up" approach to challenge discrimination. Groups such as the National Alliance for the Mentally Ill and Mental Health America have implemented commendable programs that assist consumers and their families and advocate for health policies that reduce stigma.

An Action Agenda

We recommend the following 10 actions:

1. Reframing issues of mental health to include civil and human rights and a public health approach

2. Organizing clinical records and health databases to reflect indices connected to social injustice, such as social class, gender, ethnicity, race, migrant status, and neighborhood of residence
3. Including all stakeholders, such as patients, family members, and mental health workers, in advocacy to improve mental health policies
4. Increasing recruitment of socioeconomically, ethnically, and racially diverse mental health workers, including nurses, physicians, psychologists, and social workers. Providing education and training in cultural competence for all those who treat people with mental disorders
5. Ensuring insurance coverage for mental disorders and establishing parity for care for mental disorders with care for somatic disorders
6. Providing feedback mechanisms to ensure that treatment adheres to evidence-based practices with known efficacy
7. Focusing on primary prevention by strengthening "at risk" families and communities and by reducing adverse conditions, such as poverty and discrimination
8. Increasing participation of ethnic and racial minorities in research to determine efficacy and effectiveness of treatments
9. Educating the public to reduce the stigma of mental illness
10. Developing policies that reduce the social injustice that causes mental illness

◼ REFERENCES

1. Dohrenwend B, Dohrenwend, B. Social status and psychological disorder: A causal inquiry. New York: Wiley, 1969.
2. Yu Y, Williams DR. Socioeconomic status and mental health. In: Aneshensel CS, Phelan JC, eds. Handbook of the sociology of mental health. 1st ed. New York: Kluwer Academic/Plenum Publishers, 1999:151–166.
3. Muntaner C, Ng E, Vanroelen C, et al. Social stratification, social closure, and social class as determinants of mental health inequalities. In: Aneshensel CS, Phelan JC, Bierman A, eds. Handbook of the sociology of mental health. 2nd ed. New York: Springer, 2013:205–227.
4. Bayoumi AM, Guta A. Values and social epidemiologic research. In: O'Campo P, Dunn JR, eds. Rethinking social epidemiology—Towards a science of change. New York: Springer, 2012:43–66.
5. Rawls J. A theory of justice. Cambridge, MA: Harvard University Press, 1971.
6. Sen A. The idea of justice. Cambridge, MA: Harvard University Press, 2009.
7. Eaton WW. The sociology of mental disorders. 3rd ed. London: Praeger, 2001.
8. Regier DA, Farmer ME, Rae DS, et al. One month prevalence of mental disorders in the U.S. and socio-demographic characteristics. *Acta Psychiatr Scand* 1993;88:35–47.
9. Blazer DG, Kessler RC, McGonagle KA, et al. The prevalence and distribution of major depression in a national community sample: The national comorbidity survey. *Am J Psychiatry* 1994;151:979–986.

10. Roberts RE, Lee ES. Occupation and the prevalence of major depression, alcohol and drug abuse in the U.S. *Environ Res* 1993;61:266–278.

11. Murray CJ, Lopez AD. Evidence-based health policy—Lessons from the Global Burden of Disease Study. *Science* 1996;274:740–743.

12. Eaton WW, Martins SS, Nestadt G, et al. The burden of mental disorders. *Epidemiol Rev* 2008;30:1–14.

13. Kessler RC, Aguilar-Gaxiola S, Alonso J, et al. The global burden of mental disorders: an update from the WHO World Mental Health (WMH) surveys. *Epidemiol Psychiatr Soc* 2009;18:23–33. Available at http://www.ncbi.nlm.nih.gov/pubmed?term=Chatterji%20 S%5BAuthor%5D&cauthor=true&cauthor_uid=19378696.

14. World Health Organization. The global burden of disease: 2004 update. Geneva: WHO Press, 2008.

15. Prince M, Patel V, Saxena S, et al. No health without mental health. *Lancet* 2007;370:859–877.

16. Üstün TB, Ayuso-Mateos JL, Chatterji S, et al. Global burden of depressive disorders in the year 2000. *Brit J Psychiat* 2004;184:386–392.

17. Ford DE, Erlinger TP. Depression and C-reactive protein in U.S. adults: Data from the third National Health and Nutrition Survey. *Arch Intern Med* 2004;164:1010–1014.

18. Andreasen NC, Black DW. Introductory textbook of psychiatry. 4th ed. Washington, DC: American Psychiatric Publishing, Inc., 2006.

19. McLean CP, Asnaani A, Litz BT, Hofmann SG. Gender differences in anxiety disorders: Prevalence, course of illness, comorbidity and burden of illness. *J Psychiatr Res* 2011;45:1027–1035.

20. Díaz RM, Ayala G, Bein E, et al. The impact of homophobia, poverty, and racism on the mental health of gay and bisexual Latino men: Findings from 3 U.S. cities. *Am J Public Health* 2001;91:927–932.

21. Muntaner C, Lynch J. Income Inequality, Social cohesion, and class relations: A critique of Wilkinson's Neo-Durkheimian research program. *Int J Health Serv* 1999;29:59–81.

22. Lakoff G. The political mind: Why you can't understand 21st-century American politics with an 18th-century brain. New York: Viking Adult, 2008.

23. Barry B. Why social justice matters. Cambridge, UK: Polity, 2005.

24. Haidt J. The righteous mind: Why good people are divided by politics and religion. New York: Pantheon, 2012.

25. Stiglitz JE. The price of inequality: How today's divided society endangers our future. New York: W.W. Norton & Company, 2012.

26. Krieger N. Embodying inequality: A review of concepts, measures, and methods for studying health consequences of discrimination. *Int J Health Serv* 1999;29:295–352.

27. Muntaner C, Chung H, Murphy K, Ng E. Barriers to knowledge production, knowledge translation, and urban health policy change: Ideological, economic, and political considerations. *J Urban Health* 2012;89:915–924.

28. Tyrer P, Tyrer F. Public mental health. In: Detels R, McEwen J, Beaglehole R, Tanaka H, eds. Oxford textbook of public health. 4th ed. Oxford, England: Oxford University Press, 2002:1309–1328.

29. Eaton WW, Faculty students and fellows of the Department of Mental Health Bloomberg School of Public Health. Public mental health. New York: Oxford University Press, 2012.

30. Eaton WW, Muntaner C, Sapag JC. Socioeconomic stratification and mental disorder. In: Horwitz AV, Scheid TL, eds. A handbook for the study of mental health: Social contexts, theories and systems. New York: Cambridge University Press, 1999:226–255.

31. Muntaner C, Eaton WW, Miech R, O'Campo P. Socioeconomic position and major mental disorders. *Epidemiol Rev* 2004;26:53–62.

32. Ritter C, Hobfoll SE, Lavin J, et al. Stress, psychosocial resources, and depressive symptomatology during pregnancy in low-income, inner-city women. *Health Psychol* 2000;19:576–585.

33. Danziger SK, Carlson MJ, Henly JR. Post-welfare employment and psychological well-being. *Women Health* 2001;32:47–78.

34. Eaton WW, Muntaner C, Bovasso G, et al. Socioeconomic status and depression. *J Health Soc Behav* 2001;42:277–293.

35. O'Campo P, Eaton WW, Muntaner C. Labor market experience, work organization, gender inequalities, and health status: Results from a prospective study of U.S. employed women. *Soc Sci Med* 2004;58:585–594.

36. Dalgard OS, Mykletun A, Rognerud M, et al. Education, sense of mastery and mental health: Results from a nationwide health monitoring study in Norway. *BMC Psychiatry* 2007;7:20.

37. Lorant V, Deliege D, Eaton WW, et al. Socio-economic inequalities in mental health: a meta-analysis. *Am J Epidemiol* 2003;157:98–112.

38. Fryers T, Melzer D, Jenkins R, Brugha T. The distribution of the common mental disorders: social inequalities in Europe. *Clin Pract Epidemiol Ment Health*. 2005;5:14.

39. Kurtze N, Eikemo TA, Kamphuis CB. Educational inequalities in general and mental health: differential contribution of physical activity, smoking, alcohol consumption and diet. *Eur J Public Health*. 2012. doi:10.1093/eurpub/cks055.

40. Roberts RE, Lee ES. Occupation and the prevalence of major depression, alcohol and drug abuse in the US. *Environ Res* 1993;61:266–278.

41. Quesnel-Vallée A, DeHaney S, Ciampi A. Temporary work and depressive symptoms: A propensity score analysis. *Soc Sci Med* 2010;70:1982–1987.

42. U.S. Department of Housing and Urban Development. The 2008 annual homeless assessment report to Congress, 2009. Available at https://www.onecpd.info/resources/documents/5thHomelessAssessmentReport.pdf. Accessed on March 11, 2013.

43. Vick B, Jones K, Mitra S. Poverty and severe psychiatric disorder in the U.S.: Evidence from the medical expenditure panel survey. *J Ment Health Policy Econ* 2012;15:83–96.

44. Pickett KE, Wilkinson RG. Inequality: An underacknowledged source of mental illness and distress. *Brit J Psychiat* 2010;197:426–428.

45. Messias E, Eaton WW, Grooms AN. Economic grand rounds: income inequality and depression prevalence across the United States: An ecological study. *Psychiatr Serv* 2011; 62:710–712.

46. Muntaner C, Borrell C, Chung H. Class relations, economic inequality and mental health: Why social class matters to the sociology of mental health. In Avison WR, McLeod JD, Pescosolido BA, eds. Mental health, social mirror. New York: Springer, 2007:127–141.

47. Wohlfarth T, Winkel FW, Ybema JF, et al. The relationship between socio-economic inequality and criminal victimisation: A prospective study. *Soc Psychiatry Psychiatric Epidemiol* 2000;36:361–370.

48. Wohlfarth T, van den Brink W. Social class and substance use disorders: The value of social class as distinct from socioeconomic status. *Soc Sci Med* 1998;47:51–58.

49. Wohlfarth T. Socioeconomic inequality and psychopathology: Are socioeconomic status and social class interchangeable? *Soc Sci Med* 1997;45:399–410.

50. Muntaner C, Eaton WW, Diala C, et al. Social class, assets, organizational control and the prevalence of common groups of psychiatric disorders. *Soc Sci Med* 1998;47:243–253.

51. Muntaner C, Eaton W, Diala CC. Socioeconomic inequalities in mental health: A review of concepts and underlying assumptions. *Health* 2000;4:82–106.

52. Muntaner C, Borrell C, Benach J. The association of social class and social stratification with patterns of general and mental health in a Spanish population. *Int J Epidemiol* 2003;32:950–958.

53. Borrell C, Muntaner C, Benach J, Artazcoz L. Social class and self-reported health status among men and women: What is the role of work organisation, household material standards and household labour? *Soc Sci Med* 2004;58:1869–1887.

54. Kessler R, Berglund P, Demler O, et al. National Comorbidity Survey Replication. The epidemiology of major depressive disorder: Results from the National Co-morbidity Survey Replication (NCS-R). *JAMA* 2003;289:3095–3105.

55. Kahn R, Wise PH, Kennedy BP, et al. State income inequality, household income, and maternal mental and physical health: Cross sectional national survey. *BMJ* 2000;321:1311–1315.

56. Seguin L, Potvin L, St-Denis M, et al. Socio-environmental factors and postnatal depressive symptomatology: A longitudinal study. *Women Health* 1999;29:57–72.

57. Noh S, Kaspar V. Perceived discrimination and depression: Moderating effect of coping, acculturation, and ethnic support. *Am J Public Health* 2003;93:232–238.

58. Mays VM, Cochran SD. Mental health correlates of perceived discrimination among lesbian, gay, and bisexual adults in the United States. *Am J Public Health* 2001;91:1869–1876.

59. Ory M, Kinney Hoffman M, Hawkins M, et al. Challenging aging stereotypes: Strategies for creating a more active society. *Am J Prev Med* 2003;25:164–171.

60. Pearce N, Davey Smith G. Is social capital the key to inequalities in health? *Am J Public Health* 2003;93:122–129.

61. Lynch J, Due P, Muntaner C, et al. Social capital—Is it a good investment strategy for public health? *J Epidemiol Community Health* 2000;54:404–408.

62. Dunn JR, Veenstra G, Ross N. Psychosocial and neo-material dimensions of SES and health revisited: Predictors of self-rated health in a Canadian national survey. *Soc Sci Med.* 2006;62:1465–1473.

63. Weich S, Lewis G. Material standard of living, social class, and the prevalence of the common mental disorders in Great Britain. *J Epidemiol Community Health* 1998;52:8–14.

64. Lewis G, Bebbington P, Brugha T, et al. Socio-economic status, standard of living, and neurotic disorder. *Int Rev Psychiatry* 2003;15:91–96.

65. Ferrie JE, Shipley MJ, Stansfeld SA, et al. Future uncertainty and socioeconomic inequalities in health: The Whitehall II study. *Soc Sci Med* 2003;57:637–646.

66. Ngui EM, Khasakhala L, Ndetei D, Roberts LW. Mental disorders, health inequalities and ethics: A global perspective. *Int Rev Psychiatr* 2010;22:235–244.

67. Whaley AL. Cultural mistrust and mental health services for African Americans: A review and meta-analysis. *Couns Psychol* July 2001;29:513–531.

68. Physicians for Human Rights. The right to equal treatment: An action plan to end racial and ethnic inequalities in clinical diagnosis and treatment in the United States, 2003. Available at http://www.paeaonline.org/index.php?ht=a/GetDocumentAction/i/135605. Accessed on August 15, 2012.

69. Primm AB, Vasquez MJT, Mays RA, et al. The role of public health in addressing racial and ethnic inequalities in mental health and mental illness. *Prev Chronic Dis* 2010;7:A20.

70. Corneau S, Stergiopoulos V. More than being against it: Anti-racism and anti-oppression in mental health services. *Transcult Psychiatry* 2012;49:261–282.

71. Duffy FF, Wilk J, West JC, et al. Mental health practitioners and trainees. In: Manderscheid RW, Berry JT, eds. Mental health, United States. Rockville, MD: Center for Mental Health Services, 2004:256–309.

72. Cooper-Patrick L, Gallo JJ, Gonzales JJ, et al. Race, gender, and partnership in the patient-physician relationship. *JAMA* 1999;282:583–589.

73. Lyons CJ, Pettit B. Compounded disadvantage: Race, incarceration, and wage growth. *Soc Probl* 2011;58:257–280.

74. Jencks C. The homeless. Cambridge, MA: Harvard University Press, 1994.

75. Nunez RC, Adams, M, Simonsen-Meehan A. Intergenerational inequalities experienced by homeless black families. New York: Institute for Children, Poverty and Homelessness, 2012. Available at http://www.icphusa.org/filelibrary/ICPH_Homeless%20Black%20Families.pdf. Accessed on March 11, 2013.

76. Murphy SL. Deaths: Final data for 1998. *National vital statistics reports* 2000;48:1–108. Available at http://www.cdc.gov/nchs/data/nvsr/nvsr48/nvs48_11.pdf Accessed on August 15, 2012.

77. Alegria M, Lin J, Chen CN, et al. The impact of insurance coverage in diminishing racial and ethnic inequalities in behavioral health services. *Health Serv Res* 2012;47:1322–1344.

78. Gone JP, Trimble JE. Native mental health: Diverse perspectives on enduring inequalities. *Annu Rev Clin Psychol* 2012;8:131–160.

79. Gone JP. Mental health services for Native Americans in the 21st century United States. *Prof Psychol Res Pract* 2004;35:10–18.

80. DeNavas-Walt C, Proctor BD, Mills RJ. Income, poverty, and health insurance coverage in the United States: 2003.Washington, DC: U.S. Census Bureau, 2004. Available at http://www.census.gov/prod/2004pubs/p60-226.pdf. Accessed on August 15, 2012.

81. Kataoka SH, Zhang L, Wells KB. Unmet need for mental health care among U.S. children: Variation by ethnicity and insurance status. *Am J Psychiatry* 2002;159:1548–1555.

82. Dobransky-Fasiska D, Nowalk MP, Pincus HA, et al. Public-academic partnerships: Improving depression care for disadvantaged adults by partnering with non-mental health agencies. *Psychiatr Serv* 2010;61:110–112.

83. Brown ER, Ojeda VD, Wyn R, et al. Racial and ethnic inequalities in access to health insurance and health care [report]. Los Angeles, CA: UCLA Center for Health Policy Research and the Henry J. Kaiser Family Foundation, 2000. Available at http://escholarship.org/uc/item/4sf0p1st. Accessed on August 15, 2012.

84. Chung RC-Y, Bemak F, Ortiz DP, Sandoval-Perez S. Promoting the mental health of immigrants: A multicultural/social justice perspective. *J Couns Dev* 2008; 86:310–317.

85. Parcesepe AM, Cabassa LJ. Public stigma of mental illness in the United States: A systematic literature review. *Adm Policy Ment Health* 2012; doi 10.1007/s10488-012-0430-z.

86. Prince PN, Prince CR. Perceived stigma and community integration among clients of assertive community treatment. *Psychiatric Rehabil J* 2002;25:323–331.

87. Stefan S. Unequal rights: Discrimination against people with mental disabilities and the Americans with Disabilities Act. Washington, DC: American Psychological Association, 2000.

88. Cook JA. Employment barriers for persons with psychiatric disabilities: Update of a report for the President's Commission. *Psychiatric Services* 2006;57:1391–1405.

89. Charatan F. U.S. mental health service is "highly fragmented." *BMJ* 2000;320:7.

90. Ziguras SJ, Stuart GW. A meta-analysis of the effectiveness of mental health case management over 20 years. *Psychiatric Services* 2000;51:1410–1421.

91. Everett A, Lee SY. Community and public mental health services in the United States: History and programs. In: Eaton WW; Faculty, Students, and Fellows of the Department of Mental Health, Bloomberg School of Public Health, eds. Public mental health. New York: Oxford University Press, 2012:396–414.

92. Cooper-Patrick L, Gallo JJ, Powe NR, et al. Mental health service utilization by African Americans and whites: The Baltimore Epidemiologic Catchment Area Follow-Up. *Med Care* 1999;37:1034–1045.

93. Kennedy BR, Mathis CC, Woods AK. African Americans and their distrust of the healthcare system: Healthcare for diverse populations. *J Cult Divers* 2007;14:56–60.

94. Cuffe SP, Waller JL, Cuccaro ML, et al. Race and gender differences in the treatment of psychiatric disorders in young adolescents. *J Am Acad Child Adolesc Psychiatry* 1995;34:1536–1543.

95. Zito JM, Safer DJ, dos Reis S, et al. Racial disparity in psychotropic medications prescribed for youths with Medicaid insurance in Maryland. *J Am Acad Child Adolesc Psychiatry* 1998;37:179–184.

96. Chung H, Mahler JC, Kakuma T. Racial differences in treatment of psychiatric inpatients. *Psychiatr Serv* 1995;46:586–591.

97. Flaskerud JH, Hu LT. Racial/ethnic identity and amount and type of psychiatric treatment. *Am J Psychiatry* 1992;149:379–384.

98. Briones DF, Heller PL, Chalfant HP, et al. Socioeconomic status, ethnicity, psychological distress, and readiness to utilize a mental health facility. *Am J Psychiatry* 1990;147:1333–1340.

99. Wang PS, Berglund P, Kessler RC. Recent care of common mental disorders in the United States. *J Gen Intern Med* 2000;15:284–292.

100. Young AS, Klap R, Shebourne CD, et al. The quality of care for depressive and anxiety disorders in the United States. *Arch Gen Psychiatry* 2001;58:55–61.

101. Melfi CA, Croghan TW, Hanna MP, et al. Racial variation in antidepressant treatment in a Medicaid population. *J Clin Psychiatry* 2000;61:16–21.

102. Walkup JT, McAlpine DD, Olfson M, et al. Patients with schizophrenia at risk for excessive antipsychotic dosing. *J Clin Psychiatry* 2000;61:344–348.

103. Office of the Surgeon General. Mental health: culture, race, and ethnicity—a supplement to mental health: A report of the Surgeon General. Rockville, MD: U.S. Department of Health and Human Services, Public Health Service, 2001.

104. Institute of Medicine (U.S.) Committee on Lesbian, Gay, Bisexual, and Transgender Health Issues and Research Gaps and Opportunities. The health of lesbian, gay, bisexual, and transgender people: Building a foundation for better understanding. Washington, DC: National Academies Press, 2011.

105. Cochran SD, Mays VM, Sullivan JG. Prevalence of mental disorders, psychological distress, and mental health services use among lesbian, gay, and bisexual adults in the United States. *J Consult Clin Psychol* 2003;71:53–61.

106. Jones MA, Gabriel MA. Utilization of psychotherapy by lesbians, gay men, and bisexuals: Findings from a nationwide survey. *Am J Orthopsychiatry* 1999;69:209–219.

107. Birmingham L. The mental health of prisoners. *Advances in Psychiatric Treatment* 2003;9:191–199.

108. Teplin LA, Abram KM, McClelland GM. Mentally disordered women in jail: Who receives services? *Am J Public Health* 1997;87:604–609.

109. Teplin LA. Psychiatric and substance abuse disorders among male urban jail detainees. *Am J Public Health* 1994;84:290–293.

110. Teplin LA, Abram KM, McClelland GM, Dulcan MK, Mericle AA. Psychiatric disorders in youth in juvenile detention. *Arch Gen Psychiatry* 2002;59:1133–1343.

111. Shalev S. Solitary confinement and Supermax prisons: A human rights and ethical analysis. *Journal of Forensic Psychology Practice* 2011;11: 2–3.

112. Murphy HBM. Flight and resettlement. Paris: UNESCO, 1955.

113. Pecora PJ, Jensen PS, Romanelli LH, et al. Mental health services for children placed in foster care: An overview of current challenges. *Child Welfare* 2009;88:5–26.

114. Caton CL, Dominguez B, Schanzer B, et al. Risk factors for long-term homelessness: Findings from a longitudinal review of first-time homeless single adults. *Am J Public Health* 2005;95:1753–1759.

115. Kertesz SG, Larson MJ, Horton NJ, et al. Homeless chronicity and health-related quality of life trajectories among adults with addictions. *Med Care* 2005;43:574–585.

116. Padgett DK, Gulcur L, Tsemberis S. Housing First services for people who are homeless with co-occurring serious mental illness and substance abuse. *Res Social Work Pract* 2006;16:74–83.

117. Gonzales G, Rosenheck RA. Outcomes and service use among homeless persons with serious mental illness and substance abuse. *Psychiatr Serv* 2002;53:427–446.

17 Violence

■ JAMES A. MERCY AND SARAH DEGUE

▓ INTRODUCTION

Violence can be both a consequence of social injustice and a tool used to perpetrate it. Violence against women, for example, may originate partially from customs and cultural norms that support or facilitate unjust inequities between men and women.[1] Genocide, on the other hand, such as in Nazi Germany and Rwanda, is the most extreme example of using violence as a tool to perpetrate social injustice, by attempting to deny an entire population group of its right to exist.[2] Public health workers have a fundamental role to play in preventing violence by promoting social justice[3]—a role that has expanded with heightened awareness that violence is a major contributor to premature mortality, morbidity, and disability.[4]

Public health workers have helped develop and implement strategies to prevent violence from occurring (primary prevention).[5] In addition, they have brought a multidisciplinary, scientific approach to violence prevention aimed at identifying effective preventive measures—and developed an evidence base for preventing some forms of violence.[6] They have also emphasized the need for collective action to prevent violence—involving collaboration among various scientific disciplines, organizations, and communities.

Addressing violence as a public health problem has increased dramatically since the late 1970s.[7] In 1979, *Healthy People*, a report of the U.S. Surgeon General, documented the dramatic gains made in the health of Americans during the previous 100 years and identified 15 priority areas in which, with appropriate action, further gains could be expected.[8] Among these areas was the control of stress and violent behavior. Various activities for violence prevention within the public health sector followed. In 1983, for example, the Centers for Disease Control and Prevention (CDC) established a Violence Epidemiology Branch (now the Division of Violence Prevention). In 1985, the U.S. Surgeon General held a workshop on violence and public health.[9] In 1996, the World Health Assembly—the annual gathering of all ministers of health—adopted a resolution stating that violence is a global public health priority.[3]

▓ DEFINING VIOLENCE

The World Health Organization (WHO) defines *violence* as "the intentional use of physical force or power, threatened or actual, against oneself, another person, or a group or community that either results in or has a high likelihood of resulting in injury, death, psychological harm, maldevelopment, or deprivation."[10] Therefore, violence can occur through threats or intimidation as well as physical force, and

289

may be a consequence of—or mechanism for—the exploitation of individuals or groups. The WHO definition includes outcomes beyond physical injury and death, such as psychological harm, maldevelopment, and deprivation.

Violence is defined by its effects on the health and well-being of people—not in cultural terms.[10] Some violent behavior may be consistent with prevailing cultural norms within societies. Physical violence toward spouses or children, for example, is regarded as an acceptable practice in some societies, even though these acts may have serious health consequences.[11,12]

The WHO definition includes three general types of violence: interpersonal, self-directed, and collective. Interpersonal violence includes forms perpetrated by a person or small group of people, such as child abuse and neglect by caregivers, youth violence, intimate-partner violence, sexual violence, and elder abuse.[10] Self-directed violence includes suicidal behavior as well as acts of self-abuse in which the intent may not be to take one's own life. Collective violence is the use of violence by groups—or individuals who identify themselves as members of a group—against another group or set of individuals in order to achieve political, social, or economic objectives. It includes war, terrorism, and violence sponsored by a state (nation) toward its own citizens (Box 17–1).[2]

■ THE PUBLIC HEALTH BURDEN OF VIOLENCE

Globally, in 2008 more than 4100 people, on average, died each day as a result of violence.[13] More than 90 percent of these deaths occurred in low- and middle-income countries, where violent death rates are about four times higher than in high-income countries.[13,14] About one-half of the almost 1.5 million violent deaths in 2008 were suicides, about one-third were homicides, and about one-fifth were due to war.[13] Rates of violent death vary considerably by region, country, and area within countries (Figure 17–1).

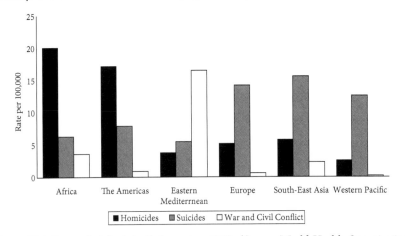

Figure 17–1 Rates of violent death by region, 2008. (*Source:* World Health Organization. Global Burden of Disease Project [2012]. Available at http://www.who.int/healthinfo/global_burden_disease/en/. Accessed on May 8, 2012.)

BOX 17-1 ■ War and Other Forms of Armed Conflict

Barry S. Levy and Victor W. Sidel

An estimated 191 million people died as a result of armed conflict, genocide, and mass murder during the 20th century—more than half of whom were civilians.[1] Many of these civilians were innocent bystanders, caught in the crossfire of opposing armies; others were specifically targeted. During the past two decades, most armed conflict has been in the form of civil wars, mainly in low-income countries, such as the civil war in the Democratic Republic of Congo, in which approximately 4 million people have died,[2] and the 30-year civil war in Ethiopia, in which 1 million people died—about half of whom were civilians.[3]

An *armed conflict*, as defined by the Stockholm International Peace Research Institute, is "a contested incompatibility between two parties—at least one of which is the government of a state—that concerns government or territory or both, where the use of armed force by the parties results in at least 25 battle-related deaths in a calendar year."[4] A *war* is "an armed conflict that results in 1000 battle-related deaths in a year."[4] During the 2001–2010 period, there were 69 armed conflicts, 30 of which were active during 2010—four of which were wars.[4]

Many people survive wars only to be physically scarred for life. Millions of survivors are chronically disabled from injuries sustained during wars or the immediate aftermath of wars. Landmines and unexploded ordnance account for many of these injuries.[5]

Millions more are psychologically impaired from wars, during which they have been physically or sexually assaulted, have been forced to serve as soldiers against their will, have witnessed the death of family members, or have experienced the destruction of their communities—or entire nations. Psychological trauma may be demonstrated in disturbed and antisocial behavior, such as aggression toward others, including family members. Many soldiers suffer from posttraumatic stress disorder (PTSD) on return from military action.[6,7]

Social chaos during war creates situations and conditions that lead to sexual violence.[8] Rape has been used as a weapon in many wars as an act of humiliation and revenge. For example, at least 10,000 women were raped by military personnel during the war in Bosnia and Herzegovina.

Children are particularly vulnerable during and after wars. Many die as a result of malnutrition, disease, or violence. Many become physically or psychologically impaired. Many are forced to become soldiers themselves or sexual slaves to military officers. Children's health during or after war suffers in many other ways, as reflected by increased infant and young-child mortality rates and decreased rates of immunization.[9]

The health-supporting infrastructure is destroyed during many wars, and therefore many civilians do not have access to food, clean water, medical care, or public health services. For example, during the Persian Gulf War in 1991 and in the first 7 years of economic sanctions that followed, there were an estimated 400,000 to 500,000 excess deaths among children,[10] mainly due to inadequate nutrition, contaminated water, and shortages of medicines—much of which was due to destruction of the health-supporting infrastructure of society (health care facilities, food and water supply systems, sewage treatment and sanitation facilities, power plants, and transportation and communication systems). Similarly, the Iraq War damaged much of the country's infrastructure.[11]

During wartime, many civilians flee to other countries as refugees or become internally displaced persons within their own countries, where it may be difficult for them to maintain their health and safety (Chapter 11). Refugees and internally displaced persons are vulnerable to malnutrition, infectious diseases, injuries, and criminal and military attacks. Substantial numbers of the global total of 10.5 million refugees and 26.4 million internally displaced persons were forced to leave their homes because of war, the threat of war, or the aftermath of war.

War and the preparation for war divert huge amounts of resources from health and human services and other productive societal endeavors.[12] This is true in many countries, including the United States, which ranks first among nations in military expenditures and arms exports, but 51st among nations in infant mortality rate. In some low-income countries, governments spend more on military expenditures than on health.

War often creates a cycle of violence, including domestic and community violence, in the countries engaged in war. War leads people, including children, to believe that violence is an acceptable method for settling conflicts. Teenage gangs mirror the activity of military forces. Former military servicemen, trained to operate with a "battlefield mentality," sometimes commit acts of domestic violence against female partners.

War and the preparation for war have profound impacts on the environment, such as the following:

- Bomb craters in Vietnam that have filled with water and provide breeding areas for mosquitoes that spread malaria and other diseases
- Destruction of urban environments by aerial carpet bombing of major cities in Europe and Japan during World War II
- Approximately 600 oil-well fires in Kuwait that were ignited by retreating Iraqi troops in 1991, which adversely affected the ecology of the area and caused acute respiratory symptoms among people exposed
- The huge amounts of non-renewable fossil fuels used by military forces
- Toxic and radioactive wastes, which can contaminate air, soil, surface water, and groundwater

New geopolitical, tactical, and technological issues concerning war are arising that have an impact on health, law, and ethics. These issues relate to new weapons, suicide bombers, policies on "preemptive" wars, and "cyber warfare."

A major concern is the U.S. use of armed drones to attack suspected terrorists in Pakistan and elsewhere—a practice that began during the George W. Bush administration and escalated during the Barack Obama administration. These drone strikes have killed innocent civilians as well as suspected terrorists. This practice has been defended by members of both administrations, but severely criticized by others.[13,14]

Some analysts believe that, due to increasing militarism and increasing power of the military-industrial complex, that the United States has drifted away from its original ideals and has become engaged in perpetual war, with its huge human and financial costs. Among the contributing factors have been the increase in presidential authority, the outsourcing of military activities to private companies, and the decreased percentage of U.S. families whose children directly participate in war.[15,16]

Box References

1. Rummel RJ. Death by government: Genocide and mass murder since 1900. New Brunswick, NJ, and London: Transaction Publications, 1994.
2. Coghlan B, Brennan R, Ngoy P, et al. Mortality in the Democratic Republic of Congo: Results from a nationwide survey. New York: International Rescue Committee and Burnet Institute, 2004.
3. Kloos H. Health impacts of war in Ethiopia. *Disasters* 1992;16:347–354.
4. Stockholm International Peace Research Institute. SIPRI Yearbook 2012. Oxford, England: Oxford University Press, 2012.
5. Stover E, Keller AS, Cobey J, et al. The medical and social consequences of land mines in Cambodia. *JAMA* 1994;272:331–336.
6. Kanter E. Post-traumatic stress disorder. In: Levy BS, Wagner GR, Rest KM, Weeks JL, eds. Preventing occupational disease and injury. 2nd ed. Washington, DC: American Public Health Association, 2005:410–413.
7. Levy BS, Sidel VW. Health effects of combat: A life-course perspective. *Ann Rev Public Health* 2009;30:123–136.
8. Ashford MW. The impact of war on women. In: Levy BS, Sidel VW, eds. War and public health. 2nd ed. New York: Oxford University Press, 2008:193–206.
9. Santa Barbara J. The impact of war on children. In: Levy BS, Sidel VW, eds. War and public health. 2nd ed. New York: Oxford University Press, 2008:179–192.
10. Ali MM, Blacker J, Jones G. Annual mortality rates and excess deaths of children under five in Iraq, 1991–98. *Popul Stud (Camb)* 2003;57: 217–226.
11. Levy BS, Sidel VW. Adverse health consequences of the Iraq War. *Lancet* 2013;381:949–958.
12. Belasco A. The cost of Iraq, Afghanistan, and other global War on Terror operations since 9/11. Washington, DC: Congressional Research Service; September 2, 2010.
13. Savage C. Top U.S. security official says "rigorous standards" are used for drone strikes. *New York Times*, April 30, 2012. Available at http://www.nytimes.com/2012/05/01/world/obamas-counterterrorism-aide-defends-drone-strikes.html. Accessed December 12, 2012.
14. Lethal force under law (editorial). *New York Times*, October 9, 2010. Available at http://www.nytimes.com/2010/10/10/opinion/10sun1.html?_r=0. Accessed December 12, 2012.
15. Maddow R. Drift: The unmooring of American military power. New York: Crown Publishers, 2012.
16. O'Connell AB. The permanent militarization of America (op-ed). *New York Times*, November 4, 2012. Available at http://www.nytimes.com/2012/11/05/opinion/the-permanent-militarization-of-america.html?pagewanted=all&_r=0. Accessed January 3, 2013.

In addition to deaths, violent behaviors—such as suicide attempts, physical and psychological abuse, sexual assault, neglect, acts of war, terrorism, and political violence—cause many non-fatal injuries and much disability. Men are disproportionately involved in violence as both perpetrators and victims; almost three-fourths of violence-related injuries occur among men.[14] Between 13 and 61 percent of women in various countries have reported that they have been physically assaulted by their male partners; between 6 and 59 percent have reported sexual violence by a partner.[11,15] Almost one-fourth of women in the United States have experienced severe physical violence by an intimate partner, and one-fifth have been raped, usually by a partner, acquaintance, or family member.[16] WHO estimates that 25 to 50 percent of children have experienced physical abuse,[13,14,17] and about 18 percent of women and 8 percent of men have experienced sexual abuse as children.[18,19]

The physical and mental health consequences of these violent behaviors often persist long after the violence has ceased. These consequences are cumulative, as victims can experience multiple episodes of different types of violence over time.[11,20,21] Permanently disabling spinal cord and brain injuries, burns, and the losses of limbs, vision, and hearing are frequent consequences of war, terrorism, and other forms of violence where powerful weapons are used.[2,17] Victims of child maltreatment, sexual violence, and intimate-partner violence suffer a variety of short- and long-term health consequences that can profoundly affect their quality of life.[11,12,20,22] Women abused by their partners, for example, are at higher risk of physical injury, depression, anxiety, suicide attempts, chronic pain syndromes, gastrointestinal disorders, infertility, sexually transmitted infections, and other consequences.[11] Exposure to maltreatment and other forms of violence during childhood contribute to (a) high-risk behaviors and conditions, such as depression, smoking, obesity, high-risk sexual behaviors, unintended pregnancy, and alcohol and drug use; and (b) as a consequence, death, disease, and disability.[20] Exposure to violence can also cause significant social and economic consequences for victims. For example, intimate-partner violence is associated with lower levels of occupational status and income attainment over time, and victims may be more likely to rely on public assistance.[23,24] Victims of child maltreatment have lower levels of educational attainment, employment, earnings, and fewer assets as adults; for example, they have a 14 percent decrease in probability of employment in middle age.[25]

War has many of the same consequences as interpersonal violence for the physical and mental health of combatants.[2,26] Modern warfare, however, has had a increasingly devastating effect on civilians, who are specifically targeted or indirectly affected during war and its aftermath.[26] The international trade in conventional weapons fuels the potential for war as well as community and domestic violence (Box 17–2). The development and possible use of nuclear weapons represent an additional form of social injustice (Box 17–3).

In those nations and communities most heavily affected, violence can have a substantial economic impact.[27] For example, estimates of the economic impact of violence between acquaintances and strangers in six Latin American countries in 1997 ranged from about 5 percent of the gross domestic product (GDP) in Peru to almost 25 percent in El Salvador.[28] The subcategories of these costs (Table 17–1), although not entirely exclusive or exhaustive, serve to illustrate the magnitude of the economic burden associated with violence. An estimate of the cost of interpersonal violence in Jamaica concluded that the direct medical costs of injuries due to interpersonal violence accounted for about 12 percent of the national health budget and about 4 percent of its GDP. The cost of injuries due to interpersonal and

---

BOX 17-2 ■ The International Arms Trade

Victor W. Sidel and Barry S. Levy

The international trade in conventional weapons puts lethal weapons into the hands of members of armies, militias, insurgent groups, and individuals throughout the world. These weapons have ultimately killed and injured many people and have led to human rights abuses, including rape and forced migration—and have contributed to destroying millions of lives.

The consequences of the global arms trade include:

- Increased availability of small arms, including handguns
- Increased resort to violence as a means of resolving disputes
- Increased community and domestic violence
- Increased occurrence—and threats—of armed conflict
- Diversion of resources

The estimated annual value of weapons in the global arms trade is approximately $60 billion (excluding domestic sales of arms). Between the 2002–2006 and the 2007–2011 periods, international transfers of major conventional weapons increased 24 percent.[1] In 2011, the 10 largest arms exporting countries exported $27 billion worth of major conventional weapons. The six largest arms exporters in 2011 were the United States ($10.0 billion), Russia ($7.9 billion), France ($2.4 billion), Germany ($1.2 billion), China ($1.4 billion), and the United Kingdom ($1.1 billion).[1] The five largest recipients of major conventional weapons were India, South Korea, Pakistan, China, and Singapore.[1]

In 2013, the United Nations General Assembly overwhelmingly approved the Arms Trade Treaty, which regulates international trade in conventional weapons. The Treaty links arms sales to the human-rights records of purchasing countries so that exported weapons do not contribute to human-rights abuses, terrorism, or organized crime. It prohibits shipments of these weapons deemed to be harmful to women or children.

Box Reference

1. Stockholm International Peace Research Institute. SIPRI Yearbook 2012. Oxford, England: Oxford University Press, 2012. Available at www.sipri.org/yearbook/2012. Accessed December 14, 2012.

---

self-directed violence have accounted for about 0.4 percent of Brazil's total health budget and 1.2 percent of its GDP.[29,30]

The high costs of violence also impact high-income nations. For example, the total lifetime economic burden resulting from new substantiated cases of child maltreatment in the United States was estimated to be at least $124 billion in 2008—almost 1 percent of GDP.[31] High rates of violence can severely limit the economic growth of countries and regions by increasing the costs of health and security services, diverting funds from socially beneficial activities to nonproductive ones and threatening the establishment and viability of businesses.[27]

BOX 17-3 ■ Nuclear Weapons and Social Injustice

Robert M. Gould and Patrice M. Sutton

Nuclear weapons have threatened the continued existence of humanity since the United States detonated atomic bombs at Hiroshima and Nagasaki in August 1945. However, thus far, the adverse impacts of nuclear weapons have been inequitably and unjustly distributed, with civilian populations, indigenous people, and future generations bearing the enormous burden of the public and environmental health consequences of the development, production, testing, and use of nuclear weapons.

Most of the 210,000 people who died by the end of 1945 from the combined effects of heat, blast, and radiation were noncombatants with little or no responsibility for the war crimes of the Japanese government. These civilians, including many women and children, also bore the brunt of subsequent radiation-induced malignancies and other chronic diseases, genetic damage, developmental disorders, and profound and persistent social and mental health consequences.

Nuclear weapons research, testing, and production has resulted in widespread contamination of the air, water, and soil in communities and ecosystems, with resultant human illness and ecosystem damage.[1] For example, atmospheric testing of over 2000 nuclear weapons globally released much radioactive material into the atmosphere—more than 12 billion curies just at the Nevada Test Site between 1951 and 1965.[2]

Unsuspecting populations downwind of atmospheric test explosions received large doses of radiation from fallout, which concentrated in the food chain. Global dissemination of radioactive fallout from all nuclear weapons tests likely produced tens of thousands of fatal cancers by 2000.[2] In the United States, children who drank fresh milk from backyard cows and goats were at high risk of being exposed to radioactive iodine-131. The National Cancer Institute has estimated that 11,300 to 212,000 additional cases of thyroid cancer will ultimately occur in the United States due to iodine-131 exposure from nuclear weapons testing.[3]

Since some fallout and other environmental releases from the nuclear-weapons cycle remain radioactive for a long time, human exposure and resultant adverse health effects will continue for thousands of years. The U.S. National Academy of Sciences has stated: "At many sites, radiological and non-radiological hazardous wastes will remain, posing risks to humans and the environment for tens or even hundreds of thousands of years. Complete elimination of unacceptable risks to humans and the environment will not be achieved, now or in the foreseeable future."[4]

Indigenous, colonized, and minority populations have disproportionately incurred the detrimental health, social, economic, cultural, and environmental impacts of the nuclear-weapons development and production cycle. Globally, indigenous lands have served as the main sites for testing nuclear weapons. The mining of uranium for nuclear weapons has relied primarily on the labor of tribal and minority workers, who have been exposed to significant occupational hazards. Workers throughout the nuclear-weapons industry have been exposed to radioactive and toxic materials, including heavy metals, silica, organic solvents, and acids. Occupational disorders due to weapons production include, but are not limited to, radiation-induced cancers, beryllium disease, and silicosis.

One of the most egregious examples of the social injustice of nuclear weapons occurred between 1946 and 1958 when the United States conducted over 65 nuclear weapons tests on or near the Bikini and Enewetok atolls in the Pacific, often vaporizing islands that had been the homeland of the Marshallese people for many generations.[5] These tests had an explosive yield 93 times that of all tests at the Nevada Test Site.[6] The approximately 6.3 billion curies of radioactive iodine that was estimated by the Centers for Disease Control and Prevention to have been released to the atmosphere from these tests was 42 times greater than the total amount emitted from the Nevada Test Site, and at least 116 times greater than the amount released in the 1986 Chernobyl meltdown.[5] Although the United States extensively documented the environmental contamination of several atolls, it hid these findings from the general public and the Marshallese people. Heavily exposed evacuees of one atoll were enrolled in a top-secret study that documented the health impacts of acute radiation exposures.[5] But research subjects were not treated adequately for radiation burns or given prophylactic antibiotics.[5,6]

Upon repatriation to their contaminated homeland in 1957, Marshallese people were secretly enrolled in an Atomic Energy Commission and Department of Defense project to determine the movement of radioactive material through humans and the food chain.[5,6] Between 1944 and 1974, the U.S. government sponsored several thousand more human-radiation experiments—many without informed consent, including secret intentional releases of radiation over populated areas.[7]

The United States spent, between 1945 and 1996, $5.5 trillion on nuclear weapons and related programs. This expenditure exceeded all other categories of government spending during this period, except for non-nuclear national defense and Social Security.[8] As expenditures for social programs have been significantly reduced, disproportionately impacting poor people and other vulnerable populations, the diversion of public resources to nuclear weapons continues unabated. Over the next decade, the United States plans to spend about $185 billion for "improving" nuclear weapons and their delivery systems—a glaring example of social injustice.

Box References

1. Sutton PM, Gould RM. Nuclear weapons. In Levy BS, Sidel VW, eds. War and public health. 2nd ed. New York: Oxford University Press, 2008:152–176.
2. International Physicians for the Prevention of Nuclear War, Inc., and Institute for Energy and Environmental Research. Radioactive heaven and earth: The health and environmental effects of nuclear weapons testing in, on and above the Earth. New York: Apex Press, 1991.
3. Institute of Medicine. Exposure to the American people to iodine-131 from Nevada nuclear-bomb tests. Review of the National Cancer Institute report and public health implications. Washington, DC: National Academy Press, 1999.
4. Wald M. Nuclear sites may be toxic in perpetuity, report finds. *New York Times*, August 8, 2000.
5. Johnston BR, Barker HM. Consequential damages of nuclear war: The Rongelap Report. Walnut Creek, CA: Left Coast Press, 2008.
6. Johnston BR. Nuclear savages. Counterpunch, June 1–3, 2012. Available at http://www.counterpunch.org/2012/06/01/nuclear-savages/. Accessed August 31, 2012.
7. U.S. Department of Energy. Final report of the Advisory Committee on human radiation experiments. Washington, DC: U.S. Government Printing Office, 1995.
8. Makhijani A, Schwartz SI. Victims of the bomb. In: Schwartz SI, ed. Atomic audit: The costs and consequences of U.S. nuclear weapons since 1940. Washington, DC: Brookings Institution Press, 1998:395–431.

TABLE 17–1 *Economic Costs of Social Violence* in Six Latin American Countries, as Percentages of Gross Domestic Product, 1997*

	Brazil	Colombia	El Salvador	Mexico	Peru	Venezuela
Health losses†	1.9	5.0	4.3	1.3	1.5	0.3
Material losses‡	3.6	8.4	5.1	4.9	2.0	9.0
Intangibles§	3.4	6.9	11.5	3.3	1.0	2.2
Transfers¶	1.6	4.4	4.0	2.8	0.6	0.3
Total	10.5	24.7	24.9	12.3	5.1	11.8

* For the purposes of this table, social violence is defined as violence that occurs between acquaintances and strangers.
†Expenditures on health services incurred as a result of the violence.
‡Private and public expenditures on police, security systems, and judicial services.
§Amount that citizens would be willing to pay to live without violence.
¶ Value of goods lost in robberies, ransoms paid to kidnappers, and bribes paid as a result of extortion.
(*Source*: Buvinic M, Morrison A, Shifter M. Technical study: Violence in Latin America and the Caribbean: A framework for action. Washington, DC: Inter-American Development Bank, 1999.)

■ SOCIAL INJUSTICE AS A CAUSE OF VIOLENCE

The forms of social injustice that often cause violence can be subdivided into three general categories: (a) the unequal access, distribution, or concentration of economic resources; (b) the influences of cultural norms, beliefs, or attitudes; and (c) the policies and practices of criminal-justice, education, social-welfare, and political institutions. However, it is difficult to reach firm conclusions about the relationship between social injustice and violence because violent behavior, in whatever form it takes, is caused by a complex interaction among a broad range of biological, psychological, social, economic, and political factors.

■ THE INFLUENCE OF ECONOMIC FORMS OF SOCIAL INJUSTICE

To varying degrees, economic resources are unequally distributed in every nation. But the presence of this unequal distribution alone does not constitute social injustice. Social injustice arises when an individual or a group takes advantage of their power to economically exploit another individual or group, or when the unequal distribution of resources interferes with the ability of individuals or groups to meet their basic human needs. In both instances, economic forms of social injustice have been associated with increased risk for violence victimization or perpetration.

Economic Exploitation

Economic exploitation is associated with violence when people or groups use force or greater power to (a) misappropriate funds or resources of other people or groups, or (b) force other people or groups to engage in behavior that economically benefits perpetrators of violence.

Human trafficking is a graphic example of economic exploitation associated with violence. At least two million people globally are exploited in forced or bonded labor, child labor, or forced sex work at any given time.[32] In the United States, at least 10,000 men, women, and children are currently engaged in forced labor as prostitutes, farm and sweatshop laborers, and domestic workers.[33] While anti-trafficking measures address this issue, many countries have not convicted anyone under anti-trafficking laws, and many lack policies or regulations to prevent the deportation of victims.[34] (See Box 21–1 in Chapter 21.)

Sex trafficking poses a major threat to the health and well-being of women and children. Women and girls throughout the world are bought and sold into prostitution and sexual slavery.[22] The U.S. Central Intelligence Agency estimates that 45,000 to 50,000 women and children are trafficked to the United States each year.[35] Women and children are often forced into sex work through physical assaults, rape, and threats of violence; working as a prostitute is associated with a high risk of violence-related injury.[36] It is estimated that globally 2.5 million prostituted children are physically assaulted, 2.5 million of them are raped, and 6900 of them are killed each year.[36]

Labor trafficking is an additional form of economic exploitation in which violence or threats of violence are used to control and coerce victims into involuntary work, frequently in unsafe conditions. Workers may be forced to work long hours for little or no pay, be deprived of health care and adequate housing, and be isolated from community resources due to physical or cultural barriers. Workers may also be exposed to physical violence by their employers or traffickers. For example, 50 percent of persons trafficked out of Kyrgyzstan reported being physically abused or tortured by their employers.[37] These victims of "modern-day slavery," by sexual and labor trafficking, are subject to severe physical and mental health impacts as well as their loss of freedom.[34,38] Although individuals of all nationalities and backgrounds can become victims of trafficking, those under significant social and economic strains may be most vulnerable to promises of legitimate employment and opportunities.

Children may be particularly vulnerable to economic exploitation. Each year, millions of children in much of the world are forced into labor, often under harsh conditions and with very low wages, often by their own desperate, impoverished parents.[39,40] In some societies, economies depend on the availability of this low-cost, unskilled labor, and official policies to end child labor are undermined by (a) the need for greater family income generated by economic inequality, and (b) the financial incentives for businesses and nations to continue these practices.[40–42] While children subjected to harsh working conditions may also suffer from coercive physical and emotional abuse by employers, the experience of dangerous work and long hours may itself constitute a form of child maltreatment. These children suffer enormous physical and mental health consequences, and may suffer from lifelong disabilities as a result of unsafe work conditions.[43]

Poverty and Relative Deprivation

Poverty is consistently found to have a strong positive correlation with interpersonal violence, especially homicide.[44] However, when other community factors distinct from, but related to, poverty are controlled for, this association is substantially weakened, suggesting that the effect of poverty on interpersonal violence may be conditional on other factors. These factors include community change associated with high residential mobility, concentrations of poverty, family disruption, high population density, and community disorganization, as reflected in weak intergenerational family and community ties, weakened social controls, and low participation in community organizations.[45,46] Poorer communities and their residents appear to be most vulnerable to interpersonal violence. This occurs when they are exposed to fundamental economic and population changes that lead to community disorganization, which, in turn, undermines their ability to exert social control over violent behavior. In the United States, for example, the shift from goods-producing industries to service-producing industries—and the associated relocation of manufacturing industries out of inner cities—is a fundamental change that has been linked to inner-city violence.[47] Similarly, rapid population growth and related economic tensions in Algeria, Senegal, and elsewhere in Africa have been associated with increases in youth violence.[48-50]

Relative deprivation—the magnitude of the gap between rich and poor people in a society or a community—is typically measured by examining economic inequality. Income inequality is strongly related to homicide rates.[51,52] Extreme social and economic inequalities, especially those between—rather than within—distinct population groups may be risk factors for collective violence.[2]

An extension of this concept involves the geographic concentration of economic deprivation. In the United States, beginning in the 1960s, many inner-city communities became increasingly isolated islands of poverty as middle- and working-class residents moved away to areas with better housing and job opportunities.[47] This exodus of more economically stable families from inner cities reduced the social and financial capital of these communities and undermined the viability of basic community institutions, such as churches and schools, which serve as social buffers against violence. The resulting concentration of poverty isolated inner-city residents—primarily African Americans—from job networks, potential spouses, quality schools, and opportunities for upward mobility. These communities developed a high concentration of factors associated with poverty and strongly related to interpersonal violence: residential instability, family disruption, and community disorganization.[44-46] This concentration of poverty in a neighborhood is associated with interpersonal violence.[53]

Poverty and inequality have also been linked to higher rates of suicide.[54-56] However, measures of social fragmentation and deprivation, including low voter turnout, low family cohesion, high proportion of manual workers, and high unemployment rate, may be better predictors of suicide rates than median income or income equality.[54,56] In addition, suicide rates may be related to periods of economic growth or recession.[57] Socioeconomic factors predict suicide rates even after controlling for cross-national differences in the *culture of suicide*—defined by shared cultural beliefs that either support or restrict suicidal behavior.[58]

▪ INFLUENCE OF CULTURAL FORMS OF INJUSTICE

Culture embodies the shared beliefs, values, customs, symbols, and behaviors that members of a society "use to cope with the world and with each other, and that are transmitted from generation to generation through learning."[59] Cultural context plays an important role in both contributing to, and protecting people from, violent behavior. Cultural sources of injustice are often entrenched in societies because they are rationalized by a body of shared knowledge and beliefs that most members of a society accept—sometimes without question. Several aspects of culture contribute toward unjust and violent treatment of specific social groups, such as women, children, and members of racial and ethnic minority groups.

Hate-Motivated Violence

Hate-motivated violence consists of acts of interpersonal or collective violence that are directed toward other people, property, or organizations because of the group they belong to or identify with.[60] These forms of violence are most commonly perpetrated against individuals or groups based on race, ethnicity, religion, and sexual orientation. Motivations for hate-related violence often emerge from cultural beliefs and attitudes that foster negative stereotypes. However, these beliefs and attitudes are often supported or exacerbated by political or economic conflicts between or among groups, such as between the Palestinians and Israelis, or among immigrant groups competing in tight job markets.

Hate-related violence has a long tradition in the United States. It is perhaps best exemplified by the lynching of African Americans by organized groups, such as the Ku Klux Klan, and unorganized lynch mobs, which escalated following the Civil War and Reconstruction.[61] Other groups have also been targets of hate-related violence in the United States. Surveys conducted between 1988 and 1991 indicated that from 9 to 24 percent of gay respondents reported that they had been punched, hit, or kicked because of their sexual orientation.[62] In addition, between 37 and 45 percent of gay respondents reported they had received threats of physical violence because of their sexual orientation.[62] In the 10 days following the terrorist attacks on New York and Washington on September 11, 2001, violent attacks on people of Middle Eastern descent or those perceived to be of Middle Eastern descent, escalated dramatically in the United States (Figure 17–2).[63]

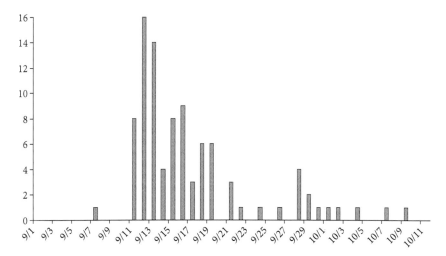

Figure 17–2 Hate-related violent attacks on Middle Easterners, United States, September 1–October 11, 2001. (*Source:* Swahn MH, Mahendra RR, Paulozzi LJ, et al. Violent attacks on Middle Easterners in the United States during the month following the September 11, 2001, terrorist attacks. *Injury Prevent* 2003;9:187–189. Reproduced with permission from the BMJ Publishing Group.)

Military actions whose primary purpose is to forcefully displace groups from their homelands based on their religious, ethnic, or national identity are a collective manifestation of hate-related violence (Chapter 11). The wars and associated "ethnic cleansing" in the former Yugoslavia and Rwanda are examples of this forced displacement. In these conflicts, the tools of ethnic cleansing were the torture and murder of noncombatant men, women, and children; the systematic use of rape to terrorize communities; the destruction of residences, farms, industries, and basic infrastructures that supply water, power, food, sanitation, and other necessities; denial of medical care; and interference with humanitarian relief efforts.[64] Other examples of "ethnic cleansing" that have received less public attention have occurred in Sri Lanka, East Timor, Armenia and Azerbaijan, Ossetia and Georgia, China and Tibet, and Iraq and Kurdistan.[64] (See Box 17–4.)

Gender Inequality

Gender inequality has many faces. For example, cultural traditions that favor male over female children, early marriage for girls, male sexual entitlement, and female "purity" place women and girls in a subordinate position relative to men and make them highly vulnerable to violent victimization.[65,66] Cultural attitudes and beliefs about gender roles that restrict women's power, freedom, and access to resources may also contribute to violence and exist, to varying degrees, everywhere.[67] Intimate-partner violence against women occurs most often in societies

Box 17–4 ■ Genocide

Victor W. Sidel and Barry S. Levy

Genocide, also known in recent years as *ethnic cleansing*, is the most far-reaching and despicable form of social injustice. In one of its first actions after its formation, the General Assembly of the United Nations on December 11, 1946, declared that genocide is a crime under international law.[1] The term was defined in 1948 in the Convention on the Prevention and Punishment of the Crime of Genocide:

Genocide means any of the following acts committed with intent to destroy, in whole or in part, a national, ethnic, racial or religious group, as such:
1. Killing members of the group;
2. Causing serious bodily or mental harm to members of the group;
3. Deliberately inflicting on the group conditions of life calculated to bring about its physical destruction in whole or in part;
4. Imposing measures intended to prevent births within the group;
5. Forcibly transferring children of the group to another group.[2]

Examples of events that are widely considered to constitute genocide include the killing of the following groups:

- An estimated one million Armenians in Turkey in 1915
- Six million Jews in the Holocaust in Europe during World War II
- 800,000 Tutsis and Hutus in Rwanda and Burundi in 1994
- Many ethnic Albanians in Kosovo in 1999 (where military intervention authorized by the United Nations was used to stop the killing)
- An estimated 80,000 Muslims in Darfur in Sudan in 2004

Genocide or threats of genocide continue in several countries.

The United Nations has permitted intervention in extraordinary humanitarian emergencies, including the use of armed force. Intervention in Kuwait in 1991 to force the withdrawal of Iraqi troops and in Kosovo in 1999 to prevent ethnic cleansing of ethnic Albanians are examples of military intervention authorized by the United Nations that have been widely accepted. On the other hand, the United States and other high-income countries—as well as the United Nations itself—have been criticized for not intervening in Rwanda in 1994.

Beginning in 2003, the government of Sudan was responsible for ethnic cleansing and other crimes against humanity in Darfur, one of the world's poorest and most inaccessible regions on Sudan's western border with Chad. The government of Sudan and the Arab militias (*janjaweed*) it armed and supported made numerous attacks on the civilian population. Government forces directly participated in massacres; summary executions of civilians, including women and children; burning of towns and villages; and uprooting of people from their homes.[3]

Debate continues about how "genocide" or "ethnic cleansing" is defined and documented, and about the authority of United Nations or individual countries to intervene when a government that has perpetrated or permitted severe, life-threatening social injustice against its own citizens refuses to permit outside intervention to protect them.[4]

Is military intervention acceptable when social injustice is so great that the dangerous consequences of armed intervention pale in comparison? Military intervention may be justified under emergency circumstances if there is strict adherence to certain conditions, such as the following:

- Failure of non-military intervention to resolve a conflict
- Preauthorization of military intervention by the United Nations Security Council
- Imposition of a strict deadline and conditions for the withdrawal of the interveners
- A plan for prompt restoration of representative government

Box References

1. United Nations General Assembly. Resolution 1946 96 (I): The Crime of Genocide, December 11, 1946.
2. United Nations General Assembly. Convention on the Prevention and Punishment of the Crime of Genocide, General Assembly Resolution 260 A (III), Article II. New York: United Nations, December 9, 1948. Available at http://www2.ohchr.org/english/law/genocide.htm. Accessed December 12, 2012.
3. Human Rights Watch. Darfur destroyed: Ethnic cleansing by government and militia forces in western Sudan. Human Rights Watch, 2004. Available at http://www.hrw.org/reports/2004/05/06/darfur-destroyed. Accessed December 12, 2012.
4. Power S. "A problem from hell": America and the age of genocide. New York: Basic Books, 2002.

where men hold household economic and decision-making power, where divorce is difficult for women to obtain, and where violence is a common and accepted tactic for conflict resolution.[68] Rape is also more common in societies where cultural traditions favoring male superiority are strong.[69] (See Chapter 4.)

Maintaining the sexual "purity" of girls is a powerful cultural value that is associated with violence in many parts of the world. Female genital mutilation, for example, is a practice usually performed on girls before puberty in many parts of Africa, some Middle Eastern countries, and immigrant communities around the world.[70] An estimated 80 to 135 million women and girls globally have undergone female genital mutilation.[70,71] Within the societies that practice it, female genital mutilation is considered essential to make a woman eligible for marriage because it is believed to reduce her desire for sex and, therefore, the likelihood that she will have sex before she is married or, later, outside of marriage.[71] *Honor killings*, another extreme outcome of cultural traditions found mainly in Middle Eastern and South Asian countries, occur when a female is killed by members of her own family after her virginity or faithfulness has been brought into question because of, for example, infidelity, rape, or disobeying religious or cultural expectations.[65,72,73] Data on this phenomenon are very limited,[74] but in Alexandria, Egypt, 47 percent of female homicide victims were killed by a relative after they had been raped by another person.[72] Honor killings appear to have increased substantially from 1989 until 2009, but that this may be due to more accurate reporting.[73]

Other forms of gender inequality are economic in nature. For example, in 2010, U.S. women earned between $0.81 and $0.86 for every $1.00 earned by their male counterparts. Women were also more likely than men to work in low-wage jobs, with single female households having the lowest average income levels.[75,76] Similar wage gaps exist between men and women globally.[77] Women's lower earning potential may increase their risk for poverty and decrease their economic independence, leading to a greater risk for violence.[78]

The cultural preference for male children is associated with high levels of female infanticide in China, some Middle Eastern countries, and India.[79] In China, the preference for sons is particularly strong in rural areas, where traditional cultural beliefs have their strongest hold.[80] The "one-couple, one-child" policy in China may have exacerbated the problem of female infanticide.[80-82] China's one-child policy has produced a dramatic demographic shift in the country, resulting in a surplus of young men who are unable to find wives. This imbalance in the gender ratio has been blamed for recent increases in sex trafficking of foreign women to China for prostitution and marriage.[81]

Suicidal behavior can be a consequence of cultural traditions that support male dominance. As an indirect consequence, women exposed to intimate-partner violence and rape are at greater risk of suicidal behavior.[11] The subordination of women has also been more directly linked to high rates of suicidal behavior, especially among women in their childbearing years.[79] In India and Nepal, for example, culturally related phenomena, such as dowry disputes and arranged marriages, have been linked with suicidal behavior among young women.[65] In China, young rural women are at especially high risk of suicide; their rates are 66 percent higher than rates among young rural men.[83] Low status, limited opportunities, and exposure to various forms of domestic violence may partially explain their elevated rates.[84]

■ INFLUENCE OF INSTITUTIONAL FORMS OF SOCIAL INJUSTICE

Social injustice often becomes incorporated into the policies and operations of key social institutions. Legal institutions, for example, can become tools of social injustice when a society creates laws that deny human rights or civil liberties to a specific social group. Violence can erupt as a response to institutionalized injustice or may be used to suppress opposition to it.

Political Repression

History is replete with examples of governments that have used their military and police powers to systematically repress their own citizens. El Salvador provides a graphic illustration of the devastating effects that violent political repression can have on a nation's population. After coming to power through a military coup in 1979, the Salvadoran government began to use its military forces to violently suppress actions by peasants and labor activists to improve living and working conditions.[85] During a civil war from 1980 through 1992, about 70,000 people—most of them unarmed—were killed by government forces and their allied death squads.[86] Torture was an officially sanctioned policy of Salvadoran government forces and was widely used on rebel combatants and their suspected supporters.[85] The political repression and associated war in El Salvador have had broad and long-lasting effects on the health and welfare of the population.[85] Similar scenarios have played out in many other places over the past few decades, including Argentina, Brazil, Chile, Colombia, Ethiopia, Guatemala, Haiti, Kashmir, Nicaragua, the Philippines, and South Africa.[64]

There may be a relationship between type of government and violent political repression that is affected by the ability of a government to respond to threats to its regime by opposition groups.[87] Democratic governments are less prone to repression because threats can be politically channeled through the more widely available official and legitimate avenues for voicing and organizing dissent and the greater accountability of political leaders to voters.[87,88] Moreover, the system of checks and balances in democracies makes it difficult to organize institutions of the state for repression. In general, autocracies also have low levels of violent political repression because demands by opposition groups are muted by the existence of state institutions that can be easily mobilized to carry out repressive actions. Governments that have intermediate levels of democracy are the most likely to engage in violent political repression because they tend to lack the institutional mechanisms for (a) addressing demands by those in opposition that exist in mature democracies, or (b) deterring opposition, as in the case of autocracies.[87]

Unfair Distribution of Justice

Criminal justice institutions—police, courts, and correctional agencies—in any society are responsible for apprehending, adjudicating, and punishing people who break the law. As part of this responsibility, they also enforce the norms of social justice that are encoded into the law. In many ways, criminal justice institutions, therefore, are a society's first line of defense against social injustice. The manner in which these institutions carry out these responsibilities has important implications for both social injustice and violence.

The ability of a state to provide social protection to its citizens is associated with violence. The presence of strong national institutions for social protection is negatively associated with homicide.[89] Inefficient or corrupt criminal justice institutions may result in an unequal distribution of justice in which disadvantaged groups are targeted with enforcement or crimes against them are ignored. In Brazil, for example, a lack of criminal justice attention to vigilante efforts to eliminate "undesirable" homeless children and adolescents through death squads, lynchings, and other forms of violence has resulted in widespread perceptions of the police as inefficient and corrupt.[90] Similarly, in post-apartheid South Africa, impunity from human rights abuses and the inability of police to change their methods may have contributed to generalized feelings of insecurity and an increasing number of extrajudicial actions involving violence.[91]

In the United States, racial bias in law enforcement and sentencing practices may have led to disproportionate incarceration rates for minority groups. For example, about one in three African American men in their 20s are under super-vision of the criminal justice system—in prison, on probation, or on parole—on any given day.[92] The incarceration rate of African Americans is almost six times that of Caucasian Americans.[93] These high rates of incarceration have significant social and health impacts on African American families and communities, includ-ing higher poverty rates, family disruption, community disorganization, broken social networks, and weakened social controls—all factors contributing to higher rates of violence in communities.[92] (See Chapter 9.)

■ WHAT NEEDS TO BE DONE

The relationship between social injustice and violence is embedded within the broader issues of political and economic development and the clash between traditional and modern culture. Interventions to reduce social injustice that contribute to violence will necessitate that public health professionals extend their attention and influence far beyond what has traditionally been consid-ered their appropriate realm. To prevent violence, we must become more cre-ative than simply calling for reductions in poverty, for greater democracy, and for the enforcement of human rights. While these are all laudable goals, their attainment requires strategies that are grounded in science and that are practical, given the clear constraints and obstacles to progress in these areas. Fortunately, there are some promising directions toward which public health measures could be directed that have health and social benefits extending beyond violence prevention. These directions all require more thorough scientific assessment, engagement with partners in other sectors, and a sustained effort.

Increasing the Cost of Injustice

Where behavior is influenced, even partly by economic considerations, increas-ing the cost of that behavior may be an effective primary prevention strategy. For example, increases in the price of beer and alcohol have been found to be associated with lower consumption and small decreases in intimate-partner vio-lence (3.1 to 3.5 percent) and child maltreatment (1.2 percent).[94,95] Because the primary motivation for sexual and labor trafficking is economic gain, strategies to increase the cost of trafficking may be useful in reducing its profitability and, hence, its frequency. Public health professionals, working together with human rights organizations, could help by (a) conducting research to make the case for more effective law enforcement intervention, and (b) using media-advocacy or social-marketing strategies to bring greater attention to the problem and greater pressure on policymakers to address it.[96]

An innovative approach to media advocacy on the issue of trafficking of women and children is illustrated by WITNESS (www.witness.org), an organization that works with local activists to use video and other communication technology to expose human rights abuses and mobilize public concern. Its advocacy has been used in Thailand, Malaysia, Indonesia, the Philippines, Taiwan, the United States, and Vietnam to encourage policymakers to enact legislation based on human rights standards that will help to increase the costs and reduce the frequency of trafficking by, for example, fully engaging law enforcement agencies in traffickers to justice.

Economic sanctions provide another opportunity to directly increase the costs of trafficking. Non-humanitarian economic sanctions by the United States government and international financial institutions, such as the World Bank, can be effective in countries that have many trafficking victims, but little governmental action to address trafficking.[34]

Prevention strategies also include reducing demand for cheap labor, goods, services, and paid sex—thereby decreasing the potential profitability of sex- and labor-trafficking.[34,97] For example, a program has reduced recidivism by men arrested for soliciting sex by enrolling them in "john schools," which increase awareness of the negative consequences of prostitution, including sex trafficking.[98]

Reducing the Impact of Poverty on Violence

The high geographic concentration and social isolation of poor people compound many problems that contribute to interpersonal and, potentially, collective violence. Interventions and policies that seek to deconcentrate poverty by dispersing poor people within more economically and socially heterogeneous communities may help to reduce their isolation from jobs, positive role models, marriage partners, and good schools. Housing voucher programs reduce violent victimization and property crime.[99] For example, a housing voucher program in the United States, in which public housing tenants are given vouchers they can use to rent housing in the private market in any location, has enabled families to move from public-housing complexes into neighborhoods with lower levels of poverty and has substantially reduced violence by adolescents.[100-102]

Microfinance programs, which provide (a) credit and savings services to the poor for income-generating projects, and (b) direct cash transfers, may also reduce poverty and risk for violence. For example, a program in Ecuador found that cash transfers to poor families delayed introduction of children into employment and increased the length of time they remained in school.[103] Similarly, a microfinance program implemented with poor women in rural South Africa found, within 2 years of participation, that their risk of physical and sexual violence by an intimate partner was reduced by half.[104]

Reducing Social Distance

Hate-motivated violence appears to flourish in societies and communities where racially or ethnically distinct groups strongly hold negative beliefs and stereotypes about each other. This type of violence may be associated with the social distance that separates such groups.[105] The greater the social distance—as reflected in the frequency of interaction, the level of functional independence, and degree of cultural disparity between two groups, the greater is the frequency and severity of collective violence.[106] The presence of strong associational forms of civic engagement, such as integrated business organizations, trade unions, political parties, and professional associations, appears to protect against outbreaks of ethnic violence.[107] In relatively peaceful communities, the existence of these forms of association creates a context that reduces the social distance among ethnic groups. Interventions and policies that support the creation and maintenance of formal mechanisms of association between social groups, otherwise at odds with one another, may be a useful tool in the prevention of collective violence, particularly where conflicting groups are in close geographic proximity.

Improving Gender Equality by Redefining Harmful Cultural Norms

Cultural norms undergo change, which can be promoted and even accelerated. Norms associated with smoking and drunk driving in the United States, for example, have undergone substantial changes over the past several decades. Although harmful traditions associated with gender inequality are, in many ways, qualitatively different from smoking- and drinking-related norms, it is possible to change them. For example, the Reproductive, Education, and Community Health Program in the Kapchorwa District of Uganda has reportedly been successful in reducing rates of female genital mutilation by enlisting the support of elders in incorporating alternatives to this practice that are consistent with their original cultural traditions.[108] Approaches based on reinforcing sentiments or beliefs within a population that run counter to a harmful norm have been successful in reducing alcohol abuse on some college campuses. These approaches are now being implemented to prevent sexual assault by engaging active bystanders to speak out against attitudes and behaviors that support sexual violence and to reinforce positive norms.[109-111] Public health programs along these lines in traditional societies must be approached with extreme sensitivity, given the passionate attachment to traditions that often exists.[10] However, these programs, which can be implemented in ways that are sensitive to cultural traditions and are likely to reduce harm, may be met with broader support than anticipated.

Other work to improve social, educational, and economic opportunities for women are also critical to ending gender inequities globally. For example, the United States has decreased the wage gap between women and men, such as by implementing the Lilly Ledbetter Fair Pay Act of 2008, which entitles women to equal pay with men for equal work.[112] Involving more women in senior management positions may have a direct impact on reducing the wage gap at the organizational level.[113] Policies and practices that improve wage parity could result in better social and health outcomes for women, including decreasing their risk of violence victimization.[78]

Strengthening Democratic Institutions

The criminal justice system provides an important form of social control within democratic societies and often functions to increase social justice and ensure access to fundamental human and civil rights. However, in some instances, the unequal application of criminal justice can lead to disparities for those directly affected and their communities. One approach that has been taken to ensure the equal distribution of justice, as well as the desired outcomes of improved community safety and organization, is sentencing reform. The United States, for example, has recently focused on identifying alternatives to incarceration for nonviolent drug offenders by redirecting them, in some cases, to specialized drug courts that offer court-supervised substance abuse treatment.[114] Other work has focused on improving sentencing parity for similar offenses. For example, the U.S. Congress has enacted legislation to reduce the disparity in minimum punishments for possession of crack and powder cocaine.[115] Previous sentencing laws resulted in much higher rates of incarceration for the mostly low-income, inner-city African American users of crack cocaine, as compared to middle- and upper-income Caucasian users of powder cocaine—contributing to the disproportionate rates of incarceration among minority groups.[115] Given the significant public health impacts of mass incarceration on communities (Chapter 9), reform of sentencing and criminal-justice system practices to ensure equitable distribution of justice for the purpose of improving community safety may also reduce rates of community disorganization and violence.[92]

Public health workers should have a greater voice in preventing political repression, which can have grave repercussions for the health of the public. Primary prevention should include the creation and support of stable democratic institutions. The probability of violent political repression is greatest in nations that are in transition from autocratic to democratic regimes—in "semi-democracies."[87] An important reason for this finding may be that in these semi-democracies the institutional framework is typically insufficient for responding to public demands and addressing threats from opposition groups.[88] A focus on assisting semi-democracies in the development of institutions, such as political-party systems, mechanisms for the peaceful transfer of power, and service systems that address basic human needs, may be the most useful for preventing repression.[87] Public health workers, in collaboration with political scientists, can use science to further understand and inform policymakers on how to prevent political repression. In addition, assistance to semi-democracies for strengthening public health services may help to forestall conditions that could contribute to political repression.

■ CONCLUSION

Social injustice is fundamentally related to violence. To have a tangible and sustained impact on violence globally, public health workers need to forthrightly address social injustice as a root cause of violence. Recognition of the role that social injustice plays in the development of violence opens up new approaches for prevention. As Bill Foege, former director of the CDC, has said, "At its base, the practice of public health is the search for social justice."[116]

■ REFERENCES

1. Heise LL. Violence against women: An integrated, ecological framework. *Violence Against Women* 1998;4:262–290.
2. Zwi A, Garfield R, Loretti A. Collective violence. In: Krug E, Dahlberg L, Mercy J, et al., eds. World report on violence and health. Geneva: World Health Organization, 2002:215–239.
3. World Health Assembly. WHA149.25: Prevention of violence: A public health priority. Geneva: World Health Organization, 1996.
4. Krug EG, Mercy JA, Dahlberg LL, Zwi AB. The world report on violence and health. *Lancet* 2002;360:1083–1088.
5. Mercy JA, Rosenberg ML, Powell KE, et al. Public health policy for preventing violence. *Health Aff* 1993;12:7–29.
6. DHHS: Youth violence: A report of the Surgeon General. Rockville, MD: U.S. Department of Health and Human Services, 2001.
7. Abad G. Violence requires epidemiological studies. *Tribuna Medica* 1962;2:1–12.
8. U.S. Department of Health, Education, and Welfare. Healthy people: The Surgeon General's report on health promotion and disease prevention. Washington, DC: US Government Printing Office, 1979.
9. Mercy JA, O'Carroll PW. New directions in violence prediction: The public health arena. *Violence and Victims* 1988;3:285–301.
10. Dahlberg LL, Krug EG. Violence—A global public health problem. In: Krug E, Dahlberg L, Mercy J, et al., eds. World report on violence and health. Geneva: World Health Organization, 2002:3–21.
11. Heise L, Garcia-Moreno C. Violence by intimate partners. In: Krug E, Dahlberg L, Mercy J, et al., eds. World report on violence and health. Geneva: World Health Organization, 2002:87–121.

12. Runyan D, Wattam C, Ikeda R, et al. Child abuse and neglect by parents and other caregivers. In: Krug E, Dahlberg L, Mercy J, et al., eds. World report on violence and health. Geneva: World Health Organization, 2002:57–86.
13. World Health Organization. Global Burden of Disease Project. Available at http://www.who.int/healthinfo/global_burden_disease/en/index.html. Accessed on May 8, 2012.
14. Herbert HK, Hyder AA, Butchart A, Norton R. Global health: Injuries and violence. *Infect Dis Clin North Am* 2011;25:653–668.
15. García-Moreno C, Jansen HA, Ellsberg M, et al. WHO multi-country study on women's health and domestic violence against women: Initial results on prevalence, health outcomes and women's responses. Geneva: World Health Organization, 2005.
16. Black M, Basile K, Breiding M, et al. The National Intimate Partner and Sexual Violence Survey (NISVS): 2010 summary report. Atlanta: National Center for Injury Prevention and Control, Centers for Disease Control and Prevention, 2011.
17. Hahm HC, Guterman NB. The emerging problem of physical child abuse in South Korea. *Child Maltreatment* 2001;6:169–179.
18. Stoltenbourgh M, van IJzendoorn M, Euser E, Bakers-Kranenburg M. A global perspective on child sexual abuse: Meta-analysis of prevalence around the world. *Child Maltreatment* 2011;16:79–101.
19. Finkelhor D. The international epidemiology of child sexual abuse. *Child Abuse Negl* 1994;18:409–417.
20. Felitti VJ, Anda RF, Nordenberg D, et al. Relationship of childhood abuse and household dysfunction to many of the leading causes of death in adults: The Adverse Childhood Experiences (ACE) Study. *Am J Prevent Med* 1998;14:245–258.
21. Follette VM, Polusny MA, Bechtle AE, Naugle AE. Cumulative trauma: The impact of child sexual abuse, adult sexual assault, and spouse abuse. *J Traumatic Stress* 1996;9:25–35.
22. Jewkes R, Sen P, Garcia-Moreno C. Sexual violence. In Krug E, Dahlberg L, Mercy JA, et al. World report on violence and health. Geneva: World Health Organization 2002:47–82.
23. Lloyd S. The effects of domestic violence on women's employment. *Law & Policy* 1997;19:139–167.
24. Riger S, Staggs SL, Schewe P. Intimate partner violence as an obstacle to employment among mothers affected by welfare reform. *Journal of Social Issues* 2004;60:801–818.
25. Currie J, SpatzWidom C. Long-term consequences of child abuse and neglect on adult economic well-being. *Child Maltreatment* 2010;15:111–120.
26. Levy BS, Sidel VW, ed. War and public health. 2nd ed. New York: Oxford University Press, 2008.
27. Mercy JA, Krug EG, Dahlberg LL, Zwi AB. Violence and health: The United States in a global perspective. *Am J Public Health* 2003;93:256–261.
28. Buvinic M, Morrison AR, Shifter M. Violence in the Americas: A framework for action. In Morrisson AR, Biehl ML, eds. Too close to home: Domestic violence in the Americas. Washington, DC: Inter-American Development Bank, 1999:3–34.
29. Bundhamcharoen K, Odton P, Mugem S, et al. Costs of injuries due to interpersonal and self-directed violence in Thailand, 2005. *J Med Assoc Thai* 2008;9(Suppl 2):110–118.

30. Butchart A, Brown D, Khanh-Huynh A, et al. Manual for estimating the economic costs of injuries due to interpersonal and self-directed violence. Geneva: World Health Organization and Centers for Disease Control and Prevention, 2008.

31. Fang X, Brown DS, Florence CS, Mercy JA. The economic burden of child maltreatment in the United States and implications for prevention. *Child Abuse Negl* 2012;36:156–165.

32. Siskin A, Wyler LS. Trafficking in persons: U.S. policy and issues for congress. *Trends in Organized Crime* 2011;14:267–271.

33. Bales K, Fletcher L, Stover E. Hidden slaves: Forced labor in the United States. Washington, DC: Free the Slaves; and Berkeley, CA: Human Rights Center, University of California Berkeley, 2004.

34. U.S. Department of State. Trafficking in persons report 2011. Washington: US Department of State, 2011: Available at http://www.state.gov/j/tip/rls/tiprpt/2011/index.htm. Accessed on April 23, 2012.

35. Richard AO. International trafficking in women to the United States: A contemporary manifestation of slavery and organized crime. Washington, DC: Center for the Study of Intelligence, 1999.

36. Willis BM, Levy BS. Child prostitution: Global health burden, research needs, and interventions. *Lancet* 2002;359:1417–1422.

37. Chauzy J. Kyrgyz Republic: Trafficking. Paper presented at International Organization for Migration (press briefing notes), Geneva, January 21, 2001.

38. Polaris Project. Available at http://www.polarisproject.org. Accessed on April 23, 2012.

39. Diallo Y, Hagemann F, Etienne A, et al. Global child labour developments: Measuring trends from 2004 to 2008. Geneva: International Labour Office, International Programme on the Elimination of Child Labour (IPEC), 2010.

40. Basu K, Van PH. The economics of child labor. *American Economic Review* 1998;88:412–427.

41. Basu K, Tzannatos Z. The global child labor problem: What do we know and what can we do? *World Bank Economic Review* 2003;17:147–173.

42. Doepke M, Zilibotti F. The macroeconomics of child labor regulation. *American Economic Review* 2005;95:1492–1524.

43. Pollack SH, Landrigan PJ, Mallino DL. Child labor in 1990: Prevalence and health hazards. *Ann Rev Public Health* 1990;11:359–375.

44. Sampson RJ, Lauritsen JL. Violent victimization and offending: Individual-, situational-, and community-level risk factors. In Reiss AJ Jr, Roth JA, eds. Understanding and Preventing Violence: Volume 3: Social Influences. Washington, DC: National Academy Press, 1994:1–114.

45. Reiss AJ, Roth JA, eds. Understanding and preventing violence. Washington, DC: National Academy Press, 1993.

46. Sampson RJ, Raudenbush SW, Earls F. Neighborhoods and violent crime: A multilevel study of collective efficacy. *Science* 1997;277:918.

47. Wilson WJ. The truly disadvantaged: The inner city, the underclass, and public policy. Chicago: University of Chicago Press, 1987.

48. Lauras-Loch T, Lopez-Escartin N. Jeunesse et démographie en Afrique [Youth and demography in Africa]. Les jeunes en Afrique: Évolution et rôle (XIXe–XXe siècles)

[Youth in Africa: its evolution and role (19th and 20th centuries)]. Paris, France: L'Harmattan, 1992:66–82.

49. Diallo Co-Trung M. La crise scolaire au Sénégal: crise de l'école, crise de l'autorité? [The school crisis in Senegal: A school crisis or crisis of authority?] In: d'Almeida-Topor HGO, Coquery-Vidrovitch C, Guitart F, eds. Les jeunes en Afrique: Évolution et rôle (XIXe-XXe siècles) [Youth in Africa: Its Evolution and Role (19th and 20th centuries)]. Paris, France: L'Harmattan, 1992:407–439.

50. Rarrbo K. L'Algérie et sa jeunesse: Marginalisations sociales et désarroi culturel. [Algeria and its youth: Social marginalization and cultural confusion]. Paris, France: L'Harmattan, 1995.

51. Fajnzlber P, Lederman D, Loayza N. Inequality and violent crime. *J Law Econ* 2002;45:1.

52. Gartner R. The victims of homicide: A temporal and cross-national comparison. *Am Sociol Rev* 1990:92–106.

53. Morenoff JD, Sampson RJ, Raudenbush SW. Neighborhood inequality, collective efficacy, and the spatial dynamics of urban violence. *Criminology* 2001;39:517–558.

54. Martikainen P, Mäki N, Blomgren J. The effects of area and individual social characteristics on suicide risk: A multilevel study of relative contribution and effect modification. *European Journal of Population/Revue européenne de démographie* 2004;20:323–350.

55. Gunnell DJ, Peters TJ, Kammerling RM, Brooks J. Relation between parasuicide, suicide, psychiatric admissions, and socioeconomic deprivation. *BMJ* 1995;311:226–230.

56. Whitley E, Gunnell D, Dorling D, Smith GD. Ecological study of social fragmentation, poverty, and suicide. *BMJ* 1999;319:1034–1037.

57. Luo F, Florence CS, Quispe-Agnoli M, et al. Impact of business cycles on U.S. suicide rates, 1928–2007. *Am J Public Health* 2011;101:1139–1146.

58. Neumayer E. Are socioeconomic factors valid determinants of suicide? Controlling for national cultures of suicide with fixed-effects estimation. *Cross-Cultural Research* 2003;37:307–329.

59. Bates D, Fratkin E. Cultural anthropology. New York: Allyn and Bacon, 2003.

60. American Psychological Association. Hate crimes today: An age-old foe in modern dress. Washington, DC: American Psychological Association, 1998.

61. Brown RM. The American vigilante tradition. In: Graham H, Gurr T, eds. The history of violence in America. Beverly Hills, CA: Sage Publications, 1969:154–226.

62. Berrill KT. Anti-gay violence and victimization in the United States. *J Interpers Violence* 1990;5:274–294.

63. Swahn M, Mahendra R, Paulozzi L, et al. Violent attacks on Middle Easterners in the United States during the month following the September 11, 2001, terrorist attacks. *Injury Prevention* 2003;9:187.

64. Annas GJ, Geiger HJ. The impact of war on human rights. In: Levy BS, Sidel VW, eds. War and Public Health. 2nd ed. New York: Oxford University Press, 2008:37–50.

65. Hayward RF. Breaking the earthenware jar: Lessons from South Asia to end violence against women and girls. Kathmandu, Nepal: UNICEF, 2000.

66. Bennet L, Manderson L, Astbury J. Mapping a global pandemic: Review of current literature on rape, sexual assault and sexual harassment of women. Melbourne: Australia University of Melbourne, 2000.

67. Dobash R, Dobash R. Violence against wives: A case against the patriarchy. New York: Free Press, 1979.

68. Levinson D. Family violence in cross-cultural perspective. Thousand Oaks, CA: Sage Publications, 1989.

69. Sanday PR. The socio-cultural context of rape: A cross-cultural study. *Journal of Social Issues* 1981;37:5–27.

70. Hosken F. The Hosken report: Genital and sexual mutilation of females. Lexington, MA: Women's International Network, 1993.

71. Walker A, Parmar P. Warrior marks: Female genital mutilation and the sexual blinding of women. New York: Harcourt Brace & Company, 1993.

72. Mercy JA, Abdel Megid LAM, Salem EM, Lotfi S. Intentional injuries. In: Mashaly AY, Graitcer PL, Youssef ZM, eds. Injury in Egypt. (PASA #263-0102-P-HI-1013-00; project # E-17-C). Cairo, Egypt: United States Agency for International Development,1993.

73. Chesler P. Worldwide trends in honor killing. *The Middle East Quarterly* 2012(Spring): 3–11.

74. Kulczycki A, Windle S. Honor killings in the Middle East and North Africa. *Violence Against Women* 2011;17:1442–1464.

75. Lips H. The gender pay gap: Challenging the rationalizations, perceived equity, discrimination, and the limits of human capital models. *Sex Roles* 2013;68:169–185.

76. U.S. Government Accountability Office. Gender pay differences: Progress made, but women remain overrepresented among low-wage workers. Washington, DC: GAO, 2011.

77. Oostendorp RH. Globalization and the gender wage gap. *World Bank Economic Review* 2009;23:141–161.

78. Aizer A. The gender wage gap and domestic violence. *American Economic Review* 2010;100:1847–1859.

79. Reza A, Mercy JA, Krug E. Epidemiology of violent deaths in the world. *Injury Prevention* 2001;7:104–111.

80. United Nations Centre for Human Rights. Harmful traditional practices affecting the health of women and children. Geneva: United Nations High Commission for Human Rights, 1996.

81. Hall AT. China's one child policy and male surplus as a source of demand for sex trafficking to China. May 2010. Available at http://nfsacademy.org/wp-content/uploads/2011/02/Hall-Chinas-One-Child-Policy.pdf. Accessed on August 27, 2012.

82. Jonson K. The politics of the revival of infant abandonment in China, with special reference to Hunan. *Population and Development Rev* 1996;22:77–99.

83. Phillips MR, Li X, Zhang Y. Suicide rates in China, 1995–99. *Lancet* 2002;359: 835–840.

84. Heise LL, Raikes A, Watts CH, Zwi AB. Violence against women: A neglected public health issue in less developed countries. *Soc Sci Med* 1994;39:1165–1179.

85. Braveman P, Meyers A, Schlenker T, Wands C. Public health and war in Central America. In Levy BS, Sidel VW, eds. War and public health. Updated ed. Washington, DC: American Public Health Association, 2000:238–253.

86. Ugalde A, SelvaSutter E, Castillo C, et al. The health costs of war: Can they be measured? Lessons from El Salvador. *BMJ* 2000; 321:169–172.

87. Regan PM, Henderson EA. Democracy, threats and political repression in developing countries: Are democracies internally less violent? *Third World Quarterly* 2002;23:119–136.

88. Davenport C. Multi-dimensional threat perception and state repression: An inquiry into why states apply negative sanctions. *Am J Poli Sci* 1995;39:683–713.

89. Pampel FC, Gartner R. Age structure, socio-political institutions, and national homicide rates. *European Sociological Review* 1995;11:243–260.

90. Scheper-Hughes N, Hoffman D. Kids out of place: Street children of Brazil. Disposable children: The hazards of growing up in Latin America. Vol. 27. New York: North American Congress on Latin America, 1994:16–23.

91. Aitchinson J. Violência e juventude na África do Sul: Caucas, lições e soluções para uma sociedade violenta [Violence and youth in South Africa: Causes, lessons and solutions for a violent society]. In: Pinheiro PS, ed. São Paulo sem medo: Um diagnóstico da violência urbana [Sao Paulo without fear: A diagnosis of urban violence]. Rio de Janeiro, Brazil: Garamond, 1998:121–132.

92. Roberts DE. The social and moral cost of mass incarceration in African American communities. *Stanford Law Review* 2004;56:1271–1305.

93. Mauer M, King RS. Uneven justice: State rates of incarceration by race and ethnicity. Washington, DC; The Sentencing Project, 2007. Available at http://sentencingproject. org/doc/publications/rd_stateratesofincbyraceandethnicity.pdf. Accessed on August 27, 2012.

94. Markowitz S. The price of alcohol, wife abuse, and husband abuse. Cambridge, MA: National Bureau of Economic Research, 1999. Available at http://www.nber.org/ papers/w6916.pdf?new_window=1. Accessed on August 27, 2012.

95. Markowitz S, Grossman M. Alcohol regulation and domestic violence towards children. *Contemporary Economic Policy* 1998;16:309–320.

96. Todres J. Moving upstream: The merits of a public health law approach to human trafficking. North Carolina Law Review 2011;89:447–506. Available at http://www. nclawreview.org/documents/89/2/todres.pdf. Accessed on August 27, 2012.

97. Raymond JG. Prostitution on demand. *Violence Against Women* 2004;10:1156–1186.

98. Shively M, Jalbert SK, Kling R, et al. Final report on the evaluation of the First Offender Prostitution Program. Cambridge, MA: Abt Associates, 2008. Available at http://www. abtassociates.com/reports/FOPP_Evaluation_FULL_REPORT.pdf. Accessed on August 27, 2012.

99. Anderson LM, Shinn C, St C, et al. Community interventions to promote healthy social environments: early childhood development and family housing. A report on recommendations of the Task Force on Community Preventive Services. *MMWR* 2002;51:1.

100. Ludwig J, Duncan GJ, Hirschfield P. Urban poverty and juvenile crime: Evidence from a randomized housing-mobility experiment. *Quarterly Journal of Economics* 2001;116:655–679.

101. Kling JR, Ludwig J, Katz LF. Neighborhood effects on crime for female and male youth: Evidence from a randomized housing voucher experiment. *Quarterly Journal of Economics* 2005;120:87–130.

102. Lindberg RA, Shenassa ED, Acevedo-Garcia D, et al. Housing interventions at the neighborhood level and health: A review of the evidence. *J Public Health Manag Pract* 2010;16:S44–S52.

103. Edmonds EV, Schady N. Poverty alleviation and child labor. *American Economic Journal: Economic Policy* 2012;4:100–124.

104. Kim JC, Watts CH, Hargreaves JR, et al. Understanding the impact of a microfinance-based intervention on women's empowerment and the reduction of intimate partner violence in South Africa. *Am J Public Health* 2007;97:1794–1802.

105. Black D. Violent structures. Paper prepared for a Workshop on Theories of Violence. Washington, DC: National Institute of Justice, 2002.

106. La Roche D, Senechal R. Why is collective violence collective? *Sociological Theory* 2001;19:126–144.

107. Varshney A. Ethnic conflict and civic life: Hindus and Muslims in India. New Haven, CT: Yale University Press, 2000.

108. Reproductive health effects of gender-based violence. In: United Nations Population Fund Annual Report. Available at http://www.uneca.org/adfvi/documents/UNFPA-RH-effects-of-GBV.pdf. Accessed on August 27, 2012.

109. Coker AL, Cook-Craig PG, Williams CM, et al. Evaluation of Green Dot: An active bystander intervention to reduce sexual violence on college campuses. *Violence Against Women* 2011;17:777–796.

110. Perkins HW, Craig DW. A multifaceted social norms approach to reduce high-risk drinking. Newton, MA: Higher Education Center for Alcohol and Other Drug Prevention, 2002.

111. Berkowitz A. How we can prevent sexual harassment and sexual assault. *Educator's Guide to Controlling Sexual Harassment* 1998;6:1–4.

112. Sorock CE. Closing the gap legislatively: Consequences of the Lilly Ledbetter Fair Pay Act. *Chi.-Kent L. Rev.* 2010;85:1199–1216.

113. Cohen PN, Huffman ML. Working for the woman? Female managers and the gender wage gap. *American Sociological Review* 2007;72:681–704.

114. O'Hear MM. Rethinking drug courts: Restorative justice as a response to racial injustice. *Stanford Law & Policy Review*, March 19, 2009;20:463–498.

115. Davis LJ. Rock, powder, sentencing—Making disparate impact evidence relevant in crack cocaine sentencing. *J Gender Race & Just* 2011;14:375–867.

116. McKenna M. The public health beat: What is it? Why is it important? Nieman Reports Spring 2003:10–11.

18 Environmental Health

■ COLIN D. BUTLER AND
ANTHONY J. MCMICHAEL

■ INTRODUCTION

Modern environmental health evolved from the concept of "miasmas," noxious vapors permeating unhealthy environments and thought to be causing illnesses, varying from cholera to bronchitis to malaria. Although this causal paradigm was discredited by the microbiological and toxicological discoveries of the 19th and 20th centuries, "miasmatic thinking" still surfaces when illnesses appear in proximity to novel environmental phenomena.

Not all miasmas were invisible. London was called the "Big Smoke" for centuries, and those with means have long tried to escape the worst contamination—whether visible, pungent, or imagined. Although not traditionally conceptualized as miasmas, interlocking social influences create patterns of clustered behavior, manifesting as cultures and customs recognizable to members and strangers. These cultures may be either conducive or resistant to the promotion of health. Many of these cultures are geographically localized, such as in neighborhoods, slums, or gated communities. Harmful behaviors exhibited by such groups range from excesses—including smoking, alcohol, junk food consumption, or the tolerance of violence—to more subtle customs, such as taboos that limit discussion of painful emotions. Practices beneficial to health include physical exercise as well as receptivity to information about diet, vaccination, or even infant sleeping position.

Many cultural practices in low-income settings perpetuate poverty and ill-health, often inadvertently. Some examples are obvious, having evolved because of lack of material resources, or the perception of a compensatory ecological benefit. Open defecation in fields, for example, helps maintain soil fertility, but increases risk of parasite transmission. Indoor air pollution in low-income countries from poorly ventilated cooking equipment[1] persists not only because of habit, but also because it is cheaper and more convenient than installing stoves with chimneys.

Some customs harmful to population health are more controversial, such as early marriage, a high fertility rate, and discrimination based on gender, ethnicity, or caste. These practices have not evolved by chance. A high fertility rate compensates for a high infant mortality rate. Large families—which result from a high fertility rate combined with a low mortality rate—can benefit groups in certain temporal and geographic niches, such as during the European colonization of North America in the 19th century. However, such gains are at the cost of other people who are displaced and/or demoralized. In many low-income countries today, a high fertility rate is still regarded as desirable—although it contributes to poverty and underdevelopment.[2,3]

In the last century, people in high-income countries increasingly recognized the health risks of living near intensely polluting processes, with consequent relocation of heavy industry—first to rural areas, then to low-income countries. Because of these concerns, heating processes and transportation became cleaner through changes such as electrification and the removal of lead from gasoline.

However, the main reason for relocating much heavy industry to low-income countries was not environmental concerns, but rather forces of neoliberalism and associated globalization. (See Box 19–1 in Chapter 19.) Large populations in low-income countries provide low-cost, compliant, non-unionized—and vulnerable—workers who attract global entrepreneurs and international corporations. Wages and other production costs in these economies are depressed, lowering consumer prices by reducing environmental and occupational safety and health standards and by having families—rather than national governments—provide safety nets. The economies in most low-income countries are permeated by long-standing, widespread, visible poverty, which reduces upward mobility. Societal structures that promote low wages and low prices enable life—although rarely health—to be maintained on incomes that are minimal by Western standards. In low-income countries, these factors combine with other elements, such as debt, to reinforce poverty and powerlessness. This collective hardship and exploitation benefits the few who are relatively affluent in low-income countries and the many who are relatively affluent in high-income countries—whose lives are virtually unknown and unknowable to poor people in low-income countries.[4,5]

Some people have repeatedly claimed that globalization is a worldwide economic boon for both rich and poor people, promising to maximize the production of goods and services at "rock-bottom" prices. The reality has been not only a global financial crisis foisted on the world by complacent bankers and corrupt officials,[6] but also oppressive and often inhumane working conditions endured by millions of workers, mainly in low-income countries. This inequality is tolerated mainly because these workers are made invisible, hidden from most consumers by vast physical, cultural, and psychological distances.

Labor disputes in places such as China and Bangladesh occur—but are rarely reported. Consumers in high-income countries speak different languages than these workers do, and rarely identify emotionally or psychologically with them. Even in low-income countries, however, affluent consumers are often indifferent to the needs of poor people within their borders. In China, a "floating population" of over 100 million poor and job-insecure people, mainly from rural areas, underpins the economy.[7,8] These people require internal passports and are, in effect, second-class citizens. In India, the ancient caste system, especially in the North, reflects and reinforces inequality—despite laws that ban it.[7] Over half of the children in the North of India are stunted.[9] In Africa, child laborers continue to form the foundation of the global cocoa industry.[10] Confidence in the counter-movement of *fair trade*—in which high-income consumers pay a premium for products produced by workers who are slightly better paid—is undermined by its transaction costs and occasional fraud.

The euphemism *guestworkers*, principally from South Asia, describes an underclass of exploited people whose sweat and subservience, far from home, make possible the glittering mega-cities of the Middle East and elsewhere.[11] These workers frequently endure sustained racial intolerance and physical insecurity, with minimal, if any, legal protections.[12] Many reside in labor camps, some in shanty towns. Even their low wages are often withheld for long periods. If they complain to officials, they may be threatened with deportation.[11] (See also Chapter 19.)

Subsistence of these workers is supported by an even poorer stratum of workers who provide goods and services to them. In a global *economic food chain*, people on successively lower income tiers struggle to cope with successively less material and freedom—in what some have called a *global claste system* (a hybrid of *class* and *caste*).[13] At the bottom of this system, almost 30 million people survive as slaves and indentured laborers, many of whom incur debt from which there is no escape.[14] Slightly higher up the ladder live the *precariat*, people who are employed, not starving, but nevertheless chronically insecure and vulnerable.[15] As one descends the economic ladder, exposure to air and water pollution, toxic wastes, and other environmental hazards increases. These costs—*negative externalities*—are rarely incorporated into the price of goods and services.

■ SCALE AND DISTRIBUTION OF ENVIRONMENTAL HEALTH HAZARDS

Quantitatively, the important environmental causes of ill health derive from microbiologically contaminated water and indoor air pollution with multiple toxic chemicals.[16] Almost the entire burden of these hazards is carried by poor populations in low-income countries. Within high-income countries, the largest environmental risks are also experienced by the poor (Figure 18–1). There have been attempts to cast doubt on the health effects of exposure to low levels of persistent hazardous pollutants.[17] Numerous methodological issues, such as assessment of exposure, chemical interactions, latency, and non-specific effects, continue to make it difficult to characterize these pollutants with epidemiological studies.[18] Nonetheless, consensus seems to be increasing that many of these toxic substances cause a wide range of disorders, including developmental defects, chronic organ dysfunction, and cancer.[19,20]

Downplaying the scale of environmental hazard has philosophical and political dimensions. In many cases, defenders of industry have used deceit, public relations, appeals to pragmatism, and corrupted scientific research to obfuscate the need for and delay the progress of reform.[21-23]

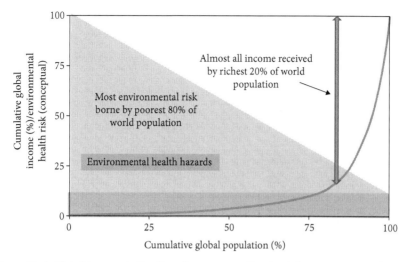

Figure 18-1 Global income is distributed very unequally; the richest 20 percent of people receive over 80 percent of global income. In contrast, most environmental hazards are experienced by the poorest 80 percent of people; however, even the richest 20 percent of people face risks from climate change. (*Note:* Data for "environmental health risk" are conceptual rather than being based on any single analysis.)

Pollution is a byproduct of the material and economic benefits of urban centers—industrial production, generation of electricity, transportation, and heating and cooking. Over time, many individuals and groups have sought to minimize their exposure to the known and perceived risks of environmental hazards. Sometimes, the invisibility of some hazards has heightened concern, making the risk more uncertain and difficult to avoid; however, for uneducated and unaware people, invisibility and ignorance probably contribute to exposure.

Those who are skeptical about environmental hazards also understate the health risk of climate change and ecosystem disruption, which together likely represent an enormous burden of future disease—perhaps exceeding that attributed to existing environmental hazards.[24] These costs are likely to be borne mainly by poor people in low-income countries, such as low-lying Bangladesh and countries in sub-Saharan Africa. Even armed conflict due to climate change may occur.[25]

■ NEW ENVIRONMENTAL HEALTH PROBLEMS

One hundred years ago, persistent organic pollutants (POPs) had not been synthesized. Greenhouse gases were accumulating in the atmosphere and ecosystems were becoming further degraded. But climate change and ecosystem disruption were not recognized as legitimate environmental health issues until the late 20th century. And some hazards, such as halogen-based chemicals that damage the stratospheric ozone layer, did not exist until then.

■ RELATIONSHIPS BETWEEN SOCIAL INJUSTICE AND ENVIRONMENTAL HEALTH

Water

The enormous progress in water safety and sanitation, which occurred in high-income countries more than a century ago,[26] has not been extended to the poorest and most vulnerable people. Almost 1 billion people still drink unimproved water.[27] An estimated 2.6 billion people lack access to improved sanitation.[28] Diarrheal disease from fecally contaminated water causes much illness and death, especially among poor children living in urban slums and rural areas of low-income countries. Chronic or repeated diarrhea in children causes physical stunting and reduced cognitive development.[29] As a result, the number of disability adjusted life-years (DALYs) lost from contaminated water is greater than mortality rates for diarrheal disease might suggest.

Access to water, even of poor quality, is also important for health. The opportunity and energy cost of carrying water limits its use for washing, with consequent adverse health effects.[30]

Indoor Air Pollution

The regular breathing of smoky air from cooking fires is almost entirely confined to poor people in low-income countries. Indoor air pollution increases the risks of acute respiratory infections in childhood—the largest cause of death among children—and chronic obstructive pulmonary disease.[1,31] Indoor air pollution is also associated with pulmonary tuberculosis, nasopharyngeal and laryngeal cancers, cataracts, and, when coal is burned, lung cancer.[32] (For a discussion of substandard housing in the United States and its impact on health, see Box 18–1.)

Outdoor Air Pollution

Outdoor air pollution, from motor vehicles, industry (Figure 18–2), and home heating, is a major human health issue in urban areas. Globally, outdoor air pollution is thought to cause approximately 1 million deaths annually, two-thirds of which occur in low- and middle-income countries. However, because most deaths occur in adults, the burden of disease, measured in DALYs, is not as high as that from indoor air pollution.[16]

Air pollution in high-income countries remains a health problem. In the Netherlands, for example, cars are thought to cause more deaths from air pollution than from trauma. Air pollution has also been linked to atopy and cardiac disease.[31] Urban outdoor air pollution is worst in the megacities of low-income countries, exacerbated by the growing use of motor vehicles, dust from

BOX 18-1 ■ Substandard Housing and Its Impact on Health

Bailus Walker, Jr.

The relationship between housing and health in the United States is illustrated by the following realities:

- More than one-fifth of all Americans (52 million people) live in neighborhoods in which at least 20 percent of the residents are poor.[1]
- Housing insecurity (high housing cost in proportion to income, poor housing quality, neighborhood instability, crowding, or homelessness) is associated with poor health, lower weight, and developmental risk in young children.[2]
- Crowded housing promotes the spread of respiratory infections.[1]
- Environmental carcinogens, such as radon and environmental tobacco smoke, are present in many homes.[3]
- Substandard housing conditions, such as leaking pipes, inadequate ventilation, and improper maintenance may increase risk of (a) mold growth; (b) infestations of mites, roaches, and insect vectors of disease; and (c) exposure to allergens.[4]
- Unintentional injuries due to structural defects in homes, resulting in about 4,000,000 emergency department visits and 70,000 hospital admissions in the United States annually.[5]

In the densely populated cities and rural villages of low-income countries, substandard housing is generally more prevalent than in the United States, with much greater adverse effects on health.

The field of public health arose largely out of concerns for the quality of human shelter, especially the living conditions of working populations. Understanding the relationships between disease occurrence and substandard housing became the basis for developing and implementing public health measures. In 1939, the American Public Health Association (APHA) Committee on Hygiene of Housing developed principles that form the basis of current housing regulations and programs to reduce health and safety hazards in housing.

The following are five types of housing factors that contribute to adverse health:

- Physical factors, such as extremes of temperature, exposure to radon, loud noise, inadequate light, and poor ventilation
- Chemical factors, such as carbon monoxide, environmental tobacco smoke, and lead
- Biological factors, such as rodents, mites, cockroaches, and mold
- Building and equipment factors, such as safety hazards that can cause injuries as well as sewage and sanitation
- Social factors, such as architectural features that influence mental health[6]

Among the most preventable housing-related health problems is childhood lead poisoning. Although progress has been made in addressing this problem, persistent major risk factors for elevated blood lead levels in children include poverty, African American racial status, and residence in older substandard housing.[7,8]

Housing policy issues—concerning location, construction, financing, upkeep, and maintenance—have profound effects on these factors. Access to healthful and safe housing is a basic right. But assurance of this right has been impeded by social injustice. For example, as suburban residents have moved into urban centers, low-income people (often minorities)—unless they have been protected by government regulations or voluntary provisions—have been forced financially to move, usually into less healthy environments.

Housing comprises four interrelated elements: house (dwelling), home (the social, cultural and economic structure created by the household), neighborhood (immediate housing environment), and social, physical, and economic character-istics within the neighborhood. Each of these elements has the potential to affect physical, social, and mental health, and the combination of two or more of these elements may have a synergistic effect. For example, the physical makeup of a neighborhood can promote health by providing:

- Safe places for children to play and adults to exercise—free of crime, vehicular traffic, and related pollution
- Landscape features that accommodate bicycling, which can promote neighbor-hood development.
- Local food stores and markets that contribute to healthy eating habits, thereby improving quality of life[9]

The interrelationship of housing and health is complex. Because residents of substandard housing have many other undesirable stressors, including low income, limited education, malnutrition, and limited job opportunities, it is difficult to dis-tinguish among multiple causes of poor health. But the absence of definitive evi-dence to support housing regulations should not discourage governmental and non-governmental work to improve the quality of housing.

What Needs To Be Done

Necessary actions include: (a) prevention of deterioration of housing and residential environments; (b) rehabilitation of substandard housing, if economically feasible; and (c) production of enough new housing to provide for population increases, to ease overcrowding, and to replace demolished and decayed structures. These activi-ties must involve many sectors and disciplines—both within and beyond the health sciences. There also needs to be an emphasis on developing policies and programs to eliminate poverty and to improve education so that all people can live in safe and healthful housing—housing that is designed, built, renovated, and maintained in ways to support the health of its residents.

Box References

1. Krieger J, Higgins DL. Housing and health: Time again for public health action. *Am J Public Health* 2002;92:758–768.
2. Joint Center for Housing Studies of Harvard University. The State of the Nation's Housing 2008. Cambridge, MA, 2008. Available at http://www.jchs.harvard.edu/research/publica-tions/state- nations-housing-2008. Accessed on June 28, 2012.
3. Shaw M. Housing and public health. *Annu Rev Public Health* 2004;25:397–418.
4. Pleis JR, Lethbridge-Cejku M. Summary health statistics for U.S. adults: National Health Interview Survey, 2006. *National Center for Health Statistics. Vital Health Stat* 10(235). 2007. Available at http://www.cdc.gov/nchs/data/series/sr_10/sr10_235.pdf. Accessed on June 28, 2012.

5. U.S. Department of Housing and Urban Development, Office of Lead Hazard Control. The Healthy Homes Initiative: A preliminary plan (full report). April 1999. Available at http://www.hud.gov/offices/lead/library/hhi/HHIFull.pdf. Accessed on June 28, 2012.

6. Bonnefo X. Inadequate housing and health: An overview. *Int J Environ Pollut* 2007;30:411–429.

7. Jacobs D. Environmental health disparities. *Am J Public Health* 2010;101:S115–S122.

8. Laumbach R, Gochfeld M. Toxicology. In: Levy BS, Wegman DH, Baron SL, Sokas RK, eds. Occupational and environmental health: Recognizing and preventing disease and injury. 6th ed. New York: Oxford University Press, 2011:527–558.

9. Robert Wood Johnson Foundation, Commission to Build a Healthier America. Where we live matters for our health: The links between housing and health. September 2008. Available at http://www.rwjf.org/files/research/commissionhousing10200.pdf. Accessed on June 28, 2012.

construction, and smoky fuels used for manufacturing and domestic purposes. Some cities, such as New Delhi and Dhaka in South Asia, are enforcing laws that encourage the use of cleaner fuels, such as compressed gas. Air pollution in China remains severe; recently, the Chinese government prohibited the U.S. embassy in Beijing from reporting levels of air pollution there.[33]

Continental Air Pollution

Haze on a continental scale is a third category of air pollution. Over South Asia, this haze is called the *atmospheric brown cloud*—caused mainly by rural

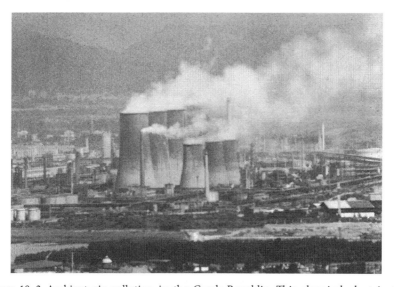

Figure 18-2 Ambient air pollution in the Czech Republic. This chemical plant in the northern part of the Czech Republic for many years accounted for much air pollution in the surrounding area. (Photograph by Barry S. Levy.)

residents burning biofuels, such as firewood, dung, and agricultural waste.[34] Continental air pollution affects agriculture (by changing regional precipitation patterns and reducing the penetration of sunlight), contributes to climate change,[35] and possibly adversely affects health in other ways. For example, during the 1970s and 1980s, sulfate-rich air that originated mainly from Central and Eastern Europe, led to reduced precipitation over the eastern Sahel in Africa—contributing to famine and conflict there.[36]

Soil and Water Contamination

Several parasitic diseases, mostly affecting poor people in low-income countries, are transmitted via contact with soil and water contaminated by human waste. The most important of these disease are schistosomiasis and hookworm. Although hookworm infestation causes few deaths, it contributes to anemia, cognitive impairment, and reduced economic output.[29] Leptospirosis, often spread through contaminated water, may be increasing in incidence from floods associated with climate change.[37]

Food

In addition to contamination with microorganisms, food can be contaminated with chemicals, such as heavy metals in fish and marine mammals, organochlorines in breast milk and farmed fish,[38] and arsenic in crops irrigated by arsenic-contaminated water. Pesticides and other chemicals, such as polychlorinated biphenyls (PCBs), can also contaminate food. Food deliberately contaminated with melamine has been a recurrent problem in China, partly due to a poor safety culture and a corrupt system, in which a senior official was executed and the parents of an affected child were imprisoned for trying to enhance awareness of the problem.[39]

Lead

On the basis of lost DALYs, lead exposure is second in importance only to indoor air pollution among environmental health problems in low-income countries.[40] There may be no "safe" concentration of lead in the body. Although lead exposures have decreased in recent decades, the total body burden of lead in Americans in the United States peaked at a concentration about 1000-fold higher than those measured in pre-industrial populations.[41]

Lead exposure has been a problem since Roman times. At high exposures, it is a systemic poison, especially affecting the central nervous system, kidneys, and bone marrow. Chronic exposure to lead is a major cause of cognitive impairment,[42,43] especially in low-income households—adding to their other health-related problems. Until recent decades, the primary environmental exposures to lead were from leaded gasoline and lead-containing paint.[41] Elimination or reduction of the lead content in gasoline has now occurred in almost all countries, with substantial health benefits.[44] Although lead-containing paint has been banned in most high-income countries, children who live in homes previously painted with lead-containing paint can be exposed to lead in dust and paint chips. In addition, children living near secondary lead smelters, battery manufacturing plants, and backyard radiator repair workshops in low-income countries remain at risk of high lead exposure.[45] Lead paint persists as a problem internationally, as demonstrated by the recall in 2007 of over 1 million toys made in China with lead-containing paint.[46]

Asbestos

In high-income countries, the health hazards of asbestos exposure and the availability of safe alternatives to asbestos are widely recognized. All forms of asbestos are banned in 52 countries, yet it is still mined in and exported by Russia, China, Kazakhstan, and Brazil. After a long campaign by activists, Canada has stopped mining asbestos.[47]

As markets in high-income countries have contracted, the asbestos industry has aggressively transferred its commercial activities—and hazards—to low-income countries.[48,49] There they attempt to justify the myth that some forms of asbestos are safe. Political and industry opposition to regulation reinforces this myth. In most low-income countries, the epidemic of asbestos-related disease (primarily asbestosis, lung cancer, and mesothelioma) is less advanced, due to the relatively recent start of asbestos use and the powerlessness of its victims.

Mercury

Mercury contamination is a global problem, caused mainly by the burning of coal,[50] gold mining, waste incineration, and other industrial processes. Mercury bioaccumulates in the food chain, especially in carnivorous fish and marine mammals.[51] The inadvertent consumption of mercury in marine animals has been recognized since the Minimata Bay disaster in Japan in the 1950s, in which birth defects and neurological disorders occurred as a result of industrial dumping of mercury into the bay and its incorporation into the food chain.[52]

Indigenous peoples of the Arctic, whose traditional diet has been based on fish and marine mammals, are probably those at greatest risk of mercury exposure. These people also absorb disproportionately high concentrations of heavy metals and chemicals, such as PCBs and other organochlorines.[53] However, their adverse health outcomes have been disputed or ignored by people in power.

Persistent Organic Pollutants

Persistent organic pollutants (POPs) are synthetic chemicals, including many pesticides, that resist environmental degradation. POPs cause many adverse health effects, and multiple POP exposures may have synergistic effects, especially to genetically vulnerable subgroups.[54] One class of POPs, organochlorines, has been suspected of having a range of adverse health effects, given their propensity to bioaccumulate, their long half-lives, and, for some, their capacity to mimic estrogen.

Farmers have been repeatedly found to have higher-than-expected rates of certain cancers, including non-Hodgkin lymphoma, probably due to their exposure to pesticides.[55] Problems with dose measurement, interactions, confounding, and lagged effects make it challenging to find strong causal relationships between POPs and specific types of cancer.

■ GLOBAL CLIMATE CHANGE AND ECOSYSTEM DISRUPTION

The focus of the debate on global climate change is shifting from whether it is really occurring to its severity and consequences. Current trends, previously viewed as far-fetched predictions, are becoming routine. The 2003 European heat wave caused the deaths of at least 35,000 people,[56] and there is increasing consensus that recent extreme weather events have been worsened by climate change, including the heat wave in Russia in 2010 and the heat wave and drought in the United States in 2011 and 2012.[57]

Direct effects of climate change on human health include increased occurrence of heat-related disorders—sometimes fatal—mainly affecting older people living alone without air-conditioning in urban areas and outdoor workers. Indirect effects include eco-climatic change, causing, for example, altered distribution of mosquitoes, ticks, and other disease-transmitting insects, with a resultant increase in malaria, dengue fever, and other vector-borne diseases.[58]

In addition, more experts are recognizing the possibility of extremely serious indirect, or "tertiary," effects on human health. These effects arise through complex multifactorial pathways, causing, for example, extreme weather events, food insecurity, famine, and conflict.[24,59] Large-scale dislocation of people may occur as a result of sea-level rise and drought.[60]

Ecosystem disruption, even without climate change, can also adversely affect development and health. For example, in 1999, Hurricane Mitch caused devastation in Central America, with a far more severe impact on human health than did Hurricane Andrew, a Category 5 storm that struck Florida in 1992. Hurricane Mitch brought about huge mudslides that killed many people, collapsed bridges, and damaged other structures; these mudslides were partly attributed to large-scale deforestation on steep hills. Lack of insurance, combined with poor emergency services, inadequate building standards, and mismanagement of relief funds, entrenched conditions of poverty for many people.

In 2005, Hurricane Katrina, which led to massive flooding in New Orleans, claimed over 2800 lives, uprooted over 100,000 people, and caused numerous long-term health effects; poor African Americans living in New Orleans suffered the most.[61-63] At the time of the storm and the resultant flooding, televised images of dead bodies and people clinging to rooftops vividly demonstrated that poverty and racism lead to profound health problems.[64] These social injustices persist and continue to adversely affect the health of poor people of color in the United States.[65,66] Other people, however, are also vulnerable to the effects of climate change, including extreme weather events, which, in turn, can weaken or damage societal infrastructure—even leading to the collapse of insurance companies.[64]

▓ ENVIRONMENTAL DISASTERS AND THE EROSION OF TRUST

Manmade disasters have magnified public suspicion of chemicals and radiation. In the Bhopal disaster in India in 1984, the Chernobyl disaster in Ukraine in 1986, and the Fukushima disaster in Japan in 2011, hazardous materials were released and adversely affected the physical and mental health of numerous people. Like many other disasters, these were characterized by initial attempts to downplay harm, denial of compensation to claimant victims, and few admissions of responsibility or guilt.[65] Collectively, these situations have eroded public trust in governments.

The worst industrial disaster occurred in Bhopal in and around a pesticide-manufacturing factory owned by a multinational company. It mainly affected thousands of people living near the plant. Estimates of the mortality and morbidity are contested, but 7000 to 10,000 people died within 3 days of the disaster, and up to 20,000 more by 2003.[66] Some studies of the health effects of Bhopal were prematurely terminated, and others were allegedly suppressed. Compensation for relatives of people who died in the explosion was delayed for many years; many victims were never even properly registered. A class-action lawsuit against the company, filed by victims of the disaster in a U.S. court, was dismissed. The former company president was designated as a "proclaimed absconder" due to his failure to appear at hearings for a criminal case filed in India.[67]

The Bhopal disaster illustrates how poor people, restricted in their choices of where they can live, are disproportionately exposed to hazardous substances, and why hazardous industrial plants and whole industries have been moved to low-income countries. Had the Bhopal disaster occurred in the United States, its victims would probably have received much more compensation. However, it is also likely that, had the plant been in the United States, the incident would never have occurred. In fact, the company operated a similar plant in the United States with greater safety precautions—reflecting a double standard.

Natural disasters also adversely impact on social justice. Populations with limited resources are, in general, less able to anticipate, cope with, resist, and recover from natural disasters. (See Box 18–2.)

BOX 18-2 ■ Impact of Natural Disasters on Social Justice

Linda Young Landesman, Micheal A. Kemp, and Kay C. Goss

A natural disaster is a human construct. The conditions for a disaster are created when humans interact with a naturally occurring event, such as a tornado, flood, hurricane, earthquake, or severe heat wave. In a disaster, societal protections break down—in a non-uniform manner. Vulnerable people, who have fewer resources, are generally unable to anticipate, cope with, resist, and recover from a disaster, compared with people with greater resources.[1-2]

Susceptibility to hazards, as in a disaster, is a function of basic demographic characteristics, access to health care, social capital, and access to lifelines.[3] Those who are most vulnerable include infants and young children, older people, people with functional needs, women, those with low socioeconomic status, and members of minority and some religious groups. To ensure social justice in response to a disaster, a community must include in its planning, preparedness, and response an understanding of the social conditions of its population.

During the severe heat wave in Chicago in 1995, economically deprived, elderly African Americans had higher mortality rates than any other demographic group. Those who were disproportionately impacted by the extreme heat were socially isolated, fearful of being criminally attacked, burdened by utility bills, and affected by several preexisting social conditions.[4]

In 1998, Hurricane Floyd swept through North Carolina and South Carolina, completely flooding Princeville and Tarboro, historically African American communities that had been established in the 1860s just after Emancipation. Initially, some response officials wanted to "buy them out" and move the people who were made homeless out of this flood plain to safety. However, the local residents successfully resisted this response, refusing to leave their communities. The attempted buyout created enormous distrust, confusion, misinformation, and stress for residents, especially those who were old, poor, or not mobile.

In 2003, a total of 14,802 largely elderly people died during a heat wave in France. Most victims had lived independently, did not know how to react, or were too impaired by the unusual heat to adapt. A refrigerated warehouse outside Paris was used to store bodies because undertakers had inadequate space to do so. As many people were on August holiday, including government ministers and physicians, bodies were not claimed for weeks. After the summer, 57 unclaimed bodies of people in the Paris area who had died were buried.

In 2005, Hurricane Katrina illustrated various forms of injustice that accompany disasters:

- People with special needs, poor people, and people who did not speak the language of emergency managers were least able to evacuate to protect themselves.
- Poor people, lacking money for transportation, physically clung to their homes.
- Women were raped.
- Some people died because they were unable to receive required medications, dialysis, or other medical treatment.
- Prisoners escaped and were present in shelters and elsewhere.

Much social injustice followed the 2010 earthquake in Haiti. People with sufficient resources left the country. Many without resources are still living there in squalor. Although government officials and representatives of non-governmental organizations in Haiti talk of reconstruction and repairing the broken infrastructure, much of the money that has been donated remains unspent and Haiti's economic recovery is still crippled. Women and other vulnerable people continue to be victimized. Meanwhile, the government now devotes its scarce resources to infrastructure building and life-and-death issues—leaving social justice to be addressed at a later time.

The U.S. government requires that vulnerable populations be addressed in community preparedness for disasters. Laws and regulations include the following:

- The Americans with Disabilities Act (1990) requires that communities assure preparedness for individuals with disabilities.
- The Pandemic and All-Hazards Preparedness Act (2006) requires communities, in preparing for emergencies, to plan for the needs of five specific vulnerable populations: those who need help maintaining independence, those who have difficulty communicating or understanding emergency orders, those without transportation, those who require supervision, and those who need medical care for unstable, terminal, or contagious diseases.
- The Post-Katrina Reform Act (2006) requires that communities provide support for individuals who need durable medical equipment or consumable medical supplies; services enabling vulnerable populations to stay in shelters that are designed for the general population; and reasonable modification of policies, procedures, and practices.

The Homeland Security Grant Program provides funding to communities for conducting assessments that identify threats, hazards, and risks within their jurisdictions. The *Comprehensive Preparedness Guide* (CPG) 101, Version 2.0, provides guidance for government agencies at all levels; it recommends incorporating risk assessments in planning for emergency operations.

To advance preparedness, communities can form emergency planning councils. In preparing for their communities, emergency management and public health agencies can coordinate with organizations serving at-risk populations to better understand their needs if a disaster should occur.[5]

Social justice can be ensured during and after natural disasters by taking the necessary measures to equally protect everyone from harm.

Box References

1. Bolin R, Stanford L. The Northridge earthquake: Vulnerability and disaster. London: Rutledge, 1998.
2. Kemp MA, Martin D. Teaching hazard mitigation. Fairfax, VA: Public Entity Risk Institute, 2011.
3. Foundation for Comprehensive Emergency Management Research Center. Community hazard risk assessment methodologies: A study of practical challenges and methodological solutions for THIRA (Threat Hazard Risk Assessment). Edwardsville, IL: Foundation for Comprehensive Emergency Management Research Center, 2012.
4. Klinenberg E. Heat wave: A social autopsy of disaster in Chicago. Chicago: University of Chicago Press, 2002.
5. Landesman LY. Public health management of disasters: The practice guide. 3rd ed. Washington, DC: American Public Health Association, 2012.

■ **GLOBALIZATION AND ENVIRONMENTAL HEALTH**

Two of the widely recognized characteristics of globalization are relevant to global environmental health: (a) the continuing drive by trade, technology, and ideology of a single global economic community, with an unprecedented sharing of culture; and (b) market deregulation. (See Box 19–1 in Chapter 19.) Previously, market forces increased environmental health risks for poor people in high-income countries. As globalization has led to the export of hazardous industries from high-income to low-income countries, poor people in these countries have experienced increased health risks, such as from exposure to lead, mercury, or other hazardous substances.

■ **NATIONAL IMPLICATIONS**

The widespread attempts to restrain capitalism that followed the Great Depression and accompanied the peak of the Soviet Union's and China's international appeal have weakened substantially in the past three decades, leading to a resurgence of market forces. Increasingly, impoverished, powerless, and vulnerable populations are appearing in high-income countries, especially in southern Europe and the United States.[68] Shanty towns, like the "Hoovervilles" of the Great Depression, are increasing in the United States.[69] Ascendancy of the so-called free market has helped to promote this inequality.

■ **WHAT NEEDS TO BE DONE**

Achieving Environmental Justice

The Environmental Justice Movement links poverty, disadvantage, and environmental health, but it has not adequately addressed the most egregious exposures to environmental hazards, which affect poor populations of low-income countries. This inadequacy results, in part, from (a) lack of awareness of the environmental risks faced by these people, (b) inadequate scientific data on these risks, (c) inadequate coverage of these risks in the news media or the scientific literature, and (d) powerlessness of these people to draw attention to these risks and to advocate that they be addressed.

Creating Greater Awareness of the Costs of Environmental Hazards

Economists use the term *negative externalities* to describe the costs of environmental hazards. These costs are poorly measured and never incorporated into the price of items. Greater awareness of these negative externalities will increase social and political pressure to reduce them. However, a full accounting of negative externalities would reduce profits and increase prices, especially in the short term—and, therefore, it is resisted, not only by those who have created these negative externalities, but also by consumers.

Harnessing Sufficient Political and Economic Will

Increasingly, economic power is distributed unequally, both within and among countries. Although the Millennium Development Goals (Table 21-7 in Chapter 21) were developed with great fanfare in 2000, few will be achieved by the target year—2015.

Much progress has been made to reduce the hazardous environmental exposures of comparatively privileged populations, but little has been achieved for the poorest populations. This disparity is due to insufficient social and political will globally to address environmental health risks faced by poor people. But, while a dramatic change of global consciousness[70] seems utopian, major changes in global thinking have occurred before, such as the birth of the United Nations in 1945 and the World Health Organization's commitment to "Health for All" in 1978.

Reducing Exposure to Hazardous Chemical Exposures

The Sanitary Revolution, which spread throughout industrialized England in the late 19th century, could provide a model for the new "Sustainability Transition."[71] Reformers and enlightened leaders with a sense of "noblesse oblige" created the Sanitary Revolution by utilizing improved technology and generated competition among cities to improve sanitation. Its costs were outweighed by many economic benefits, including the stimulus it gave to new industries, and reduced illness in the population. Similarly, in the Sustainability Transition, cleaner technologies will stimulate new industries and health and economic productivity will increase.

There are numerous examples of how people have averted environmental damage, improved global public health, and generated vast numbers of new jobs. In most high-income countries, use of lead and asbestos has been banned or restricted, stimulating the development and use of alternative substances. In many countries, acid rain has decreased. So has the use of substances that deplete stratospheric ozone. In some high-income countries, such as Germany and Spain, measures are being taken to substantially lower domestic greenhouse gas emissions. And the cost of solar technology has markedly decreased.[72]

Performing Epidemiological Research

Investigation of environmental health hazards in most low-income countries is rudimentary for several reasons, including inadequate resources. Vested-interest groups may oppose such investigation, such as by opposing funding for in-country research. However, the need for countries to replicate research that has been done elsewhere is usually not necessary.

As globalization advances, enlightened funding bodies and philanthropists are increasing their support for research projects in low-income countries. This support could increase local capacity and public awareness, and eventually facilitate legal and social reform. Advocacy for these goals by epidemiologists based in high-income countries could promote this work.

Reforming Organizations and Institutions

Consumers and shareholders support corporations because the goods they supply are the cheapest and the profits they deliver are the highest. Citizens in high-income countries support, implicitly, the policies of the World Bank and the International Monetary Fund because they feel their own lives are made richer and more secure by so doing.

Therefore, the attitudes and values of middle-class people globally need to be transformed. They need to be convinced that their acquiescence to policies that are unsustainable as well as being socially and environmentally exploitative places the future of their children and grandchildren at serious risk. A transformation in their attitudes and values would likely lead to changes in global values and resultant changes in technology, advertising, and economic policy.

■ CONCLUSION

Reducing environmental hazards globally requires ambitious and innovative strategies to address socioeconomic disparities, overconsumption of natural resources, population growth, and unfair economic policies, and to develop environmentally friendly technologies. Effectively addressing these challenges also requires better education and information dissemination, fair trade policies, and more democracy globally. When these goals are achieved, the Sustainability Transition will be complete.

■ ACKNOWLEDGEMENTS

We thank Susan Butler and Colin Soskolne for their editorial assistance.

■ REFERENCES

1. Fullerton DG, Bruce N, Gordon SB. Indoor air pollution from biomass fuel smoke is a major health concern in the developing world. *Trans R Soc Hop Med Hyg* 2008;102:843–851.
2. Campbell M, Cleland J, Ezeh A, Prata N. Return of the population growth factor. *Science* 2007;315:1501–1502.

3. Ezeh AC, Bongaarts J, Mberu B. Global population trends and policy options. *Lancet* 2012;380:142–148.

4. Raina V, Chowdhury A, Chowdhury S, eds. The dispossessed. Victims of development in Asia. Hong Kong: ARENA Press, 1997.

5. Labonté R, Schrecker T, Gupta AS. Health for some? Death, disease and disparity in a globalizing era. Toronto: Centre for Social Justice, 2005.

6. Taibbi M. The great American bubble machine. Rolling Stone, 2009. Available at: http://www.rollingstone.com/politics/news/the-great-american-bubble-machine-20100405. Accessed March 7, 2013.

7. Butler CD. Environmental change, injustice and sustainability. *J Bioethical Inquiry* 2008;5:11–19.

8. Wang J-W, Cui Z-T, Cui H-W, et al. Quality of life associated with perceived stigma and discrimination among the floating population in Shanghai, China: A qualitative study. *Health Promot Int* 2010;25:394–402.

9. Black RE, Allen LH, Bhutta ZA, et al. Maternal and child undernutrition: Global and regional exposures and health consequences. *Lancet* 2008;371:243–260.

10. Athreya B. White man's "burden" and the new colonialism in West African cocoa production. *Race/Ethnicity:Multidisciplinary Global Contexts* 2011;5:51–59.

11. Walters TN, Kadragic A, Walters LM. Miracle or mirage: Is development sustainable in the United Arab Emirates? *Middle East Review of International Affairs* 2006;10:80–91.

12. Ehrenreich B, Hochschild AR, editors. Global woman: Nannies, maids and sex workers in the new economy. New York: Henry Holt and Company, 2002.

13. Butler CD. Inequality, global change and the sustainability of civilisation. *Global Change and Human Health* 2000;1:156–172.

14. Bales K. Disposable people: New slavery in the global economy. Berkeley, Los Angeles, London: University of California Press, 1999.

15. Standing G. The Precariat: The new dangerous class. New York: Bloomsbury USA, 2011.

16. Ezzati M. Indoor air pollution and health in developing countries. *Lancet* 2005;366:104–106.

17. Ames B. Paracelsus to parascience: The environmental cancer distraction. *Mutation Research* 2000;447:3–13.

18. Briggs D. Environmental pollution and the global burden of disease. *Br Med Bull* 2003;68:1–24.

19. Grandjean P, Bellinger D, Bergman Å, et al. The Faroes statement: Human health effects of developmental exposure to chemicals in our environment. *Basic Clin Pharmacol Toxicol* 2007;102:73–75.

20. Vineis P, Xun W. The emerging epidemic of environmental cancers in developing countries. *Ann Oncol* 2009;20:205–212.

21. Warren C. Brush with death: A social history of lead poisoning. Baltimore, MD: Johns Hopkins University Press, 2000.

22. Oreskes N, Conway EM. Merchants of doubt: How a handful of scientists obscured the truth on issues from tobacco smoke to global warming. New York: Bloomsbury Press, 2010.

23. Michaels D. Doubt is their product: How industry's assault on science threatens your health. New York: Oxford University Press, 2008.

24. Butler CD, Harley D. Primary, secondary and tertiary effects of the eco-climate crisis: The medical response. *Postgrad Med J* 2010;86:230–234.
25. Morisetti N. Climate change and resource security. *BMJ* 2012;344. doi:10.136/bmj.e.
26. Szreter S. Economic growth, disruption, deprivation, disease and death: On the importance of the politics of public health. *Population and Development Review* 1997;23:693–728.
27. Dar OA, Khan MS. Millennium development goals and the water target: Details, definitions and debate. *Trop Med Int Health* 2011;16:540–544.
28. UNICEF and World Health Organization. Progress on drinking water and sanitation: 2012 update. New York and Geneva: UNICEF and WHO, 2012:14. Available at http://www.unicef.org/media/files/JMPreport2012.pdf. Accessed on August 22, 2012.
29. Dillingham R, Guerrant RL. Childhood stunting: Measuring and stemming the staggering costs of inadequate water and sanitation. *Lancet* 2004;363:94–95.
30. White GF, Bradley DJ, White AU. Drawers of water: Domestic water use in East Africa. Chicago: The University of Chicago Press, 1972.
31. Brook RD, Rajagopalan S, Pope CA, et al. Particulate matter air pollution and cardiovascular disease. *Circulation* 2010;121:2331–2378.
32. Dherani M, Pope D, Mascarenhas M, et al. Indoor air pollution from unprocessed solid fuel use and pneumonia risk in children aged under five years: A systematic review and meta-analysis. *Bulletin of the World Health Organization* 2008;86:390–398.
33. Bradsher K. China asks other nations not to release its air data. *New York Times*, June 5, 2012. Available at http://www.nytimes.com/2012/06/06/world/asia/china-asks-embassies-to-stop-measuring-air-pollution.html. Accessed on August 22, 2012.
34. Schmidt CW. Black carbon: The dark horse of climate change drivers. *Environ Health Perspect* 2011;119:A172–A175.
35. Shindell D, Kuylenstierna JCI, Vignati E, et al. Simultaneously mitigating near-term climate change and improving human health and food security. *Science* 2012;335:183–188.
36. Lelieveld J, Berresheim H, Borrmann S, et al. Global air pollution crossroads over the Mediterranean. *Science* 2002;298:789–791.
37. Lau CL, Smythe LD, Craig SB, Weinstein P. Climate change, flooding, urbanisation and leptospirosis: Fuelling the fire? *Trans R Soc Trop Med Hyg* 2009;104:631–638.
38. Hites RA, Foran JA, Carpenter DO, et al. Global assessment of organic contaminants in farmed salmon. *Science* 2004;303:226–229.
39. Reuters. China court sentences melamine milk activist to jail. November 10, 2010. Available at http://af.reuters.com/article/worldNews/idAFTRE6A914Y20101110. Accessed on August 22, 2012.
40. Chen J, Tong Y, Xu J, et al. Environmental lead pollution threatens the children living in the Pearl River Delta region, China. *Environmental Science and Pollution Research* 2012:19:3268–3275.
41. Tong S, von Schirnding YE, Prapamontol T. Environmental lead exposure: A public health problem of global dimensions. *Bull WHO* 2000;78:1068–1077.
42. McMichael A, Baghurst P, Wigg N, et al. Port Pirie Cohort Study: Childhood blood lead history and neuropsychological development at age four years. *N Engl J Med* 1988;319:468–475.
43. Lanphear BP, Hornung R, Khoury J, et al. Low-level environmental lead exposure and children's intellectual function: An international pooled analysis. *Environ Health Perspect* 2005;113:894–899.

44. Tsai PL, Hatfield TH. Global benefits from the phaseout of leaded fuel. *J Environ Health* 2011; 74:8–14.

45. Gottesfeld P, Pokhrel AK Review: Lead exposure in battery manufacturing and recycling in developing countries and among children in nearby communities. *J Occup Environ Hyg* 2011;8:520–532.

46. Hanser A. Yellow peril consumerism: China, North America, and an era of global trade. *Ethnic and Racial Studies* 2012;35:1–19.

47. LaDou J, Castleman B, Frank A, et al. The case for a global ban on asbestos. *Environ Health Perspect* 2010;118:897–901.

48. Joshi TK, Gupta RK. Asbestos-related morbidity in India. *Ind J Occup Environ Health* 2003;9:249–253.

49. Joint Policy Committee Societies of Epidemiology. Position statement on asbestos from the Joint Policy Committee of the Societies of Epidemiology (JPC-SE), June 4, 2012. Available at http://www.jpc-se.org/position.htm. Accessed on August 22, 2012.

50. Zhang MQ, Zhu YCZ, Deng RW. Evaluation of mercury emissions to the atmosphere from coal combustion, China. *Ambio* 2002;31:482–484.

51. Bjerregaard P, Hansen JC. Organochlorines and heavy metals in pregnant women from the Disko Bay area in Greenland. *Science of the Total Environment* 2000;245:87–102.

52. McNeill JR. Something new under the sun: An environmental history of the twentieth-century world. New York: W. W. Norton, 2000.

53. Brown TN, Wania F. Screening chemicals for the potential to be persistent organic pollutants: A case study of Arctic contaminants. *Environmental Science & Technology* 2008;42:5202–5209.

54. Satake W, Nakabayashi Y, Mizuta I, et al. Genome-wide association study identifies common variants at four loci as genetic risk factors for Parkinson's disease. *Nature Genetics* 2009;41:1303–1307.

55. Alavanja MCR, Bonner MR. Occupational pesticide exposures and cancer risk: A review. *J Toxicol Environ Health, Part B* 2012;15:238–263.

56. Kosatsky T. The 2003 European heat waves. *Eurosurveillance* 2005;10:148–149.

57. Stott P, Peterson TC, Herring S. Explaining extreme events of 2011 from a climate perspective. *Bulletin of the American Meteorological Society* 2012;93:1041–1043.

58. Alonso D, Bouma MJ, Pascual M. Epidemic malaria and warmer temperatures in recent decades in an East African highland. *Proc R Soc B* 2011;278:1661–1669.

59. Butler CD, ed. Climate change and global health. Wallingford, UK: CABI, in press.

60. Hansen J. Scientific reticence and sea level rise. *Environmental Research Letters* 2007;2:doi:10.1088/1748-9326/2/2/024002.

61. Atkins D, Moy EM. Left behind: The legacy of Hurricane Katrina. *BMJ* 2005;331:916–918.

62. Toldson IA, Ray K, Hatcher SS, Straughn LL. Examining the long-term racial disparities in health and economic conditions among Hurricane Katrina survivors: Policy implications for Gulf Coast recovery. *Journal of Black Studies* 2011;42:360–378.

63. Weber L, Hilfinger Messias DK. Mississippi front-line recovery work after Hurricane Katrina: An analysis of the intersections of gender, race, and class in advocacy, power relations, and health. *Soc Sci Med* 2012;74:1833–1841.

64. Mills E. Insurance in a climate of change. *Science* 2005;309:1040–1044.

65. Smith JT, Comans RNJ, Beresford NA, et al. Pollution: Chernobyl's legacy in food and water. *Nature* 2000;405:141.

66. Sharma DC. Bhopal: 20 years on. *Lancet* 2005;365:111–112.

67. Editorial. Has the world forgotten Bhopal? *Lancet* 2000;356:1863.

68. Ehrenreich B. Nickel and dimed: On (not) getting by in America. New York: Metropolitan Books, 2001.

69. McKinley J. Cities deal with a surge in shanty towns. *New York Times*, March 2 5, 2009. Available at http://www.nytimes.com/2009/03/26/us/26tents.html?_r=1&partner=rss&emc=rs. Accessed on August 22, 2012.

70. Raskin P, Gallopin G, Gutman P, et al. Great transition: The promise and lure of the times ahead. Boston, MA: Stockholm Environment Institute, 2002.

71. McMichael AJ, Smith KR, Corvalan CF. The sustainability transition: A new challenge. *Bull WHO* 2000;78:1067.

72. Global Energy Assessment. Global energy assessment—Towards a sustainable future. Cambridge, UK, and New York: Cambridge University Press and Laxenburg, Austria: International Institute for Applied Systems Analysis, 2012. Available at http://www.iiasa.ac.at/Research/ENE/GEA/doc/GEA-Summary-web.pdf. Accessed on August 22, 2012.

19 Occupational Health and Safety

■ ANDREA KIDD TAYLOR AND
LINDA RAE MURRAY

■ INTRODUCTION: HISTORICAL OVERVIEW AND SCOPE OF THE PROBLEM

Occupational disease and injury must be considered in the context of the relationship between capital and labor, as urged by President Abraham Lincoln in his first annual message to Congress in 1861, when he said: "Labor is prior to, and independent of, capital. Capital is only the fruit of labor, and could never have existed if labor had not first existed. Labor is the superior of capital and deserves much the higher consideration." The patterns of occupational injury and disease are determined by the power relations reflected in systems of production.[1-3]

Since work-related injury and disease are socially produced, they can be prevented—the mission of occupational health and safety programs. The global annual burden of occupational injury and disease is estimated to be 2.3 million deaths and 337 million non-fatal diseases and injuries.[4] In 2007, occupational injuries and diseases cost the United States an estimated $250 billion in medical expenses and indirect costs, such as lost wages and benefits. Workers' compensation programs pay for only about one-fourth of this total cost. This total cost is about the same annual cost as cancer and more than the cost of diabetes, stroke, or coronary heart disease.[5] Nevertheless, the resources and attention allocated to addressing and preventing work-related injury and disease is minuscule compared to that for other diseases.

Work offers significant life-sustaining benefits. Throughout history, work has been a basic requirement of human survival. How work is organized, who does what, and who reaps the benefits of work largely determine the nature and level of social justice in a society.

Social injustice in the workplace is demonstrated by health disparities and disproportionate representation of workers of color in the most hazardous jobs. It is also demonstrated by the lack of workplace democracy—the ability of workers to control their work environments and thereby to shape their lives. Social injustice in the workplace also reflects the absence of justice in other spheres of society—and it is a major structural determinant of social injustice in most spheres of human activity.

The nature of work has a profound impact on the social status, well-being, and health of individuals and populations. Wages, economic inequality, working conditions, the structure of the workforce, and occupational segregation—all of which in the United States exacerbate and perpetuate class, racial/ethnic, and gender inequalities—contribute to the social determinants of health inequity.[6]

The founding of the United States was, in part, based on expropriation of land from Native Americans, the colonists' practice of indentured servitude, and development of the slavery-based economy of the South. The lack of workplace democracy in the United States can be traced to the time of slavery or earlier, when every aspect of some individuals' existence was overshadowed by compulsory labor.[7] When slavery ended after the Civil War, sharecropping became an economic surrogate for slavery; through indebtedness, the former slaves—then tenant farmers—became as tied to the land as they were under slavery. A conscious campaign to imprison African Americans in order to use their labor in chain gangs and other enterprises characterized African American labor in the South for decades after the Civil War.[8]

Waves of immigrants continued to supply cheap labor to industry in the United States. Whether immigrant workers were Irish immigrants working in steel mills or Asian immigrants building railroads, they were denied basic rights and exposed to extreme hazards. Racism against Asian Americans, Mexican Americans, Native Americans, and African Americans led to inhumane treatment and dangerous occupational exposures.

Job discrimination starts when people are denied the right to freely compete for the kinds of jobs to which they aspire and for which they are qualified. It continues in the workplace. Historically, within manufacturing, there was (a) discrimination in applying seniority rules and in denying opportunities for in-plant training and industrial courses, and (b) "Jim Crow"* segregation barriers in many unions.[9] The industrial boom of World War II forced a temporary breach in the pattern of Jim Crow laws, when, in 1942, President Franklin D. Roosevelt by executive order established the Fair Employment Practice Committee (FEPC). The FEPC was created to promote the fullest employment of all available persons and to eliminate discriminatory employment practices.

During this period, the "job ceiling" was slightly raised and thousands of African American men and women entered areas of skilled employment from which they had traditionally been barred. However, a report issued by the FEPC indicated that (a) nearly two-thirds of all African American women workers remained in service occupations, (b) close to one-half still held domestic-service jobs, and (c) almost one-half of the African American men continued working as unskilled laborers or as farm workers. While African Americans gained a foothold in industry, this foothold has always been a precarious one. And the overall strategy of the U.S.

---

* Jim Crow laws, passed by states and localities between 1876 and 1965, mandated racial segregation in public facilities in states in the South that had been part of the Confederacy.

free-market enterprise system has been designed to hold poor workers, African Americans, and other workers of color in perpetuity as a special reserve of cheap and underprivileged labor—an instrument for undercutting the standards of white workers and a deterrent to working-class unity.[9]

The role that "migrant labor" has played historically helps define the context for today's inequities in occupational injury and disease. The war between the United States and Mexico from 1846 to 1848 resulted in the seizure of the northern portion of Mexico, making an estimated 86,000 to 116,000 Mexicans U.S. residents. By 1900, much of the land owned by Mexicans had been taken over by Anglo Americans. The dispossession of land and the displacement of many skilled artisans forced Mexican workers into low-skilled and low-paid jobs. Mexicans were employed in production of cotton, fruit, and vegetables; sheep and cattle ranching; and large-scale mining of gold, silver, copper and lead. Mexicans replaced Chinese workers as low-skilled labor on the railroads following the passage of the Exclusion Act of 1882. By 1900, Mexican laborers were being recruited across the border, and, by the 1920s, an average of 50,000 Mexican immigrants came to the United States each year.

In the 1930s and 1940s, the traditional tactic for any major U.S. industry was to use African American sharecroppers of the South and the poorest peasants of Europe, Mexico, and Asia as "wage-cutters" and "strike-breakers"— thereby limiting workplace democracy. As a result, racism was used to drive a wedge in the American working class. White workers were persuaded to believe that these "inferior" groups had wages and living standards that undercut their own.

We cannot artificially "silo" the impact of different societal sectors; they are all interrelated. For example, it is difficult to underestimate the role of residential segregation in urban areas of the United States. From the 1970s through the 1990s, industry relocated from inner cities to suburban areas. Because of racism and segregation, African American workers were not as mobile as white workers, and therefore they found it difficult to obtain jobs in suburban areas.[10]

During the youth rebellions of the 1960s, young factory workers, newly recognizing their civil rights in society, reacted against authoritarianism in their workplaces. A free market economy could not survive as a social system, given the increased security and equality for workers. Working-class victories and concessions from business were raising expectations and threatening profits, class power, and class rule. What were earlier viewed as measures of progress—such as better wages, better social programs, and greater security—were redefined as barriers that blocked the needs of a free-market system.[11] The drive for the success and stability of free trade globally has led to a decline over time in social justice in the workplace and to poor health, especially for those workers who have remained in low-wage and high-hazard jobs.

Work-related injuries and occupational exposure to toxic chemicals, physical hazards, and poor and risky working conditions are generally related to low wages, and are increased among workers of low socioeconomic status and among racial and ethnic minorities.[12,13] Historically, each group that arrived in the United States worked in the most dangerous jobs in industry, and each was followed in these jobs by the next immigrant group. During the post–World War II economic boom, expanding membership made organized labor a powerful political constituency, but much of the leadership remained white and male, with little inclination to broaden the labor movement to include underrepresented workers. Although some unions made significant gains in organizing female workers and workers of color, most of these workers remained unorganized through the 1950s. Among rank-and-file members of the unions and their leadership, racial and sexual discrimination and discriminatory hiring and employment patterns in many industries have prevented African Americans, Latino Americans, Asian Americans, and Native Americans from moving out of entry-level, low-wage, and hazardous jobs.[14,15] (See Chapters 3 and 4.)

In the 1960s, unions mobilized to support national legislation, which led to the passage in 1970 of the Occupational Safety and Health Act, which established the Occupational Safety and Health Administration (OSHA). The most important consequence of the Act was to place workplace safety and health issues on the agendas of unions, workers, health professionals, and the general public—thereby improving workplace democracy. With increasing pressure from their membership, unions formed health and safety committees to teach their members how to identify and control workplace hazards.[5,16]

■ THE IMPACT OF OSHA

OSHA regulations have been promulgated very slowly, and, in recent years, very few new regulations have been adopted. OSHA regulations have been weakened by lack of strict enforcement, layers of government bureaucracy, and very influential industry lobbyists. Employers were never very enthusiastic about the prospect of oversight by a centralized government bureaucracy; therefore, it was no surprise that attacks on OSHA began not long after it started promulgating and enforcing standards in the 1970s. Since then, OSHA enforcement and promulgation of new standards have been principally guided by electoral politics.[17] Despite a need to strengthen the enforcement authority of OSHA and to increase funding of the occupational safety and health research through the National Institute for Occupational Safety and Health, OSHA can be credited with saving at least 400,000 lives in its first 40 years.[18]

Although substantial gains have occurred in many workplaces since the establishment of OSHA, many disparities remain, due to unchecked hazardous working conditions. One example of such a disparity was the devastating fire that occurred in 1991 at a poultry plant in Hamlet, North Carolina, a poor rural community. Twenty-five workers were killed when locked safety doors prevented them from escaping the fire (Figure 19–1).

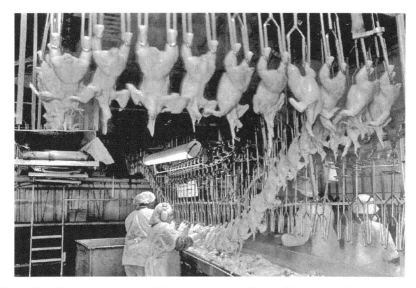

Figure 19–1 Workers processing chickens on an assembly line. Minority workers and women are over-represented in entry-level jobs like this one, in which safety and health hazards are prevalent. Twenty-five workers in a similar chicken-processing plant died in Hamlet, North Carolina, in 1991, when few workers were able to escape a fire that swept through the plant because the employer had locked most of the exit doors. (Photograph by Earl Dotter.)

▨ THEORETICAL FRAMEWORK FOR HEALTH INEQUITIES

Disparities in health status in the United States have been observed for centuries. Strategies to reduce or eliminate these differences must be based on a conceptual theoretical framework about how these inequities are created. (See Chapter 2.)

In the United States, the standard medical thinking well into the 20th century was that African Americans (and other minorities) were biologically inferior.[19] W.E.B. DuBois refuted this standard notion when he wrote: "The undeniable fact is, then, that in certain diseases the Negroes have a much higher rate than whites...(T)he differences can be explained on other grounds than race....If the population were divided as to social and economic conditions the matter of race would almost be entirely eliminated."[20] He demonstrated that a wide range of social and economic conditions produced the observed health disparities. He further noted:

The matter of sickness is an indication of social and economic position...(T)he Negro death rate and sickness are largely matters of condition and not due to racial traits and tendencies....With the improved sanitary condition, improved education and better economic opportunities, the mortality of the race may and probably will steadily decrease until it becomes normal.[20]

Today, ecosocial models, such as the model prepared by Nancy Krieger (Figure 19–2), have gained currency.[21] (See Chapter 26.) She has summarized the essential questions that should be addressed:

- What is and isn't known about the magnitude of and trends in occupational health inequities?
- Who is most burdened by these adverse health outcomes (and in relation to what referent group)?
- Who is most adversely affected by lack of knowledge about these health inequities and their causes?
- How are determinants of occupational health inequities—and potential confounders and effect mediators—conceptualized, measured, and modeled in empirical analyses (including at what level, and in relation to lifecourse and historical generation)?
- What kinds of actions and by whom are needed to reduce both the occurrence of work-related hazards and their inequitable distributions?[22]

The Commission on Social Determinants of Health of the World Health Organization proposed a broad theoretical framework to consider social injustice, work, and production of health inequities. This framework forces one to consider workplace conditions in a much wider context, as a reflection of power relationships in society. (See Chapter 2.) It is these power relationships that define public policy, the existence (or absence) of a welfare state, and the nature of the labor market.

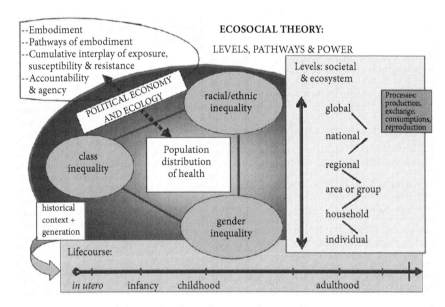

Figure 19–2 Ecosocial theory: Levels, pathways, and power. (*Source:* Krieger N. Proximal, distal, and the politics of causation: What's level got to do with it? *Am J Public Health* 2008;98[2]:224.)

▪ INCOME DISPARITIES IN THE UNITED STATES

Income inequalities in the United States—a reflection of structural factors in the workforce and the general economy—are greater than in other industrialized nations. These disparities have been increasing during the past 30 years, even when tax and benefit policies are considered. The growth of income of the top quintile—especially the top 1 percent—far outpaces that of the rest of the population.[23]

Personal income inequality in the United States peaked twice during the 20th century—just before World War I and just before the Great Depression. Between the end of World War II and 1970, the average U.S. worker made significant gains in income, with those on the bottom rungs making greater progress. During the 1970s, these trends stagnated.

Since the 1980s, the United States has experienced a steady increase in income disparities. Between 1947 and 1979, the average annualized rate of growth for family income increased in all strata of society, with the lower quintiles experiencing more growth than the upper quintiles. Between 1979 to 2007, the poorest quintiles experienced little or no growth in family income, while the top quintiles experienced the largest growth.

Between 1947 and 1969, black median family income rose as a percentage of white median family income—from 51 to 61 percent. During the 1970s and 1980s, this declined to 56 percent. By 2000, the relative income of African American families rose to 64 percent and that of Latino families to 65 percent, but fell to 61 and 63 percent, respectively, by 2010.

All quintiles saw a decrease in average family income between 2007 and 2010 with the lowest quintile experiencing the greatest decrease (11 percent). This decrease varied by race and ethnicity: Caucasians (5 percent), Latinos (7 percent), Asian Americans (8 percent), and African Americans (10 percent). Possible explanations for the increasing income disparities have included:

- Changes in workforce composition, such as the impact of workers of the "Baby Boom" generation (78 million Americans born between 1946 and 1964), more women workers, and new waves of immigrants, especially immigrant workers of color
- A decline in the manufacturing sector
- An increase in the service sector
- Globalization (Box 19–1)

These income disparities, in combination with poverty, discrimination, and other factors, have had a profoundly adverse impact on morbidity and mortality.[24]

▪ UNEMPLOYMENT AND JOB INSECURITY

Unemployment remains the most prevalent "occupational disease" in the United States and it causes many adverse effects on physical and mental health.[25-33]

BOX 19-1 ■ Economic Globalization

Ellen R. Shaffer and Joseph E. Brenner

Economic globalization refers to the increasing pace and volume of (a) international trade in goods and services among interconnected multinational corporations, (b) the flow of capital across borders, and (c) the related migration of populations, facilitated by technological changes in communication and transportation. It also includes changes in policies favoring the privatization of public enterprises and the reduction of government's right to regulate corporate activity in the public interest. While increasing wealth for some corporations, these policies contribute to social inequality and instability.

Public health workers can help ensure that the world's economy supports social justice and sustainable development. The most effective modes of action are through networks of like-minded colleagues. Relevant listservs and websites as well as meetings and publications sponsored by professional organizations can stimulate thinking and facilitate interactions among individuals and groups with similar concerns.

Basic to any action are (a) analyses of policies, principles, and institutions that shape economic globalization—and their implications for population health and for health care services, and (b) an understanding of where opportunities exist to address problems created by globalization.

International financial institutions (IFIs)—the World Trade Organization (WTO), the International Monetary Fund (IMF), and the World Bank—play an important role in establishing policies that govern the global economy. The IMF and the World Bank, which orchestrate loans and enforce economic policies on such matters as interest rates and public budget deficits, also fund programs and set policies in health. The WTO, established in 1995, sets the framework for multinational trade agreements. Regional and bilateral (country-to-country) trade agreements are increasingly influential.

Drawing on the wealth, power, and influence of high-income countries, the IFIs have prescribed for low-income countries controversial measures that rely on (a) market forces to regulate all economic activity, (b) fiscal discipline by states, (c) privatization, (d) deregulation, and (e) liberalization of rules restricting foreign trade. Policies of the IFIs aim to accomplish the following:

- Reduce the role of governments by restricting their ability to regulate
- Encourage competition from private companies to own and produce services and goods
- Reduce public funding and allocate public subsidies to private corporations
- Shift the burden of raising revenues for services from public subsidies to individuals, through cost recovery, user fees, or co-payments
- Target remaining public subsidies to the poorest, which generally creates a two-tiered system in which people who can afford to pay receive a higher level of services than those who cannot
- Decentralize administrative and financial procedures to the state and local level, thereby weakening control at the national level

Trade agreements impose these rules and curtail the right and ability of nations to determine whether they wish to abide by them, challenging the role that democratically elected public officials and civil society leaders play in determining the rules of trade and their own policy priorities. The WTO is empowered to impose substantial financial penalties on member nations that it determines do not comply with its rules.

In addition, many regional and bilateral agreements include *investor-state* rules that allow corporations to sue governments directly, as the tobacco industry has done to challenge restrictions on marketing. Disputes about compliance are adjudicated by tribunals that deliberate without public scrutiny. Government intervention in trade in the interests of social, environmental, and health policy objectives can be disallowed by WTO tribunals. For example, the WTO has overridden prohibitions against importing tuna caught with a method that also snares dolphins.

These policies and the commercialization of vital human services, such as health care and provision of water, adversely affect population health. While the stated goal of privatization and deregulation is to increase prosperity through trade, analysts increasingly contend that they contribute to the increase in global poverty and economic inequality and instability—and, therefore, to increased preventable illness and death.

For many years, liberalization of trade meant reducing barriers to international trade, such as tariffs and other measures that discouraged competitive trade from foreign producers, relating primarily to goods. However, the WTO has added agreements on intellectual property, services, and agriculture. Agreements such as Trade-Related Aspects of Intellectual Property Rights (TRIPS) and the General Agreement on Trade in Services (GATS) apply trade rules to a wide range of regulations regarding affordable medicines, tobacco control measures, and vital human services (including health care, education, and provision of water and sanitation) for all 158 member nations of the WTO. These agreements broaden the range of public health protections that can be struck down by trade panels.

These agreements could limit the ability of federal, state, or local governments to adopt and enforce public health standards concerning, for example, health care facilities, health insurance, health professional training and licensing, access to medications, environmental protection, occupational health and safety, tobacco control, alcohol, firearms, and provision of water and sanitation.

Public health workers can influence international trade agreements and their adverse impacts on health by taking actions such as the following:

1. *Write a journal or a newspaper article exploring the tensions between commercial and health interests.* What rules regulate tobacco companies, the health insurance industry, or hospitals? How do those rules contribute to economic productivity and human well-being? How do human rights treaties, international environmental agreements, and trade agreements address the value of life?

2. *Promote assessments of the impact of international trade agreements on population health.* One could examine why trade rules on intellectual property protect pharmaceutical companies from price competition, which would otherwise make essential medicines affordable to people with HIV/AIDS and other diseases.

3. *Write a resolution for your professional association explaining the role of trade rules in determining health protections.* Establish a committee to develop and implement an advocacy program that brings the public health perspective to policymakers. (See item 6, below.)

4. *Ask your member of Congress or Senator to designate you and your colleagues as her or his public health advisory committee.* In this way, you could provide a

public health perspective on proposed trade agreements and on the implementation of existing ones. You could hold public hearings to inform your community and the news media. Ask her or him to recommend that the U.S. Trade Representative establish a similar committee.

5. Support enforceable commitments to advancing population health and to achieving universal access to health care, to affordable medications, and to safe, affordable water in the United States and other countries. Link your daily work with advocacy campaigns to ensure that safe and affordable health care, medicines, and water are not eroded by trade agreements.

6. Participate in the network of the Center for Policy Analysis on Trade and Health (CPATH) (www.cpath.org). Enroll in the CPATH listserv to stay informed and to participate in campaigns to contact policymakers regarding pending decisions in Congress and at trade summits. Ask your professional association to endorse CPATH's Call for Public Health Accountability in Trade.

Workers of various economic strata who lose their jobs experience adverse health effects even if they are re-employed.[34] Unemployment leads to relative poverty, social isolation, loss of self-esteem, and unhealthy behaviors—and increased mortality for many diseases. Workers with chronic diseases fare even worse when they are unemployed or under-employed.[35,36] Being unemployed correlates with increased consumption of sugary and salty snacks and decreased consumption of fruits and vegetables.

Unemployment and job insecurity are not evenly distributed among workers—they are higher among low-wage workers, workers of color, and women workers. Some studies also demonstrate the adverse health impact of temporary employment, job instability, and restructuring of jobs.[37]

▪ GENDER, RACE, ETHNICITY, AND CLASS

There is a complex and nuanced relationship in the United States among race/ethnicity, gender, and class in causing poor health and health disparities. Since most studies on these issues have focused on only one factor, it is difficult to adequately understand these relationships.[38]

In the United States, as in much of the world, women are employed and segregated in lower-paying, more-insecure industries. (See Chapter 4.) In addition, women still perform most of the unpaid labor in the home related to day-to-day family life. Occupational hazards and exposures that are specific to nursing, the garment industry, and other occupations and industries dominated by women, differentially impact the women who work in them. Bullying and discrimination on the job occurs more frequently among low-paid and hourly workers.[39]

The role of structural racism in the workplace is important. For example, studying the underground and illegal garment industry, in which Latina workers predominate, cannot be done without considering that they are women of color, often "undocumented immigrants" (Box 22–1 in Chapter 22), whose ability to exercise power in the workplace is extremely limited. Occupational segregation by gender and race/ethnicity causes increased exposures to hazards and higher rates of occupational diseases and injuries among women and workers of color. Such labor segregation has caused some of the worst industrial disasters in U.S. history, such as the horrific Gauley Bridge/Hawk's Nest disaster in the 1930s in which black workers disproportionately died of acute silicosis.[3,40-43]

■ PRISON LABOR: SLAVERY BY ANOTHER NAME

Mass incarceration in the United States represents a crisis of public health and social justice. (See Chapter 9.) While the United States has 5 percent of the world's population, it has 25 percent of incarcerated people. In 2008, there were 2.3 million people incarcerated in the United States, a rate of 753 inmates per 100,000 population—a 254 percent increase from 1980.[44] Sixty percent of people now in prison in the United States are people of color. Among the 1.6 million inmates in federal and state facilities in 2010, the rate of imprisonment for African American men (3074 inmates per 100,000 population) was almost seven times greater than that of white men (459 inmates per 100,000 population)— with Latinos having an intermediate incarceration rate (1258 inmates per 100,000 population). An estimated 7 percent of African American men between 30 and 34 years of age have been incarcerated in state or federal prison.[45,46]

The use of prison labor in the United States dates back to the early 1800s—then mainly in jails in the North. While the 13th Amendment abolished slavery, it contained a critical clause: "except as a punishment for crime whereof the party shall be duly convicted." This clause was used throughout the South to incarcerate Blacks and exploit their labor as convicts. The Hawes-Cooper Act (1929), the Walsh-Healy Act (1936), and several other laws controlled and severely restricted prison labor to the production of goods for federal needs and a few other purposes.

Prison labor in the United States has increased in the past three decades under the 1979 Prison Industry Enhancement Certification Program. The program is theoretically designed to reduce recidivism. However, incarcerated workers under the Program receive very low wages, and their workplaces are not subject to OSHA standards.[47] Today, a wide range of industries use prisoners, thereby undercutting their competitors who use private-sector labor, contributing to unemployment.[48] Some economists estimate that prison labor lowers the wages of people who have dropped out of high school (but are not incarcerated) by at least 5 percent.

■ CHILD LABOR

Child labor is a major public health problem, especially in low-income countries. Even in the United States, for many years, children of lower-working-class families were expected to work—in mines, in factories, and on the streets of urban centers. Federal and state regulations decreased much child labor in the United States during the 20th century. In spite of 20th-century reforms, some communities and industries in the United States continue to represent occupational health and safety dangers for adolescent and child workers.

In the early 1980s, President Ronald Reagan proposed several policy changes concerning child labor—an extension of the number of hours of work allowed, permission for children to work in jobs previously considered to be hazardous, and permission for some full-time students to be employed at less than the minimum wage. While these proposals were not adopted, child labor protections were gradually reduced during the 1980s and 1990s.[49]

The U.S. Institute of Medicine (IOM) has documented the health and safety issues of child workers in the United States. Most adolescents who work do so in the retail sector, such as in fast-food restaurants; only about 8 percent work in agriculture. As of 2004, approximately 70 children under age 18 died each year at work; of those under age 20 killed at work, 45 percent were under age 16, and 10 percent under age 10.[50] The IOM recommended improving occupational health surveillance systems for child and adolescent workers, stressed that education should be the primary activity of children and adolescents, and recommended occupational health and safety training as part of the K–12 curriculum.[51]

In the United States, businesses and farms owned by families can employ children of these families. Therefore, children can be "hired" to work in agriculture. Farms are dangerous places for children; many children are injured or killed not directly by work, but by being in dangerous settings.

■ IMMIGRANT WORKERS

The work of immigrants and internal migrants—including African Americans, Mexicans and others from Latin America, and European and Asian immigrants—has played a critical role in building the wealth of the United States. These workers have faced increased risks for occupational injury and illness. Each new wave of immigrant workers has had inadequate information—often due to language and cultural challenges—concerning their work and workplaces.[52,53] Immigrant workers have historically been hired into jobs that are dangerous and demanding. Inadequate education, lack of legal status, and racism and other forms of discrimination have led to new immigrants' working in the worst and often most dangerous jobs.[54] "Job ghettos" in the garment, poultry, meatpacking, and other industries have developed in many locations and historical periods.[55,56]

The share of the civilian workforce comprised of immigrants increased from about 5 percent in 1970 to 16 percent in 2010. Immigrant workers are bimodally concentrated in (a) specific industries, such as information technology and "high-tech" manufacturing, which require highly skilled workers; and

(b) construction, agriculture, food services, and private household work, which require low-skilled workers.[57]

Unauthorized immigrants composed about 5 percent of the U.S. workforce in 2008. This workforce is concentrated in some states: Nevada, for example, has the highest proportion of unauthorized immigrant workers (12 percent). About 25 percent of farmworkers, 19 percent of building-and-grounds workers, 17 percent of construction workers, and 12 percent of food-preparation and food-service workers are estimated to be unauthorized (undocumented) immigrants.[58] The working conditions of immigrant workers—and especially those without legal documents—will continue to be a serious problem until the United States passes comprehensive immigration reform designed to protect their rights. (See Box 22–1 in Chapter 22.)

■ WHAT NEEDS TO BE DONE

Educating Workers and Communities To Take Power

Worker education is an important tool in creating stronger workplace democracy and equipping workers to increase their power on the job and in the broader society. This education should focus not only on occupational health and safety, but also on electoral politics, labor union organizing, and coalition building. Recognizing that language and cultural barriers often exist, worker education programs should be designed appropriately, be presented in languages spoken by the workers involved, and specifically address the workers' needs. Worker education can help build effective leadership and active participation of workers who otherwise might feel disenfranchised in addressing poor working conditions and other health and safety problems at their worksites.

Education alone is not sufficient. Also necessary is *community empowerment*, a social-action process by which individuals, communities, and organizations gain mastery over their lives in the context of changing their political and social environment to improve equity and quality of life.[59] Therefore, when there is workplace democracy, the community is represented—it has a seat at the table. Community empowerment—as opposed to a "top-down" approach—emphasizes partnership and collaboration. Workers and the others in their communities, in order to defend themselves against attacks on their rights, need to prepare to engage in debate and policy discussions—a prerequisite to effective democracy. (See Chapter 24.)

Addressing Structural Racism and Preventing Discrimination

Greater workplace democracy and social justice depend on preventing discrimination against workers of color, immigrant workers, women workers, child laborers, and older workers. Structural racism, sexism, and job discrimination are major obstacles to workers and communities in strategizing, organizing, and forming coalitions to fight together for better workplace protections and to establish mechanisms to prevent corporate negligence and indifference. Acknowledging, understanding, and recognizing these obstacles are critical for identifying and resolving issues that are the root causes of hostility among different racial and ethnic populations and the root causes of socioeconomic disparities.

Promoting Workplace Democracy and Environmental Justice

Occupational health and safety are linked to the movement for better workplace democracy—workers' democratic ability to control their work environment and to shape their own lives. Shared principles include equity and empowerment of workers, individuals, and communities. To improve the overall health of workers and promote healthier communities, labor unions, public interest groups, community activists, and public health practitioners should join forces to (a) organize workers and members of the community to fight for equal justice and protection under occupational and environmental laws and regulations, and (b) rally together against corporate interests. Achieving workplace democracy and environmental justice will depend on the sharing of expertise and resources.[17]

Improving Surveillance and Research

In order to eliminate health inequities in occupational health and safety, the scope and nature of problems need to be clearly understood. Improvement of occupational exposure and health surveillance and development of reliable data sources need to become a national priority. Surveillance systems and research studies should gather and analyze data not only on occupation, but also on socioeconomic class and race/ethnicity to help develop hypotheses about the interactions between occupational exposures and both class and race/ethnicity.[43]

Reforming OSHA

In the early 1990s, labor unions organized campaigns promoting OSHA reform. The legislation they proposed, which was not passed by Congress, would have mandated (a) joint labor-management health and safety committees at all worksites, (b) more OSHA compliance officers, (c) more targeted inspections of hazardous workplaces, (d) criminal arrests for employers who willfully violate OSHA standards and cause employee deaths, and (e) the worker's right to refuse hazardous work. Such OSHA reform legislation is still needed today. It could substantially enhance workplace democracy by providing workers with direct participation and a voice "at the table" on health and safety matters at their workplaces.

Public health workers and students should join with labor leaders in advocating for OSHA reform by lobbying Congress and holding their elected officials accountable for protecting the health and safety and for ensuring the rights of all workers. In the midst of globalization and a pro-business, anti-regulatory climate, more strategic actions and plans are needed to provide increased worker participation in the political process, better worker education, and recruitment of workers to increase union membership, thereby providing more workers with a united voice to fight for stronger and more effective workplace protections.

Reforming Workers' Compensation

The United States does not have a unified workers' compensation system. Each state has its own standards and practices. The burden of proof that disease is occupationally related lies with workers and their physicians. Judges who hear contested cases must be unbiased and open to the possibility that workers' illnesses and injuries are related to their work.[60] A national workers' compensation system with uniform benefits should be established. Employers should bear the burden of proof if they believe that workers' illnesses and injuries are not related to work. Workers' compensation should also not be the "exclusive remedy" for workers seeking to recover damages from employers; "pain-and-suffering" awards should be allowed. More importantly, industry should not be allowed to shift costs that it generates to Medicare, Medicaid, and Social Security Disability Insurance (SSDI). All of this will require abolishing expensive and inefficient state workers' compensation systems and requiring industry to pay for the damages it causes.[61]

Promoting the Role of Organized Labor

Workers who can be fired at the whim of their employers cannot be very insistent in demanding safer working conditions. This situation is especially true in (a) workplaces where there is no union, and (b) jobs where employees can easily be replaced and for which alternative safer jobs at marginally lower wage rates are not available. In addition, the costs associated with switching jobs— such as loss of health care benefits, pension rights, and seniority; the need to become familiar with a new employer; and the expense and personal disruption of relocation—may be too high a price for many workers to pay.

Labor unions have been a powerful market force to protect workers' rights and to assist workers in confronting employer market power. Starting in the 1980s, however, the power of many labor unions diminished to the point where workers in many industries were forced to accept wage concessions. In other industries, prominent companies replaced unionized workers with nonunion workers. And the overall percentage of unionized workers in the U.S. workforce declined from 22 percent in 1982 to less than 10 percent in 2012.

Union organizing has become the principal rallying cry for unions in the AFL-CIO. Unions at every level are being asked to shift resources to help workers organize. Unions are recruiting and training new organizers whose diversity reflects that of workers in the United States.[62] Forming a labor organization in the workplace is still a fundamental right. Now, more than ever, workers need a strong and countervailing voice to corporate power—to speak out against the social injustice of an unhealthy work environment. Due to liberalized trade practices, free market economic policies, and the elimination or weakening of protective labor legislation, the risks and costs to workers attempting to organize have increased. Public policies protecting the right to form unions and providing incentives for unionized workplaces, such as tax credits, would help increase the percentage of unionized workers in the United States. Unions can win organizing drives—even in hostile organizing climates—if they implement more comprehensive and multifaceted organizing strategies. Humility, class unity, persistence, and determination—combined with commitments to better wages, better workplace health and safety protection, and fair contracts—form a strong foundation for organizing workers.[63]

▪ CONCLUSION

Work profoundly defines the well-being of individuals and populations. The structure of the workplace is a reflection of both general social conditions in the society at large and the organization within the specific workplace. It is in the context of the workplace that the fundamental determinants of health, such as class, gender, and race/ethnicity, and the power relationships that determine the distribution of resources are most clearly played out.

The workplace remains the crucible where social justice must be established. The increase in socioeconomic and health disparities in the United States represents a major barrier to achieving social justice. Inequities in working conditions must be addressed if occupational injuries and illnesses are to be prevented.

To achieve health and safety goals, a large, militant, and principled labor movement is needed—the major tool to achieving democracy in the workplace. Upon that foundation, we believe, rest all measures to expand democracy in general, and to eliminate social injustice based on class, race, ethnicity, and gender.

▪ REFERENCES

1. Friedman-Jimenez G, Claudio L. Disparities in environmental and occupational health. In: Rom WN, Markowitz SB, eds. Environmental and occupational medicine. 4th ed. Philadelphia: Lippincott, Wilkins & Williams, 2007:1747–1763.
2. Slatin C. Environmental and occupational health and human rights. *New Solutions* 2011;21:177–195.

3. Abrams HK. A short history of occupational health. *Journal of Health Policy* 2001;22:34–80.
4. Al-Tuwaijri S, Fedotov I, Feirshans I, et al. Introductory report—Beyond death and injuries: The ILO's role in promoting safe and healthy job. XVIII World Congress on Safety and Health at Work, Seoul, Korea, 2008. Geneva: International Labour Office, 2008.
5. Leigh JP. Economic burden of occupational injury and illness in the United States. *Milbank Q* 2011;89:728–772.
6. Baron SL, Wilson S. Occupational and environmental health equity and social justice. In: Levy BS, Wegman DH, Baron SL, Sokas RK, eds. Occupational and environmental health: Recognizing and preventing disease and injury. 6th ed. New York: Oxford University Press, 2011:69–97.
7. Davis A. Women, race and class. New York: Vintage Books, 1981.
8. Blackmon DA. Slavery by another name: The re-enslavement of black Americans from the Civil War to World War II. New York: Anchor Books, Random House, 2008.
9. Haywood H. Negro liberation. Chicago: Liberator Press, 1976.
10. Harvey D. Social justice and the city. Rev. ed. Athens, GA: University of Georgia Press, 2009.
11. Gindin S. Social justice and globalization: Are they compatible? *Monthly Review Press,* 2002. Available at http://monthlyreview.org/2002/06/01/social-justice-and- globalizati on-are-they-compatible. Accessed November 21, 2012.
12. Evans G, Kantrowitz E. Social status and health: The potential role of environmental risk exposure. *Annu Rev Public Health* 2002;23:303–331.
13. Taylor A, Murray L. Minority workers. In: Levy BS, Wegman DH, eds. Occupational health: Recognizing and preventing work-related disease and injury. 4th ed. Philadelphia: Lippincott, Williams & Wilkins, 2000:679–687.
14. Green J. The world of the worker: Labor in the twentieth century America. New York: Hill and Wang, 1980.
15. Morris R, ed. A history of the American worker. Princeton, NJ: Princeton University Press, 1983.
16. Berman D. Why work kills: A brief history of occupational safety and health in the United States. *Int J Health Serv* 1977;7:63–88.
17. McGarity T, Shapiro S. Workers at risk: The failed promise of the Occupational Safety and Health Administration. Westport, CT: Greenwood Publishing Group, 1993.
18. AFL-CIO. Death on the job: The toll of neglect: A national and state-by-state pro-file of worker safety and health in the United States. 20th ed. Washington, DC: AFL-CIO, 2011.
19. Gamble VN, Stone D. U.S. policy on health inequities: The interplay of politics and research. *Journal of Health Politics Policy and Law* 2006;31:99–108.
20. DuBois WEB, ed. The health and physique of the Negro American. Report of a social study made under the direction of Atlanta University: Together with the Proceedings of the Eleventh Conference for the Study of the Negro Problems. Held at Atlanta University, on May the 29th, 1906.
21. Krieger N. Proximal, distal, and the politics of causation. *Am J Public Health* 2008;98:221–230.
22. Krieger N. Workers are people too: Societal aspects of occupational health disparities: An ecosocial perspective. *Am J Indust Med* 2010;53:104–115.

23. Mishel L, Bivens J, Gould E, Shierholz H. Overview: Policy-driven inequality blocks living-standards growth for low- and middle-income Americans. In: Economic Policy Institute. The state of working America. 12th ed. Available at: http://stateofworkingamerica.org/subjects/overview/?reader. Accessed December 10, 2012.

24. Subramanian S, Kawachi I. Wage poverty, earned income inequality, and health. In: Heyman J, ed. Global inequalities at work: Work's impact on the health of individuals, families, and societies. Oxford, England: Oxford University Press, 2003.

25. Deaton A, Paxson CH. Aging and inequality in income and health. *American Economic Review* 1998;88:248–253. Available at: http://www.princeton.edu/~deaton/downloads/Aging_and_Inequality_in_Income_and_Health.pdf. Accessed December 10, 2012.

26. Elo I, Preston S. Educational differentials in mortality: United States, 1979–85. *Soc Sci Med* 1996;42:47–57.

27. Pappas G, Queen S, Hadden W, Fisher G. The increasing disparity in mortality between socioeconomic groups in the United States, 1960–1986. *N Engl J Med* 1993;329:103–115.

28. Korpi T. Accumulating disadvantage: Longitudinal analyses of unemployment and physical health in representative samples of the Swedish population. *Eur Sociol Rev* 2001;17:255–273.

29. Saegert S, Libman K, Fields D. An interdisciplinary and social-ecological analysis of the U.S. foreclosure crisis as it relates to health. In: Freudenberg N, Klitzman S, Saegert S, eds. Urban health and society. San Francisco, CA: Jossey-Bass, 2009.

30. Wadsworth ME, Montgomery S, Bartely MJ. The persisting effect of unemployment on health and social well being in men early in working life. *Soc Sci Med* 1999;48:1491–1499.

31. Artazcoz L, Benach J, Borrell C, Cortes I. Unemployment and mental health: Understanding the interactions among gender, family roles and social class. *Am J Public Health* 2004;94:82–88.

32. Burgard S, Brand J, House J. Perceived job insecurity and worker health in the United States. *Soc Sci Med* 2009;69:777–785.

33. Dave D, Kelly I. How does the business cycle affect eating habits? NBER Working Paper 16638. National Bureau of Economic Research, December 2010.

34. Strully K. Job loss and health in the U.S. labor market. *Demography* 2009;46:221–246.

35. Bartely M. Unemployment and ill health: Understanding the relationship. *J Epidemiol Community Health* 1994;48:333–337.

36. Bartley M, Owen C. Relationship between socioeconomic status, employment, and health during economic change, 1973–93. *BMJ* 1996;313:445–449.

37. Landsbergis P, Grzywacz JG, LaMontagne AD. Work organization, job insecurity, and occupational health disparities: An issue paper for discussion at the Eliminating Health and Safety Disparities at Work Conference. Chicago, IL, September 14 and 15, 2011. Available at http://www.aoecdata.org/conferences/healthdisparities/whitepapers/work-organization.pdf. Accessed December 10, 2012.

38. Artazcoz L, Borrel C, Cortes I, et al. Occupational epidemiology and work related inequalities in health: A gender perspective for two complementary approaches to work and health research. *J Epidemiol Community Health* 2007;61(Suppl II):ii39–ii45.

39. Clougherty J, Souza K, Cullen M. Work and its role in shaping the social gradient in health. *Ann NY Acad Sci* 2010;1186: 102–124.

40. Cherniack M. The Hawk's Nest Incident: America's worst industrial disaster. New Haven, CT: Yale University Press, 1986.

41. Frumkin H, Walker E, Friedman-Jimenez G. Minority workers and communities. *Occup Med* 1999;14:495–517.

42. Krieger N, Waterman P, Hartman C, et al. Social hazards on the job: Workplace abuse, sexual harassment, and racial discrimination—A study of black, Latino and white low-income women and men workers in the United States. *Int J Health Serv* 2006;36:51–85.

43. Murray L. Sick and tired of being sick and tired: Scientific evidence, methods, and research implications for racial and ethnic disparities in occupational health. *Am J Public Health* 2003;93:221–226.

44. Schmitt J, Warner K, Gupta S. The high budgetary cost of incarceration. Center for Economic and Policy Research, June 2010. Available at http://www.cepr.net/documents/publications/incarceration-2010-06.pdf. Accessed December 10, 2012.

45. Alexander M. The new Jim Crow: Mass incarceration in the age of colorblindness. New York: New Press, 2010.

46. Guerino P, Harrison P, Sabol W. Prisoners in 2010. December 2011, NCJ 236096 (revised September 2, 1912). U.S. Department of Justice. Bureau of Justice Statistics Bulletin. Available at http://bjs.ojp.usdoj.gov/content/pub/pdf/p10.pdf. Accessed December 10, 2012.

47. Cox R. An economic analysis of prison labor (dissertation). Georgia State University, 2009.

48. Elk M, Sloan B. The hidden history of ALEC and prison labor. *The Nation*, August 1, 2011. Available at: http://www.thenation.com/article/162478/hidden-history-alec-and-prison-labor. Accessed March 8, 2013.

49. Whittaker WG. Child labor in America: History, policy, and legislative issues. Washington, DC: Congressional Research Service; 2005. Available at http://digitalcommons.ilr.cornell.edu/cgi/viewcontent.cgi?article=1204&context=key_workplace. Accessed December 10, 2012.

50. Goldcamp M, Hendrick K, Myers J. Farm fatalities to youth 1995–2000: A comparison of age groups. *J Safety Research* 2004;35:151–157.

51. Committee on the Health and Safety Implications of Child Labor, National Research Council, and Institute of Medicine. Protecting youth at work: Health, safety, and development of working children and adolescents in the United States. Atlanta, GA: National Academies Press, 1998.

52. Schenker M. A global perspective of migration and occupational health. American *J Indust Med* 2010;53:329–337.

53. Smith J. Immigrant workers and worker's compensation: The need for reform. *Am J Indust Med* 2012;55:537–544.

54. Orrenius P, Zavodny M. Do immigrants work in riskier jobs? *Demography* 2009;46:535–551.

55. Quandt S, Arcury-Quandt A, Lawlor E, et al. 3-D jobs and health disparities: The health implications of Latino chicken catcher's working conditions. *Am J Indust Med* 2013;56:206–215.

56. Marin A, Grzywacz J, Arcury T, et al. Evidence of organizational injustice in poultry processing plants: Possible effects on occupational health and safety among Latino workers in North Carolina. *Am J Indust Med* 2009;52:37–48.

57. Brookings Institute Report. Immigrant workers in the U.S. labor force. Available at www.renewoureconomy.org/sites/all/themes/pnae/img/Immigrant_Workers_Brookings.pdf. Accessed December 7, 2012.

58. Passel J, Cohn D. A portrait of unauthorized immigrants in the United States. Pew Hispanic Center Report, 2009. Available at http://www.pewhispanic.org/2009/04/14/a-portrait-of-unauthorized-immigrants-in-the-united-states/. Accessed December 10, 2012.
59. Wallerstein N. Empowerment to reduce health disparities. *Scand J Public Health* 2002;30(suppl 59):72–77.
60. Boden LI, Barth PS, Leifer NT, et al. Legal remedies. In: Levy BS, Wegman DH, Baron SL, Sokas RK, eds. Occupational and environmental health: Recognizing and preventing disease and injury. 6th ed. New York: Oxford University Press, 2011:664–696.
61. LaDou J. Workers' compensation reform. *Int J Occup Environ Health* 2012;18:92–95.
62. Sweeney J. Public addresses: Building a labor movement strategy for the new century. *Georgetown J Poverty Law Policy* 2000;VII:163–172.
63. Taylor A. Organizing marginalized workers. *Occup Med State Art Rev* 1999; 14:687–695.

20 Oral Health

■ MYRON ALLUKIAN, JR.,
ALICE M. HOROWITZ, AND
CHLOE A.WONG

■ INTRODUCTION

Oral diseases are often called a "neglected" or "silent epidemic."[1-8] They are largely due to social injustice in which private wealth overrides the public's health.

With billions of dollars at stake, the food and tobacco industries and organized dentistry have profound impacts on oral health and access to dental services. Although oral diseases affect almost everyone, prevention of them and access to dental services have not been high priorities in the United States. In fact, adult dental services have recently been limited or entirely eliminated from dental Medicaid programs in most states, resulting in increased emergency department visits for dental care—a giant step backwards.[9] The most vulnerable populations have become even more vulnerable, while politicians, entertainers, and others who are in the public eye spend much money to achieve an ideal image: a healthy mouth and a healthy smile.

Why is oral health given such low priority in the United States? Oral health is generally not viewed as an integral component of overall health. Since the first dental school was established in 1840, dentistry has developed as a profession separate from medicine. Most dental schools teach little about overall health. And most medical schools teach little about oral health. Leaders in medicine have had a dominant influence in the development of U.S. health policy, from which leaders in oral health have usually been excluded. It is therefore not surprising that, in the United States, only 10 percent of dental care is publicly financed, compared with 35 percent of medical care.[10]

■ DEFINING ORAL HEALTH

Oral health is being able to eat, chew, talk, smile, kiss, sleep, read, think, study, and work without oral pain, discomfort, or embarrassment. Oral health is having a smile that helps you feel good about yourself and gives others a healthy and positive image of you. Oral health is essential and integral to overall health and well-being. As the late C. Everett Koop, a former U.S. Surgeon General, said, "You're not healthy without good oral health." The maintenance of oral health is important for all of the following:

- Freedom from pain, infection, suffering, and even death[11]
- Ability to eat and chew, as well as proper digestion and nutrition

- Ability to speak properly
- Social mobility
- Employability
- Self-image and self-esteem
- Overall quality of life

▓ A NEGLECTED EPIDEMIC

Oral diseases are lifelong problems for most Americans. Although oral health in the United States has markedly improved since the 1970s—due to fluoridation of community water supplies, use of fluorides and dental sealants, technological advances, dental insurance, and better education, oral diseases remain a neglected epidemic, as reflected in the following data:

- Among teenagers 16 to 19 years old, more than 67 percent have had tooth decay, with an average of six affected tooth surfaces.[12]
- Among people 50 to 64 years old, 96 percent have had tooth decay, with an average of 54 affected tooth surfaces.[12]
- Among those older than 65 years of age, 23 percent have no teeth.[13]
- Among children 2 to 4 years old, dental caries in primary teeth increased by 33 percent between 1988–1994 and 1999–2004.[12]
- Among children 6 to 12 years old, about 13 percent have suffered a toothache in the previous 6 months.[14]
- Among those 35 to 44 years old, about 17 percent have destructive periodontal disease.[12]
- From 2006 to 2009, there was a 16 percent increase in emergency department visits for dental care.[9]
- More Americans die from oral and pharyngeal cancer than from cervical cancer.[15]

There are great disparities in oral health between the "haves" and "have-nots." People who are educated and have adequate financial resources use personal preventive procedures and receive dental services on a regular and periodic basis. For everyone else, dental services are crisis-oriented.

Increasingly less money is being spent on oral health in the United States. In 2010, the total cost for dental care, about $104.8 billion, represented only 4 percent of all health care expenditures, compared with 6 percent in 1970—a 37 percent decrease.[16]

▓ PRIVATE WEALTH VERSUS THE PUBLIC'S HEALTH

Unfortunately, private financial gain often takes precedence over the public's health, resulting in unnecessary cases of oral disease and limitations to accessing dental care. For example, the food and tobacco industries, while profiting financially, create unnecessary oral disease and poor oral health. Organized dentistry, which has made many positive contributions to oral health, has also limited access to dental care.

▓ THE FOOD INDUSTRY

The food industry in the United States—a $1.5 trillion business in 2011—spends about $30 billion a year promoting its products.[17,18] Processed foods adversely affect the health, including the oral health, of most Americans, because of high concentrations of sugar, salt, and fat. Nearly 96 percent of adults in the United States have had tooth decay, and about 69 percent of adults and 33 percent of children are overweight or obese.[12,19,20]

In 2004, the average American consumed more than 22 teaspoons of added sugar a day.[21] Daily, over 50 percent of Americans consume sugary beverages—25 percent consume at least one 12-ounce can.[22] Children consume an average of six cans of soda per week.[23] Each 12-ounce serving of a sweetened soft drink contains 10 teaspoons of sugar. Consuming one can of soda a day can lead to an annual 15-pound weight gain.[24]

Soft-drink consumption among children 6 to 17 years of age increased from 37 percent in 1977–1978 to 56 percent in 1994–1998. During this period, the average daily intake increased from 5 to 12 fluid ounces.[25] However, although soda sales in the United States increased about 3 percent annually during the 1990s, they decreased 0.5 percent in 2010 and 1 percent in 2011.[26]

Increased consumption of sugary drinks has resulted from aggressive marketing campaigns to target children. In 2010, beverage companies spent $948 million to advertise high-sugar drinks and energy drinks through media, a 5 percent increase since 2008.[27] Social media and mobile marketing have also been used to market high-sugar drinks and energy drinks; interactive interfaces engage children and teenagers. To increase sales, beverages are packaged in single-serving, easy-to-open, reclosable containers that facilitate immediate and continued consumption—in portion sizes that have more than tripled in recent decades.[27]

Several years ago, there was an outcry by parents, educators, and health care providers against the soft drink industry's practice of "buying schools"—giving money to schools in exchange for exclusive rights to sell high-sugar drinks there. Approximately 16 percent of school districts in the United States made such an arrangement. Because most schools were experiencing severe budget cuts, this supplement to their income—totaling more than $20 million—had a huge impact on what their students drink at school.[28,29] In recent years, access to soda in schools has decreased—from 54 percent of students having access in 2006–2007 to 25 percent in 2010–2011.[30] Nevertheless, high-sugar beverages, such as fruit juices, coffees, and sports drinks, are widely available at school—83 percent of high-school students and 55 percent of middle-school students have access to sports drinks at school.[30]

People now know more about the adverse health impact of high-sugar drinks. These drinks cause tooth decay and contribute to the United States having the highest percentage of overweight and obese school-age children—33 percent—of any country.[20] This has stimulated policymakers to take action. For example, in 2012, the New York City Board of Health approved a ban on the sale of sugary drinks in containers larger than 16 ounces from restaurants, street vendors' carts, and movie theaters.[31] However, the ban was invalidated by a State Supreme Court judge 1 day before it was to go into effect. And New York State proposed a one-cent-an-ounce tax on sodas in 2010—which failed when the soda industry spent $13 million to lobby the state legislature.[32]

Public health campaigns, such as New York City's "Pour on the Pounds" and Philadelphia's "Get Healthy Philly," educate young people and their parents about the consequences of consuming high-sugar drinks, but these campaigns have been challenged by larger organizations representing the beverage industry. For example, in 2011, the American Beverage Association filed a lawsuit against New York City for its campaign.[27]

Confectionary companies generate about $29 billion annually in retail sales.[33] Candy is frequently sold at schools to raise money for team uniforms, recreational equipment, and computers. Children's television shows and fast-food restaurant chains promote high-fat and high-sugar products, often with toys or gifts. Enticing children to eat these products is a social injustice because many of them do not know enough to make healthy food choices. The amount of money the food industry spends for advertisements aimed at children far outweighs public money spent to educate children about healthy food choices. Since high-sugar products are usually less expensive than healthy food choices, this situation is even more inequitable for low-income families.

■ **THE TOBACCO INDUSTRY**

Tobacco use adversely affects oral health in several important ways. Smoking (cigarettes, cigars, or pipes) and the use of smokeless tobacco cause oral cancer (cancers of the lip, tongue, mouth, and throat). Tobacco use also causes periodontitis (inflammation of the tissue around teeth), gum recession, loss of teeth, leukoplakia (white plaques and patches on the oral mucosa), staining of teeth, halitosis (bad breath), and loss of taste sensation. Tobacco use is highly addictive, and it is very difficult for cigarette smokers and other tobacco users to quit.

More than 443,000 people die each year in the United States from cancer and other tobacco-related diseases—about 20 percent of all deaths.[34] And each day, 3800 American children and teenagers (under age 18) begin smoking.[34] The tobacco industry annually spends more than $10 billion—about $27 million a day—to promote smoking.[35] (In addition, the tobacco industry spends about $17 million annually to lobby Congress.[36]) In contrast, all U.S. states annually spend about $500 million for tobacco control.

Tobacco use among teenagers—and even younger children—represents an important example of social injustice. About 23 percent of 12th-graders use tobacco.[37] There may be an even higher percentage of teenagers not attending high school who use tobacco. Some schools still allow the tobacco industry to support sporting events, and some school districts continue to allow the use of tobacco on school grounds. Many coaches and teachers are tobacco users. And the tobacco industry continues to promote its product directly to teenagers, although often in subtle ways. Some tobacco companies have increased advertising in youth-directed magazines.[38] Smokeless tobacco is promoted to circumvent smoking bans. Those people who are most disadvantaged are often those who are most attracted to tobacco use—in 2009, 49 percent of Americans who had obtained a General Educational Development (GED) certificate smoked, compared with 6 percent of those with a graduate degree.[39]

Although cigarette consumption in the United States decreased by 33 percent from 2000 to 2011, combustible tobacco consumption (such as loose tobacco and cigars) increased from 3 to 10 percent.[37] From 2008 to 2011, roll-your-own tobacco use decreased from 10.7 billion to 2.6 billion units (a 76 percent decrease), while pipe tobacco consumption increased from 2.6 billion to 17.5 billion units (a 573 percent increase).[40] Use of smokeless tobacco and cigars declined during the late 1990s, but has changed little since then.

Although comprehensive tobacco control programs decrease tobacco use, relatively little funding is available to implement these programs. From 1998 to 2010, states received $244 billion in settlement funds from tobacco litigation and cigarette excise tax revenue, but less than 3 percent of all of this money was used for tobacco control. Recently, tobacco use has declined at a slower rate than before, probably because of inadequate funds for tobacco control, especially media campaigns to discourage teenagers from smoking.[37]

▨ ORGANIZED DENTISTRY AND ACCESS TO CARE

Although organized dentistry has done much to improve oral health in the United States, it also has limited access to dental care for millions of Americans. Its continued opposition to offering dental services within Medicare has denied millions of older people access to dental care. Its continued opposition to mid-level dental providers (dental therapists) and to expanded duties for dental hygienists and dental assistants has limited access to dental care for additional millions of people. For example, in 2006, the American Dental Association and the Alaska Dental Society sued individual Alaska Native and American Indian dental therapists and their organization (the Alaska Native Tribal Health Consortium). These properly trained dental therapists, whose profession provides care in 50 other countries, were simply doing their job in a nonprofit dental program in rural Alaska, a 570,000-square mile area with no roads, public transportation, or dentists. This suit was settled in 2007 after the Alaska Superior Court upheld the decision of the Alaska Attorney General, who had previously ruled in favor of the dental therapist program.[41] Organized dentistry should become more accountable—and have a more realistic response—to people who need access to dental care.

◾ VULNERABLE POPULATIONS

Laws, regulations, policies, customs, marketing practices, and inadequate understanding of oral health can serve as barriers to social justice in oral health. Social injustice especially affects the oral health of vulnerable populations, including children, older people, migrants, immigrants, people who have low income or low health literacy, and people who are poorly educated, developmentally disabled, medically compromised, homebound, homeless, infected with HIV, uninsured, institutionalized, residents of inner cities and rural areas, or members of racial, ethnic, and linguistic minorities.

Vulnerable populations have greater oral health needs, less understanding of how to avoid preventable dental diseases, and less access to resources to respond to these needs. Data illustrating the oral health needs of vulnerable people in the United States include the following:

- Oral disease represents the most prevalent unmet health problem of children.[42]
- Low-income children have almost 14 times more days missed from school due to dental conditions than do higher-income children.[43]
- About 19 percent of children in poor and near-poor families have unmet dental needs, compared with 4 percent of higher-income children.[44]
- The oral cancer mortality rate of African American males is almost double that of white males.[45]
- Among non-Hispanic African Americans 5 to 19 years of age, 17 percent use preventive dental sealants, compared to 30 percent of non-Hispanic white people.[13]
- Uninsured children are six times more likely to have unmet dental needs as children with private health insurance, and four times more likely to have unmet dental needs, compared to children with Medicaid or other public coverage.[46]
- The average cost of a Medicaid enrollee's inpatient hospital treatment for dental problems is 10 times more expensive than the cost of preventive care.[47]
- Among adults who did not earn a high school diploma, 15 percent have lost all their natural teeth, compared with 3 percent of adults who completed college.[48]

There are strong relationships between both low utilization of dental care and poor oral health status and (a) low education, (b) low income, (c) nonwhite racial status, and (d) lack of health insurance coverage. (Tables 20–1 and 20–2 and Box 20–1.) For example, only about 46 percent of people 18 years or older who did not complete high school have visited a dentist during the

TABLE 20-1 *Percentage of Persons Age 18 or Older Who Had Visited a Dentist or Dental Clinic in the Past Year by Sex, Education, Income, Race, and Ethnicity, United States, 2008*

Category	Percentage of Persons Who Had a Dental Visit in the Past Year
Sex	
Male	66
Female	71
Education	
Less than high school	46
High school or General Educational Development (GED) certificate	62
Some post-high school	69
College graduate	81
Income	
Less than $15,000	47
$15,000–$24,999	52
$25,000–$34,999	60
$35,000–$49,999	68
$50,000 +	81
Race and Hispanic Origin	
White, non-Hispanic	72
Black, non-Hispanic	59
Hispanic	60

Source: National Oral Health Surveillance System, Dental visits. Atlanta, GA: National Center for Chronic Disease Prevention and Health Promotion, Centers for Disease Control and Prevention, 2010.

past year, compared with about 81 percent of those who are college graduates (Table 20-1). About 60 percent of children 2 to 17 years old from low-income households have not been to a dentist in the past year, compared with

TABLE 20-2 *Percentage of Children Ages 2–17 with a Dental Visit by Race/Ethnicity, Income, and Insurance, 2008*

Category	Percentage of Persons Who Had a Dental Visit in the Past Year
Family Economic State	
Poor	37
Low-income	41
Middle-income	51
High-income	64
Race	
White, non-Hispanic	54
Black, non-Hispanic	40
Hispanic	43
Dental Insurance Coverage	
With private insurance	57
With public insurance	41
Not insured	26

Source: Agency for Healthcare Research and Quality, Medical Expenditure Panel Survey, 2002–2008. Rockville, MD: U.S. Department of Health and Human Services, 2010.

BOX 20-1   ■   **Oral Health Inequalities in Developing Countries**

Most oral diseases can be prevented or controlled, yet they often are rampant, especially in low-income countries. The food and tobacco industries often have fewer restrictions or laws governing their products and marketing strategies in low-income countries; therefore, it is easier for them to promote and sell their disease-producing products. Social injustice in oral health in low-income countries often mirrors that among lower socioeconomic groups in the United States. The people who are least educated and informed about the adverse health effects of products are those most likely to buy them, especially in low-income countries where these products, such as cigarettes and high-sugar beverages, are glamorized and readily available with no laws or restrictions. Globally, one in four smokers first tried smoking before the age of 10.[1]

Many poor people in low-income countries do not realize they can live without dental pain or infection. Few can go to a dentist or use a fluoride toothpaste. All too often, oral health is not considered important or part of overall health. Myths about oral health are perpetuated.

Community water fluoridation is often not feasible—but fluoridated salt, a proven method of ensuring adequate levels of systemic fluoride, could be used in countries where central water supplies are sparse.[2] This method of preventing dental caries is an effective and equitable approach because virtually all people buy and use salt. In Central and South America, the Pan American Health Organization (PAHO) has promoted fluoridated salt, which usually costs the same as non-fluoridated salt. Fluoride toothpaste and other sources of fluoride may not be available in these countries or may be too expensive. Even toothbrushes are often not available or affordable.

In addition, in many low-income countries there are few, if any, sources of dental care. The dental personnel-to-population ratio in these countries varies (such as 1:100,000 in Zambia and 1:33,000 in Afghanistan), compared to a dentist-to-population ratio of about 1:2000 in the United States.[3]

U.S. industries export huge quantities of sugar-laden products, especially sugary drinks. These products contribute to tooth decay and obesity. The World Health Organization (WHO) developed a strategic plan to help countries address obesity, but the United States attempted to derail it because of pressure from food and sugar industries that wanted to continue selling their products in other countries.[4]

In many low-income countries, young children who are malnourished and have poor oral hygiene develop noma or cancrum oris, a form of gangrene that destroys the mouth and face. Ninety percent of affected children die without having been treated. This disease is preventable, but the WHO budget for preventing it and other oral health disorders is inadequate.[5]

Although tobacco use is decreasing in high-income countries, its use is rapidly increasing in low- and middle-income countries. Tobacco-induced oral diseases include periodontitis and oral and pharyngeal cancers, which rank among the three most common cancers in South Central Asia.[5,6] Use of tobacco also is associated with congenital defects, such as cleft lip and palate, in children whose mothers have smoked during pregnancy.

In 2003, the World Health Assembly agreed on a treaty to control tobacco supply and consumption.[6] Because there are increasing restrictions on tobacco use in the United States, multinational tobacco industries have increasingly targeted other countries where there are few restrictions. In most Asian countries, children have easy access to cigarette machines, and there is little public education about the dangers of tobacco use. About 20 percent of students own an object with a cigarette-brand logo, and 10 percent have been offered free cigarettes by a tobacco company representative.[1]

Implementing the following measures would improve oral health in low-income countries:

- The United States should be more responsive to the oral health needs in other countries and should not support the export of U.S. products deleterious to oral health.
- Low-income countries should place a higher priority on oral health and implement community-based primary prevention programs, such as fluoridation of community water supplies, salt fluoridation, and school-based dental programs.
- WHO and PAHO should make oral health a much higher priority, especially in low-income countries.

Box References

1. Centers for Disease Control and Prevention. Global youth tobacco surveillance 2000–2007. *MMWR Morb Mortal Wkly Rep* 2008; 57(SS01), 1–21.
2. Estupinan-Day S. Promoting oral health: The use of salt fluoridation to prevent dental caries. Washington, DC. PAHO, 2005.
3. World Health Organization. World health statistics 2012. p 120–137. Available at http://www.who.int/gho/publications/world_health_statistics/EN_WHS2012_Full.pdf. Accessed on March 15, 2013.
4. Stein R. U.S. says it will contest WHO plan to fight obesity. *Washington Post*, 2004, pA3.
5. Petersen PE. The World Oral Health Report 2003: Continuous improvement of oral health in the 21st century—The approach of the WHO Global Oral Health Program. *Community Dent Oral Epidemiol* 2003;31(suppl 1):3–24.
6. Petersen PE. Tobacco and oral health—The role of the World Health Organization. *Oral Health Prev Dent* 2003;1:309–315.

36 percent of those from high-income households (Table 20–2). About 40 percent of Hispanic Americans age 18 and older have not been to a dentist in the past year, compared with 28 percent of Caucasians (Table 20–1). A U.S. national study showed that Mexican American children and adults had greater unmet dental needs, less dental insurance, and fewer dental visits than other Hispanics or Latinos.[49]

■ HEALTH LITERACY AND SOCIAL INEQUALITY

Higher levels of education are generally associated with better overall health status. Health literacy is recognized as an essential skill not only for managing disease, but also for preventing disease and navigating the health care system to facilitate access.[50] Oral health literacy is associated with knowledge about oral health,[51] dental visits,[52] severity of dental caries,[53] failed appointments,[54] and higher oral-health-related quality of life.[55,56] An estimated 80 million U.S. adults are challenged to obtain, process, and understand basic health information needed to make informed health decisions.[57] They may not be able to read or understand directions on prescriptions and over-the-counter medicines; interpret bus schedules, which may preclude getting to dental care appointments; understand that most oral diseases can be prevented; complete Medicaid forms to determine if their children are eligible for oral health care; and understand what their health care providers tell them.[50]

Meanwhile, most health care providers have not been trained to communicate with patients so that patients or their caregivers understand how to improve their health. Although most people report getting their oral health information from dentists, routine use of recommended communication techniques by dentists is low.[58] In addition, if decision-makers are not aware of the impact of health literacy on health outcomes, the health programs they support are probably less effective and more expensive.

Adults generally do not know much about many aspects of oral health, especially about preventing dental caries,[6] although methods to eliminate or control dental caries are well established.[59] Often people with low income and low education have the least access to science-based information on oral health and are unable to navigate the dental care system.[50] Improving oral health literacy can improve oral health and decrease oral health disparities.

▪ NATIONAL ISSUES

The U.S. government has not adequately responded to oral health needs, as illustrated by the following:

- Medicare does not include dental services, except for trauma or cancer.
- Medicaid dental programs serve only 38 percent of eligible children.[60]
- Most state Medicaid programs do not provide dental care to adults.[61]
- About 25 percent of federally funded community and migrant health centers do not include dental services.
- There are more than 4300 dental health professional shortage areas with more than 44 million residents needing almost 9000 dentists.[62]

Federal agencies have documented the oral health needs, in publishing reports such as *Healthy People 2020* and *Oral Health in America: A Report of the Surgeon General*. Implementation of the Patient Protection and Affordable Care Act will enable more children to be eligible for dental care under Medicaid. However, extended Medicaid benefits for adults who are at or below 138 percent of the federal poverty level will be determined by individual states.

■ STATE AND LOCAL ISSUES

Additional problems at the state and local level include the following:

- Only 23 percent of state and local health agencies serving more than 250,000 people have a dental professional with public health training, and most of them are inadequately funded and understaffed.[63]
- Many states have restrictive state practice acts that limit who may practice dentistry and what scope of services may be provided by dental hygienists and dental assistants.
- Most state and local boards of health do not include a dentist or dental hygienist.
- Many local boards of health in non-fluoridated communities have not attempted to fluoridate their water supplies, although it is the most cost-effective measure for improving oral health—and was designated by the Centers for Disease Control and Prevention as one the of 10 greatest public health achievements of the 20th century.[64]
- Only a few local health departments have dental programs.

■ SCHOOL PROGRAMS

Many school-age children in the United States do not have access to basic, preventive, and primary dental care—even though they may qualify for free school meals. They would benefit from school-based health clinics that include oral health services, that include preventive measures, use of fluorides and sealants, and dental care.[65,66] Basing these services in schools reduces students' time lost from classes and parents' time lost from work. School-based programs should be part of larger community-based dental systems.[66] There are more than 1900 school-based health centers in the United States, of which only 12 percent have dental care providers on site.[67] Schools are excellent sites not only for providing oral health services, but also for increasing oral health literacy skills.[68]

Many schools have replaced high-sugar beverages with healthier options, but these beverages remain available to one-third of students in public elementary school.[69]

Despite national improvements, 21 states and the District of Columbia still place unnecessary hurdles, like restrictive state practice acts, on school-based sealant programs for low-income children.[70]

■ DENTAL PUBLIC HEALTH INFRASTRUCTURE

Most of the more than 2800 local health departments in the United States do not employ dentists or dental hygienists who are trained in public health.

Although most state health departments employ full-time dentists or dental hygienists, they generally have very limited funding and few staff members. Of the approximately 155,000 dentists in the United States, only 159 are certified by the American Board of Dental Public Health.[71,72] Public health dentists are trained to improve and protect the oral health of communities and population groups at the community, town or city, state, region, or national level—focusing on children, low-income people, homeless people, older people, and other vulnerable populations.

Although dentists trained in public health can better improve the oral health of a population than dental clinicians or private practitioners, they are often not valued by our society. Although they have had more education and training than most dental clinicians, their income is much less because they do not treat individual patients. It seems that the reward system is the reverse of what it should be.

▨ DENTAL WORKFORCE

The dental workforce does not mirror the U.S. population. Although 12 percent of the U.S. population is composed of African Americans, they represent only 3 percent of practicing dentists—and the future does not look promising.[73] In 2010, about 6 percent of all dental school graduates were African American.[74] Twelve of the 58 dental schools in the United States did not have *any* entering African American students, and six schools had only one entering African American.[75] Hispanic and Native American dentists also are sorely needed.

▨ WHAT NEEDS TO BE DONE

National initiatives could help sensitize policymakers and the general public about the need for better oral health. The publication of *Healthy People 2010* and *Healthy People 2020*, the *Leading Health Indicators, Oral Health in America: A Report of the Surgeon General*, and the *Surgeon General's National Call to Action*[76] have been steps in the right direction. But they have led to relatively little action.

Healthy People 2020

This report on U.S. national health objectives for 2020 includes oral health—one of 42 topic areas with almost 600 objectives and 1200 measures. These national objectives provide a strategic management tool for local, state, and national government agencies and organizations to develop their own health plans with objectives specific to their needs. They have helped to provide guidance to interested parties concerning national needs and priorities. Oral health has 17 objectives with 26 measures in areas such as children and adults, access to preventive services, interventions, surveillance, and infrastructure.[63,77]

Healthy People 2020 leverages information technology to help communities develop innovative approaches for prevention and to monitor their progress to reduce disparities through a determinants of health approach. However, there has been no significant funding to achieve these objectives at the national, state, or local level.

Leading Health Indicators

Oral health is one of the 12 leading health indicators—the high-priority health issues of *Healthy People 2020* that will be used to assess the health status of Americans, promote collaboration, and initiate action. This work should lead to the development and implementation of a national prevention program for oral health.

Oral Health in America: A Report of the Surgeon General

The first U.S. Surgeon General's report on oral health, published in 2000,[6] raised the visibility of the "silent epidemic of oral diseases" and documented the importance of oral health as essential to overall health and well-being. The report documented great disparities between the "haves" and "have-nots." It also stressed the importance of effective community-based prevention programs and the need for a strong dental public health infrastructure. Its major findings were as follows:

- Oral diseases and disorders affect health and well-being throughout life.
- Safe and effective measures exist to prevent the most common dental diseases—dental caries and periodontal diseases.
- Neither the general public nor health care providers know how to prevent dental caries.
- Lifestyle behaviors that affect general health, such as tobacco use, excessive alcohol use, and poor dietary choices, also adversely affect oral health.
- There are profound and consequential oral health disparities within the U.S. population.
- More information is needed to improve oral health and eliminate health disparities.
- The mouth reflects general health and well-being; oral diseases and conditions are associated with other health problems.
- Scientific research is key to further reduction in the burden of diseases and disorders that affect the face, mouth, and teeth.

Although this report was beneficial, it was not accompanied by any legislation, executive orders, or funding to respond to unmet dental needs. In 2012, David Satcher, who had been Surgeon General at the time of this report, stated that there is still an oral disease epidemic in the United States.[8]

The Patient Protection and Affordable Care Act

The Patient Protection and Affordable Care Act (ACA) may improve access to dental services for children.[73] About eight million additional children are eligible for dental coverage through state plans, which will increase demand for services. The Act includes metrics to assess oral health programs for children. However, extended Medicaid benefits for adults who are at or below 138 percent of the federal poverty level will be determined by individual states.

A National Call to Action to Promote Oral Health

In 2003, U.S. Surgeon General Richard Carmona released *A National Call to Action to Promote Oral Health*,[76] as recommended in the Surgeon General's Report on Oral Health. It envisioned advancing "the general health and well-being of all Americans by creating partnerships at all levels of society to engage in programs to promote oral health and prevent disease." Its three goals were to promote oral health, to promote quality of life, and to eliminate oral health disparities. It recommended the following actions:

1. Change perceptions of oral health
2. Overcome barriers by replicating effective programs and proven efforts
3. Build a science base and accelerate transfer of science
4. Increase the diversity, capacity, and flexibility of the oral health workforce
5. Increase collaborations

The Surgeon General has recommended that action plans be written throughout the United States, each by a consortium of stakeholders at the local, regional, and state level, using the Healthy People objectives to establish goals and to guide needs assessments and outcome measures. However, the Call to Action consists primarily of guidance—without substantive funding or legislation for programs that can make a difference in lives of people, especially vulnerable populations. Implementation of the ACA will help support some of the objectives of the Call to Action.[11,77]

▪ CONCLUSION

The neglected epidemic of oral disease is a social injustice for many people, especially vulnerable populations. Millions of people have unnecessary oral diseases because cost-effective, population-based preventive measures, such as community water fluoridation, have not been implemented—and the private wealth of the food and tobacco industries and organized dentistry have overridden the interests of the public's health.

Institutions, agencies, and organizations should recognize and promote the concept that oral health is an integral part of total health. People are much more likely to have poor oral health if they have low health literacy or are low-income, uninsured, developmentally disabled, homebound, homeless, medically compromised, or members of minority groups or other high-risk populations who do not have access to oral health services. Although oral health disparities are well documented, oral health will not improve without improved funding and new legislation.

We recommend the following actions:

- Establishing a national health program with a meaningful comprehensive oral health component for people of all ages that stresses prevention and primary dental care
- Making oral health a higher priority, focusing on increasing oral health literacy of the public, health care providers, and policymakers
- Making effective prevention programs, initiatives, and services, such as water fluoridation and school-based prevention programs, the foundation for all dental programs at the local, state, and national levels
- Ensuring that federal, state, and local government agencies and non-governmental organizations and institutions give a much higher priority to oral health by making it an integral component of all health programs
- Ensuring that all public schools provide (a) comprehensive health education, with an oral health component, for all children in kindergarten through grade 12; and (b) dental care services in all school health clinics and centers for high-risk children
- Promoting more realistic state practice acts so that the oral health workforce has greater diversity, flexibility, sensitivity, and expertise in population-based, oral health prevention programs and services for vulnerable populations

Implementing these recommendations and monitoring their impact can lead to social justice for better oral health.

■ REFERENCES

1. Allukian M. The neglected American epidemic. *Nation's Health* 1990;May–June:2.
2. Allukian M Jr. Oral diseases: The neglected epidemic. In: Scutchfield FD, Keck CW, eds. Principles of public health practice. 2nd ed. Albany, NY: Delmar Publishers, 2003:387–408.
3. The Dental Health Foundation. The oral health of California's children: A neglected epidemic. San Rafael, CA: Dental Health Foundation, 1997.
4. Gotsch AR. The neglected epidemic. *Nation's Health* 1999; September:2.
5. Allukian M Jr. The neglected epidemic and the Surgeon General's Report: A call to action for better oral health (editorial). *Am J Public Health* 2000;90:843–845.
6. U.S. Department of Health and Human Services. Oral health in America: A report of the Surgeon General. Rockville, MD: National Institute of Dental and Craniofacial Research, National Institutes of Health, 2000.
7. Krisberg K. Call to action issued on oral health diseases. *Nation's Health* 2003:2,19.

8. Affordable dental care: Former Surgeon General David Satcher says oral health epidemic persists. *Dental Health Magazine*, July 17, 2012. Available at http://worldental.org/dental-news/affordable-dental-care-surgeon-general-david-satcher-oral-health-epidemic-persists/7571/. Accessed on September 11, 2012.

9. Agency for Healthcare Research and Quality. Healthcare Cost and Utilization Project (HCUP)—The Nationwide Emergency Department Sample for the year[s] 2009 and 2006. Available at http://hcupnet.ahrq.gov. Accessed on September 11, 2012.

10. Centers for Medicare and Medicaid Services, Office of the Actuary, National Health Statistics Group; U.S. Department of Commerce, Bureau of Economic Analysis, and U.S. Bureau of the Census. Table 4. National health expenditures, by source of funds and types of expenditure: Calendar years 2004–2010, 2012. Available at http://www.cms.gov/Research-Statistics-Data-and-Systems/Statistics-Trends-and-Reports/NationalHealthExpendData/downloads/tables.pdf. Accessed on September 11, 2012.

11. Otto M. Boy's death fuels drives to fund dental aid to poor. *Washington Post*, March 3, 2007, pp. B1 & B4. Available at http://www.washingtonpost.com/wp-dyn/content/article/2007/03/02/AR2007030200827.html. Accessed on September 11, 2012.

12. Dye BA, Tan S, Smith V, et al. Trends in oral health status: United States, 1988–1994 and 1999–2004. National Center for Health Statistics. *Vital Health Stat* 2007;11:1–92.

13. Dye BA, Li X, Beltran-Aguilar ED. Selected oral health indicators in the United States, 2005–2008. NCHS data brief no 96. Hyattsville, MD: National Center for Health Statistics, 2012.

14. Lewis C, Stout J. Toothache in U.S. children. *Arch Pediatr Adolesc Med* 2010;164: 1059–1063.

15. Ahmedin J, Siegel R, Xu J, et al. Cancer statistics, 2010. *CA Cancer J Clin* 2010;560: 277–300.

16. Centers for Medicare and Medicaid Services, Office of the Actuary, National Health Statistics Group. National health expenditure projections, Table 2: National health expenditures amounts, and annual percent change by expenditure: Calendar years 2006–2012. Available at https://www.cms.gov/Research-Statistics-Data-and-Systems/Statistics-Trends-and-Reports/NationalHealthExpendData/Downloads/Proj2011PDF.pdf. Accessed July 5, 2012.

17. Plunkett Research, Ltd. Introduction to the food & beverage industry. Available at http://www.plunkettresearch.com/food-beverage-grocery-market-research/industry-and-business-data. Accessed July 5, 2012.

18. Kaiser Permanente. The weight of the nation: Community activation kit topics, 2012. Available at http://info.kaiserpermanente.org/communitybenefit/html/our_work/global/weightofthenation/docs/topics/WOTNCommActTopic_Food_Marketing_F.pdf. Accessed on September 11, 2012.

19. Ogden CL, Carroll MD, Kit BK, Flegal KM. Prevalence of obesity and trends in body mass index among U.S. children and adolescents, 1999–2010. *JAMA* 2012;307:483–490.

20. Centers for Disease Control and Prevention. Childhood obesity facts. Available at http://www.cdc.gov/healthyyouth/obesity/facts.htm. Accessed on March 8, 2013.

21. American Heart Association. Association recommends reduced intake of added sugars: American Heart Association scientific statement, August 24, 2009. Available at http://newsroom.heart.org/pr/aha/800.aspx. Accessed on September 11, 2012.

22. Odgen CL, Kit BK, Carroll MD, Park S. Consumption of sugar drinks in the United States, 2005–2008. Available at http://www.cdc.gov/nchs/data/databriefs/db71.pdf. Accessed July 3, 2012.

23. Sturm E, Powell LM, Chriqui JF, Chaloupka FJ. Soda taxes, soft drink consumption, and children's body mass index. *Health Aff* 2010;29:1052–1058.

24. Apovian CM. Sugar-sweetened soft drinks, obesity, and type 2 diabetes. *JAMA* 2004;292:978–979.

25. French SA, Lin BH, Guthrie JF. National trends in soft drink consumption among children and adolescents age 6 to 17 years: Prevalence, amounts, and sources. *J Am Diet Assoc* 2003;103:1326–1331.

26. Berk CC. Drop in soda sales accelerates as healthier options grow. March 20, 2012. Available at http://www.cnbc.com/id/46796332/Drop_in_Soda_Sales_Accelerates_as_Healthier_Options_Grow. Accessed on September 11, 2012.

27. Sugary drink F.A.C.T.S.: Food advertising to children and teens score. New Haven, CT: Rudd Center for Food Policy and Obesity, 2011. Available at http://www.sugardrinkfacts.org/resources/SugaryDrinkFACTS_Report.pdf. Accessed on October 30, 2012.

28. Nestle M. Soft drink pouring rights. *Public Health Rep* 2000;115:308–319.

29. American Academy of Pediatrics. Policy statement. Soft drinks in schools. *Pediatrics* 2004;113:152–154.

30. Healy M. At-school sales of soda drop, but other sugary drinks remain. *Los Angeles Times,* August 6, 2012. Available at http://www.latimes.com/health/boostershots/la-heb-soda-schools-20120806,0,448515.story. Accessed on September 11, 2012.

31. Grynbaum M. Health panel approves restriction on sale of large sugary drinks. *New York Times,* September 14, 2012, p. A24. Available at http://www.nytimes.com/2012/09/14/nyregion/health-board-approves-bloombergs-soda-ban.html. Accessed on October 8, 2012.

32. Grynbaum M. Soda makers begin their push against New York ban. *New York Times,* July 1, 2012, p. A10. Available at http://www.nytimes.com/2012/07/02/nyregion/in-fight-against-nyc-soda-ban-industry-focuses-on-personal-choice.html?_r=1&pagewanted=all. Accessed on September 11, 2012.

33. National Confectioners Association. 2009 Industry review: United States confectionary market. Available at http://www.candyusa.com/Sales/content.cfm?ItemNumber=1440&navItemNumber=2685. Accessed on September 11, 2012.

34. U.S Department of Health and Human Services. Preventing tobacco use among youth and young adults: A report of the Surgeon General. Rockville, MD: Public Health Service, Office of the Surgeon General, 2012.

35. Campaign for Tobacco-Free Kids. Toll of tobacco in the United States of America, 2012. Available at http://www.tobaccofreekids.org/research/factsheets/pdf/0072.pdf. Accessed on September 11, 2012.

36. Center for Responsive Politics. Tobacco. March 4, 2013. Available at http://www.opensecrets.org/lobby/indusclient.php?id=a02&year=2012. Accessed on March 13, 2012.

37. Centers for Disease Control and Prevention. Current tobacco use among middle and high school students—United States, 2011. *MMWR Morb Mortal Wkly Rep* 2012;61:581–585.

38. Healton C, Nelson K. Reversal of misfortune: Viewing tobacco as a social justice issue. *Am J Public Health* 2004;94:186–191.

39. Centers for Disease Control and Prevention. Vital signs: Current cigarette smoking among adults aged ≥ 18 years—United States, 2009. *MMWR Morb Mortal Wkly Rep* 2010;59:1135–1140.

40. Centers for Disease Control and Prevention. Consumption of cigarettes and combustible tobacco—United States, 2000–2011. *MMWR Morb Mortal Wkly Rep* 2012;61:565–569.

41. Alaska Superior Court. *Alaska Dental Society, et al. v. State of Alaska, et al.* Order Case No. 3AN-06-04797 CI, June 27, 2007.

42. Children's Dental Care Access in Medicaid. The role of medical care use and dentist participation. Child Health Insurance Research Initiative (CHIRI™) issue brief 2. Agency for Healthcare Research and Quality (AHRQ) Publication No. 03-0032, June 2003. Agency for Healthcare Research and Quality, Rockville, MD. Available at http://www.ahrq.gov/chiri/chirident.htm. Accessed on September 11, 2012.

43. Adams PF, Hendershot GE, Marano MA. Current estimates from the National Health Interview Survey, 1996. National Center for Health Statistics. *Vital Health Stat* 1999;10:1–203.

44. National Center for Health Statistics. Summary Health Statistics for U.S. Children: National Health Interview Survey, 2009. *Vital and Health Statistics* 2010;10(247). Available at http://www.cdc.gov/nchs/data/series/sr_10/sr10_247.pdf. Accessed on September 11, 2012.

45. Howlader N, Noone AM, Krapcho M, et al., eds. Surveillance Epidemiology and End Results (SEER) Cancer Statistics Review, 1975–2009 (vintage 2009 populations). August 20, 2012. National Cancer Institute. Bethesda, MD. Available at http://seer.cancer.gov/csr/1975_2009_pops09/index.html. Accessed on September 11, 2012.

46. Bloom B, Cohen RA, Freeman G. Summary health statistics for U.S. children: National Health Interview Survey, 2010. National Center for Health Statistics. *Vital Health Stat* 2011;10:1–80.

47. Pettinato E, Webb M, Seale SN. A comparison of Medicaid reimbursement for nondefinitive pediatric dental treatment in the emergency room versus periodic preventative care. *Pediatric Dentistry* 2000;22:463–468.

48. Pleis JR, Lethbridge-Çejku M. Summary health statistics for U.S. adults: National Health Interview Survey, 2006. National Center for Health Statistics. *Vital Health Stat* 2007;10:1–153.

49. Scott G, Simile C. Access to dental care among Hispanic or Latino subgroups: United States 2000–2003. Advance data from vital and health statistics. Hyattsville, MD: National Center for Health Statistics, May 12, 2005.

50. Rudd RE, Moeykens BA, Colton TC. Health and literacy: A review of medical and public health literature, National Center for the Study of Adult Learning and Literacy annual review of adult learning and literacy. Vol. 1. New York: Jossey-Bass, 2000.

51. Jones M, Lee JY, Rozier RG. Oral health literacy among adult patients seeking dental care. *J Am Dent Assoc* 2007;138:199–208.

52. White S, Chen J, Atchinson R. Relationship of preventive health practices and health literacy: A national study. *Am J Health Behavior* 2008;32:227–242.

53. D. Miller E, Lee JY, DeWalt DA, Vann WF Jr. Impact of caregiver literacy on children's oral health outcomes. *Pediatrics* 2010;126:107–114.

54. Holtzman J, Gironda M, Atchison, K. The relationship between patients' oral health literacy and failed appointments. Presentation at the National Oral Health Conference, Milwaukee, WI, April 29, 2012.

55. Lee JY, Rozier RG, Lee SY, et al. Development of a word recognition instrument to test health literacy in dentistry: The REALD-30—A brief communication. *J Public Health Dent* 2007;67:94–98.

56. Richman JA, Lee JY, Rozier RG, et al. Evaluation of a word recognition instrument to test health literacy in dentistry: The REALD-99. *J Public Health Dent* 2007;67:99–104.

57. Kutner M, Greenberg E, Jin Y, Paulsen C. The health literacy of American's adults: Results from the 2003 National Assessment of Adult literacy (NCES 2006-483). U.S. Department of Education. Available at http://nces.ed.gov/pubs2006/2006483.pdf. Accessed on September 11, 2012.

58. Rozier RG, Horowitz AM, Podschun G. Dentist-patient communication techniques used in the United States: The results of a national survey. *J Am Dent Assoc* 2011;142:518–530.

59. Horowitz AM: The public's oral health: The gaps between what we know and what we do. *Adv Dent Sci* 1995;9:91–95.

60. Centers for Medicare and Medicaid Services. Medicaid/ CHIP oral health services: Fact sheet, October 2010. Available at http://www.medicaid.gov/Medicaid-CHIP-Program-Information/By-Topics/Benefits/Downloads/2010-Dental-Factsheet.pdf. Accessed on September 11, 2012.

61. Centers for Medicare and Medicaid Services. Dental care. March 4, 2013. Available at http://www.medicaid.gov/Medicaid-CHIP-Program-Information/By-Topics/Benefits/Dental-Care.html. Accessed on March 13, 2013.

62. U.S. Department of Health and Human Services, Health Resources and Services Administration. Shortage designation: Health professional shortage areas and medically underserved areas/populations, July 2012. Available at http://bhpr.hrsa.gov/shortage/. Accessed on September 11, 2012.

63. U.S. Department of Health and Human Services, Office of Disease Prevention and Health Promotion. Healthy People 2020. Washington, DC. Available at http://www.healthypeople.gov/2020/faqs.aspx#g. Accessed on September 11, 2012.

64. Centers for Disease Control and Prevention. Ten great public health achievements— United States, 1900–1999. *MMWR Morb Mortal Wkly Rep* 1999;48:241–243.

65. Horowitz AM, Harris NO. Creating effective, school-based oral health programs. In: Harris NO, Garcia-Godoy F, eds. Primary preventive dentistry. 6th ed. Upper Saddle River, NJ: Pearson Prentice-Hall, 2004:521–553.

66. Behrens D, Graham Lear J. Strengthening children's oral health: Views from the field. *Health Aff* 2011;30:2208–2213.

67. The Center for Health and Health Care in Schools. Dental and mental health services. Available at http://www.healthinschools.org. Accessed on September 11, 2012.

68. Braun B, Horowitz AM, Kleinman DV, et al. Oral health literacy: At the intersection of K–12 education and public health. *Cal Dent Assoc* 2012;40:323–330.

69. Turner L, Chaloupka F. Encouraging trends in student access to competitive beverages in U.S. public elementary schools, 2006–2007 to 2010–2011. *Arch Pediatr Adolesc Med* 2012;166:673–675.

70. Pew Center on the States. The state of children's dental health: Making coverage matter. Exhibit D: Pew Center on the States analysis of eight key policy indicators, May 2011. Available at http://fha.dhmh.maryland.gov/oralhealth/docs1/cdh-entire_pew_report.pdf. Accessed on September 11, 2012.

71. Bureau of Labor Statistics, U.S. Department of Labor. Occupational outlook handbook, dentists, 2012–13 edition. Available at http://www.bls.gov/ooh/healthcare/dentists.htm. Accessed on September 11, 2012.

72. Council on Dental Education and Licensure. Report of national certifying boards for special areas of dental practice: Report of the ADA-recognized dental specialty certifying boards. Chicago, IL: American Dental Association, April 2012.

73. Institute of Medicine. Improving access to oral health care for vulnerable and underserved populations. Washington, DC: The National Academies Press, 2011.

74. American Dental Association. 2009–2010 survey of dental education: Academic programs, enrollment, and graduates. Vol. I. April, 2011. Available at http://www.agd.org/files/webuser/website/membership/vol.%201_academic%20programs_enrollment_graduates.pdf. Accessed on September 11, 2012.

75. American Dental Education Association. U.S. dental school applicants and enrollees, 2010 entering class (ADEA AADSAS Application Cycle 2010–11). Table 10: Race/ethnicity of applicants and enrollees by school, 2010. Available at http://www.adea.org/publications/library/ADEAsurveysreports/Documents/ADEADental SchoolAppEnrollees2010ClassExecSummaryTables.pdf. Accessed on September 11, 2012.

76. U.S. Department of Health and Human Services. A national call to action to promote oral health. Rockville, MD: U.S. Department of Health and Human Services, Public Health Service, Centers for Disease Control and Prevention and the National Institutes of Health, National Institute of Dental and Craniofacial Research (NIH publication no. 03-5303), May 2003.

77. Institute of Medicine. Advancing oral health in America. Washington, DC: The National Academies Press, 2011.

21 International and Global Health

■ BARRY S. LEVY AND VICTOR W. SIDEL

■ INTRODUCTION

Social injustice anywhere reflects social injustice everywhere. This chapter focuses on social injustice in low-income, or developing, countries. In many other chapters of this book, social injustice in low-income countries is partially addressed—as it affects specific population groups (Chapters 2 to 11) and as it affects aspects of public health (Chapters 12 to 20). This chapter discusses extreme poverty, failure to protect human rights, inadequate foreign assistance, external debt, corruption, and globalization as well as human trafficking, hunger and malnutrition, and export of hazardous substances from developed to developing countries. It also addresses the impact of social injustice on public health in these countries and what needs to be done.

Widespread social injustice leads to profoundly increased rates of illness and premature death in low-income countries—related to inadequate public health services and medical care, as well as other internal and external factors.

Internal factors include:

- Extreme poverty
- Discrimination against women, indigenous peoples, racial and ethnic minorities, physically and mentally disabled people, and other vulnerable groups
- Unrepresentative, unaccountable governments and often widespread corruption
- Failure to protect human rights

External factors—many of which result from the policies of high-income countries, multinational corporations, and international financial institutions—include:

- High external debt
- *Structural adjustment policies* (see below), which reduce health and other human services
- Trade barriers that limit exports from low-income to high-income countries
- Export of hazardous substances—and sometimes hazardous industries—from high-income to low-income countries
- Inadequate financial and technical assistance from high-income to low-income countries

- The "brain drain" of educated people from low-income to high-income countries
- The international trade in guns and other conventional arms (see Box 17–2 in Chapter 17)

The World Health Organization (WHO), in 2003, categorized 132 of the 192 countries as *developing* (or *less-developed*) *countries,* the better-off of which are sometimes considered *industrializing countries* or *countries in transition.* It classified 72 of these countries as *high-mortality developing countries* (46 of them in Africa) and 60 of them as *low-mortality developing countries.*[1] It classified the other 60 countries as *developed countries,* including the United States, Canada, Japan, Australia, New Zealand, and all European nations.[1] (In most of this book, we also use the term *high-income countries* to designate developed countries, and *low-income countries* to designate developing countries. We also recognize that some countries that are industrializing or in transition can be designated as *middle-income countries.*)

■ EXTREME POVERTY

Developing countries are characterized by profoundly low levels of income, high population density, and high fertility rates (Table 21–1).[2,3] There are wide gaps between the very few people who are rich and the many people who are poor.[4] In 2008, approximately 1.3 billion people lived on less than the equivalent of US$1.25 per day—almost all in developing countries.[5] Many people in developing countries cannot meet their basic needs for food, clothing, shelter, and health care. Such extreme poverty—often due to multiple forms of social injustice—has a huge impact on health as a result of poor nutrition, limited access

TABLE 21–1 *Characteristics of Selected Developing Countries and, for Comparison, the United States, 2010*

Country	Population (in millions)	Gross National Income per Capita (converted to U.S. dollars)	Population Density (per square kilometer)	Fertility Rate (births per woman)
Afghanistan	34.4	410	53	6.3
Guatemala	14.4	2740	131	4.0
Haiti	10.0	650	363	3.3
Iraq	32.0	2380	74	4.7
Kenya	40.5	810	71	4.7
Pakistan	173.6	1050	225	3.4
Peru	29.1	4900	23	2.5
Sierra Leone	5.9	340	82	5.0
South Africa	50.0	6090	41	2.5
Vietnam	86.9	1160	280	1.8
United States	309.3	47,350	34	2.1

Source: The World Bank. World development indicators. Washington, DC: The World Bank. Available at data.worldbank.org/indicator/. Accessed December 17, 2012.

TABLE 21-2 *Expenditures on Health in Selected Developing Countries and, for Comparison, the United States, 2010*

Country	Annual Total Per-Capita Expenditures on Health (in current U.S. dollars)	Public Expenditures on Health (percentage of total health expenditures)
Afghanistan	38	12%
Guatemala	196	36%
Haiti	46	21%
Iraq	247	81%
Kenya	37	44%
Pakistan	22	39%
Peru	269	54%
Sierra Leone	43	11%
South Africa	649	44%
Vietnam	83	38%
United States	8362	53%

Source: The World Bank. World development indicators. Washington, DC: The World Bank. Available at data.worldbank.org/indicator/. Accessed December 17, 2012.

to medical care and public health services, and increased exposure to health and safety hazards. Individuals and governments in developing countries spend far less money per capita on health than in developed countries (Table 21–2).[3]

Education and employment opportunities are extremely limited in developing countries. Primary school completion rates are much lower and adult literacy rates are much higher than in developed countries (Table 21–3).[3] Inadequate economic development restricts opportunities for individuals and entire countries. As a result, highly educated individuals, including many physicians, nurses, and other health professionals, often leave their home countries—creating a *brain drain*—to seek better educational and employment opportunities in developed countries.[6] For example, in 2002, there were at least 5334 non-federal physicians licensed to practice medicine in the United States who had been trained in African medical schools.[7]

TABLE 21-3 *Primary-School Completion Rate and Adult Literacy Rate for Men and Women, in Selected Developing Countries*

Country	Primary-School Completion Rate (year)	Adult Literacy Rate (year)
Afghanistan	NA*	NA
Guatemala	84% (2010)	74% (2009)
Haiti	NA	NA
Iraq	65% (2007)	78% (2009)
Kenya	NA	87% (2009)
Pakistan	67% (2010)	56% (2008)
Peru	100% (2010)	90% (2007)
Sierra Leone	74% (2011)	41% (2009)
South Africa	NA	89% (2007)
Vietnam	NA	93% (2009)

*NA: Not available in World Bank Indicators.
Source: The World Bank. World development indicators. Washington, DC: The World Bank. Available at data.worldbank.org/indicator/. Accessed December 17, 2012.

▪ FAILURE TO PROTECT HUMAN RIGHTS

In low-income countries, protection of human rights is often limited or non-existent. Threats to human rights include (a) large-scale abuses, such as genocide[8] and ethnic cleansing (Box 17–4 in Chapter 17), torture (Box 27–1 in Chapter 27), and forced migration (Chapter 11); and (b) chronic, systemic problems that deny people their basic rights, including access to safe food and water, health care, security, and a safe workplace and healthful home environment; freedom of religion, speech, and assembly; and protection against arbitrary use of governmental power. Human rights problems also include:[9]

- Discrimination based on gender, age, racial and ethnic status, political opinion, sexual orientation, and health and disability status
- Child labor, with more than 250 million children between the ages of 5 and 14 working—approximately half of them working full-time
- Human trafficking (Box 21–1)
- Design and implementation of health policies that adversely affect health
- Civil wars and international armed conflicts (Box 17–1 in Chapter 17)

Women provide a substantial amount of health care in low-income countries. They head many households in these countries, especially in Africa and Latin America. And, in many low-income countries, they grow a high percentage of food consumed domestically and grown for export. Nevertheless, women face widespread and serious discrimination in these countries (Chapter 4). A substantial proportion become mothers before reaching age 20. Many girls are subjected to genital mutilation. And many women and girls die of pregnancy-related complications—the lifetime risk of maternal death is 1 in 150 in developing countries.[10]

▪ INADEQUATE FOREIGN ASSISTANCE

Many developed countries are providing less financial aid and technical assistance to developing countries than they did 20 years ago. This has occurred for a variety of reasons, including the end of Cold War competition in foreign assistance between the United States and the Soviet Union. The United Nations has recommended that developed countries contribute 0.7 percent or more of their gross domestic product (GDP)—almost equivalent to gross national income (GNI)—for official development assistance. In 2011, only five countries—Denmark, Luxembourg, Norway, the Netherlands, and Sweden—met this standard. Although the United States contributed more than 0.7 percent of its GNI for foreign assistance in the early 1960s, this percentage has substantially declined; in 2011, for example, it was only 0.20 percent[11] (Figure 21–1).

BOX 21-1 ■ Trafficking in Persons

Trafficking in persons, or *human trafficking*, is the "recruitment, transportation, transfer, harboring or receipt of persons," by threat or use of force or other coercion, abduction, fraud, deception, abuse of power or position of vulnerability, or giving or receiving of payments or benefits in order to achieve the consent of a person having control over another person for the purpose of exploitation.[1]

From Himalayan villages to Eastern European cities, people—especially women and girls—are attracted by the prospect of a well-paid job as a domestic servant, waitress, or factory worker. Traffickers recruit victims through false advertisements, mail-order bride catalogs, and casual acquaintances.

Upon arrival at their destinations, victims are placed in conditions controlled by traffickers, while they are exploited to earn illicit revenues. Many are physically confined, their travel or identify documents are taken away, and they or their families are threatened if they do not cooperate. Women and girls who have been forced to work as prostitutes are blackmailed by the threat that traffickers will tell their families. Trafficked children are dependent on the traffickers for food, shelter, and other basic needs. Traffickers also play on victims' fear that police or other government officials in a strange country will prosecute or deport them if they ask for help. Ironically, victims of trafficking are often not identified as such and instead are considered to be people who have violated laws concerning migration, labor, and/or prostitution.

As a result of trafficking, an estimated 2.5 million people at any given time are in sexual exploitation and other forms of forced labor—56 percent of them in Asia and the Pacific region. Beyond the sex trade, other forms of human trafficking include forced or bonded labor, forced marriage, domestic servitude, organ removal, and exploitation of children in begging and warfare.[2]

Virtually every country is a place of origin, transit, or destination of trafficked persons. Most trafficked persons are between the ages of 18 and 24. About 1.2 million children are trafficked annually. Almost all trafficking victims experience sexual or other physical violence during trafficking. It is estimated that 43 percent of victims (98 percent of whom are women and girls) are exploited through forced commercial sex work.[2]

Trafficking is lucrative: In 2005, global profits were estimated at about $32 billion per year—about half in industrialized countries.[3] Yet few traffickers are prosecuted or convicted; for example, in 2006, globally there were only about 5800 prosecutions and 3200 convictions—one conviction for about every 800 trafficking victims.[2]

Addressing the Problem

Deterrence and criminal punishments are important elements, but addressing the underlying conditions that drive both supply and demand are also necessary. Another important preventive measure is public information to mobilize support for effective laws, raise the awareness of key law-enforcement and other officials, and inform socially marginalized groups from which victims are often recruited about trafficking so they will be less likely to be deceived when approached by traffickers.

The Protocol to Prevent, Suppress and Punish Trafficking in Persons,[1] which came into effect in 2003, was established to prevent trafficking in persons, assist victims of trafficking, and promote international cooperation. As of 2010, there were 177 state signatories to the Protocol.

Since the Protocol came into effect, there has been substantially increased attention and response to human trafficking. As of 2008, there were 98 countries that had passed legislation against trafficking in persons that addressed the major forms of trafficking, and another 15 had passed less-comprehensive anti-trafficking legislation. In addition, more than 80 countries have set up anti-trafficking police units, and a similar number have developed national action plans addressing human trafficking. All of these actions have led to an increased number of prosecutions and convictions.[4]

The United Nations Global Program Against Trafficking in Human Beings aims to shed light on the involvement of organized criminal groups in human trafficking and to promote the development of effective criminal justice–related responses. At the country level, this program raises awareness; trains law enforcement officers, prosecutors, and judges; advises on drafting relevant legislation; advises on and assists in strengthening anti-trafficking programs; and improves victim and witness support. At the international level, this program assists agencies, institutions, and governments in designing effective programs and measures against trafficking in persons.

Trafficking in persons in the United States began with the slave trade. The Trafficking Victims Protection Act, which was passed by Congress in 2000 and amended in 2003 and 2005, is the legislation in the United States that criminalizes human trafficking. Between 2008 and 2010, the U.S. Department of Justice investigated about 2500 suspected cases of human trafficking, 82 percent of which involved sex trafficking and about half of which involved victims under the age of 18. About five-sixths of sex-trafficking victims were U.S. citizens, but about two-thirds of labor-trafficking victims were undocumented immigrants.[5] The Federal Bureau of Investigation (FBI) and Immigration and Customs Enforcement (ICE) are the two federal agencies that are primarily involved with investigating trafficking in persons. In fiscal year 2010, the most recent year for which statistics are available, there were 119 human trafficking arrests made by the FBI, 95 indictments made in FBI trafficking cases, and 79 convictions made (some from earlier years).[6] ICE initiated 651 trafficking investigations in Fiscal Year 2010 and had 144 convictions.[6]

Acknowledgment

We acknowledge the assistance of Mark Sidel, JD, who reviewed an earlier draft of this box and made helpful suggestions.

Box References

1. United Nations Office on Drugs and Crime. The protocol to prevent, suppress and punish trafficking in persons. In: United Nations Convention Against Transnational Organized Crime and the protocols thereto. 2004. Available at http://www.unodc.org/documents/treaties/UNTOC/Publications/TOC%20Convention/TOCebook-e.pdf. Accessed December 19, 2012.
2. Global Initiative to Fight Human Trafficking. Human trafficking: The facts. Available at http://www.unglobalcompact.org/docs/issues_doc/labour/Forced_labour/HUMAN_TRAFFICKING_-_THE_FACTS_-_final.pdf. Accessed December 19, 2012.

3. United Nations Office on Drugs and Crime. Factsheet on human trafficking. Available at http://www.unodc.org/documents/human-trafficking/UNVTF_fs_HT_EN.pdf. Accessed December 19, 2012.
4. United Nations Office on Drugs and Crime. Global report on trafficking in persons. Geneva: United Nations, 2009. Available at http://www.unodc.org/unodc/en/human-trafficking/global-report-on-trafficking-in-persons.html. Accessed December 19, 2012.
5. U.S. Department of Justice. Characteristics of suspected human trafficking incidents, 2008–2010. Available at http://bjs.ojp.usdoj.gov/content/pub/pdf/cshti0810.pdf. Accessed December 28, 2012.
6. U.S. Department of Justice. Attorney General's annual report to Congress and assessment of U.S. Government activities to combat trafficking in persons, Fiscal Year 2010. Available at http://www.justice.gov/ag/annualreports/tr2010/agreporthumantrafficking2010.pdf. Accessed December 28, 2012.

▓ EXTERNAL DEBT BURDENS AND STRUCTURAL ADJUSTMENT POLICIES

Developing countries suffer the effects of huge external debt. By 2011, for example, 47 heavily indebted poor countries in Africa had a total debt of more than $330 billion.[12] This debt began to grow substantially during the 1970s and 1980s as a result of high interest rates and recessions in developed countries, weak commodity prices, the high price of oil, and domestic factors within these countries, including high trade and budget deficits, low savings rates, poor public sector management, weak economic policies, and protracted civil wars.[13]

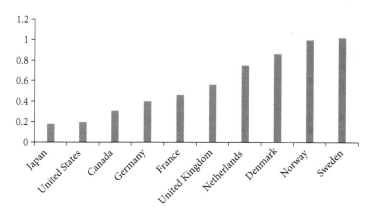

Figure 21–1 Official development assistance as a percentage of gross national income (GNI), in selected countries, preliminary data for 2011. (*Source*: Organization for Economic Co-operation and Development. Net official development assistance from selected OECD members in 2011: Preliminary data for 2011. Available at http://www.oecd.org/dac/aidstatistics/50060310.pdf. Accessed December 18, 2012.)

Structural adjustment policies (SAPs) are economic policies that countries must adopt to qualify for new loans from the World Bank and the International Monetary Fund (IMF) and to receive assistance in repaying previous debts to the World Bank, other governments, and commercial banks. These SAPs often require debtor nations to devalue their currencies against the dollar, lift import and export restrictions, balance their budgets, and remove price controls and state subsidies. This devaluation leads to both these countries' exported goods becoming cheaper for other countries to buy and other countries' imported goods becoming more expensive for these countries to purchase. The IMF encourages affected nations to balance their budgets by reducing government spending, which often leads to sharp reductions in health and other human services, which, in turn, have their most adverse effects on poor people.[14,15]

■ UNREPRESENTATIVE GOVERNMENTS AND CORRUPTION

In many developing countries, the general population has only a limited role in political and economic decisions. In addition, because civil society is disorganized in many developing countries, there are relatively few non-governmental organizations (NGOs)—and those that do exist have less influence on government decisions than NGOs in developed countries. Corruption and mismanagement of resources are widespread in many developing countries, with government officials often using corrupt policies and practices to stay in power and to siphon off funds for their own personal gain. This corruption goes unchecked in many countries where public participation in decision-making is limited and NGOs are weak.

Major sources of corruption in the health sector include contracting and procurement, petty theft, the sale of accreditations or positions, disappearance of public funds, absence of physicians and other health professionals from their government jobs, and the need for *informal payments* (charges for services or supplies that are supposed to be free) by patients or their families to obtain services.[16] For example, a World Bank survey published in 2003 reported that, in 10 of 22 developing countries and countries in transition, the health sector was perceived as being among the top four most corrupt sectors. In this survey, absentee rates among health care workers in several countries was about 30 percent, and the frequency of informal payments by patients or their families for hospital services ranged from 15 to 65 percent.[16]

Some practical elements encountered in the implementation of human rights in developing countries include bad governance and embezzlement of public funds, poverty and underdevelopment, the burden of external debt, the absence of law and order in countries where a civil war is occurring, and the absence of legitimate government or democratic systems based on the protection of human rights.[17] (See Chapter 22.)

▪ ECONOMIC GLOBALIZATION

Economic globalization has benefited some individuals in some developing countries, but it has often undermined governments, social structures, and national cultures. Free-enterprise zones have been established in some developing countries, where low-wage jobs are available, but organization of workers into labor unions is restricted or prohibited, and many occupational health and safety problems exist. Often, very hazardous industries have flourished in these zones. (See Box 19–1 in Chapter 19.)

▪ IMPACT OF SOCIAL INJUSTICE ON PUBLIC HEALTH IN DEVELOPING COUNTRIES

Endemic and Epidemic Diseases

Life expectancy is significantly lower in developing countries[3] (Table 21–4). While infectious diseases, such as lower respiratory infections, diarrheal diseases, HIV/AIDS, malaria, and tuberculosis, continue to account for a substantial proportion of deaths in low-income countries (Chapter 13), ischemic heart disease and cerebrovascular disease are among the 10 leading causes of death[18] (Figure 21–2 and Chapter 15). HIV/AIDS has had, and continues to have, a catastrophic impact on developing countries; for example, in 2012, there were about 23 million people living with HIV/AIDS in sub-Saharan Africa, accounting for approximately 69 percent of all people living with HIV/AIDS in the world.[19] A similar percentage of all AIDS deaths globally occur in sub-Saharan Africa. In addition, depression and other mental disorders are widespread and people who suffer from them are typically stigmatized. (See Chapter 16.)

TABLE 21–4 *Years of Life Expectancy at Birth, Males and Females, in Selected Developing Countries and, for Comparison, the United States, 2010*

Country	Males	Females
Afghanistan	48	48
Guatemala	67	74
Haiti	61	63
Iraq	65	72
Kenya	55	58
Pakistan	64	66
Peru	71	76
Sierra Leone	47	48
South Africa	51	53
Vietnam	73	77
United States	76	81

Source: The World Bank. World development indicators. Washington, DC: The World Bank. Available at data.worldbank.org/indicator/. Accessed December 17, 2012.

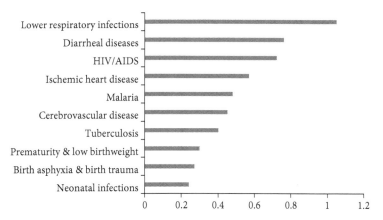

Figure 21-2 The 10 leading causes of death in low-income countries, in millions of deaths by cause, 2008. (*Source*: World Health Organization. Fact sheet: The top ten causes of death. 2011. Available at http://www.who.int/mediacentre/factsheets/fs310_2008.pdf. Accessed December 18, 2012.)

Social injustice has a profoundly negative impact on children's health, leading to much malnutrition, illness, and premature death that could otherwise be prevented. Three-fourths of all child deaths are primarily due to preventable causes: neonatal conditions, pneumonia, diarrhea, malaria, and measles.[20] Malnutrition contributes to high rates of childhood mortality, as a result of dietary deficiencies of protein, energy, and micronutrients; it also inhibits children's ability to fight infection and adversely affects their physical and mental development[21] (Table 21-5, Box 21-2, and Chapters 5 and 14).

Inadequate prenatal and maternity care accounts for poor birth outcomes, including high infant mortality rates from perinatal conditions and high maternal

TABLE 21-5 *Infant Mortality Rate (Infant Deaths per 1000 Live Births), Under-5 Mortality Rate (Deaths per 1000 Children), and Under-5 Malnutrition Prevalence, in Selected Developing Countries and, for Comparison, the United States, 2011*

Country	Infant Mortality Rate (2011)	Under-5 Mortality Rate (2011)	Under-5 Malnutrition Prevalence, based on weight for age (year)
Afghanistan	73	101	NA
Guatemala	25	30	13% (2009)
Haiti	68	70	NA
Iraq	31	38	NA
Kenya	50	73	16% (2009)
Pakistan	60	72	31% (2011)
Peru	15	18	5% (2008)
Sierra Leone	121	185	21% (2008)
South Africa	36	47	9% (2008)
Vietnam	18	22	20% (2008)
United States	7	8	NA

Source: The World Bank. World development indicators. Washington, DC: The World Bank. Available at data.worldbank.org/indicator/. Accessed December 17, 2012.

BOX 21-2 ■ Hunger and Malnutrition in Developing Countries

The United Nations Food and Agriculture Organization (FAO) estimated that the number of hungry (chronically undernourished) people globally in 2006–2008 was approximately 850 million, and in 2010–2012 approximately 870 million—almost all in developing countries.[1] Even if the Millennium Development Goal of halving, between 2000 and 2015, the number of people who suffer from hunger were achieved, there would still be about 600 million undernourished people in developing countries.[1] (See Chapter 14.)

Several factors have accounted for the continuing—and increasing—large numbers of hungry and undernourished people, including high food prices and volatility of food prices, food losses (especially in post-harvest processing), rapid population growth, inadequacy of social safety nets, prolonged drought in some areas and more frequent extreme weather events, and growth in the production and use of biofuels that reduces available land to grow food crops. Discrimination against women (Chapter 4) has been an important contributing factor leading to less education and literacy, less paid employment and lower income, and malnutrition during pregnancy and breastfeeding. The underlying cause of much hunger in the world is the lack of political will to adequately address this problem.[1]

Poor health, such as from HIV/AIDS, contributes to hunger and malnutrition in several ways. HIV/AIDS victims often die in young adulthood, when they could be highly productive agricultural workers. Their surviving relatives are often too young or too old to have the strength, resources, and ability to grow enough food to survive. These survivors often migrate from rural to urban areas, where their risks of HIV/AIDS are usually increased.

Approaches to addressing hunger and malnutrition in developing countries include:

- Long-term investment in the agricultural sector that respects human rights, benefits local communities, promotes food security and environmental sustainability, and helps them adapt to and to mitigate the consequences of climate change
- Improvement of social safety nets to reduce short-term food insecurity and its consequences
- Promotion of cost-effective irrigation, improved land management, and research to develop better seeds
- Promotion of education, job training, and employment opportunities for women and protection of their rights
- Provision of health services for malnourished mothers and children
- And, perhaps most important, the development of the political will to reduce, and ultimately eliminate, hunger

Box Reference

1. Food and Agriculture Organization. The state of food insecurity in the world 2012. Rome: FAO, 2012.

TABLE 21-6 *Percentage of Low Birthweight Infants, Percentage of Births Attended by Skilled Health Staff, and Maternal Mortality Ratio (Maternal Deaths per 100,000 Live Births, Modeled Estimates), in Selected Developing Countries and, for Comparison, the United States*

Country	Percentage of Low Birthweight Babies, as a percentage of all births (year)	Percentage of Births Attended by Skilled Staff (year)	Maternal Mortality Ratio (2010)
Afghanistan	NA	24% (2008)	460
Guatemala	11% (2009)	51% (2009)	120
Haiti	NA	NA	350
Iraq	NA	80% (2007)	63
Kenya	8% (2009)	44% (2009)	360
Pakistan	32% (2007)	39% (2007)	260
Peru	8% (2007)	84% (2010)	67
Sierra Leone	14% (2008)	42% (2008)	890
South Africa	NA	NA	300
Vietnam	5% (2009)	NA	59
United States	NA	NA	21

Source: The World Bank. World development indicators. Washington, DC: The World Bank. Available at data.worldbank.org/indicator/. Accessed December 17, 2012.

mortality ratios[3] (Table 21-6). Childhood immunization rates, while increasing, are still lower in developing countries than in developed countries. Measles, pertussis, and tetanus still account for thousands of childhood deaths in developing countries.

Access to Adequate Medical Care and Public Health Services

People in developing countries generally have inadequate access to effective medical care and public health services.[22] Many governments in developing countries spend less than the equivalent of US$5 per capita on health. Facilities, equipment and supplies, and human resources are grossly inadequate. And the numbers of physicians, nurses, midwives, dentists, and pharmacists are inadequate in many developing countries. For example, in Afghanistan, there are about 21 physicians per 100,000 population; in Pakistan, about 81; and in Sierra Leone, about 2—compared with 242 in the United States.[23] In Afghanistan, there are about 50 nurses and midwives per 100,000 population; in Pakistan, about 56; and in Sierra Leone, about 17—compared with 982 in the United States.[23] (WHO recommends a minimum of 20 physicians and 100 nurses per 100,000 population.)

Greater Impact on Poor People

Throughout developing countries, there are serious inequalities in health status and health care. The poorest women and children face the greatest risks to their health, and they are far less likely to use necessary health services than richer people. For example:

- Poorer women have more children and have them earlier in their lives.
- The poorest adolescents aged 15 to 19 are three times more likely to give birth than are the richest in this age group.
- The poorest children are three times more likely to be stunted (low height-for-age) and twice as likely to die as the richest children.
- The poorest women are twice as likely to be malnourished, one-fourth as likely to use contraceptives, and one-fifth as likely to have medically trained assistants present during labor and delivery.[24]
- In developing countries, poor people generally lack almost all of the factors necessary for good health, such as education, knowledge related to health, nutrition, and access to health services. For example, the poorest women are, on average, one-ninth as likely to have a fifth-grade or higher education compared with the richest women.[24]

Environmental Health Issues

Developing countries face a wide range of environmental health issues.[25] Water contamination with microorganisms and toxic chemicals, such as pesticides, occurs frequently in developing countries. Approximately 900 million people globally, mainly in developing countries, lack access to an *improved water supply*, such as a household connection to a water supply, a protected deep well or spring, or a rainwater collection system.[26] About 2.6 billion people lack access to *improved sanitation*, such as a connection to a public sewer or septic system or a pour-flush, simple-pit, or ventilated improved-pit latrine.[26] Water contamination with microorganisms contributes to much diarrheal disease and to many of the approximately 4000 deaths that occur daily due to diarrheal disease, the vast majority of which occur in developing countries.[27] Exposure to heavy metals, such as lead, represents another significant environmental hazard, especially to children.[28] Climate change is likely to increase vector-borne disease, heat-related disorders, food and water shortages, flooding, and extreme weather in developing countries—with adverse effects on health.[29,30] (See Chapter 18.)

Living Conditions

Relatively few people in developing countries have access to adequate housing. Although most people in developing countries live in rural areas, many people live in urban slums (Figure 21–3). Often, young men leave their wives and children behind in rural areas as they seek jobs in cities. In urban slums, housing is typically overcrowded and often lacks safe water and sanitation.[31] Within developing countries, millions of people are internally displaced, often

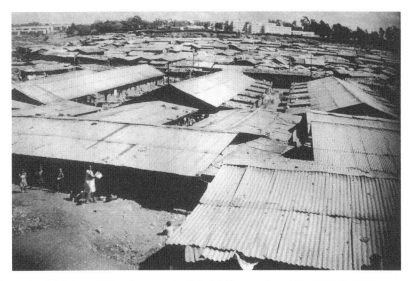

Figure 21-3 Mathare Valley slum area in Nairobi, Kenya, pictured in 1989. In 2013, approximately 600,000 people lived in this 3-square-mile area in crowded housing with no electricity and little running water. (Photograph by Barry S. Levy.)

due to civil war in their countries or neighboring countries; their basic needs are usually not met. In addition, about 11 million refugees—the vast majority from developing countries—have left their homes seeking political or economic asylum elsewhere. (See Chapter 11.)

Occupational Health and Safety Issues

Many developing countries face serious problems in occupational health and safety (Chapter 19).[32,33] These problems reflect their lower level of industrial development and their import of hazardous substances, such as pesticides, from developed countries (Figure 21-4 and Box 21-3). Many countries are in such need of economic development and "hard cash" to pay off their external debt that they are willing to establish or import hazardous industries. Similarly, many people in developing countries are so desperate for work that they are willing to take unsafe and hazardous jobs. In addition, these countries have less infrastructure for diagnosing, treating, and preventing occupationally-related illnesses and injuries and fewer workplace health and safety laws and regulations—that are less stringently enforced.[34]

Violence

Many people in developing countries face the consequences of war and other forms of armed conflict, especially civil wars, which continue in several

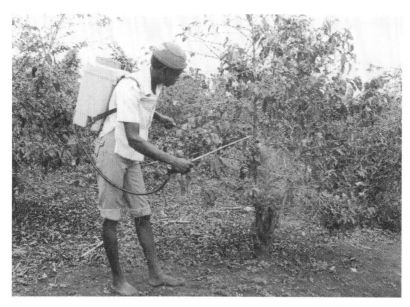

Figure 21-4 Pesticide applicator in Kenya. Workers in developing countries are often exposed to pesticides that have been banned or restricted for use in developed countries, where these pesticides are manufactured. This worker was exposed, both by inhalation and skin absorption, to captafol, a fungicide that was banned in the United States and in the United Kingdom, where it was produced. (Photograph by Barry S. Levy.)

developing countries.[35] War not only causes immediate morbidity and mortality, but also leads to long-term physical and mental health consequences among survivors and their families. War causes widespread damage to the health-supporting infrastructure and environment. War forcibly displaces people from their homes and communities. War violates human rights. War—and the preparation for war—sap economic, human, and other resources that could otherwise be used for health and human services. Domestic and community violence, often byproducts of war, continue to take a heavy toll, especially in developing countries. (See Box 17-1 in Chapter 17.) The import of arms, both legally and illegally, into developing countries exacerbates violence. (See Box 17-2 in Chapter 17.)

▪ WHAT NEEDS TO BE DONE

The Millennium Development Goals provide a framework for addressing the problems discussed in this chapter. (See Table 21-7 and Chapter 29.) A multisectoral approach to achieving these goals is needed, in which health professionals and others can play important roles.

BOX 21-3 ■ **Export of Hazardous Substances from Developed Countries to Developing Countries**

The export of hazardous substances, hazardous waste, and even entire hazardous industries from developed to developing countries represents a major challenge to social justice and public health. Tobacco and pesticides are among the hazardous substances most frequently exported from developed to developing countries.

Tobacco

There are more than 1 billion smokers globally, with about 800 million living in developing countries. Large multinational tobacco companies that are based in the United States and Great Britain are mainly responsible for increased smoking in developing countries. Almost three-fourths of all tobacco is grown in developing countries. Multinational tobacco companies exploit developing countries in several ways. They make loans to small farmers, often trapping them in a cycle of debt. Tobacco production contributes to deforestation, erosion, and desertification. Multinational tobacco companies have often strengthened their presence in developing countries by becoming involved in their economies and communities, such as by building schools and hospitals, which has enabled tobacco companies to have a presence in educational and health facilities. As a result, many developing countries are likely to look favorably on the tobacco industry.[1]

By 2030, tobacco is anticipated to be the single largest cause of death globally, accounting for about 8 million deaths a year. In some countries, tobacco consumption has a direct impact on the health of poor households, with some poor people spending less on food, which may result in malnutrition of children. Poor people who are smokers could each add more than 500 calories daily to the diet of one or two children if they stopped smoking.

An important step toward controlling tobacco globally is the World Health Organization's Framework Convention on Tobacco Control (FCTC). Adopted by the World Health Assembly in 2003 and in force since 2005, this international treaty is legally binding in 176 countries. It addresses issues of tobacco advertising and promotion, agricultural diversification, smuggling, taxes, and subsidies.[2] It focuses on the dangers of tobacco and on limiting its use, with regulations on production, sale, distribution, advertising, and taxation of tobacco. Much more progress is needed. Less than 11 percent of the global population is protected by comprehensive national smoke-free laws, and national comprehensive health-care services supporting smoking cessation are present in only 19 countries, in which only 14 percent of the global population lives.

Pesticides

The export of banned and restricted pesticides from the United States and other developed countries to developing countries accounts for much unnecessary illness and death. During 2001–2003, the United States exported 1.7 billion pounds of pesticide products—28 million pounds of which were pesticide products whose use was forbidden in the United States and more than 500 million pounds of which were pesticides that are known or suspected causes of cancer.[3]

Although there has been a decline in the export of hazardous pesticides from developed to developing countries, this export continues. In developing countries, many agricultural workers who are women and children are exposed to these pesticides, some of which can cause cancer and adverse reproductive effects.[4] Several international measures have contributed to the decline in the export of hazardous pesticides, such as the Stockholm Convention on Persistent Organic Pollutants, which was signed in 2001 and went into force in 2004.[5] As of late 2012, there were 178 states parties to the Convention. The primary goal of this treaty is to eliminate or restrict the production and use of persistent organic pollutants (POPs), by requiring developed countries to provide new and additional financial resources and measures to eliminate production and use of intentionally produced POPs, eliminate unintentionally produced POPs wherever possible, and manage and dispose of wastes from POPs in ways that are environmentally sound. The Convention initially addressed 12 chemicals: aldrin, chlordane, dieldrin, endrin, heptachlor, hexachlorobenzene, mirex, toxaphene, polychlorinated biphenyls (PCBs), DDT, dioxins, and polychlorinated dibenzofurans. However, it specifically allows the use of DDT to control the mosquitoes that transmit malaria.

Box References

1. Action on Smoking and Health. Fact sheet no. 21: Tobacco in the developing world. 2001. Available at http://www.ash.org.uk/html/factsheets/html/fact21.html. Accessed on December 31, 2012.
2. World Health Organization. WHO Framework Convention on Tobacco Control. 2003. Available at http://www.who.int/tobacco/areas/framework/en. Accessed on December 31, 2012.
3. Smith C, Kerr K, Sadripour A. Pesticide exports from U.S. ports, 2001–2003.*Int J Occup Environ Health* 2008;14:176–186.
4. Levy BS, Levin JL, Teitelbaum DT, eds. DBCP-induced sterility and reduced fertility among men in developing countries: A case study of the export of a known hazard. *Int J Occup Environ Health* 1999;5:115–153.
5. Stockholm Convention on Persistent Organic Pollutants. 2004. Available at http://chm. pops.int. Accessed on December 31, 2012.

Promoting Approaches That Focus on Poor People

Resources should be directed to areas of greatest need. Measures that focus on poor people include:

- Adopting policies in education, labor, and primary health care that promote the flow of benefits of growth and development to poor people
- Investing in education to decrease health inequalities by enabling people to obtain better and safer jobs, improve health literacy, take preventive measures, avoid risky behaviors, and demand higher quality health services
- Directing programs toward the health problems and residential environments of poor people
- Providing all people with a basic package of cost-effective health services
- Increasing and improving primary care facilities and services
- Developing partnerships between governments and NGOs

TABLE 21-7 *Millennium Development Goals (1990–2015)*

Goal 1: *Eradicate extreme poverty and hunger*
Target 1.A: Halve the proportion of people whose income is less than $1 a day
Target 1.B: Achieve full and productive employment and decent work for all, including women and young people
Target 1.C: Halve the proportion of people who suffer from hunger
Goal 2: *Achieve universal primary education*
Target 2.A: Ensure that children everywhere, boys and girls alike, will be able to complete a full course of primary schooling
Goal 3: *Promote gender equality and empower women*
Target 3.A: Eliminate gender disparity in primary and secondary education and in all levels of education
Goal 4: *Reduce child mortality*
Target 4.A: Reduce by two-thirds the under-5 mortality rate
Goal 5: *Improve maternal and reproductive health*
Target 5.A: Reduce by three-quarters the maternal mortality ratio
Target 5.B: Achieve universal access to reproductive health
Goal 6: *Combat HIV/AIDS, malaria, and other diseases*
Target 6.A: Halt and begin to reverse the spread of HIV/AIDS
Target 6.B: Achieve universal access to treatment for HIV/AIDS for all those who need it
Target 6.C: Halt and begin to reverse the incidence of malaria and other major diseases
Goal 7: *Ensure environmental sustainability*
Target 7.A: Integrate the principles of sustainable development into country policies and programs and reverse the loss of environmental resources
Target 7.B: Reverse biodiversity loss, achieving a significant reduction in the rate of loss
Target 7.C: Halve the proportion of the population without sustainable access to safe drinking water and basic sanitation
Target 7.D: By 2020, achieve a significant improvement in the lives of at least 100 million slum dwellers
Goal 8: *Develop a global partnership for development*
Target 8.A: Develop further an open, rule-based, predictable, non-discriminatory trading and financial system
Target 8.B: Address the special needs of least-developed countries
Target 8.C: Address the special needs of landlocked developing countries and small-island developing states
Target 8.D.: Deal comprehensively with the debt problems of developing countries
Target 8.E: In cooperation with pharmaceutical companies, provide access to affordable essential drugs in developing countries
Target 8.F: In cooperation with the private sector, make available benefits of new technologies, especially information and communications

---

Source: The United Nations. Millennium Development Goals. Available at www.un.org/millenniumgoals/. Accessed December 18, 2012.

- Mobilizing community resources, including training community-based health workers, involving traditional healers, and ensuring that services are provided at the local level (see Box 24–1 in Chapter 24)
- Establishing prepayment for health care through taxes or insurance, based on people's ability to pay[36]

Promoting and providing microcredit programs for the poorest of poor people is extremely important. Microcredit, the extension of small loans to entrepreneurs too poor to qualify for traditional bank loans, is an effective and popular measure in reducing poverty. For example, the Grameen Bank Project, established in

1976 in Bangladesh, has lent over $8 billion to more than 8 million borrowers, of whom 97 percent are women. The Bank, which has over 2500 branches in almost 80,000 villages, has a loan recovery rate of almost 97 percent. Loans have been made not only for small enterprises, but also for housing and education, enabling many extremely poor people to substantially improve their lives. The Grameen system, which promotes credit as a human right, is not based on any collateral in contracts; it is based on trust. It provides service where poor people live, based on the principle that people should not have to go to the bank; rather the bank should go to the people. The Grameen system believes that (a) poverty is not created by poor people, but rather by the institutions and policies that surround poor people; and (b) in order to reduce poverty, it is necessary to make appropriate changes in the institutions and policies and to develop new ones.[37]

Promoting and Protecting Human Rights and Reducing Discrimination and Its Impact

Human rights—especially for indigenous people, as well as women, children, older people, and other vulnerable populations—need to be promoted and pro-tected.[38] The Universal Declaration of Human Rights (Appendix to Chapter 1) provides a strong foundation for these initiatives.[39] The United Nations and its component agencies and committees play a vital role in building global part-nerships for human rights, preventing human rights violations, responding to emergencies, promoting human rights along with democracy and development as guiding principles for lasting peace, and strengthening the United Nations Human Rights Program.[40]

Human rights are monitored for six international treaties: the International Covenant on Civil and Political Rights; the International Covenant on Economic, Social, and Cultural Rights; and international conventions concerning racial dis-crimination, discrimination against women, the rights of children, and torture and other cruel, inhumane, or degrading treatment or punishment.[40] The work of the United Nations and individual countries for promoting and protecting human rights depends on a global network of partnerships, with NGOs and other repre-sentatives of civil society, such as academic institutions and citizens' groups, play-ing critically important roles. (See also Chapter 22.)

Many specific suggestions have been made to improve respect for human rights in developing countries, including:

- Improving democratic institutions and the rule of law
- Establishing massive campaigns to explain human rights to the general pub-lic and policymakers
- Identifying areas where rapid progress can be made
- Establishing free legal procedures concerning human rights in the context of elections

- Increasing development assistance and making it more effective
- Strengthening national and international mechanisms for the protection of human rights

Much needs to be done to reduce discrimination and its impact. For example, to address discrimination against women and its adverse effect on health, the World Bank recommends a package of essential health services for women, including:

- Prevention and management of unwanted pregnancies
- Provision of safe pregnancy and delivery services
- Prevention and management of sexually transmitted infections
- Promotion of positive health practices, such as public education and individual counseling to encourage delayed childbearing, safe sex, and adequate nutrition
- Prevention of practices harmful to health, such as gender discrimination, domestic violence, rape, and female genital mutilation[41]

In addition, the World Bank recommends a wider choice of family planning methods, nutrition assistance for women before and beyond reproductive age, cervical and breast cancer screening and treatment, and greater attention to the health problems of women beyond reproductive age.[41] (See Chapter 4.)

Improving Health Care Systems

Health care systems in developing countries are critically important for reducing social injustice and its impact on health. New facilities need to be developed to widen access to medical care.

More professionals need to be trained—not only physicians, but also nurses, physician's assistants, nurse-midwives, community health workers, and other health personnel. Incentives need to be strengthened to encourage these health professionals to serve where they are most needed. In addition, policies need to be designed and implemented to encourage health professionals who train abroad to return to their home countries. Discriminatory practices in medical care need to be eliminated so that all people have adequate access to medical care. In addition, there needs to be a greater emphasis on prevention—not only clinical preventive services that are designed to detect and treat disease at an early stage, but also community-based public health services to improve individual and community health. In addition, capabilities in developing countries need to be improved for manufacturing essential medicines, including antiretroviral drugs to treat HIV/AIDS.

Improving Education and Health Literacy

Because literacy and educational status are so closely linked to health status, access to and quality of education in developing countries must be improved. So must *health literacy*, the ability of people "to obtain, process, and understand basic health information and services needed to make appropriate health decisions."[42] As a result of low health literacy, people lack knowledge about medical care and medical conditions, do not understand or use preventive services, and have poorer health status.[43] Health literacy can be improved by improving the readability of health education materials and medical care information, and by training health care providers.

Increasing Foreign Assistance

Increased foreign assistance from developed countries can provide critically important financial and human resources to reduce social injustice and improve health in developing countries. Foreign assistance should promote sustainable policies and programs that rely on local resources, and promote policies and programs that are culturally, politically, and socioeconomically appropriate. Health professionals and others need to enable government officials and the general public in developed countries to recognize that it is in their enlightened self-interest to provide adequate financial assistance to developing countries.

Reducing the Export of Hazards from Developed to Developing Countries

Development and enforcement of international treaties and other agreements can do much to reduce the import of hazardous products and wastes and industries that are hazardous. The agreements of the World Health Assembly on the international tobacco trade[44] and on persistent organic pollutants (POPs), which initially targeted elimination of 12 toxic chemicals,[45] provide excellent models for restricting exports of hazardous substances from developed to developing countries.

Preventing War and Other Forms of Violence

The potential for war and other forms of violence can be minimized by reducing the international arms trade; promoting nonviolent means of conflict resolution; strengthening international treaties and conventions concerning antipersonnel landmines as well as nuclear, chemical, and biological weapons[46]; and promoting a culture of peace. A reduced potential for war would likely decrease military expenditures, which drain scarce financial and human resources—an especially tragic situation in many developing countries. (See Boxes 17–1 and 17–2 in Chapter 17.)

Promoting Representative Government and Reducing corruption

Policies and programs must be developed to promote more representative governments in developing countries that are accountable to the populations they serve. Public participation needs to be improved in many ways. The United

Nations Development Program is playing an important role in promoting democratic governance by strengthening parliamentary oversight, representation, and law-making; electoral systems and processes; access to justice and human rights; access to information; local government; and public administration and civil service.[47] In addition, NGOs need to be strengthened so they can influence decisions at all levels of government and help to reduce corruption in government. Various remedies have been proposed to reduce corruption in developing countries and its adverse effect on health, including implementing anticorruption policies, promoting a culture of public service, adopting and enforcing procurement and contracting rules, adopting public standards of conduct and oversight, improving the public management of health services, and appropriately compensating health care providers for their work. Fiscal oversight—with enforcement of penalties for unlawful practices—needs to be improved.[16]

Changing International Economic Policies

International lending institutions, including the World Bank, need to continue to reduce the debt burden on developing countries, which restricts their ability to promote sustainable human development.[48] Governments relieved of external debt will have substantially more money to support delivery of needed health services. In addition, structural adjustment policies by the World Bank and the IMF, which decrease health and other human services, need to be modified or eliminated.

Developed countries need to reduce their import tariffs that make it difficult or impossible for farmers and others in developing countries to sell their crops or other products in the United States and other developed countries. These tariffs have been disastrous in many developing countries, such as by preventing farmers and others from fairly competing in world markets. Measures by developed countries to reduce tariffs would help reduce poverty and improve health in developing countries.

Promoting Sustainable Development

Reducing social injustice and resultant poor health in developing countries requires sustained economic growth to increase productivity and income in these countries. (See Chapter 29.) However, development involves more than economic growth. Sustainable development also requires attention to environmental and social issues. As stated in *Sustainable Development in a Dynamic World: Transforming Institutions, Growth, and Quality of Life*, a World Development Report of the World Bank:

> Lack of assets, opportunity and effective voice for large segments of the population blocks the emergence of general welfare-enhancing policies, impedes growth and

undermines the potential for positive change. At the national level, it robs us of the talents of those left out in society. And at the international level, it deprives us of the contribution poor countries can make to a more just and sustainable future. A more sustainable development path is more socially inclusive. It enables societies to transform and solve collective problems. The challenge, now and in the future, is to develop the courage and commitment to manage the processes that underpin human life and well-being and to bring about a transformation that improves the quality of the environment, strengthens our social fabric, and enhances the quality of people's lives. The more people heard, the less assets wasted.[49]

■ CONCLUSION

There is much to be done to ensure social justice for people in developing countries. Health professionals in both developing and developed countries have important roles to play in education and training, in advocacy for improved national and international policies to promote social justice and to protect human rights, and in consultation and technical assistance to reduce social injustice in these countries and to minimize its health consequences. Social justice in developed countries cannot be achieved until it is also achieved in developing countries.

■ REFERENCES

1. World Health Organization. The World Health Report 2003: Shaping the future. Geneva: WHO, 2003.
2. World Health Organization. Global Health Observatory: World health statistics 2012.Geneva: WHO, 2012. Available at http://www.who.int/gho/publications/world-health-statistics/2012/en/. Accessed January 1, 2013.
3. The World Bank. World development indicators. Washington, DC: The World Bank. Available at data.worldbank.org/indicator/. Accessed December 17, 2012.
4. Sarin R. Rich–poor divide growing. In: The Worldwatch Institute. Vital signs 2003: The trends that are shaping our future. New York: W.W. Norton & Company, 2003:88–89.
5. The World Bank. Poverty reduction & equity: Poverty. Washington, DC: The World Bank. Available at http://web.worldbank.org. Accessed January 1, 2013.
6. Physicians for Human Rights. An action plan to prevent brain drain: Building equitable health systems in Africa (a report by Physicians for Human Rights).Boston: Physicians for Human Rights, 2004.
7. Hagopian A, Thompson MJ, Fordycel M, et al. The migration of physicians from sub-Saharan Africa to the United States: Measures of the African brain drain. *Human Resources for Health* 2004;2:17.
8. Power S. "A problem from hell": America and the age of genocide. New York: Basic Books, 2002.
9. Mann JM, Gruskin S, Grodin MA, Annas GJ, eds. Health and human rights: A reader. New York: Routledge, 1999.

10. World Health Organization. Maternal mortality: Fact sheet no. 348. Geneva: WHO, 2012. Available at http://www.int/mediacentre/factsheet/fs345/en/index.html. Accessed January 1, 2013.

11. Organization for Economic Cooperation and Development. Net official development assistance from DAC and other OECD members in 2011: Preliminary data for 2011. Available at http://www.oecd.org/dac/aidstatistics/50060310.pdf. Accessed December 18, 2012.

12. U.S. Central Intelligence Agency. The World Factbook. Available at https://www.cia.gov/library/publications/the-world-factbook/rankorder/2079rank.html. Accessed December 18, 2012.

13. International Monetary Fund Staff. The logic of debt relief for the poorest countries. Washington, DC: International Monetary Fund, 2000. Available at http://www.imf.org/external/np/exr/ib/2000/092300.htm. Accessed December 17, 2012.

14. The Whirled Bank Group. Structural adjustment program. 2003 Available at http://www.whirledbank.org/development/sap.html. Accessed December 17, 2012.

15. Shah A. Structural adjustment: A major cause of poverty, November 28, 2010. Available at http://www.globalissues.org/article/3/structural-adjustment-a-major-cause-of-poverty. Accessed December 17, 2012.

16. Lewis M. Corruption and health in developing and transition economies. Eleventh International Anticorruption Conference, Seoul, Republic of Korea, May 25–28, 2003.

17. Kobila JM. Comparative practice on human rights: North–South. In: Coicaud JM, Doyle MW, Gardner AM, eds. The globalization of human rights. Tokyo, Japan: United Nations University Press, 2003:89–115.

18. World Health Organization. Fact sheet: The top ten causes of death. 2011. Available at http://www.who.int/mediacentre/factsheets/fs310_2008.pdf. Accessed December 18, 2012.

19. World Health Organization. HIV/AIDS: Fact sheet No. 360, November 2012. Available at http://www.who.int/mediacentre/factsheets/fs360/en/index.html. Accessed March 22, 2013.

20. World Health Organization. Child health epidemiology. 2011.Available at http://www.who.int/maternal_child_adolescent/epidemiology/child/en/index.html. Accessed December 18, 2012.

21. West KP Jr, Caballero B, Black RE. Nutrition. In: Merson MH, Black RE, Mills AJ, eds. International public health: Diseases, programs, systems, and policies. Gaithersburg, MD: Aspen Publishers, 2001:207–291.

22. Mills AJ, Ranson MK. The design of health systems. In: Merson MH, Black RE, Mills AJ, eds. International public health: Diseases, programs, systems, and policies.Gaithersburg, MD: Aspen Publishers, 2001:515–557.

23. World Health Organization. Global Health Observatory Data Repository: Aggregated data: Density per 1000. Available at http://apps.who.int/gho/data/?vid=92100. Accessed December 18, 2012.

24. Population Reference Bureau. The wealth gap in health: Data on women and children in 53 developing countries.Washington, DC: Population Reference Bureau, 2004.

25. Shahi GS, Levy BS, Binger Al, et al, eds. International perspectives on environment, development, and health: Toward a sustainable world. New York: Springer Publishing Company, 1997.

26. UN Water. Drinking water and sanitation. Available at http://www.unwater.org/statistics_san.html. Accessed December 18, 2012.

27. World Health Organization. Diarrhoeal disease. 2009. Available at http://www.who.int/mediacentre/factsheets/fs330/en/index.html. Accessed December 18, 2012.

28. Meyer PA, McGeehin MA, Falk H. A global approach to childhood lead poisoning prevention. *Int J Hyg Environ Health* 2003; 206: 363–369.

29. McMichael AJ, Campbell–Lendrum DH, Corvalan CF, et al, eds. Climate change and human health: Risks and responses. Geneva: World Health Organization, 2003.

30. Shuman EK. Global climate change and infectious diseases. *Int J Occup Environ Med* 2011; 2:11–19.

31. Birn A, Pillay Y, Holtz TH. Textbook of international health: Global health in a dynamic world, 3rd ed. New York: Oxford University Press, 2009.

32. LaDou J. International occupational and environmental health. In: Rom WN, Markowitz SB, eds. Environmental and occupational medicine. 4th ed. Philadelphia: Lippincott Williams & Wilkins, 2007:1720–1735.

33. Levy BS, Wegman DH, Baron SL, Sokas RK, eds. Occupational and environmental health: Recognizing and preventing disease and injury. 6th ed. New York: Oxford University Press, 2011.

34. Heymann J, ed. Global inequalities at work: Work's impact on the health of individuals, families, and societies. Oxford: Oxford University Press, 2003.

35. Levy BS, Sidel VW, eds. War and public health. 2nd ed. New York: Oxford University Press, 2008.

36. Carr D. Improving the health of the world's poorest people (Health bulletin 1). Washington, DC: Population Reference Bureau, 2004.

37. Grameen Bank. Bank for the poor. 2009. Available at http://www.grameen-info.org/index.php?option=com_content&task=view&id=177&Itemid=503. Accessed December 17, 2012.

38. Kim JY, Millen JV, Irwin A et al., eds. Dying for growth: Global inequality and the health of the poor.Monroe, ME: Common Courage Press, 2000.

39. General Assembly, United Nations. The Universal Declaration of Human Rights. New York: United Nations, December 10, 1948.

40. United Nations. A United Nations priority: Human rights in action. New York: United Nations. Available at http://www.un.org/rights/HRToday/action.htm. Accessed December 17, 2012.

41. The World Bank. A new agenda for women's health and nutrition. Washington, DC: The World Bank, 1994.

42. Centers for Disease Control and Prevention. Learn about health literacy. Available at: http://www.cdc.gov/healthliteracy/Learn/. Accessed March 25, 2013.

43. Sorensen K, Van den Broucke S, Fullam J, et al. Health literacy and public health: A systematic review and integration of definitions and models. *BMC Public Health* 2012; 12:80.doi.10.1186/1471–2458–12–80.

44. World Health Organization. WHO Framework Convention on Tobacco Control. 2003. Available at http://www.who.int/tobacco/areas/framework/en/. Accessed December 17, 2012.

45. Stockholm Convention on Persistent Organic Pollutants. 2004. Available at http://chm.pops.int. Accessed on December 31, 2012.

46. Levy BS, Sidel VW, eds. Terrorism and public health: A balanced approach to strengthening systems and protecting people. 2nd ed. New York: Oxford University Press, 2012.

47. United Nations Development Programme. Democratic governance. Available at http://www.undp.org/content/undp/en/home/ourwork/democraticgovernance/overview.html. Accessed December 17, 2012.

48. The World Bank. Global development finance: External debt of developing countries, 2012. Available at: data.worldbank.org/sites/default/files/gdf_2012.pdf. Accessed March 25, 2013.

49. The World Bank. World Development Report 2003. Sustainable development in a dynamic world: Transforming institutions, growth, and quality of life. New York: Oxford University Press, 2003.

PART IV

An Agenda for Action

22 Addressing Social Injustice in a Human Rights Context

■ SOFIA GRUSKIN AND PAULA BRAVEMAN

▓ INTRODUCTION

The violation or neglect of human rights jeopardizes health directly by interfering with physical, mental, and social well-being.[1] In this chapter, we consider the relevance of human rights to public health in three major spheres: (a) as legal standards and obligations of governments, (b) as a conceptual framework for analysis and advocacy, and (c) as guiding principles for designing and implementing policies and programs.

Core Concepts

Human rights are internationally recognized norms and standards that apply equally to people everywhere and that define obligations of governments toward individuals and groups. International human rights law is based on legal agreements to which governments have agreed for the purpose of promoting and protecting these rights. Governments are accountable, as signatories of human rights treaties, to set targets and show good-faith movement toward the full realization of all human rights. Signatory nations are responsible for reporting periodically to the relevant international monitoring bodies on their compliance with human rights treaties.

International human rights law not only prohibits direct violations of rights, but also holds governments responsible for progressively ensuring conditions that enable individuals to realize their rights as fully as possible. Governments are responsible for progressively removing the obstacles to individuals achieving all of their rights, with particular attention to those individuals or groups that have more obstacles to realizing their rights, such as the poor, the marginalized, and the excluded.[1,2]

The term *human rights* within the United States generally calls to mind civil and political rights, such as freedoms of speech, assembly, and religion, as well as freedom from torture or arbitrary arrest. However, human rights norms and agreements also span entitlements that are economic, social, and cultural in nature. This wide scope of human rights has tremendous implications for those committed to social justice.

While it is possible to identify different categories of rights, it is also critical to rights discourse and action to recognize that all rights are interdependent and interrelated, and that individuals rarely suffer from the neglect or violation of one right in isolation. For historical reasons, the rights described in human rights documents were divided into two categories: (a) civil and political rights, including, among others, the rights to liberty, to security of person, to freedom of movement, and to vote; and (b) economic, social, and cultural rights, including, among others, the rights to the highest attainable standard of health, to work, to social security, to adequate food, to clothing, to housing, to education, and to enjoyment of the benefits of scientific progress and its applications. (See also Chapter 27.)

Although the Universal Declaration of Human Rights (1948)[3] contains both categories of rights, these rights were artificially split into two treaties due to Cold War politics, with the United States focusing on civil and political rights and the former Soviet Union mainly focusing on economic, social, and cultural rights. Since the end of the Cold War, the indivisibility and interdependence of rights has again been acknowledged. The Convention on the Rights of the Child (1989),[4] the first human rights treaty to be opened for signature since the end of the Cold War, includes civil, political, economic, and social rights considerations—not only within the same treaty, but also within the same right. (The United States and Somalia remain the only countries not to have ratified the Convention on the Rights of the Child.)

Perhaps the right most relevant to social injustice and public health is the *right to health*, defined as the right to the highest attainable standard of health[5-7]—in practice, that experienced by the most privileged social stratum in a society.[8] The right to health reinforces government responsibility for prevention, treatment, and control of disease and for the creation of conditions necessary to ensure access to health care facilities, goods, and services that are essential for health.[9,10]

However, in addition to the right to health—and of equal importance in pursuing the right to health—are human rights to water; food; shelter; safe working conditions; education; information; participation in social, economic, and political life; and enjoyment of the benefits of scientific progress. Because human rights principles hold that all rights—economic, social, cultural, civil, and political—are interdependent and indivisible, governments are accountable for progressively addressing conditions that may impede not only the realization of the "right to health," but also the realization of related rights.[11] Every country is now party to at least one treaty that addresses health-related rights.[12,13]

The principle of non-discrimination, the overarching principle that cuts across all rights, is of great relevance for social justice. It covers not only explicit or direct discrimination, but also structural discrimination—the discrimination inherent in societal structures that subtly, but systematically, keeps some groups at a disadvantage. Governments can be understood to be obligated to remove barriers, such as linguistic or cultural obstacles, that can (a) discourage groups that have historically experienced discrimination from making appropriate use of health care services or from receiving necessary education, or (b) track marginalized groups into health-damaging jobs and neighborhoods.

▩ HUMAN RIGHTS AS LEGAL STANDARDS AND OBLIGATIONS OF GOVERNMENTS

Human rights and ethical principles related to health are strongly consonant. In particular, equal opportunities to be healthy (distributive justice) and the human rights obligation to remove barriers so that individuals and groups can realize their right to health seem to be closely related. However, human rights instruments provide a unique and powerful contribution for achieving social justice in public health by removing the concerns for improving the health of disadvantaged groups from the voluntary realms of ethics, charity, and solidarity to the realms of law and entitlement.

Human rights standards and legal obligations relevant to social justice are, unfortunately, not being sufficiently fulfilled in many places, demonstrating that the existence of entitlements and laws is not sufficient to guarantee their reality. However, the enforcement of human rights and the effectiveness of accountability mechanisms to ensure human rights could be greatly strengthened if they were used routinely by leaders in public health and other development and social sectors committed to social justice.

Official and unofficial mechanisms now exist to monitor compliance with international and regional human rights norms and standards. At the international level, governments that ratify human rights treaties are obliged to report every several years to the specific body responsible for monitoring government action under a given treaty. They are responsible for demonstrating how they are—or are not—in compliance with treaty provisions. They must show constant improvement in respecting, protecting, and fulfilling specific rights. Each of the treaty bodies meets several times each year to assess the government reports that have been submitted and to provide concluding comments and observations as to what must be improved. There are nine international bodies that monitor human rights treaties monitoring bodies—each corresponding to a major human rights treaty (Table 22–1). In addition, international political bodies of the United Nations, most notably the General Assembly, are charged with following up on agreements made at major summits, such as the Millennium Development Goals (Table 21–7).

All of these bodies have expressed a commitment to exploring government obligations under the treaties for health and for specific issues raised by HIV/AIDS, disabilities, health systems, and reproductive and sexual health. Health-oriented United Nations agencies, such as the World Health Organization (WHO), UNAIDS, and the United Nations Children's Fund (UNICEF), are invited to provide information on the state of health and the performance of health systems in the countries under review. Non-governmental organizations (NGOs) can also submit informal reports—often termed *shadow reports*—providing additional information and stating their views on specific situations and issues. NGOs (such as Amnesty International, Oxfam, the Center for Reproductive Rights, and

TABLE 22-1 *Human Rights Treaties and Their Monitoring Bodies*

Treaty	Monitoring Body
International Convention on the Elimination of All Forms of Racial Discrimination	Committee on the Elimination of All Forms of Racial Discrimination
International Covenant on Economic, Social, and Cultural Rights	Committee on Economic, Social, and Cultural Rights
International Covenant on Civil and Political Rights	Human Rights Committee
International Convention on the Elimination of All Forms of Discrimination Against Women	Committee on the Elimination of All Forms of Discrimination Against Women
Convention Against Torture, and Other Cruel, Inhuman or Degrading Treatment or Punishment	Committee Against Torture
Convention on the Rights of the Child	Committee on the Rights of the Child
International Convention on the Protection of the Rights of All Migrant Workers and Members of Their Families	Committee on the Protection of the Rights of All Migrant Workers and Members of Their Families
Convention on the Rights of Persons with Disabilities	Committee on the Rights of Persons with Disabilities
International Convention for the Protection of All Persons from Enforced Disappearances	Committee on Enforced Disappearances

Physicians for Human Rights) and the news media, through their public statements, also play major, though unofficial, roles in monitoring compliance with human rights norms and agreements.

Nevertheless, these formal mechanisms need to be strengthened. Health workers committed to social justice could play important roles, such as by (a) institutionalizing routine processes to review data on health and health care from a social justice and human rights perspective, using relevant concluding comments and observations of the monitoring bodies to guide their analyses; and (b) using this review to stimulate public debate and consideration by national-level bodies that monitor human rights and/or the implications for health and human rights of government actions.

The recognition of human rights norms as entitlements and legal standards can also be a powerful tool to influence national policies. For example, affirmative action—preferential action in favor of historically disadvantaged or disenfranchised groups, such as racial and ethnic minorities, as well as women—has been a potentially important tool for social justice. Affirmative action has had important implications for health, such as in ensuring a diverse health workforce to serve disadvantaged populations and in focusing attention and resources on reducing health disparities. However, affirmative action in the United States continues to face many legal and other challenges. Reference to human rights principles may be helpful in building consensus for the legitimacy of affirmative action. Particularly relevant are (a) the cross-cutting human rights principle of non-discrimination, and (b) human rights agreements that call for concerted action by governments to remove obstacles for women and marginalized groups, including indigenous peoples.

■ HUMAN RIGHTS AS A CONCEPTUAL FRAMEWORK FOR ANALYSIS AND ADVOCACY

Human rights principles can provide a useful, systematic framework for analyzing health and social justice issues and advocating effectively for social justice in public health. This framework can focus attention on how violations or lack of attention to human rights can have serious health consequences and how the design or implementation of health policies, programs, and practices can promote or violate rights. A human rights focus brings attention not only to the technical and operational aspects of health-related interventions, but also to their civil, political, economic, social, and cultural contexts.[14] For strategies to achieve social justice in public health, human rights principles and standards provide guidance about (a) who should be considered disadvantaged, and (b) the importance of addressing the non-medical, as well as the medical, determinants of health. Human rights norms also provide a framework—and forums—for institutionalizing a social justice perspective in all health-sector actions.

Who is disadvantaged? According to human rights norms, the disadvantaged are those with underlying obstacles affecting their ability to realize all of their rights. A human rights perspective can thus provide a universal frame of reference for identifying social justice concerns. For example, whether a given disparity constitutes an injustice may be a matter of dispute. Privileged groups have, at times, claimed that health disparities adversely affecting the health of, for example, a disenfranchised ethnic group merely reflect different "cultures" or "lifestyles." Privileged groups have claimed that poor people have poorer health because they engage in health-damaging behaviors, such as smoking and eating less-nutritious food; implicitly, privileged groups view these behaviors as entirely freely chosen— rather than shaped by the conditions in which disadvantaged groups live because of their social position. Such a view provides a rationale for not committing more public resources to addressing the conditions in disadvantaged communities that support health-damaging behaviors.

By contrast, human rights norms assert rights to living standards needed for optimal health and expressly prohibit discrimination on the basis of such factors as gender, racial or ethnic group, national origin, religion, disability, sexual orientation, and gender identity. Especially where certain groups, such as women and disenfranchised racial and ethnic groups, are systematically excluded from decision-making, human rights standards can play a crucial role in setting agendas for action by strengthening consensus about the existence of inequities in health and the need to reduce them. For example, in some western European countries during the past 30 years, systematic monitoring and public discussion of socioeconomic inequalities in health have played an important role in building consensus among people in the more-advantaged segments of society about the need to address those inequalities.

As another example, the 2010 Arizona Senate Bill 1070, one of the broadest and strictest anti-immigrant measures in recent U.S. history, has been a source of much controversy due to concerns about racial profiling and unconstitutional detention—each with the potential to drive people away from health services and to violate many other rights. The bill was appealed all the way to the U.S. Supreme Court, in part because of a provision that allows law enforcement officers to demand immigration papers from anyone they suspect of being illegally in the country. (In June 2012, the Supreme Court ruled on the case, *Arizona v. United States*, upholding the provision requiring immigration status checks, but striking down three other provisions as violations of the Supremacy Clause of the U.S. Constitution.) While human rights perspectives were not explicitly invoked in bringing attention to the harmful provision of this bill, we believe that future work on similar issues would be strengthened by explicit reference to human rights principles—and education of the public on these principles and their application. (See Box 22–1.)

Are non-medical determinants of health, including poverty and lack of education, appropriate concerns for health workers who care about social justice? Both social justice principles and human rights principles dictate striving for equal opportunity for health for groups who have experienced discrimination or social marginalization. Achieving equal opportunities for health for all groups in society entails buffering the health-damaging effects of poverty and marginalization by providing health services. But it also includes reducing disparities among groups in the underlying conditions necessary to be healthy, such as access to clean water and sanitation, nutritious food, adequate shelter, education, and a healthful and safe environment. Addressing these underlying determinants of health and health care requires attention to both social justice principles and human rights perspectives. Human rights perspectives provide an especially compelling rationale for government responsibility—not only to provide health services, but also to alter the conditions that create, exacerbate, and perpetuate economic poverty, social and economic deprivation, and marginalization or social exclusion.

Economic poverty—with and without its associated social disadvantages—plays a central role in creating, exacerbating, and perpetuating ill health. Even in the absence of absolute deprivation, relative inequalities in economic resources may have damaging effects on the health of all members of a society—including the most advantaged.[15-19]

Although poverty is not, in and of itself, a violation of human rights, government action or inaction leading to poverty and government failure to adequately address the conditions that create, exacerbate, and perpetuate poverty and marginalization often reflect—or are closely connected with—violations or denials of human rights.[20] For example, lack of access to education, especially primary education, can be understood as both the denial of a right, in and of itself, and inextricably connected with poverty and ill health. Education, which fosters empowerment and participation in informed decisions about health-related behaviors, is crucial

BOX 22-1 ■ Promoting the Rights of "Undocumented Immigrants"

Carmen Rita Nevarez

The history of the United States is a history of immigration. After centuries during which Native Americans alone inhabited much of North America, waves of immigrants came from England, Northern Europe, Southern and Eastern Europe, Latin America, and Asia. In addition, centuries ago, many Africans were brought here forcibly as slaves, followed more recently by many other people coming from Africa. Many immigrants came here from countries where armed conflict, tyrannical government, abject poverty, and absence of human rights protections make life unlivable.

Immigration supports the economic and social growth of the United States. In 2010, for example, the U.S. population included almost 40 million people born in other countries[1]—of whom 44 percent were naturalized citizens, 24 percent, legal permanent residents, 29 percent, unauthorized migrants; and 3 percent, temporary legal residents.[2] By far the largest number of immigrants (12 million) came from Mexico, although, in the past few years, more people may have moved from the United States to Mexico than from Mexico to the United States.[3]

Immigrants come to the United States to work. For example, of the 11.2 million Mexican immigrant men, 94 percent work. And newly arrived immigrants tend to work in hazardous jobs that pay low wages—mostly in service, construction, and agriculture. In the United States, 40 percent of dishwashers, 36 percent of roofers, and 35 percent of gardeners are Mexican immigrant men.[4] In addition, immigrants have a profound impact on business. For example, between 2002 and 2007, Hispanic-owned businesses increased by 44 percent to 2.3 million.[5]

Nevertheless, immigrants repeatedly suffer indignities. They suffer from punitive social policies that drive them further under the radar, and therefore make it difficult to document their plight.

Immigrants understandably fear the intentions of government. State governments have increasingly attempted to establish and enforce laws that violate the civil rights of immigrants and their descendants. Arizona's SB 1070 law flagrantly invites racial profiling against Latinos, Asian Americans, and others who appear foreign by authorizing police to demand citizenship or immigration-status papers from anyone they stop and suspect of being in the United States unlawfully. Alabama, Georgia, Indiana, South Carolina, and Utah have passed similar laws. Although courts have struck down many elements of these laws, finding them to be unconstitutional, these laws have had a chilling impact on immigrants and their communities. This type of legislation is not only unfair and unjust against immigrants, but it also suppresses lawful activity by people who "look like" immigrants and do not wish to be scrutinized because of their appearance.

At the local, state, and national levels, immigrants suffer from fiscal policies that have lowered the quality of public schools. They are often denied voting rights by the intimidation of "voter ID" legislation. And they are denied the benefits of the Patient Protection and Affordable Care Act (ACA). With these policies, the United States is disinvesting in the future of its youth, upon whom older people rely—so their health and well-being may also be at risk.

Public health workers need to understand and address regressive policies that adversely affect immigrants, such as by supporting the DREAM Act.*

Immigrants' children brought to the United States without legal status should not be held accountable for actions of their parents. High-achieving immigrant students should be rewarded with a path to citizenship and should be supported in pursuing higher education. And public health workers should support immigrants' being covered under the ACA.

Immigrants' undocumented status can restrict their job opportunities and lead to lives in poverty, with substandard housing and unhealthful food. And the undocumented status of immigrants can adversely affect their health and population health in many other ways, as illustrated by the following two examples. Immigrants experienced poor working conditions or observed poor sanitation at a meat-packing plant where they worked, but they did not complain or report these problems to government agencies, fearing deportation if they did. In another situation, many stable workers had physical contact with a rabid horse, but declined to receive free injections to prevent rabies.

Because undocumented immigrants often have to disguise their status in many situations, they decline opportunities to protect their own health—and in so doing, threaten the health of others. Public health workers should approach these situations with much care and sensitivity. They should acknowledge the courage of these immigrants to live under conditions in which they daily face the risk of being uprooted from family and friends. When addressing the health risks of immigrants, they should assure immigrants that their goal is only to protect their health and the health of others—sometimes by enlisting the support of respected community members or friends. In situations where legal action may be necessary, such as in treating a recalcitrant patient with multiple-drug-resistant tuberculosis, they should seek the advice of an attorney sympathetic to and expert in immigration issues. Public health workers should scrupulously protect the confidentiality of immigrants. They should perform case-finding activities, when necessary, with personal respect, while pointing out that this work supports not only individual health, but family and community health as well.

Public health workers, who are committed to assuring the conditions in which all people can be healthy, have a civic and moral obligation to support policies and programs that enable immigrants to contribute and to fully participate in society.

Box References

1. Grieco E, Acosta YD, de la Cruz GP, et al. The foreign-born population in the United States: 2010: American community survey reports. *United States Census Bureau*, May 2012. Available at http://www.census.gov/prod/2012pubs/acs-19.pdf. Accessed December 3, 2012.
2. Motel, S. Statistical portrait of the foreign-born population in the United States, 2010. *Pew Research Center*, February 21, 2012. Available at http://www.pewhispanic.org/2012/02/21/statistical-portrait-of-hispanics-in-the-united-states-2010/. Accessed December 3, 2012.
3. Passal J, Cohn D, Gonzalez-Barrera A. Net migration from Mexico falls to zero—and perhaps less. *Pew Research Center*, May 3, 2012. Available at http://www.pewhispanic.

* The Development, Relief, and Education for Alien Minors Act, which was first proposed in the U.S. Senate in 2001, and, if passed, would provide conditional permanent residency to some undocumented residents of good moral character who graduated from high schools in the United States, arrived in the country as minors, and lived in the United States continuously for at least 5 years before the passage of the Act.

org/2012/04/23/net-migration-from-mexico-falls-to-zero-and-perhaps-less/?src=prc-headli
ne. Accessed December 3, 2012.
4. Health Initiative of the Americas, the University of California, and the California
Endowment. Migration work & health: The facts behind the myths. Los Angeles:
University of California, Berkeley, 2007. Available at http://www.ailadownloads.org/advo/
UniversityOfCalifornia-MigrationHealth.pdf. Accessed December 3, 2012.
5. United States Census Bureau. Census Bureau reports Hispanic-owned businesses increase
at more than double the national rate. September 21, 2010. Available at http://www.census.
gov/newsroom/releases/archives/business_ownership/cb10–145.html. Accessed December
3, 2012.

to breaking the poverty–ill health cycle. Health workers can play an important
role in advocating for policies to improve education and to eliminate poverty by
addressing the health implications of these policies.

▓ AN AGENDA FOR ACTION

Integrating Social Justice and Human Rights in All Health-Sector Actions

Most public health work is intended to benefit entire populations—but often it
is targeted to especially benefit the disadvantaged; however, a strategic approach
is necessary to overcome the tendency for poor or marginalized people to benefit too little from even the best-intentioned activities.[19,21] Work on social justice and human rights must be integrated as an ongoing priority—not as an
afterthought—in all health-sector actions. This approach will require the use
of simple, practical tools that health workers perceive as helpful to their work,
as well as training and ongoing support.[22,23] Presenting social justice principles
within a human rights framework could reinforce their importance, in part by
showing that they reflect a broad global consensus. Social justice principles and
human rights norms should routinely be used to frame discussions on assessments of health disparities. And these assessments should then be presented in
forums for monitoring of human rights.

Monitoring Social Justice and Human Rights Implications of Policies That Affect Health

Using human rights norms, routine assessment of potential health implications
for people in different social strata should become standard practice in the
design, implementation, and evaluation of all development policies that could
conceivably affect health—not only policies within the health sector.[24] Social
justice and human rights principles suggest that routinely collected population
data on health—and on health care and other determinants of health—should

be disaggregated by degree of social advantage. For example, relevant data should be analyzed by gender, race, ethnicity, income, education, and other factors that reflect social position. Without monitoring, there is no accountability for the potentially different impact of policies on population groups with different degrees of social disadvantage.[8,25,26] The fact that most societies have far less tolerance for social disparities in health than for disparities in wealth or other social privileges can provide health workers with opportunities to influence public opinion and mobilize public action.[27]

Strengthening Arguments and Building Public Consensus for Achieving Equitable Financing of Health Care

Equitable financing means that those with the least resources pay the least, both in absolute terms and as a proportion of their total resources. It also means that lack of personal resources does not restrict an individual from receiving needed services that are recommended on the basis of prevailing norms and scientific knowledge. Equitable financing would increase access to health care, which—if health care services are effective—should improve people's health and, thus, their ability to earn a living, which is essential to realizing many rights. Equitable financing of health care could also reduce poverty more directly by protecting those who are most vulnerable from impoverishment resulting from health care expenditures. Equitable financing is likely to be sustainable with such measures as risk pooling.[28] Implementation of this strategy requires building public consensus regarding commitment to social justice, which could be strengthened by demonstrating the linkages to the human rights obligations of governments.

Using Human Rights Principles to Design and Implement Policies and Programs

Human rights principles require that health workers—and their agencies and organizations—systematically consider how the design or implementation of policies and programs may affect social marginalization, disadvantage, vulnerability, or discrimination. For example, improving the geographic and financial accessibility of preventive health services may not alleviate disparities in their use without active outreach and support for the groups most likely to be under-utilizers, despite equal or greater need.[20,29] Health workers need to identify and address obstacles—including unconscious and de facto discrimination—such as language, cultural beliefs, racism, gender discrimination, and homophobia—that keep disadvantaged groups from receiving the full benefits of health initiatives. Although many policies and programs to reduce poverty and improve the health of the poor routinely consider and address these concerns, still many do not.[21] Explicit adoption of human rights approaches can help bring systematic attention to social disadvantage, vulnerability, and discrimination in health policies and programs.[28,30]

Human rights principles require that public health institutions ensure that health care services effectively address the major causes of preventable ill health— and associated impoverishment—among disadvantaged people. This approach requires systematic and sustained efforts to build infrastructure, to overcome the complex barriers to receiving health care that often accompany low social position, and to achieve comprehensive and high-quality universal services.[31] Access and quality are inseparable; perceived low quality is a widespread barrier to use of available services by the disadvantaged.[32]

Especially among agencies supporting health programs in low-income countries, resource constraints are at times cited as a rationale for focusing on a limited number of conditions that disproportionately affect poor people, such as malaria, tuberculosis, HIV/AIDS, and maternal morbidity and mortality. The current financial crisis has resulted in calls for quick wins rather than longer-term solutions, which may appear more costly in the short term—with potentially negative implications for strengthening health systems and responding to HIV/AIDS and other diseases. A human rights commitment to "progressive realization" of all rights requires that such a narrowed focus only be temporary. Targets should be set within a long-range plan in order to ensure that, over time, increasingly comprehensive, high-quality services relevant to the health needs of the entire population are provided.[28]

Strengthening and Extending Public Health Functions to Address the Social Determinants of Health

The health sector can make a major contribution to addressing social justice and human rights concerns by strengthening and extending those crucial public health functions—beyond health care services—that address the basic conditions needed to achieve health and to escape from the vicious cycle of poverty and ill health. These functions include setting and enforcing standards for water and sanitation, food and drug safety, tobacco control, child care, and working, housing, and environmental conditions. These functions benefit society as a whole, and they especially benefit disadvantaged people.

The health sector, however, has little or no direct control over most of the underlying conditions necessary for health. Therefore, traditional public health functions need to be expanded through collaboration with other sectors to develop strategic plans addressing these conditions in light of both social justice and human rights concerns. Reflecting human rights norms, these expanded public health functions could include:

- Promotion of an adequate food supply
- Education that permits full economic, social, and political participation
- Housing and neighborhood environments that promote health
- Dignified, safe employment[5-7]

Such measures require collaboration with a range of sectors that have not traditionally collaborated with the health sector, such as those sectors addressing economic, social, political, educational, environmental, and general development activities. These expanded public health functions would enable the health sector—within social justice and human rights frameworks—to help shape public policy.

▪ CONCLUSION

Health workers should be aware that human rights principles, norms, standards, laws, and accountability mechanisms are relevant tools to help achieve social justice in health. Human rights treaties and other agreements can provide important mechanisms to strengthen accountability of governments for social justice in health. Their increased use by health workers could be a major step toward this goal. In addition, human rights principles and norms can strengthen advocacy for social justice in health, in part by emphasizing a broad international consensus on (a) key issues, such as the need to eliminate gender, racial, and ethnic discrimination; and (b) the right to health and related rights to water, food, shelter, information, education, and the benefits of scientific progress. Human rights perspectives and instruments can also strengthen the analytical frameworks that are used to develop strategies to achieve social justice, especially in addressing the non-medical determinants of health. Finally, human rights principles and norms can provide guidance on how to shape the design of health programs to reduce obstacles to achieving the right to health and related rights—with explicit attention to the human rights principle of non-discrimination. This principle provides a crucial framework for achieving social justice in health.

Human rights principles and standards can be used to ensure that governments do not directly violate human rights—and that they promote and ensure the realization of the conditions needed to enable individuals and groups to achieve all of their rights. Health workers need to advocate that governments address underlying unjust societal conditions and structures—not just buffer their health-damaging effects by providing health services. Human rights principles provide a framework that can guide health workers and others in achieving social justice in health.

■ ACKNOWLEDGMENTS

The authors wish to acknowledge Eva Wallstam and Eugenio Villar Montesinos of the World Health Organization (WHO), who developed the idea to address the linkages between human rights and social justice in relation to health. The authors are solely responsible for the opinions and perspectives expressed in this chapter.

■ REFERENCES

1. Gruskin S, Mills EJ, Tarantola D. History, principles, and practice of health and human rights. *Lancet* 2007;370:449–455.
2. Gruskin S, Tarantola D. What does bringing human rights into public health work actually mean in practice? In: Heggenhougen K, Quah S, eds. International encyclopedia of public health. Vol. 3. San Diego: Academic Press, 2008:137–146.
3. United Nations. Universal Declaration of Human Rights, General Assembly Resolution 217A (III), United Nations Document A/810 at 71, 1948. Available at http://www.un.org/en/documents/udhr/history.shtml. Accessed on August 8, 2012.
4. United Nations. Convention on the Rights of the Child. United Nations General Assembly Document A/RES/44/25, 1989. Available at http://www.un.org/documents/ga/res/44/a44r025.htm. Accessed on August 8, 2012.
5. WHO. Constitution of the World Health Organization, as adopted by the International Health Conference, New York, June 19–22, 1946. Available at: http://whqlibdoc.who.int/hist/official_records/constitution.pdf. Accessed on August 8, 2012.
6. United Nations. International Covenant on Economic, Social and Cultural Rights, General Assembly Resolution 2200 (XXI), United Nations Document A/6316, 1966. Available at: http://www1.umn.edu/humanrts/instree/b2esc.htm. Accessed on August 8, 2012.
7. United Nations Committee on Economic, Social and Cultural Rights. The right to the highest attainable standard of health. Geneva: United Nations, 2000.
8. Braveman P, Gruskin S. Defining equity in health. *J Epidemiol Commun Health* 2003;57:254–258.
9. Yamin AE. Will we take suffering seriously? Reflections on what applying a human rights framework to health means and why we should care. *Health Human Rights* 2008;10:45–63.
10. Leary V. The right to health in international human rights law. *Health Human Rights* 1994;1:24–56.
11. Eide A. Economic, social and cultural rights as human rights. In Eide A, Krause C, Rosas A, eds. Economic, social and cultural rights: A textbook. Dordrecht, the Netherlands: Martinus Nijhoff, 1995.
12. Tomasevski, K. Health rights. In: Eide A, Krause C, Rosas A, eds. Economic, social and cultural rights: A textbook. Dordrecht, the Netherlands: Martinus Nijhoff, 1995.
13. United Nations. Manual on human rights reporting. Geneva: United Nations Center for Human Rights, 1996 (UN document no. HR/PUB/96/1).
14. Tarantola D, Gruskin S. Human rights approaches to public health policy. In Heggenhougen K, Quah S, eds. International encyclopedia of public health. Vol. 3. San Diego: Academic Press, 2008:477–486.

15. Wilkinson R, Pickett KE. The spirit level. London: Allen Lane/Penguin, 2009.
16. Wilkinson RG, Pickett KE. Income inequality and population health: A review and explanation of the evidence. *Soc Sci Med* 2006;62:1768–1784.
17. Lynch JW, Kaplan GA. Understanding how inequality in the distribution of income affects health. *J Health Psychol* 1997;2:297–314.
18. Kawachi I, Kennedy BP. Health and social cohesion: Why care about income inequality? *BMJ* 1997;314:1037–1040.
19. Lynch J, Smith GD, Harper S, Hillemeier M. Is income inequality a determinant of population health? Part 2: U.S. national and regional trends in income inequality and age- and cause-specific mortality. *Milbank Q* 2004;82:355–400.
20. Hart JT. The inverse care law. *Lancet* 1971;1:405–412.
21. Gwatkin DR. How well do health programmes reach the poor? *Lancet* 2003;361: 540–541.
22. Cottingham J, Kismodi E, Hillber AM, et al. Using human rights for sexual and reproductive health: Improving legal and regulatory frameworks. *Bull WHO* 2010;88:7.
23. Gender, Human Rights and Culture Branch of the UNFPA, Harvard School of Public Health Program on International Health and Human Rights. A human rights-based approach to programming: Practical implementation manual and training materials. New York: UNFPA, 2010.
24. Gruskin S, Ferguson L. Using indicators to determine the contribution of human rights to public health efforts: Why? What? And how? *Bull WHO* 2009;87:714–719.
25. Braveman P. Monitoring equity in health and healthcare: A conceptual framework. *J Health Popul Nutr* 2003;21:273–287.
26. Braveman PA, Tarimo E. Social inequalities in health within countries: Not only an issue for affluent nations. *Soc Sci Med* 2002;54:1621–1635.
27. Whitehead M, Dahlgren G. Concepts and principles for tackling social inequities in health: Levelling up (Part 1). Copenhagen: WHO Regional Office for Europe, 2006.
28. Davies P, Carrin G. Risk-pooling—Necessary but not sufficient. *Bull WHO* 2001; 79:587.
29. Aday LA, Andersen RM. Equity of access to medical care: A conceptual and empirical overview. *Med Care* 1981;19:4–27.
30. Gruskin S, Bogecho D, Ferguson L. Rights-based approaches to health policies and programs: Articulations, ambiguities, and assessments. *J Public Health Policy* 2010;31:129–145.
31. Gruskin S, Ahmed S, Bogecho D, et al. Human rights in health systems frameworks: What is there, what is missing and why does it matter? *Global Public Health* 2012;7: 337–351.
32. Haddad S, Fournier P, Machouf N, Fassinet Y. What does quality mean to lay people? Community perceptions of primary health care services in Guinea. *Soc Sci Med* 1998;47:381–394.

23 Promoting Social Justice Through Public Health Policies, Programs, and Services

■ ALONZO L. PLOUGH

▓ INTRODUCTION

Public health policies, programs, and services—collectively termed *public health practice*—in the United States have been the subject of a series of reports by the Institute of Medicine (IOM)[1,2] and considerable commentary by the federal government, professional associations, and academic institutions.[3-5] However, social injustice is rarely discussed as a focus of public health practice.

Most assessments of the state of public health practice have dealt with such issues as organizational structure, funding shortfalls, and capacity limitation. They have typically focused on defining functional capacity (to provide the 10 essential public health services*) and the growing gaps between challenges to population health and the resources invested in the public health system.[6]

The public health system has reportedly been described as being in disarray, especially at the local level. National- and state-level attempts to bring coherence to public health practice through standards and performance measures have been presented as remedies for systemic dysfunction. The relatively new national process for voluntary accreditation in public health translates the 10 essential public health services into standards that can be measured in all public health jurisdictions. It also establishes, as a standard, community engagement, which, if substantial and sustained, can be a pathway to addressing social injustice in order to improve population health.[7] Strategic planning by the Centers for Disease Control and Prevention (CDC), which supports improved coordination among state, local,

---

* The 10 essential public health services are: monitoring health status to identify community problems; diagnosing and investigating health problems and health hazards in the community; informing, educating, and empowering people about health issues; mobilizing community partnerships and action to identify and solve health problems; developing policies and plans that support individual and community health efforts; enforcing laws and regulations that protect health and ensure safety; linking people to needed personal health services and assuring the provision of health care when otherwise unavailable; assuring a competent public health and personal health care workforce; evaluating the effectiveness, accessibility, and quality of personal and population-based health services; and researching for new insights and innovative solutions to health problems.

and territorial health departments, now focuses on community engagement.[8] These contexts of community engagement imply that public health departments need to participate in improving the social conditions that have a profound influence on health and well-being. Components of public health practice concerning community engagement include social determinants of health, community-based public health, community-based participatory research, and the social/ecological model.* However, focusing on social determinants does not necessarily lead to analyses and actions to improve social justice. And, while evolving national standards and performance measures address community engagement, they do not explicitly deal with the promotion of social justice as a core capacity in public health practice.

To make social justice a goal of public health practice, one must recognize that public health practice is overwhelmingly a government activity—in the way services are organized, financed, and delivered—and one must refute conventional wisdom that public health practice is in disarray. Government public health practice is placed in a challenging context, because work to promote social justice identifies social injustice as a cause of poor health status of specific communities and challenges the broad political economy. How a health department approaches this problem will depend on (a) the level of government—federal, state, or local—at which the agency is located; (b) the political ideology of elected officials who oversee the department; (c) the capacity and commitment of public health officials; (d) the ability of staff members to meaningfully engage community residents in collaborative endeavors; and (e) competing challenges in public health, such as H1N1 influenza, emergency preparedness planning, outbreaks of disease, inspections of various facilities, and mandates for service delivery. An operational focus on root causes of poor health, such as poverty, inequalities in income and wealth, and racism, requires public health capacity to manage the urgent demands of public health practice, while simultaneously understanding—for both current practice and strategic planning—the social context and root causes of the poor health of populations.

▪ PUBLIC HEALTH AGENCIES AND SOCIAL JUSTICE

Federal Agencies

The capacity to address social injustice in public health practice—or the ability to develop it—varies with the level of government in which a health agency operates. Federal agencies, such as CDC and the Health Resources and Services Administration (HRSA), operate with a national scope, provide many grants and contracts, and perform intramural research—all of which could

* The social/ecological model describes how social, physical, and genetic factors influence health status. This includes contextual and relational influences on health, such as social and community networks, living and working conditions, institutional influences, and political and economic policies—all of which interact to shape population and individual health.

focus public health practice on social injustice. But they do so infrequently. Even when they do focus on social injustice, as they did during the Bill Clinton administration with HRSA's 100 Percent Access and Zero Disparities initiative and the environmental justice focus of CDC's National Center for Environmental Health, funding has been limited and programs have not been adequately developed. During the George W. Bush administration, initiatives focusing on social justice were significantly reduced or eliminated. During the Barack Obama administration, many policies to address the root causes of poor health have been implemented, such as community-based prevention programs funded by the Patient Protection and Affordable Care Act (ACA). And overall, since each president's administration has had a different vision of the government's role in addressing social injustice, there has been little or no continuity in policies and programs.

State Health Departments

State-level public health practice has faced similar challenges, with frequent changes in governors, high turnover of public health officials, and no ongoing political support for public health initiatives to address social injustice. And most state health departments do not interact with community-based public health practice. Public health practice at the state level includes pass-through of federal funds to local health agencies and organizations, general development of statewide policies, and regulatory activities. Advocacy and activism by public health officials—essential for policies to address social injustice—are constrained.

The average tenure of state public health directors is only 2.9 years.[9] As a result, they have usually been unable to provide leadership in addressing social injustice as a key function of public health practice. Based on a review of the websites of all state health departments, it appears that only the Minnesota Department of Health has extensively incorporated social justice as a standard of practice.[10] The website of the Association of State and Territorial Health Officials (ASTHO) reflects an increased focus in state health departments on health equity and the social determinates of health.[11] ASTHO collaborates on the National Partnership for Action, whose goal is to reduce health disparities for racial and ethnic minority groups and other underserved communities.

A social justice strategy links health disparities to root causes in the political economy and suggests policy changes and social actions to create fundamental changes in these root causes. Policy strategies of state health departments that focus on health equity and health disparities generally restrict their programmatic and action focus to data analysis of the proximate causes of disparities and to services to reduce disparities through conventional public health services.

Federal and state public health agencies could address social injustice indirectly by influencing the development and implementation of key policies by other state agencies in such areas as education, taxation, housing, and economic development. Progressive public health officials have embraced this strategy, sometimes termed a *health-in-all-policies approach*, to take advantage of opportunities to promote health across a wide range of state policies. The size and complexity of government bureaucracy, the "silo" structure and function of government agencies, and the political divisiveness of some public health issues make this type of collaboration difficult.

Nevertheless, federal and state public health agencies can help address social injustice at the local level through funding that is flexible enough for community-driven preventive measures based on the social determinants of health. For example, CDC's Racial and Ethnic Approaches to Community Health (REACH) grants program has funded local coalitions to address disparities in HIV/AIDS, diabetes, and infant mortality, and has enabled community-level interventions that have addressed root causes of poor health in a social justice framework. The U.S. Department of Health and Human Services, through the Community Transformation Grants program (a component of the ACA), has awarded more than $103 million to government agencies and non-governmental organizations in 61 states and communities.[12]

These grants, which support capacity-building and implementation of preventive measures, focus on tobacco-free living, active living and healthy eating, evidence-based prevention and control of hypertension and hypercholesterolemia, social and emotional wellness, and healthy and safe physical environments.

The Community Transformation Grants, through community-based programs with mandated community participation, aim to reduce disparities in risk factors for, and the occurrence of, chronic diseases by addressing low-income populations, people enrolled in food or housing assistance programs, low-wage employees, and Medicaid enrollees.[13] Funded activities may include eliminating "food deserts" (districts with little or no access to food items required to maintain a healthy diet, but often served by many "fast-food" restaurants) and increasing access to healthy food options, such as by improving nutrition in school food services and bringing healthier food to local grocery stores in urban areas.[14]

Local Health Departments

Public health practice is best situated to explicitly address social injustice at the local level. Local health departments are the backbone of the government public health system. But they have been poorly represented in studies and reports on the current and projected status of public health practice.[15] Reports of the Institute of Medicine in 1988 and 2002 have assessed the public health system—in terms of both conventional standards and technical capacity—as being in disarray. They especially cite local health departments as having limited capacity. The 2002 report, while appropriately focusing on dysfunctional funding for population health, describes public health practice as organizationally fragmented.[16]

There are several flaws, however, in this analysis of local public health capacity.[17] Seventy percent of the U.S. population, and almost all large urban areas, which are characterized by health disparities by race, ethnicity, and socioeconomic status, are served by city or county health departments with effective policies, programs, and services. These health departments, which are closely connected with the communities they serve, explicitly address social injustice.

The best examples of a commitment to social justice in public health practice are associated with the policy commitment to social justice of the National Association of County and City Health Officials (NACCHO). The NACCHO website, which serves as a technical resource for local public health practitioners, has numerous references to social justice.[18] In 2001, NACCHO formed the Health and Social Justice (HSJ) Partnership with the Center for the Advancement of Health, a private organization that accelerates the application of new research on prevention to improve health policy; America's Health Together, a university-based entity that coordinates research and service activities to eliminate racial and ethnic disparities in health; and the Center for Minority Health at the University of Pittsburgh, an advisory organization that raises awareness of the relationship of social inequality to health. The goal of the Partnership is to eliminate disparities in health status by raising awareness about (a) the relationship of these disparities to socioeconomic inequalities, and (b) what can be done to address the conditions that produce these disparities. Through op-ed pieces, magazine articles, and other media-related strategies, the HSJ Partnership creates a national dialogue and proposes public policies for eliminating the root causes and the consequences of these disparities.[19]

NACCHO's strategic plan defines, as a core strategic action of local public health practice, the capacity "to address issues of health equity and social justice, oppose racism, and support diversity and cultural competence." In addition, through its Health Equity and Social Justice initiatives, NACCHO provides local health departments with resources to examine the causes of health disparities and to develop policies to reduce them. These initiatives include:[20]

- The Roots of Health Inequity: A Web-Based Course for the Public Health Workforce, which enables health department staff members to investigate the relationship between social injustice and everyday public health practice
- The Local Health Department National Coalition for Health Equity, an online network that aims to eliminate the fundamental causes of health disparities through public health practice
- The Health Equity Campaign, sponsored by the California Endowment, which hosts community discussions about health equity and facilitates these discussions with the Public Broadcasting Service documentary film series *Unnatural Causes: Is Inequality Making Us Sick?*
- The Health Equity and Social Justice Toolkit, a searchable database of health equity tools, publications, and resources, available in NACCHO's "toolbox"

- Publications tailored to local health departments, including the anthology *Tackling Health Inequities Through Public Health Practice: A Handbook for Action*,[21] and NACCHO's *Guidelines for Achieving Health Equity in Public Health Practice*.[22]

NAACHO has had a profound effect with its explicit support for social justice as a core competency in public health practices, and its provision of tools, trainings, workshops, and other technical assistance to local public health practitioners. NAACHO has provided grants and other resources for building strategic action in many communities throughout the United States. The framework for public health practice that NAACHO provides gives legitimacy for advocacy work at the local level. When a member of a local board of health or a city official questions why the health department is engaged in land-use or environmental-justice issues, the ability of health department officials to cite NAACHO's strategic plans and practice guidelines can demonstrate that this type of engagement is consistent with national standards of public health practice.

Local public health practice, grounded in specific communities, is part of a local network of community-based organizations, government agencies, and private-sector institutions that share a local geographic and governmental context. Social conditions that adversely influence health outcomes—such as unemployment, poverty, disinvestment in public education, neighborhood crime, and suburban sprawl—have a day-to-day immediacy in local public health practice.

With the leadership and commitment to engage with communities in challenging social injustice, local public health departments can be social enterprises that combine the technical tools of epidemiology and health assessment with advocacy skills and community partnerships. The relatively long tenure of local public health officials enables them to be long-term leaders for sustained policies and programs to address social justice. Since staff members of local health departments are members of the communities that they serve, they can help link other community members who suffer health problems related to social injustice with programs and services of the department—and help their departments become more accountable to these communities.

Government public health agencies, including local health departments, are challenged in establishing authentic community partnerships. For public health agencies to be effective in a community-linked approach to addressing social injustice, they need to incorporate new approaches to collaboration that go far beyond the traditional expert-driven approach to public health practice.[23] Effective collaboration between communities and public health agencies requires empowerment, community building (the bridging of social ties), and community engagement—all of which are essential activities of public health practice. All too often, public health agencies use the policy language of "the social determinants of health" and the need to "reduce health disparities," but, at the same time, they have not transformed internally in order to address social injustice. (See Chapter 24.)

The major challenge of public health practice is to translate knowledge of the impact of social injustice on public health into sustainable changes in policies and practices. These changes include (a) providing support and training to staff members in the development of community partnership, and (b) extending public health practice to develop partnerships with initiatives in other sectors, such as economic development, land use planning, housing, transportation, and education.

Local public health practitioners can broaden public awareness of the impacts of social injustice on community health by generating and communicating local data on the impact of specific socioeconomic factors on health. Effective use of local media is an essential tool of public health practice. Evidence-based presentations to local elected officials and board of health members are an essential component of public health practice addressing social injustice.

Local public health practice depends largely on (a) building on a broad base of community partnerships, some of which are not focused on health; (b) identifying root causes of problems and opportunities for change; and (c) selecting the most effective tools and strategies to address social injustice. Root causes of social injustice are often best addressed by focusing on policies concerning labor and employment, taxation, environmental conditions, housing, land use, and child development and support. In order to address social injustice, public health practice needs to recognize the broader context of causation—not limiting policies, programs, and interventions to those based on individual behavior or a small number of diseases.

■ PUBLIC HEALTH PRACTICE ORIENTED TO SOCIAL JUSTICE

This section examines two examples of how public health policies, programs, and practices can highlight the relationship between social injustice and the public's health. Each example provides some practical insights into how community partnerships can be used to deepen knowledge of root causes of poor health, mobilize and activate political and community leadership, and make initial efforts sustainable. The case studies are drawn from local public health agencies in San Francisco and Seattle. Each case study focuses on a health-related problem with significant social determinants, with each public health agency and its community partners deploying different strategies to link the broader social justice problem with a specific approach to health improvement at the community level. Each of these case studies illustrates different scales of impact and degrees of potential sustainability of programs. They highlight the complexities of addressing social injustice through public health practices and policies that are primarily based in government.

Case Study 1

The San Francisco Department of Public Health, a city and county health department serving a diverse metropolitan population, promotes social justice through public health practice in a framework that is linked to national strategies. For example, its environmental health section operates the Program on Health, Equity, and Sustainability, the goal of which is "to make San Francisco a livable city for all residents and to foster environmental, community, and economic conditions that allow residents to achieve their human potential."[24]

In 2002, the Department addressed disparities in the occurrence of asthma, especially focusing on exposure of low-income children to indoor air of poor quality. Recognizing that their neighborhoods had much substandard housing, and drawing on studies that related to poor indoor-air quality to the presence of mites, cockroaches, and mold, the Department raised community awareness about childhood asthma by presenting data and mobilizing communities. The Department stated that about 54,000 residents had asthma, and that people of color had more severe outcomes.[24]

Development of the San Francisco Asthma Task Force mobilized the community. It was chaired by a representative of a local non-governmental organization that provided social services. Its composition reflected the diversity of the community, including representatives of nonprofit organizations and community-advocacy organizations as well as other community members, many of whom had asthma in their families. The Task Force developed focused working groups that, in order to develop a community-based definition of the problem, obtained information from tenants with asthma, property owners and managers, and builders and contractors. Then teams from the Department and the Task Force applied interdisciplinary tools of environmental health, environmental epidemiology, enforcement of building and housing codes, and tenant organizing to further define policies and interventions to address asthma in the community. Through an open community process, which included retreats, the Task Force developed recommendations that focused on improving indoor-air quality for lower-income tenants. The final report of the Task Force highlighted the structural deficiencies of buildings, which lead to exposure to mold, fumes, and other hazards that exacerbate asthma. The Task Force recognized that low-income people have few housing options and are disproportionately exposed to these hazards.[25]

Recommendations from this locally driven public health partnership reflect insights gained and action strategies developed when public health workers and community partners create dynamic collaboration to address social injustice. The major action strategies that it developed to address environmental determinants of asthma included the following:

1. *Establishing a cross-agency group to inspect public-housing properties and to create accountability mechanisms that brought conditions into compliance with*

the housing code. This strategy involved creating interagency collaboration among the health department, the housing agency, and agencies involved with enforcement of the housing code, the police, and the legal and judicial systems—all of which focused on improving underlying social conditions that account for income-based disparities in asthma.

2. *Establishing comprehensive standards and guidelines for healthy housing, including roles for property owners.* This strategy required government entities to strengthen the relationship between building codes and landlords' legal obligation to tenants to reduce housing-related health risks.

3. *Instituting a legal housing-advocacy program for low-income patients with asthma.* This monitoring and engagement strategy raised awareness about environmental determinants of asthma and provided low-income asthma patients using hospital emergency departments with information and linked them with housing advocates.

This case study demonstrates how many elements of a public health practice oriented to social justice can be developed and implemented. While the overall project recognized the clinical and disease-control issues, its thrust addressed the root causes of asthma in housing and economic policies. The Department of Public Health was a key participant, but the project was broadly based in the community and led by community organizations. Finally, recommendations addressed the social context of risk and incorporated non-traditional approaches for providing public health programs and services. In 2011, the San Francisco Asthma Task Force was transformed into a community coalition, while retaining the Department as a key partner in proposing policies to increase health equity among communities. Now with broader goals, the Task Force advocates for improved child care, education, medical care, and housing to reduce asthma in low-income communities.[26]

Case Study 2

Public Health–Seattle and King County, a large metropolitan health department serving nearly two million people, has long recognized the critical importance of social justice in public health practice—as reflected in its mission and value statements and its organizational structure. Its Community-Based Public Health Practice (CBPHP), an interdisciplinary unit, was established in 1998 to develop community-driven activities based on a deep understanding of the social determinants of health.[27] A major focus of CBPHP has been improving the poor health status of communities of color.

The department initiated surveys and studies that documented growing disparities between economically marginalized racial and ethnic groups and other populations in King County. Investigation of disparities in infant mortality, teen pregnancy, diabetes, and other health outcomes led to an examination of root causes of these disparities.[28] The results of these studies were published in an easily accessible form and made widely available on the Internet and through other communication channels. Health department staff members worked closely with advocates to increase community awareness of these problems and to engage community members in strategies to improve underlying socioeconomic factors that had led to poor health outcomes. This work involved community-driven assessment of health as well as examination of critical social contexts in specific groups, including American Indians and Alaska Natives, African Americans, specific Asian and Pacific Island groups, and Hispanics.

The King County Ethnicity and Health Survey revealed that discrimination influenced the occurrence of all health disparities. For example, 32 percent of African Americans thought that they had been discriminated against at some time when receiving health care services.[29] Lower percentages of other groups reported experiencing this type of discrimination. Department leaders believed that a broader strategy was required for effective advocacy and change. Community partners and Department staff members recognized that racism was the root cause of health disparities and that they had to address how racism influenced health status and health-seeking behavior of specific minority populations. In a clinical setting, perceptions of discrimination can powerfully impact health-seeking behavior and health status. Giving a voice to individuals who had experienced racism in clinical settings provided a vivid picture of the problem. By presenting the issues in human terms, the report presented a dramatic and compelling sense of the problem—much more than could have been achieved by presenting statistical data. As a result, the strategy was likely to improve the behavior of clinicians in institutions where discrimination had occurred.

The health department contracted with a community-based organization to develop and conduct the Racial Discrimination in Health Care Interview Project.[30] The results were reported in community and public health reports that were widely distributed among health care providers and their institutions, as well as political and community leaders.[31] The reports highlighted the extensive range and frequency of perceived discrimination experienced by those interviewed. The discrimination events, which had taken place at nearly 30 public and private health care facilities throughout King County, included racial slurs and blatant examples of rude behaviors and differential treatment. As the report stated, most interviewees reported changing their behaviors as a result of discrimination they had experienced. Some reported delaying treatment because of this discrimination and their not knowing where else to seek care.

These descriptive and experience-based examples from the survey were presented in numerous public settings, including press conferences with the county executive, community meetings, conferences of health professional associations, and Board of Health meetings. They generated much media attention. The results of the studies were presented to the chief executives of major hospitals and health plans in the region. A call to action was delivered in all of these settings, seeking a broad community consensus to adopt the recommendations of the reports, including training health care providers, establishing uniform institutional policies to prevent discrimination, and collecting data and performing monitoring by including questions regarding discrimination on patient satisfaction surveys. Many of the recommendations were implemented by local institutions.

The work to eliminate discrimination continues. The Health Department has established more programs in the community and internally that aim to prevent disparities and to frame policies to ensure health equity. These include programs aimed at preventing chronic diseases and infant mortality as well as promoting good nutrition and healthy living. The Department's development and implementation of these programs launched, in 2008, the Equity and Social Justice Initiative Plan for Public Health, which created a framework in which public health policies, programs, plans, and strategies will be driven by social justice.[32] The Initiative addresses inequities throughout King County—by focusing not only on health-related issues, such as access to health care and safe neighborhoods, but also on affordable housing, quality education, and other challenges that minority and low-income communities face. In 2010, King County including the Initiative into its countywide 2010–2014 strategic plan.[33] In the same year, the plan was incorporated into an ordinance that broadly integrated the "fair and just" principle into county government.[34]

▪ ADDITIONAL EXAMPLES OF PUBLIC HEALTH PRACTICE THAT ADDRESS SOCIAL INJUSTICE

These two case studies provide good examples of how public health practice can incorporate a social justice framework that influences policies and services. There are many other ways that government-based public health practice, especially at the local level, can address social injustice. One example is using public health surveillance data to identify the adverse health effects of social injustice. Public health agencies can closely monitor a set of social indicators—such as measures of poverty, income inequality, housing costs, unemployment, and even the number of parents who read to young children—that are strongly associated with health and human development. It is increasingly important to link these types of social indicators to the traditional vital statistics and health status measures, and to use census tracts and ZIP codes as sociodemographic units of analysis. By this approach, public health departments can develop, with their community partners, neighborhood-focused assessments that can assist communities in advocating to improve socioeconomic conditions that underlie health disparities. Monitoring can also focus on preventive services, such as prenatal care for low-income women at community and public health clinics.

Addressing factors such as inadequate housing, lack of jobs with a livable wage, unsafe workplaces, and community exposures to environmental hazards are often more important than providing traditional, client-focused public health services. With widespread budget cuts for public health services, it is unlikely that public health agencies can directly ensure that all appropriate services are available and accessible. However, they can align funded services to populations with the greatest needs and aggressively present the political and social context for the critical gaps in access to preventive services.

▪ AN ACTION AGENDA FOR A SOCIAL JUSTICE CORE COMPETENCY IN PUBLIC HEALTH PRACTICE

For public health practice to better address social injustice, there will need to be a fundamental shift in what is currently viewed as core (or essential) public health functions. Evolving local, state, and federal standards for public health practice in the United States focus on traditional roles of disease prevention and health promotion, achieved by a traditional array of services and other activities. Community involvement and engagement, although seen as core public health activities, are contextualized in behavior change of individuals to reduce conventional risk factors for disease. For example, it is often said community assessment and partnership activities cause more people to eat healthy diets and to exercise regularly, or to enable more teenagers to understand the risk factors associated with drug use.

A public health practice competency that addresses the impact of social injustice on health goes beyond affecting individual behavior change and improving the effectiveness of health services. It instead focuses on making more accountable the people who make decisions concerning those who have poor health due to discrimination based on race, income, language, ethnicity, or sexual orientation. Its outcomes can be measured by sustainable reductions in the social determinants of this discrimination.

Three Barriers to Wide Acceptance of a Core Public Health Competency of Demonstrating Ability to Reduce Social Injustice

As reflected in curricula of schools of public health and other academic public health programs, public health educators are developing courses in skills and methods for reducing the impact of social injustice on health. While the number of courses on health disparities, minority health, and social determinants of health are increasing, they focus on describing problems—generally not on engaging with communities to address the root causes of health disparities. This is the first of the three barriers. Courses on community-based public health practice should go beyond community-based assessment of conventional risk factors and focus on community organizing and empowering actions to address the root causes of social injustice. These courses could link to public health practice settings, where people who have suffered poor health due to social injustice could share their experiences in order to educate students.

A second and closely related barrier to wider acceptance of this core competency is the lack of sustainable federal funding to support developing public health practice approaches to address social injustice. This inadequacy includes limited funding for partnerships among local health departments, communities, and academic institutions to develop and disseminate best practices. More federal funding to local health departments could enable their staff members to understand how to develop effective community partnerships and how to develop expertise in non-traditional areas of practice. Government mandates are needed to facilitate authentic community partnerships in policy and program development. The promises of both community transformation grants and the prevention components of the ACA are great, but also politically fragile. A social movement will be necessary to sustain these and other activities that promote prevention and social justice.

State health departments need to recognize that, because the social determinants of health are community-based, a decentralized focus on community development and local leadership is required. Such a focus would move away from aggregated state plans for reducing disparities to legislative and regulatory policy approaches to reduce the impact of social injustice on the public's health. It would require that legislators and other policymakers at all levels of government understand that, for example, housing and land-use/zoning decisions have a major influence on the public's health.

The third barrier to wider acceptance of this core public health competency is inadequate financial support for it. Therefore, public health practitioners will need to use data on the social determinants of health creatively in order to inform and influence decisions of elected officials. The greatest challenge may be the perception that social injustice is rarely eliminated by public health services alone—although these services can reduce the impact of social injustice on the people who receive them. A public health practice commitment to incorporating social justice as a core capacity means going far beyond providing services. It means being a catalyst for sustainable structural changes to reduce social injustice.

■ REFERENCES

1. Institute of Medicine. The future of public health. Washington, DC: National Academy Press, 1988.
2. Institute of Medicine. The future of the public's health in the 21st century. Washington, DC: National Academies Press, 2002.
3. Fraser M. State and local health department structures implications for systems change. Transformations for public health. *Turning Point Newsletter* 1998;1(4).
4. National Association of County and City Health Officials. Local public health agency infrastructure: A chartbook. October 2001. Available at http://www.naccho.org/topics/infrastructure/research/upload/chartbook_COMPLETE.pdf. Accessed October 1, 2012.

5. Freund CG, Liu Z. Local health department capacity and performance in New Jersey. *J Public Health Manag Pract* 2000;6:42–50.
6. Mays GP, Miller CA, Halverson PK (eds.). Local public health practice: Trends and models. Washington, DC: American Public Health Association, 2000.
7. Public Health Accreditation Board. Accreditation process. Available at http://www. phaboard.org/accreditation-process. Accessed September 20, 2012.
8. Center for Disease Control and Prevention. Office for State, Tribal, Local and Territorial Support. Available at http://www.cdc.gov/OSTLTS. Accessed September 20, 2012.
9. Meit MB. I'm OK, but I'm not too sure about you: Public health at the state and local levels. *J Public Health Manag Pract* 2001;7:vii–viii.
10. Minnesota Department of Health. Benefits of community engagement. Available at http://www.health.state.mn.us/communityeng/index.html. Accessed October 1, 2012.
11. Association of State and Territorial Health Officials. Health equity. Available at: http:// www.astho.org/programs/health-equity. Accessed September 20, 2012.
12. Center for Disease Control and Prevention—Division of Community Health. Community Transformation Grants (CTGs). Available at http://www.cdc.gov/ communitytransformation. Accessed September 13, 2012.
13. U.S. Department of Health & Human Services. Community Transformation Grants: Addressing health disparities and improving opportunities for health, September 27, 2011. Available at http://www.healthcare.gov/news/factsheets/2011/09/disparities 09272011a.html. Accessed September 17, 2012.
14. U.S. Department of Health & Human Services. News release: $100 million in Affordable Care Act grants to help create healthier U.S. communities, May 13, 2011. Available at http://www.hhs.gov/news/press/2011pres/05/20110513b.html. Accessed September 13, 2012.
15. Barry MA, Centra L, Pratt E, et al. Where do the dollars go? Measuring local public health expenditures. 1998. Submitted to the Office of Disease Prevention and Health Promotion, Department of Health and Human Services, by National Association of City and County Health Officials, National Association of Local Boards of Health, and Public Health Foundation. Available at http://www.phf.org. Accessed January 28, 2005.
16. Institute of Medicine. For the public's health: Investing in a healthier future. Available at http://www.iom.edu/Reports/2012/For-the-Publics-Health-Investing-in-a-Healthier-Future.aspx, April 10, 2012. Accessed September 20, 2012.
17. Plough AL. Understanding the financing and functions of metropolitan health departments: A key to improved public health response. *J Public Health Manag Pract* 2004;10:421–427.
18. National Association of County and City Health Officials. Creating health equity through social justice. Washington, DC: NACCHO; September 2002.
19. National Association of County and City Health Officials. Health and social justice partnership 2001. Available at http://www.naccho.org/general577.cfm. Accessed January 28, 2005.
20. National Association of County and City Officials. Health equity and social justice. Available at http://www.naccho.org/topics/justice. Accessed September 17, 2012.
21. Hofrichter R, ed. Tackling health inequities through public health practice: A handbook for action. Washington, DC: NACCHO; and Lansing, MI: The Ingham County Health Department, 2006.
22. National Association of County and City Officials. Guidelines for achieving health equity in public health practice. Washington, DC: NAACHO; April 2009.

23. Plough AL. Common discourse but divergent actions–Bridging the promise of community health governance and public health practice. *J Urban Health* 2003;80:53–57.

24. San Francisco Department of Public Health. Program on health, equity and sustainability 2004. Available at http://www.sfphes.org/. Accessed October 3, 2012.

25. The San Francisco Asthma Task Force. Strategic plan on asthma for the city and county of San Francisco. San Francisco, CA: San Francisco Board of Supervisors; June 2003:3.

26. San Francisco Asthma Task Force. Advocating to reduce asthma's impact. Available at http://www.sfgov3.org/index.aspx?page=706. Accessed September 17, 2012.

27. Public Health–Seattle and King County. Strategic direction: A guide to public health programs over the next 5 years. September 1999.

28. Public Health–Seattle and King County. Data watch: Racial disparities in infant mortality 1980–1998. August 2000. Available at: http://www.kingcounty.gov/healthservices/health/data/~/media/health/publichealth/documents/data/infantmortality_1980_98.ashx. Accessed March 20, 2013.

29. Public Health–Seattle and King County. The King County ethnicity and health survey for King County. October 1998. Available at http://www.kingcounty.gov/healthservices/health/data/~/media/health/publichealth/documents/reports/EthnicityHealth1998.ashx. Accessed March 20, 2013.

30. Public Health–Seattle and King County. Racial discrimination in health care interview project. January 2001. Available at: http://www.kingcounty.gov/healthservices/health/data/~/media/health/publichealth/documents/data/discriminationinterviews.ashx. Accessed March 20, 2013.

31. Public Health–Seattle and King County. Public health special report: Racial and ethnic discrimination in health care settings. January 2001.Available at: http://www.kingcounty.gov/healthservices/health/data/~/media/health/publichealth/documents/data/discriminationinhealthcare.ashx. Accessed March 20, 2013.

32. King County Equity and Social Justice. 2008 equity and social justice report. Available at http://www.kingcounty.gov/exec/equity/toolsandresources.apsx. Accessed September 18, 2012.

33. King County Office of the Executive. King County strategic plan. May 6, 2011. Available at http://www.kingcounty.gov/exec/PSB/StrategicPlan/CountyStratPlan.aspx. Accessed September 18, 2012.

34. King County Equity and Social Justice. Ordinance 16948. October 11, 2010. Available at http://www.kingcounty.gov/exec/equity/vision.aspx. Accessed September 18, 2012.

24 Strengthening Communities and the Roles of Individuals in Building Community Life

■ ROBERT E. ARONSON, KAY LOVELACE,
JOHN W. HATCH, AND
TONY L. WHITEHEAD

▧ INTRODUCTION

Strengthening communities and the roles of individuals in building community life can help prevent disease and disability and expand resources for promoting social justice. In this chapter, we focus on addressing race and socioeconomic-related disparities experienced by persons living in geographically defined communities. We recognize that "communities" can take many forms, not all of which are tied to location, and that different strategies may be required for different types of communities. Communities have strengths, such as individual members, social networks, social support, social capital, and their capacity to identify and solve their own problems. Communities also have potentially harmful factors, such as oppressive social controls, limited connection to social resources in the wider society, and hazardous environmental factors. Understanding both the protective and the potentially harmful factors of communities is critical to a practice of public health that builds communities and the roles of individuals as builders and sustainers of them.

Individuals are essential to community life and, when engaged collectively, can be the engines of community transformation and social change. Therefore, our focus is not on individualism, but rather on engaged individuals who recognize their interdependence. *Social networks* are the set of social connections among people; these networks can be characterized by their size, the qualities of ties among members, and the characteristics of members. Social networks have been linked to health outcomes through behavioral, psychological, and physiological pathways.[1]

Social networks may influence health by providing emotional, informational, instrumental, and appraisal support. Emotional support may affect health through the love and caring that people experience. Informational, instrumental, and appraisal support may help individuals' health by improving their access to material goods, resources, and services. Networks are a source of social influence—both by the influence of one person on another and by the influence of shared norms concerning health. Networks promote social participation and social engagement, and thus define and reinforce societal roles as well as provide opportunities for companionship. Networks also affect health by providing or preventing exposure to infectious diseases. In addition to affecting health directly, networks, through their patterns of associations, may afford opportunities for individuals to work in concert to solve problems and to take action. Therefore, social networks may be the mechanisms through which much community capacity for change is achieved.

Social capital pertains to the aspects of a social structure that facilitate action,[2] such as norms of reciprocity and civic engagement, social trust, and networks of social relations that can be mobilized for civic action.[3] Research linking social capital to health, though still in its early stages, may explain some differences in health outcomes.[4-6] However, a major problem in drawing conclusions from current research in this area is the lack of consensus on an operational definition of *social capital*, including the level at which it should be measured and the measures to be used in studies.[7]

The emphasis given to *social cohesion*—one aspect of social capital—and its relationship to health outcomes has been criticized for diverting attention from such structural determinants of health as income inequality, discrimination, and institutional racism.[8,9] Another critique is that social capital, when defined as social cohesion, can have both negative and positive social effects.[10] For example, social capital can be quite strong within antisocial groups, such as white-supremacy organizations, the militia movement, and neighborhood gangs.

Community capacity comprises the characteristics of a community that enable it to mobilize, identify, and solve community problems.[11] Researchers have identified numerous dimensions of community capacity. Some of these dimensions have been linked to improved program implementation and health outcomes, both theoretically and empirically.[12,13] Community-level traits, leadership, resources, and patterns of association can be identified and utilized to solve community problems and contribute to community health improvement.[14] Mobilizing community capacity to identify and solve problems is a fundamental ingredient of changing oppressive social structures and patterns of meanings. Transformative changes cannot be sustained without engaged and mobilized citizens.

Optimism plays an important role in protecting individuals and their communities from the effects of chronic stressors. Hope and optimism at the individual level positively influence health and protect against the effects of stress.[15,16] In contrast, hopelessness is thought to diminish health.[17] In his essay "Nihilism in Black America," Cornel West, an American philosopher, activist, and author of *Race Matters* and other books, discusses the problem of hopelessness in black America and its deeply ingrained effects on culture and society.[18] Optimism has not been investigated as a community-level construct, but it is a critical component of individual—and possibly community—transformation. Mediating structures, such as churches and community associations, may provide a means for oppressed communities to build hope and optimism by meeting some of their needs—such as the need to exercise leadership—beyond the needs met by resources provided through either government agencies or market forces. By working in partnership with communities in ways that build individual skills, strengthen organizations and institutions that communities control, and avoid paternalistic approaches that extract power from communities, community organizing can build hope and optimism.

The protective aspects of community life are beneficial to community health and can be enhanced through community-organizing and community-building strategies.[19] Health workers and community development workers, working with community members, have successfully addressed issues such as infant mortality, crime, violence, teenage pregnancy, and gang-related activities. These community-building participatory approaches aim to strengthen the capacity of communities to deal with these issues and others.[19] Identifying and strengthening community resources—as opposed to focusing solely on community risks—is essential to bringing about the kind of community-based change that is needed to improve health outcomes.[19-21]

■ ADDRESSING SOCIAL INJUSTICE THROUGH COMMUNITY TRANSFORMATION

Multiple multilevel strategies are needed to repair the fallout from social inequalities and social injustice and to stop the societal perpetuation of these problems. As public health workers, we need strategies to assist individuals and communities in their own transformation as they address health disparities and the root causes of these disparities. We need strategies to improve access to—and the quality of—facilities and services, including public health programming. We also need strategies to stimulate macroeconomic, political, and cultural change.[22]

During the past few decades, public health has emphasized developing and implementing effective approaches to reduce the burden of disease in populations, especially by primary prevention (which aims to prevent the occurrence of illness or injury before it occurs). Primary prevention strategies have focused almost exclusively on influencing behavioral risk factors of individuals, using policies and programmatic strategies with individuals and communities.

As we examine the *social* production of health disparities, we must ask, "How can we stop this injustice?" We believe the answer lies in community transformation and social change.

Building on the understanding of the relationship between individuals and societies proposed by Anthony Giddens,[23] a British sociologist known for his holistic view of modern socieites, we believe society is transformed when individuals and communities change the routinized patterns of social organization and meaning. In order to eliminate health disparities, individuals and communities need to come together to change these patterns in ways that alter the power structures that enable social inequalities to persist. This approach is not new; it has long been part of professional practice in the fields of community development, community organizing for health, and even some forms of comprehensive community-oriented primary health care. Examples appear in the literature of approaches that were viewed as real threats to the status quo, the political elite, and international interests.[24,25]

In considering strategies to address social injustice and its effects on the health of communities and population groups, community health workers must partner with local communities, recognize and build upon community strengths, and use public health approaches that address the root causes of health disparities—while being cautious about potential dangers of their work. We propose the following set of principles, based on the work of one of us (J.W.H.) during almost five decades in the Mississippi Delta, Boston, and North Carolina. Building on his mentorship, the other three of us have applied these principles to our work in Baltimore, Washington, DC, and North Carolina.

■ DEVELOP AUTHENTIC PARTNERSHIPS WITH COMMUNITIES

Do Not Extract Power from Communities

Altruistic motives and zeal for addressing health disparities and the social injustices that create and perpetuate these disparities often take the shape of paternalistic solutions. In poor communities, outside institutions exert decision-making power and control over the defining of problems, the identification of solutions, the implementation of programs, and the evaluation of success. Without the power to make these important decisions, the only choice that remains for community members is whether or not to utilize the services being offered. Public health programs are not the only ones that extract power from communities; so does virtually every governmental and non-governmental entity, including those in education, law enforcement, social services, health care, city planning, housing, and entertainment, as well as media organizations, religious institutions, charities, and private foundations. We must employ new approaches that respect the need for people to have control over the decisions that affect their lives.

Start Where the People Are

Public health workers and their organizations can address social injustice and health problems by joining with communities to address their concerns. Public health workers in communities need to start "where the people are."[26] This principle is important from the perspectives of both ethics and practicality.[27] From an ethical perspective, starting "where the people are" acknowledges a community's right to self-determination, liberty, and actions based on the values of the community members. From a practical perspective, problems and solutions defined by outside consultants or health workers have a long history of failure and mismatch with community motivations and concerns. Although health workers may be responding from a population perspective to critical health issues, such as cardiovascular disease, diabetes, or infant mortality, these concerns are rarely the same as those of community members. Therefore, when health workers focus solely on their concerns or the concerns raised by data, they may have difficulty getting community members involved. In contrast, when health workers join with community members in addressing their concerns, it is often possible to address not only community concerns, but eventually also the concerns of the health workers or funding agencies.

Understand the Local Context and Listen to the Community

In order to understand the role that the local context plays in the lives and health of community members, we must look beyond numbers and rates to the stories and experiences of community members. But, in order to be granted the privilege to hear these stories, we must enter into authentic relationships with people and institutions in the community. If disenfranchised populations are not having their concerns heard and addressed, it may be because no one is listening or no one is trusted. How can we listen if we do not interact in meaningful ways with the populations we serve? By listening to and hearing the voices of the people we serve, public health researchers and practitioners can better understand the social issues that most significantly affect their lives and their health. For example, one of us (R.E.A.) has explored, through focus groups, community concerns and notions of what makes a community a good place in which to live for women and children. Figure 24–1 depicts the contrasts between the broad set of concerns voiced by community residents and the narrow focus taken by typical programs for prevention of infant mortality. The residents' concerns listed in this figure should be priorities for our shared action agenda to address.

Nurture a Sense of Optimism and Hope

The erosion of dignity, of self-worth, and of a useful role in society have led many people to believe that their lives and their communities will never

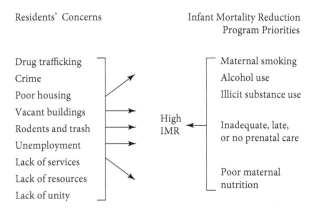

Figure 24–1 Contrasting community and program priorities. (IMR = infant mortality rate)

improve. This lack of hope can also be seen when some people in groups in the community believe that other people or groups are beyond being helped. The loss of hope can be threatening to the survival of a sense of morality and community among African Americans.[18,19]

Paulo Freire, a Brazilian educator and philosopher, described the dehumanization that occurs as a result of oppression and social injustice and the impact of this dehumanization on self-esteem:

> Self-deprecation is another characteristic of the oppressed, which derives from their internalization of the opinion the oppressors hold of them. So often do they hear that they are good for nothing, know nothing and are incapable of learning anything— that they are sick, lazy, unproductive—that in the end they become convinced of their own unfitness.[28]

According to Paulo Freire, the first step in surmounting oppression is critically recognizing its causes. In doing so, the oppressed can begin to see themselves and their humanity more fully. Public health strategies to restore dignity, self-respect, and regard for others are needed to repair the damage caused by societal oppression. Only when individuals see themselves as fully human can they act to end their oppression.

▪ RECOGNIZE AND BUILD ON COMMUNITY STRENGTHS

Recognize the Resources That Exist Within Communities

Communities are built on strengths and assets—not on problems.[29] Understanding the community context in which health problems arise should include an assessment of community assets and ways they have helped solve previous problems. Public health workers are not the default source of information and advice regarding health in most communities. Local opinion leaders, trusted community members, and natural helpers tend to serve in this role. In African American communities, institutions parallel to those of the wider society have served as bases of belonging, self-esteem, leadership development, and social activism.[30] Because blacks were often not able to gain access to broader societal institutions or were not treated equally to whites when such access was gained, they were left to develop and nurture parallel institutions,[31] including fraternal organizations, clubs, and secret societies; economic and educational institutions, such as historically black colleges and universities; and—of great importance—black churches. These parallel institutions have facilitated the survival of African Americans, led the civil rights movement, and nurtured individual and community capacity.

Lay health advisor programs build on the strengths of African American churches and natural helpers to reduce health disparities.[32,33] Among the projects conducted by these programs in conjunction with these churches that have been aimed to reduce health disparities are those that have focused on nutrition,[34,35] breast health,[36] prostate cancer,[37] diabetes,[38] and physical activity.[39]

Strengthen the Capacity of Local Institutions, Networks, and Community Groups

Addressing health problems through local institutions, networks, and community groups is an important strategy to help people to live healthy lives in their communities. According to *The Future of the Public's Health in the 21st Century*, a 2002 report of the Institute of Medicine:

> Government public health agencies, as the backbone of the public health system, are clearly in need of support and resources, but they cannot work alone. They must build and maintain partnerships with other organizations and sectors of society, working closely with communities and community based organizations, the health care delivery system, academia, business, and the media.[40]

Although formal public health institutions are in need of resources and support, community-based institutions they partner with may have even greater needs. As public health professionals work with community-based institutions, they must bring resources from the wider public health system to build the capacity of these institutions. Needs for capacity-building may include the development of basic technical skills, such as in budgeting and proposal writing, leadership, and financial and human resources. Strengthening local institutions, networks, and community groups makes it more likely that work to address health disparities will be sustainable. An important outcome of past community building has been the development of individuals who return to serve their communities after gaining additional training and education.

Strengthen and Expand Social Networks in Communities and Beyond Communities

Social networks influence the health of individuals in many ways.[4] They can produce adverse effects related to social control and reduced behavioral options that may encourage risky behaviors that are harmful to health. Social networks may provide redundant types of social support with less access to the goods and services of society if the members of the network are relatively homogeneous in terms of education, occupation, and social class.[41] We do not recommend an approach that simply tries to encourage community members to interact with one another, thereby expanding social networks in communities. Rather, we encourage strategies that build networks of support for community and societal change and for greater access to the goods and services of society.

In a 13-county area in eastern North Carolina, two of us (R.E.A. and J.W.H.) worked with a network of 105 churches in a major African American denomination. To develop the churches' role in promoting health among their members, the existing networks within churches needed to expand outside these churches' walls and into their communities. The training of lay health educators involved a combination of (a) dialogue/problem-posing workshops on the nature of community health problems, and (b) lectures led by local representatives of public health departments, health associations, and other community agencies. Involving professionals from outside the churches helped create connections between the churches and these professionals. The churches' networks expanded to include service providers with access to goods and services not routinely available. The connections were mutually beneficial. Church networks developed larger pools of resources for assistance on important community issues and the network of service providers, including county health departments and nonprofit organizations, such as the American Heart Association and the American Red Cross. As a result, they had greater access to the populations that they were seeking to serve.

▓ USE PUBLIC HEALTH APPROACHES THAT ADDRESS THE ROOT CAUSES OF HEALTH DISPARITIES

Use Ameliorative and Fundamental Approaches

In order to effectively address health disparities, we need to use both ameliorative and fundamental approaches to public health practice.[42] Ameliorative approaches target specific risk factors that are associated with health outcomes in a given community context, and facilitate development of protective factors to enhance the health of individuals, communities, and larger populations.[42] In contrast, fundamental approaches seek to transform the elements of society that give rise to inequalities and health disparities. We need to use both of these approaches at the individual, community, and societal levels. It should not be assumed that societal-level approaches will necessarily be addressing root causes.[42]

Maintain a Long-Term Perspective on Fundamental Issues

By maintaining a long-term vision while addressing immediate needs, public health workers and communities can contribute to reducing the social injustices that contribute to poor health. Communities may be better able to advocate and demand change when local public health work strengthens community leadership, expands social networks, and fosters community problem-solving. One of us (J.W.H.), reflecting on his work in the Mississippi Delta, described how a perspective on long-term social change was always a part of his framework, even when addressing immediate needs in ways that were non-confrontational.

The focus of much of the action was on practical concerns, such as digging wells, building outdoor sanitary toilets, and reducing health risks in the local environment. Small successes nurtured the belief that change was possible through collective action. Many who doubted the possibility of positive change began to attend meetings related to the health council and the farm cooperative. For many, this was a political awakening. People involved with these organizations were recruited by civil rights groups, such as Delta Ministry and the Mississippi Democratic Freedom Party, to lead voter-registration campaigns. Organizing strategies used to educate, recruit, and involve people in the farm cooperative enabled organizers to develop skills similar to those required for political action.

While Addressing These Important Issues, Build Race, Class, and International Bridges

William Julius Wilson, a noted Harvard sociologist, contends that the political muscle needed to address some of the social problems facing the United States cannot be achieved without a broad-based, multiracial coalition—one that focuses on issues that are important to most Americans and emphasizes their interdependence.[43] Among these issues are government policies to assist vulnerable families, trade policies that do not reduce employment opportunities or displace workers, monetary policies that promote full employment, livable-wage policies, and policies to restore American cities.

Many economic forces that have disproportionately affected African Americans have arisen from global economic forces that are non-racial in origin. For example, trade policies such as those of the North American Free Trade Agreement (NAFTA) have resulted in a decline in lower-skilled, low-wage jobs in the United States. Nearly half of recent job losses among less-educated blacks have resulted from the loss of manufacturing jobs.

The importance of building bridges among citizens of the United States and those of other nations is particularly relevant for environmental issues and trade agreements. Free-trade and investment agreements have undermined public health by increasing social inequalities, depleting natural resources, and increasing environmental pollution.[44] The importance of building bridges with activists from other countries has been demonstrated in the tobacco-control movement.[45] Stricter tobacco-control legislation in the United States has resulted in more aggressive international marketing of tobacco-control products. Partnerships among tobacco-control organizations in various countries have helped groups to frame tobacco issues in an international context and provide information, advice, and resources across borders. In addition, examples of egregious behavior by tobacco companies in other countries can be used sometimes to address their behavior in the United States. (See Box 21–3 in Chapter 21.)

Support Actions That Build Participatory Democracy and Engaged Citizens

Community-based strategies to address public health problems are most effective when the population is mobilized and engaged in the identification of problems and the development of solutions. Developing broad-based coalitions of existing community-based organizations, agencies, associations, and concerned citizens can be a powerful way to mobilize and engage communities. (See Box 24–1, which addresses strengthening communities in low-income countries.)

Democracy in the United States is threatened by corporations and wealthy people who purchase access to government officials, especially since the *Citizens United* decision by the Supreme Court. As public health professionals working with disenfranchised communities to address health disparities, we need to use participatory strategies that maximize the potential for individual and community learning, empowerment, citizen engagement, and mobilization. Lessons learned and power gained through such strategies—multiplied across communities—can help to strengthen democracy and address social injustices. Geni Eng, a professor of health behavior at the University of North Carolina, and her colleagues have found that communities with higher rates of participation in addressing health issues are more likely to address other community issues.[13]

Work with Other Organizations to Address the Public's Health

Now that we are gaining an increased awareness of the power that context wields in the health of populations, public health professionals should embrace comprehensive approaches to improving the context of people's lives. This may mean that we become involved in issues not typically seen as part of public health. It may mean that we need to expand our set of partners to include those from other organizations seeking to improve the context of people's lives. The public health system does not always need to be the lead in local work to improve community health. Addressing the social determinants of health may require other agencies and/or communities to take the lead.

In addition, many of the upstream causes of health disparities are addressed by organizations in the community beyond the local public health agency, and therefore require action by everyone concerned with the public's health.[46] For example, public organizations, business organizations, government entities, and communities could develop fruitful partnerships to address health disparities resulting from the built environment. Together, transdisciplinary groups representing environmental health, community planning, economic development, housing, transportation, social services, public health, justice, and community health could collaboratively address issues associated with low-income neighborhoods.

BOX 24-1   ■   **Strengthening Communities in Developing Countries**

Gail Snetro-Plewman and Angie Brasington

Community capacity enables a community to reflect on its strengths and needs in order to improve its well-being and that of its residents. Strengthening community capacity can lead to better outcomes in health and social change. Participation in health and development programs can strengthen the voice of ordinary citizens and ensure their involvement in decisions that affect their lives and the life of their communities. Participation of community members also increases the impact of health and development programs and can lead to long-term sustainability. In response, individuals and groups who are actively involved become committed to—and feel increasingly capable of—improving their health and living conditions.[1]

The Community Action Cycle[2] (CAC) is a common method for strengthening community capacity and mobilizing communities towards collective action. Use of the CAC fosters a community-led process through which those people most affected by a problem organize, explore, set priorities, plan, and act collectively for improved health and development outcomes. The CAC is based on a social-systems approach to individual and social change—a process by which people "define who they are, what they want, and how they can get it."[3] The CAC and other empowering processes are grounded in the following principles:

- Sustainability of social change is more likely if the individuals and communities most affected "own" the change.
- Communities should be the agents of their own change.
- Persuasion and unidirectional transmission of information from external technical experts should be replaced by dialogue, debate, and negotiation among community members.
- Improving development outcomes should focus on social norms, culture, policies, and improvement of the supportive environment—especially where individual decision-making power is limited by strong cultural and gender norms.
- Community members who have been previously silent, inactive, or marginalized should be given a voice and encouraged to participate.

Participation should engage people in the decisions that affect their lives and promote self-reliance. In the context of health and development programs, self-reliance means creating and strengthening appropriate forms of interdependence among communities and governments, service providers, or other external agents.

There is a continuum of levels of participation and self-reliance. Attending a meeting without expressing opinions, for example, can be an important first step—especially for those without experience in having their voices heard. Later, these people can become more actively involved. In some cases, involving those who are most marginalized is not possible at the start of a project; their involvement may require additional work to enable them to believe that they are capable of participating. A step-by-step approach to participation may be more appropriate for individuals and groups who have been reluctant to participate in development programs or who mistrust external interventions.

The following examples represent the application of these principles in projects sponsored by Save the Children, a nonprofit organization that works to strengthen community capacity in more than 50 low-income countries, serving more than 33 million children and 19 million adults.

In Ethiopia, a network of care and support for 500,000 orphans and vulnerable children was established by linking and building the capacity of six international organizations, 36 in-country non-governmental organizations, and 575 community-based organizations. Community-based groups were strengthened to explore the issues affecting vulnerable children; to plan and act together to access, demand, and deliver services; and to mobilize and manage financial and human resources.

In South Africa, in an area where health services were underutilized and a wide sociocultural gap existed between service providers and community members, these two groups came together to jointly define "quality of care." Community access to health services was improved by having ongoing dialogue, setting common priorities, and planning together.

In Bangladesh, community leaders in underserved areas are organizing and empowering men's and women's groups to develop ways to improve care and support of pregnant women and newborns. Community leaders receive training and support to facilitate dialogue within peer groups that enables participants to better understand why mothers and infants have been dying during childbirth, and to address local barriers by planning and acting together.

By strengthening community capacity, communities (a) learn how to apply political pressure to improve the quality of services, (b) generate and contribute additional resources not previously available to the health system, (c) facilitate changes in social strategies, structures, and norms to increase access to information and services for those who need them most, and (d) strengthen their ability to claim their right to respectful treatment. Through this process, community members' abilities to address many underlying causes of health problems, such as poverty and discrimination, are developed.

The following measures for strengthening community capacity may also increase participation:

- Supporting ongoing dialogue among community members regarding development issues, including health
- Strengthening the capacity of community-based groups in leadership, group maintenance, resource mobilization and management, external links to services, and use of data for decision-making
- Working in partnership with communities in all phases of project management to promote co-learning, in which "teachers" and "students" work together in the quest for knowledge, understanding, and wisdom

Box References

1. Tapia M, Brasington A, Van Lith L. Involving those directly affected in health and development communication programs. Baltimore, MD: Health Communication Partnership, Johns Hopkins Bloomberg School of Public Health, 2007.
2. Howard-Grabman L, Snetro G. How to mobilize communities for health and social change: A health communication partnership field guide. Baltimore, MD: Health Communication Partnership, Johns Hopkins Bloomberg School of Public Health, 2003.
3. Grey-Felder D, Dean J. Communication for social change: A position paper and conference report. New York: Rockefeller Foundation Report, 1999.

Further Reading

Minkler M. Community organizing and community building for health. 2nd ed. New Brunswick, NJ: Rutgers University Press, 2004.
Gibbon M, Labonte R, Laverack G. Evaluating community capacity. *Health Soc Care Community* 2002;10:485–491.

Partners might include local architects, developers, and nonprofit organizations such as Habitat for Humanity. Built-environment features that emphasize physical activity, such as parks and sidewalks, also strengthen community life by making social connections easier. Parks provide contact with other people and with nature—features of our environment that promote health.[47]

Funding for Community-Based Research and Public Health Practice Should Emphasize Community Building

With the increased attention given to the importance of context in population health, funding for research and public health practice should contribute to the process of improving people's lives. Greater emphasis should be placed on participatory research strategies, such as community-based participatory research (CBPR), that engage communities in the process of defining research priorities and developing research strategies. The community brings an understanding of the context, including issues of concern and knowledge of how the community "gets things done." Participation by community members helps to restore trust in the public health system and builds skills and community capacity that are important for an engaged citizenry. Funding for public health programs, likewise, should emphasize comprehensive and community-building strategies to improve the context in which people live. Changing behavior without changing the context in which it occurs is not likely to be sustainable. State and national funding agencies should consider requiring research staff members and project personnel to complete an orientation to ethics of community-based research and practice—similar to the online training required for research involving human subjects.

Continue to Exert Pressure from Outside the Community

The production of social injustice and health disparities is global. Addressing social injustice and health disparities therefore requires global coordination on such issues as environmental degradation, greenhouse gas emissions, biodiversity loss, water shortages, fishery declines, poverty, financial instability, taxation, food insecurity, trade in health-damaging products, and armed conflict—as well as governance.[48] What happens in our local communities has global effects, and what happens globally has local effects. For example, policies of the World

Trade Organization result in disinvestment in small, family-based, sustainable agriculture, which, in turn, reduces food security.[44] Addressing these issues effectively will take joint action from both within and outside communities and across borders from members of community-based organizations, academic and scientific institutions, and government agencies.

▦ SOME CAUTIONS

As public health workers, we often do not live in the communities where we work. Therefore, our understandings of these communities are likely to be tinted by our own cultural lenses. Furthermore, if organizing efforts go awry, we can leave these communities and escape many of the physical and social consequences of our actions. Therefore, it is critical for us to:

- Reflect on and understand our own relationships with the communities with which we work and our own relationships with power
- Be aware of the dangers of organizing among oppressed people
- Know when the challenges of addressing social injustice exceed our capacities as individuals

Working with poor communities to eliminate social injustice requires that we, as public health workers, think reflectively about our own views of the community, our own privileges, and our own comfort level with different roles in promoting health. Such reflection is critical when organizing or working with communities that are different than our own. Without intending to do so, we may demonstrate personally-mediated racism.[49] For example, devaluation of individuals based on race, which is one form of personally mediated racism, may be demonstrated by either an expression of surprise at someone's competence or by an attempt to stifle a person's aspirations. It occurs when we have a view of a community as "half empty" rather than "half full." Acting naïvely and with good intentions, we might do more for the community than necessary and therefore increase—rather than decrease— the dependency of community members. Communities have a vital life force and ways of doing things that may not be apparent to us as outsiders. It takes concentrated and sustained listening over time to discover how things work in communities and the ways in which communities get things done. Given our education and training, we might not challenge our own views of what the community has to offer and might believe that our way of doing things is more informed and more effective. All of these actions devalue what community members might be able to do.

As public health workers with professional training, we have a different relationship with power than do members of the poor communities with whom we work. Examining our relationships with power will help us avoid unintentionally holding the status quo in place. We must develop an ability and comfort to work with community partners to conduct a structural analysis of the conditions that enable disparities to persist. Powerful persons and institutions with which we work may be challenged by such an analysis. But, without this analysis, we may not see the ways in which we have privileges not held by the community members with whom we work. If we lack self-knowledge, our ability to work in partnership with the communities will be hampered.

Because using community and social transformation for eliminating health disparities involves upsetting and changing routinized patterns of power, it is usually accompanied by conflict. Root causes of health disparities, such as income and wealth inequalities, racism, and sexism, persist because of powerful interests, which must lose some power if meaningful change is to occur. As health workers and organizers, we face several dilemmas. Organizing is often dangerous, leading to backlash, exploitation, and oppression. Historically, in the civil rights movement, local leaders sometimes were beaten, jailed, or forced to leave after outside organizers moved on. At other times, local leaders and organizers were killed.

There are differing views about how the dangers in organizing should be addressed. One approach would be to temper social activism by having the community decide how far to take confrontation-based tactics—because the community is often left to address the fallout from these tactics. Building on an analysis of the root causes of injustice and of the powers that sustain it can enable us to enter situations with our eyes open and to anticipate potential backlash.

Not everyone is comfortable with this type of work. To grow as people and public health workers, we need to better understand ourselves and our work. Sometimes, we will recognize that we do not have the capacity for this work, or that, because of other circumstances, we must choose to work more indirectly with communities. In these roles, we still can choose to be supportive allies with communities and health workers. As examples, we can support community businesses, associations, and cultural activities; we can speak up for the rights and perspectives of communities in the organizations in which we work; and we can refuse to support or approve of organizations or individuals who undermine these communities.

■ CONCLUSION

Health disparities suffered by poor and minority populations are socially produced. They result largely from current and historical social injustice. Addressing these disparities requires approaches that are both ameliorative and fundamental, addressing both current problems and root causes. Comprehensive approaches are needed that work across the wide domain of social ecology—individuals, families, communities, organizations, institutions, and the broader society. Communities possess strengths and assets that can be used to address the health problems that they face. Communities can be strengthened in their capacity to address their current health problems and the root causes of these problems. Public health research studies and interventions in communities should be designed and implemented in ways that build community capacity and the skills of individuals to contribute to community problem-solving. Engaged and critically conscious people are needed to sustain work for social change.

Public health workers need new skill sets and intervention strategies to assist communities in meeting the challenges they face. Our understanding of the effects of contexts on health must include insight into how health problems are experienced by people living within these contexts. This understanding should lead us to consider broader approaches to improving the context of people's lives by working collaboratively with communities.

■ REFERENCES

1. Berkman L, Glass T, Brissette I, et al. From social integration to health: Durkheim in the new millennium. *Soc Sci Med* 2000;51:843–857.
2. Coleman J. Social capital in the creation of human capital. *Am J Sociol* 1988;94:S95–S120.
3. Putnam R. The strange disappearance of civic America. *Am Prospect* 1996;24:34–48.
4. Kawachi I, Kennedy BP, Lochner K, et al. Social capital, income inequality, and mortality. *Am J Public Health* 1997;87:1491–1498.
5. Kreuter M, Lezin N, Baker B. Social capital: When best practices aren't enough. Indianapolis, IN: 48th Annual Meeting of the Society of Public Health Education, 1997.
6. Sampson R, Raudenbush S, Earls F. Neighborhoods and violent crime: A multilevel study of collective efficacy. *Science* 1997;277:918–924.
7. Macinko J, Starfield B. The utility of social capital in research on health determinants. *Milbank Q* 2001;79:387–427.
8. Lynch J. Income inequality and health: Expanding the debate. *Soc Sci Med* 2000;51:1001–1005.
9. Muntaner C, Lynch JW. Income inequality and social cohesion versus class relations: a critique of Wilkinson's neo-Durkheimian research program. *Int J Health Serv* 1999;29:59–81.
10. Kreuter M, Lezin N. Social capital theory. In: DiClemente R, Crosby RA, Kegler MC, eds. Emerging theories in health promotion practice and research. San Francisco: Jossey-Bass, 2002.
11. McLeroy K. Community capacity: What is it? How do we measure it? What is the role of the prevention centers and CDC? Atlanta, GA: Sixth Annual Prevention Centers Conference, Centers for Disease Control and Prevention, National Center for Chronic Disease Prevention and Health Promotion, 1996.
12. Goodman R, Speers M, McLeroy K, et al. An initial attempt at identifying and defining the dimensions of community capacity to provide a basis for measurement. *Health Educ Behav* 1998;25:258–278.
13. Eng E, Briscoe J, Cunningham A. Participation effect from water projects on EPI. *Soc Sci Med* 1990;30:1349–1358.
14. Norton B, McLeory KR, Burdine JN, et al. Community capacity: Concept, theory, and methods. In: DiClemente R, Crosby RA, Kegler MC, eds. Emerging theories in health promotion practice and research. San Francisco: Jossey-Bass, 2002.
15. Scheier M, Carver CS. Optimism, coping, and health: Assessment and implications of generalized outcome expectancies. *Health Psychol* 1985;4:219–247.

16. Snyder C, Harris C, Anderson JR, et al. The will and the ways: Development and validation of an individual-differences measure of hope. *J Personality Soc Psychol* 1991;60: 570–585.

17. Scheier M, Carver CS. Effects of optimism on psychological and physical well-being: Theoretical overview and empirical update. *Cogn Therapy Res* 1992;16:201–228.

18. West C. Race matters. New York: Vintage Books, Random House, 2001.

19. Minkler M, Wallerstein N. Improving health through community organization and community building: A health education perspective. In: Minkler M, ed. Community organizing and community building for health. New Brunswick, NJ: Rutgers University, 1997.

20. McKnight J. Two tools for well-being: Health systems. In: Minkler M, ed. Community organizing and community building for health. New Brunswick, NJ: Rutgers University, 1997.

21. Walter C. Community building practice. In: Minkler M, ed. Community organizing and community building for health. New Brunswick, NJ: Rutgers University, 1997.

22. Benezeval M, Judge K, Whitehead M. Tackling inequalities in health: An agenda for action. London: King's Fund, 1995.

23. Giddens A. The constitution of society. Los Angeles: The University of California Press, 1984.

24. Heggenhougen H. Will primary health care efforts be allowed to succeed? *Soc Sci Med* 1984;19:217–224.

25. Morgan L. International politics and primary health care in Costa Rica. *Soc Sci Med* 1990;30:211–219.

26. Nyswander, D. Education for health: Some principles and their applications. *Health Educ Monogr* 1956;14:65–70.

27. Minkler M, Pies C. Ethical issues in community organization and community participation. In: Minkler M, ed. Community organizing and community building for health. New Brunswick, NJ: Rutgers University, 1997.

28. Friere P. Pedagogy of the oppressed: New revised 20th-anniversary edition. New York: The Continuum Publishing Company, 1993.

29. McKnight J. The careless society: Community and its counterfeits. New York: Basic Books, HarperCollins Publishers, 1995.

30. Hatch J, Lovelace K. Involving the southern rural church and students of the health professions in health education. *Public Health Rep* 1980;95:23–26.

31. Whitehead TL. Health disparities among African Americans: A history of social injustice and processes of environmental stress and adaptation. Working Document of the Cultural Systems Analysis Group, University of Maryland, College Park, MD, 2003.

32. Campbell MK, Demark-Wahnefried W, Symons M, et al. Fruit and vegetable consumption and prevention of cancer: The Black Churches United for Better Health Project. *Am J Public Health* 1999;89:1390–1396.

33. Eng E, Hatch J, Callan A. Institutionalizing social support through the church and into the community. *Health Educ Q* 1985;12:81–92.

34. Ammerman A, Washington C, Jackson B, et al. The PRAISE! project: A church-based nutrition intervention designed for cultural appropriateness, sustainability, and diffusion. *Health Promot Pract* 2002;3:286–301.

35. Resnicow K, Jackson A, Wang T, et al. A motivational interviewing intervention to increase fruit and vegetable intake through black churches: Results of the Eat for Life Trial. *Am J Public Health* 2001;91:1686–1693.

36. Derose KP, Fox SA, Reigadas E, et al. Church-based telephone mammography counseling with peer counselors. *J Health Commun* 2000;5:175–188.

37. Weinrich S, Holdford D, Boyd M, et al. Prostate cancer education in African American churches. *Public Health Nurs* 1998;15:188–195.

38. McNabb W. The PATHWAYS church-based weight loss program for urban African-American women at risk for diabetes. *Diabetes Care* 1997;20:1518–1523.

39. Hatch J, Cunningham A, Woods W, et al. The Fitness Through Churches project: Description of a community-based cardiovascular health promotion intervention. *Hygiene* 1986;5:9–12.

40. Institute of Medicine. The future of the public's health in the 21st century. Washington, DC: National Academies Press, 2002.

41. Granovetter M. The strength of weak ties. *Am J Sociol* 1973;78:1360–1379.

42. Geronimus A. To mitigate, resist, or undo: Addressing structural influences on the health of urban populations. *Am J Public Health* 2000;90:867–872.

43. Wilson WJ. The bridge over the racial divide: Rising inequalities and coalition politics. Berkeley, CA: University of California Press, 1999.

44. Labonte R. International governance and World Trade Organization (WTO) reform. *Critical Public Health* 2002;12:65–86.

45. White A. Global partnerships for tobacco control. Boston, MA: 2003 National Conference on Tobacco and Health, 2003.

46. Halverson PK. Embracing the strength of the public health system: Why strong government public health agencies are vitally necessary but insufficient. *J Public Health Manag Pract* 2002;8:98–100.

47. Frumkin H. Healthy places: Exploring the evidence. *Am J Public Health* 2003;93:1451–1456.

48. Labonte R, Spiegel J. Setting global health research priorities: Burden of disease and inherently global health issues should both be considered. *BMJ* 2003;326:722–723.

49. Jones C. Levels of racism: A theoretic framework and a gardener's tale. *Am J Public Health* 2000;90:1212–1215.

25 Promoting Social Justice Through Education in Public Health

■ ROBERT S. LAWRENCE

▨ INTRODUCTION

This chapter examines the opportunity to promote social justice through education programs for students in schools of public health, medical school departments of community and preventive medicine, and elsewhere. It also examines how education can equip public health practitioners, researchers, and educators with a social-justice perspective that will guide their future work.

Two major developments of the past seven decades provide crucial information and values for developing and implementing social justice curricula. First, the evolution of human rights law since the end of World War II and the emergence of the health and human rights movement have provided new ways of thinking about the right to health and an expanded ethical framework for considering the health of populations and the interdependency of human rights—civil, political, economic, social, and cultural rights (Chapters 22 and 27). Second, great progress has occurred in the quantitative and qualitative analyses of the social determinants of health and how inequalities and inequities are among the most potent determinants of premature morbidity and mortality (Chapter 2). Together, richer and deeper reflections on the right to health and the social determinants of health provide the material for placing education to promote social justice at the heart of the public health curriculum.

▨ PRINCIPLES OF SOCIAL JUSTICE AND EDUCATION IN PUBLIC HEALTH

By framing the issue of social justice in the context of risk factors for premature morbidity and mortality caused by unjust treatment of subgroups within the population, public health practitioners can apply the core population-health tools of epidemiology, biostatistics, social and behavioral sciences, environmental and occupational health, and policy analysis to (a) identify key determinants of risk, (b) prioritize policies or interventions to lower risk, and (c) evaluate and communicate the results. Analysis of health status by population groups identified by race, ethnicity, gender, sexual orientation, religious beliefs and practices, country of origin, insurance and employment status, social status, or class often reveals profound differences. These differences, in turn, usually reflect the inequitable distribution of society's resources—in the form of (a) material benefits of better housing or safer worksites, or (b) in the amount of control people have over their lives and their opportunities for social engagement, tolerance, respect, and development of their full potential.

John Rawls, considered by many to be the most important political philosopher of the second half of the 20th century, further developed, in his theory of justice as *fairness*, the traditional idea of the social contract to introduce the concept of *distributive justice*.[1] Distributive justice emerges when, behind a "veil of ignorance" about what status we might have in a theoretical society, we establish as our "original position" the circumstances we would be willing to accept if we were among the least-favored members of society. As science advances our understanding of the social determinants of health, the necessary elements of the "original position," from a population health perspective, emerge more clearly, reinforcing with detail the more general statements rooted in the language of the right to health found in the United Nations Charter, the Universal Declaration of Human Rights, and the International Covenant on Economic, Social and Cultural Rights.[2]

In 1992, at a ceremony celebrating the 75th anniversary of the founding of the Johns Hopkins School of Hygiene and Public Health (now the Bloomberg School of Public Health), faculty and students at the school embodied these concepts of social justice and the right to health in the International Declaration of Health Rights (Box 25–1).[3] Executive Director of the United Nations Children's Fund (UNICEF) James Grant, Director General of the World Health Organization (WHO) Hiroshi Nakajima, Dean Alfred Sommer, and hundreds of others in attendance signed the declaration, which is read aloud each year by a graduating student at the school's commencement exercises.

Several other schools of public health have adopted the International Declaration of Health Rights for use in their commencement exercises, and similar pledges to uphold the right to health are included in the mission statements of many schools of public health. These encouraging developments are among the predisposing conditions for including social justice issues in educational programs for public health. The moral development of students in the professions occurs when they move beyond the stage of basing their behavior on the values and norms of those around them to a "more principled stage where they identify and attempt to live by personal moral values."[4] Public health educators have a duty to assist in this transformation by being examples in word and action of the centrality of social justice to the ideals of public health.

■ LOGIC OF SCIENCE ADDED TO MORAL AND ETHICAL REASONS FOR SOCIAL JUSTICE

Recent contributions from epidemiology, social and behavioral sciences, economics, and human rights studies have strengthened and clarified the scientific

---

BOX 25-1 ■ **International Declaration of Health Rights**

We, as people concerned about health improvement in the world, do hereby commit ourselves to advocacy and action to promote the health rights of all human beings.

The enjoyment of the highest attainable standard of health is one of the fundamental rights of every human being. It is not a privilege reserved for those with power, money or social standing.

Health is more than the absence of disease, but includes prevention of illness, development of individual potential, a positive sense of physical, mental and social well-being.

Health care should be based on dialogue and collaboration between citizens, professionals, communities and policy makers. Health services should be affordable, accessible, effective, efficient and convenient.

Health begins with healthy development of the child and a positive family environment. Health must be sustained by the active role of men and women in health and development. The role of women, and their welfare, must be recognized and addressed.

Health care for the elderly should preserve dignity, respect and concern for quality of life and not merely extend life.

Health requires a sustainable environment with balanced human population growth and preservation of cultural diversity.

Health depends on the availability to all people of basic essentials: food, safe water, housing, education, productive employment, protection from pollution, and prevention of social alienation.

Health depends on protection from exploitation without distinction of race, religion, political belief, economic or social condition.

Health requires peaceful and equitable development and collaboration of all peoples.

(*Source:* International Declaration of Health Rights. Baltimore, MD: Bloomberg School of Public Health, Johns Hopkins University, 1992. Available at http://www.jhsph.edu/about/school-at-a-glance/international-declaration-of-health-rights/. Accessed June 10, 2012.)

---

basis for the relationship between health and well-being. Advocacy for social justice in the past was often predicated on the link between the elimination of discrimination and prejudice and the fulfillment of civil and political rights. Public health professionals were among the first to connect the realization of human rights to the ability to shape the social and economic forces that create the conditions for improved health. Now a growing body of empirical data adds the logic of science to the moral and ethical reasons for demanding greater social justice.[5–8]

Integration of human rights with public health provides the essential elements for transforming the education of public health professionals. Values clarification and commitment to the principle of the right to health and the knowledge of the social gradient will equip graduates to help them fulfill their professional obligation to address root causes of ill health. These root causes include social injustices that determine so much of the burden of preventable morbidity and premature mortality among marginalized groups in society and create the health disparities that are present in all countries.

■ HISTORICAL CONTEXT

The epidemiology of scrotal cancer among London chimney sweeps was one of the earliest observations in the West of the association among socioeconomic status, occupational exposure, and health. Percival Pott, a London physician, described in 1776 the incidence of scrotal cancer in young chimney sweeps, who were usually nutritionally stunted orphans or abandoned children prized for their small size and in desperate need of employment of any kind. The House of Lords finally approved an Act of Parliament in 1864, after many years of campaigning by child advocates, to outlaw the use of children for climbing inside chimneys. The delay of almost nine decades between the scientific observation of the problem and the implementation of a policy to protect children established what became a familiar pattern of delay in building sufficient political will to correct an injustice. The Industrial Age (from about 1760 to about 1830) did bring a growing awareness of the link between health and conditions of work and living subject to public-sector regulation. In 1848, Parliament passed the Public Health Act to address poor labor conditions, and over the next 50 years, it adopted additional laws to protect the public from risks in the workplace.

In the first half of the 20th century, progress was slow in developing a coherent view of the social determinants of health. Most regulations protecting the health of the public in the United States focused on safety in the workplace, control of infectious diseases by vaccines and quarantine, and protecting the purity of food and water supplies. The increasing definition of health as a public matter—as well as a personal matter—led to the establishment of the Pan American Health Organization (PAHO) in 1902, the Office International d'Hygiène Publique in 1907, the International Labor Organization in 1919, and WHO in 1946.[9] WHO developed the idea of *health* as "a state of complete physical, mental and social well-being and not merely the absence of disease or infirmity."[10] This broadened definition of health included the concept of *well-being*, which depends on a physical and social environment that creates the conditions necessary to achieve health.

WHO is one of several United Nations agencies rooted in the post–World War II renunciation of war and violence as a means of resolving conflict between nations. The Preamble of the Charter of the United Nations includes among the purposes for establishing the United Nations in 1945 the following:[11]

to reaffirm faith in fundamental human rights, in the dignity and worth of the human person, in the equal rights of men and women and of nations large and small, and to establish conditions under which justice and respect for the obligations arising from treaties and other sources of international law can be maintained, and to promote social progress and better standards of life in larger freedom.

In 1948, the Universal Declaration of Human Rights declared, in Article 25:[12]

Everyone has the right to a standard of living adequate for the health and well-being of himself and of his family, including food, clothing, housing and medical care and necessary social services, and the right to security in the event of unemployment, sickness, disability, widowhood, old age or other lack of livelihood in circumstances beyond his control.

Similar language later appeared in the International Covenant on Economic, Social and Cultural Rights, which entered into force in 1976.[13] (As of early 2013, 160 of the 193 United Nations member countries were states parties to the Covenant. The United States has signed, but not ratified, the treaty.) The right to health—and the other economic, social, and cultural rights—falls within the category of positive, aspirational, and nonjusticiable rights, in contrast to those articulated in the International Covenant on Civil and Political Rights. States are urged to respect, protect, and fulfill these economic and social rights to the "maximum of [their] available resources, with a view to achieving progressively the full realization of the rights."[13] Some have argued that these rights have no real meaning without the power of legal recourse, and that closer attention to civil and political rights would be more likely to ensure conditions of social justice and therefore improve well-being. But the declaration of the right to health had struck responsive chords in many countries, leading to the widespread endorsement of the Declaration of Alma-Ata, adopted at the 1978 International Conference on Primary Health Care, which set as a goal by the year 2000 for all peoples of the world a level of health that would "permit them to lead a socially and economically productive life—Health for All."[14]

"Good health is the bedrock on which social progress is built. A nation of healthy people can do those things that make life worthwhile, and as the level of health increases so does the potential for happiness."[15] These opening words of *A New Perspective on the Health of Canadians* ("The Lalonde Report") speak to the close links between social justice and health. Forty years ago, Canadian Prime Minister Pierre Trudeau identified health disparities among different racial and ethnic groups as one of the important problems to address as part of his new administration's commitment to promoting social justice. He appointed Marc Lalonde, Minister of National Health and Welfare Canada, as chair of a commission to review the determinants of health and prepare recommendations for actions and policies to improve health and reduce disparities.

The commission grouped the determinants of health in four "fields"—human biology, environment, lifestyle, and health care organization. Contrary to their initial assumptions, the members of the commission concluded that health care organizations contributed only a modest amount to the health status of Canadians, and that much more attention needed to be given to environmental and lifestyle factors to reduce health disparities. Lack of education, substandard housing, inadequate environmental protections, food insecurity, and poverty emerged as the critical factors leading to health disparities of premature morbidity and mortality among indigenous people and other marginalized groups in Canada.[16] The idea of using social policy as an explicit tool to improve health status became part of Health Canada's strategy to reduce disparities.

Douglas Black, Chief Scientist to the United Kingdom's Department of Health from 1973 to 1977, described the concept of "disparities in health status" and their relationship to the above demographic variables in 1980 in a report commissioned by the Labour government of the United Kingdom in 1977 and suppressed by the Conservative government of Margaret Thatcher,which had just come to power.[17] Only several hundred photocopies were distributed, but the report had a great impact on political thought. Both WHO and the Organization for Economic Co-operation and Development (OECD) used it to examine health inequalities in 13 other countries. The report provided robust data showing that the poorest in the United Kingdom had the highest rates of poor health and premature death. Dr. Black argued that income, education, and lifestyle alone could not explain the disparities. He asserted that the disparities were also the result of a lack of a coordinated policy that would provide for more equitable provision of services, health goals, increased benefits, and restrictions on tobacco.

In 1988, the U.S. Institute of Medicine (IOM) released a report entitled *The Future of Public Health,* which stated that the mission of public health is to "fulfill society's interest in assuring conditions in which people can be healthy."[18] The report also described the three functions of public health—assessment, policy formulation, and assurance—that have become an important organizing principle for education in public health.

In 2002, the IOM published *The Future of the Public's Health in the 21st Century,*[19] revisiting many of the themes in the earlier report. New language had appeared, however, influenced by the discourse on the right to health. The report called for government and a broad spectrum of society to "work effectively together as a public health system and individually to create the conditions that allow people in the United States to be as healthy as they can be. Such a commitment will require political will that has yet to be mobilized." Education of the future public health workforce to advocate for social justice is an important part of generating that political will.

■ USING EDUCATION IN PUBLIC HEALTH TO PROMOTE SOCIAL JUSTICE

Although recent trends include increasing numbers of undergraduate public health programs or majors, the following section focuses on graduate education. Education in public health in the United States occurs mainly at the graduate-school level in the 49 schools of public health, which are members of the Association of Schools of Public Health (ASPH), and in the 83 medical schools and other health sciences schools with departments offering the master of public health (MPH) degree accredited by the Council on Education for Public Health (CEPH).[20] In the 2010–2011 academic year, 26,340 students were enrolled in the 46 schools of public health then accredited.

Diversity among students in public health is an essential component of an educational environment that prepares students to be effective in working for social justice. In 2010, a total of 8957 students graduated.[21] Of the U.S. students newly enrolled in schools of public health in 2010, 3168 (33 percent) belonged to minority groups: Asian, 14 percent; African American, 11 percent; Hispanic, 8 percent; and Native American/Alaskan Native, 0.7 percent. In the past decade, the percentage of newly enrolled students in schools of public health who are minorities has plateaued, with slight declines in the percentages of Hispanic and African American enrollees. Much earlier, a study of 45,000 students matriculating at U.S. universities from the early 1970s to the early 1990s revealed that race-sensitive admissions created a learning environment that improved the capacity of both minority and majority students to live and work with persons of different races and to have more successful careers.[22]

Courses in the core disciplines of public health—epidemiology, biostatistics, environmental health sciences, behavioral sciences/health education, and health services administration—are required for a school of public health or an MPH program housed in a school of medicine or health sciences school to meet CEPH standards for accreditation. These core courses should be enriched to include case studies and problem sets with a social justice perspective to demonstrate the important relationship between inequities and inequalities in social and economic status and health disparities.

"Public Health Problem Solving," for example, is a core course at the Bloomberg School of Public Health in which case studies are used to stimulate analysis of key determinants of health—biological, socioeconomic, environmental, behavioral, and health services—from the perspective of the social gradient in health. Faculty members introduce concepts of *quintile spread*, the *Gini coefficient*, and *fairness and justice in the distribution of goods and services*. Students work in small groups to examine important public health problems, using a stepwise methodology—problem definition, magnitude of problem, key determinants, policy and intervention options, priority setting, implementation, evaluation, and communication—to prepare written reports and make presentations in the form of briefings to a legislative body. The written report includes an analysis of the human rights impact of the policy or program being implemented, using the methodology developed by Lawrence Gostin and Jonathan Mann.[23] Use of this analysis provides an excellent pedagogical method to educate public health students about the linkage between (a) "least restrictive policies" from a human rights perspective, and (b) the promotion of social justice and protection against unintended policy consequences that might exacerbate inequalities or compromise human rights.

In a seminar on health and human rights, faculty members at the school have used readings, discussions, and case studies to explore topics—including structural violence, the health impacts of conflict, violations of human rights (civil, political, social, economic, and cultural rights)—and their health effects; complex humanitarian emergencies; gender-based violence; refugee health; environmental justice; the Human Poverty Index; and the role of advocacy in promoting health for marginalized populations. The seminar is part of the requirement for the Certificate in Health and Human Rights offered at the School since 1996. Capstone projects for MPH students qualifying for the certificate include a broad range of topics addressing social justice and human rights challenges, ranging from sexual violence against Sudanese refugees in Uganda to the development of a new index of social inequalities to be used in Baltimore.

The CEPH requirement for capstone or practicum experiences has stimulated links with organizations working to promote social justice through service to vulnerable groups. The Albert Schweitzer Fellowship provides service-learning opportunities for graduate students in the health professions and law in 12 cities or regions of the United States. Albert Schweitzer fellows in Baltimore work with safety-net organizations in the poorest neighborhoods of the city, learning first-hand the lessons of the close relationship between social injustice and poor health. The 200 hours of service during the fellowship year are a transforming experience, reinforcing the fellows' commitment to use their professional training to advocate for social justice.

Participation in research provides students the opportunity to acquire skills and methods to expand knowledge about the social gradient, to design and implement programs to reduce health risk among vulnerable populations, and to influence policy. Doctoral students are conducting dissertation research on health disparities in most schools of public health in the United States.

Students can participate in advocacy for social change at the local or regional level through groups such as student chapters of Physicians for Human Rights and the American Medical Student Association. The American Public Health Association, Physicians for Social Responsibility, Physicians for a National Health Program, and other professional organizations provide excellent opportunities for students to learn about and engage in advocacy for social justice.

■ AN AGENDA FOR ACTION

The ultimate goal is to have all career education and training programs in public health include a perspective on human rights and the social determinants of health. Social justice should become central to the educational mission of public health. The strategy most likely to succeed is to influence the accreditation criteria used by CEPH. An explicit requirement that social justice be included in the curriculum of all schools of public health—and all MPH programs sponsored by schools of medicine or other health sciences schools (which are accredited by organizations other than CEPH)—would stimulate the development of new courses and improve existing courses. Specific goals could include:

- Developing and sharing curricular materials and instructional modules—in acute and chronic disease epidemiology, environmental health, health policy, maternal and child health, nutrition, mental health, and international health—that demonstrate the connection between social injustice and poor health

- Designing methodology courses for research and analysis to increase understanding of the importance of social justice to improvements in health status (In promoting social justice, it is important to bring disparities to public attention so they can be appropriately addressed.[24])

- Mobilizing ASPH to sponsor and support activities in the pedagogy of social justice through its Council on Education, its Council on Minority Health, and its other units

- Sponsoring workshops for training in advocacy skills for communicating the growing body of knowledge about the social gradient in health to policymakers at the local, state, and federal level (Long-term goals would be to increase social and political will for support of policies that would address structural barriers to achieving social justice.)

- Partnering with other private groups and government agencies engaged in the analysis of the determinants of health inequalities to provide internships, practicum experiences, or other opportunities for education and training (Examples include participation in the project on health disparities at the Agency for Healthcare Research and Quality, evaluation of progress toward the goals of *Healthy People 2020* that address disparities, and continued monitoring by Physicians for Human Rights of the goals outlined in *The Right to Equal Treatment*.[25])

■ CONCLUSION

Rudolf Virchow, the great German pathologist who fought on the side of the democrats in the 1848 revolution in Germany, combined passion for social justice with scientific rigor. After the revolution, he established and edited the journal *Medicinische Reform* (The Reform of Medicine). In an early issue, he introduced the terms *public health* and *public health care* into the scientific literature, arguing that it is the responsibility of the state to create healthy conditions for the public and to provide public health services. He wrote:

> Should medicine ever fulfill its great ends, it must enter into the larger political and social life of our time; it must indicate the barriers which obstruct the normal completion of the life-cycle and remove them. Should this ever come to pass, Medicine,

what ever it may then be, will become the common good of all. It will cease to be medicine and will be absorbed into that general body of knowledge which is identifiable with power.[26]

As the gaps between rich and poor people and rich and poor countries continue to grow, the barriers obstructing "the normal completion of the life-cycle" loom large to those of us in public health. Like Albert Schweitzer, we may think and feel that our "knowledge is pessimistic, but my willing and hoping are optimistic."[27] His pessimism came from feeling the "full weight of what we conceive to be the absence of purpose in the course of world events." His optimism derived from his confidence that "the spirit generated by truth is stronger than the force of circumstances."

Our duty to the next generation of public health professionals is to provide them as students and younger colleagues with ample opportunities to learn the truth about social justice and the social determinants of health in order to help them surmount the barriers to equity in health. The challenge to educators in public health is to provide curricula and practicum experiences in supportive educational environments that enable students to grow into their ideals.

■ REFERENCES

1. Rawls J. A theory of justice. Cambridge, MA: Belknap Press of Harvard University Press, 1971 (Reissued 2005).
2. Office of the High Commissioner on Human Rights. The International Bill of Human Rights. December 1948. Available at http://www.ohchr.org/Documents/Publications/FactSheet2Rev.1en.pdf. Accessed June 10, 2012.
3. International Declaration of Health Rights. Baltimore, MD: Bloomberg School of Public Health, Johns Hopkins University, 1992. Available at http://www.jhsph.edu/about/school-at-a-glance/international-declaration-of-health-rights/. Accessed June 10, 2012.
4. Branch WT Jr. Supporting the moral development of medical students. *J Gen Intern Med* 2000;15:503–508.
5. Adler NE, Boyce T, Chesney M, et al. Socioeconomic status and health: The challenge of the gradient. *Am Psychol* 1994;49:15–24.
6. Marmot M. Inequalities in health. *N Engl J Med* 2001;345:134–136.
7. Marmot M. Economic and social determinants of disease. *Bull WHO* 2001;79:988–989.
8. Adler, NE. Looking beyond the borders of the health sector: The socioeconomic determinants of health. In: Rubin ER, Schappert SL, eds. Meeting health needs in the 21st century. Washington, DC: Association of Academic Health Centers, 2003.
9. University of Minnesota Human Rights Library. The Right to Health. Available at http://www1.umn.edu/ humanrts/edumat/IHRIP/circle/modules/module14.htm. Accessed June 25, 2012.
10. World Health Organization. WHO definition of health, 1948. Available at http://www.who.int/about/definition/en/. Accessed June 25, 2012.
11. United Nations. Charter of the United Nations, 1945. Available at http://www.un.org/en/documents/charter/. Accessed June 10, 2012.

12. United Nations. Universal Declaration of Human Rights, 1948. Available at http://www.un.org/en/documents/udhr/. Accessed June 10, 2012.

13. International Covenant on Economic, Social and Cultural Rights, 1966. Available at http://www2.ohchr.org/english/law/cescr.htm. Accessed June 10, 2012.

14. Declaration of Alma-Ata, 1978. Available at http://www.euro.who.int/en/who-we-are/policy-documents/declaration-of-alma-ata,-1978. Accessed June 10, 2012.

15. Lalonde M. A new perspective on the health of Canadians: A working document. Ottawa: Health Canada, 1974.

16. Frohlich KL, Potvin L. Transcending the known in public health practice. The inequality paradox: The population approach and vulnerable populations. *Am J Public Health* 2008;98:216–221.

17. Gray AM. Inequalities in health: The Black Report: A summary and comment. *Int J Health Serv* 1982;12:349–380.

18. Committee for the Study of the Future of Public Health, Institute of Medicine. The future of public health. Washington, DC: National Academies Press, 1988.

19. Institute of Medicine. The future of the public's health in the 21st century. Washington, DC: National Academies Press, 2002.

20. Council on Education for Public Health. Accredited schools and programs, 2013. Available at http://ceph.org/accredited/. Accessed March 11, 2013.

21. Association of Schools of Public Health. Annual Data Report 2010. Available at http://www.asph.org/UserFiles/DataReport2010.pdf. Accessed June 10, 2012.

22. Bowen WG, Bok D. The shape of the river: Long-term consequences of considering race in college and university admissions. Princeton, NJ: Princeton University Press, 1998.

23. Gostin LO, Mann J. Towards the development of a human rights impact assessment for the formulation and evaluation of public health policies. *J Health Hum Rights* 1994;1:59–80.

24. Healton C, Nelson K. Reversal of misfortune: Viewing tobacco as a social justice issue. *Am J Public Health* 2004;94:186–191.

25. The right to equal treatment. A report by the Panel on Racial and Ethnic Disparities in Medical Care. Boston, MA: Physicians for Human Rights, 2003.

26. Virchow R. De Einheitsbestrebunger in der Wissenschaftlichen, quoted in Strauss MB. Familiar medical quotations. Boston, MA: Little, Brown and Company, 1968.

27. Schweitzer A. Out of my life and thought. Baltimore, MD: Johns Hopkins University Press, 1998.

26 Researching Critical Questions on Social Justice and Public Health: An Ecosocial Perspective

■ NANCY KRIEGER

> When I give food to the poor, they call me a saint.
> When I ask why the poor have no food, they call me a communist.
> —DOM HELDER CAMARA (1909–1999), Archbishop of Recife, Brazil[1]

■ INTRODUCTION

Questioning the existence of injustice is central to work for social justice. Asking about its causes and consequences is at once both a practical necessity and a vital act of imagination and hope, premised on the insight that what *is* need not always *be*. Once the question is raised, critical and creative work can and must be done to expose why the injustice exists, including who gains and who loses and how it wreaks its woe, thereby generating knowledge useful for both rectifying harm and creating just and sustainable solutions.

Translated into issues of social justice and public health, critical research questions necessarily focus on two concerns:

What is the evidence that social injustice harms health?
What can be done to prevent this harm?

Straightforward as these questions may seem, the answers are far from simple. As shown in Figure 26–1, important debates swirl around the existence and magnitude of and solutions to social inequalities in health. While many of these disputes are polarized between "right" and "left" political analyses, as exemplified by arguments about individualistic versus structural explanations for social inequalities in health,[2–5] or risk associated with various commercial products, such as tobacco[5–7] or organochlorines,[8] not all of them are. Critical debates also occur among proponents of social justice deeply concerned about social inequalities in health, as evident in controversies over how to study the contribution of socioeconomic deprivation to racial/ethnic disparities in health[9,10] and whether income inequality harms health, and if so, why.[11–15] The complexities of problems encompassed in social injustices in health and of conducting valid research on their causes means that both legitimate and manufactured disagreements can give rise to conflicting claims.

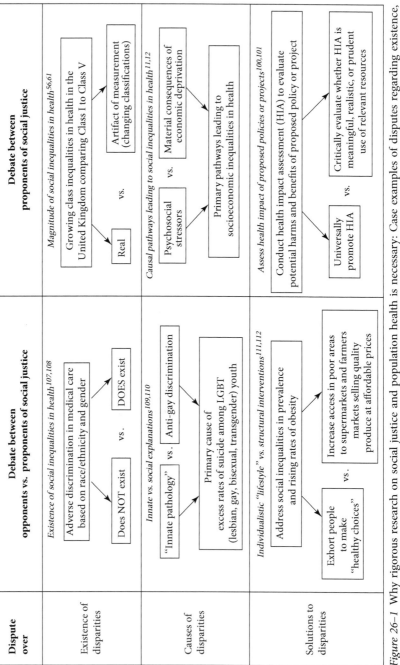

Figure 26–1 Why rigorous research on social justice and population health is necessary: Case examples of disputes regarding existence, causes, and solutions to social inequalities in health.

Complexity, however, is not an excuse for inaction—especially because "inaction" inevitably translates into shoring up the status quo. The challenge instead is to devise a useful research agenda for social justice in public health. Four key reasons to develop such an agenda are as follows:

Ignorance forestalls action. Two adages suffice: "If you don't ask, you don't know," and "If you don't know, you can't act." The converse is: "No data, no problem."[16]

The "facts" never "speak for themselves." Instead, research findings must be critically evaluated in relation to (a) the theoretical frameworks that researchers use; (b) the rigor with which we—both researchers and those who read the research—conceptualize, operationalize, analyze, and interpret the relevant constructs and data; and (c) the intellectual honesty we muster to address thoughtfully the likely limitations of any given study and implications for the conclusions reached.[2–4,17–19]

Specificity matters. The overarching hypothesis that social injustice harms health in no way implies that each and every type of injustice is causally related to each and every type of health outcome, or that such relationships are static.[2,4] Consider, after all, the marked class shift in smoking over the course of the 20th century in industrialized nations, which went from being concentrated chiefly among more affluent sectors of the populations to becoming most prevalent among more impoverished groups.[6,7,20] Explaining the actual current and changing population distributions of disease, including social inequalities in health, thus constitutes a core test of both etiologic hypotheses and the efficacy of policies and interventions intended to improve the public's health.[2,17,18]

Research can exacerbate and even generate, rather than help rectify, social inequalities in health. This sorry statement is readily illustrated by the blatant examples of scientific racism and eugenics.[2,17,21] Also of concern are more subtle and insidious examples whereby studies focus on characteristics of the dispossessed but not their context—as has occurred, for example, in research on homelessness and health that identifies causes of homelessness in characteristics of homeless people without considering the characteristics of the housing market.[22,23]

Testing claims about the causes and consequences of and solutions to social inequalities in health is thus necessitated by both the problematic legacy and critical potential of public health research.

In this chapter, I discuss a proposal for a public health research agenda that advances issues of social justice and includes four components: theory, monitoring, etiology, and prevention. Drawing on ecosocial theory[2,17,18] and the proposition that social justice is the foundation of public health,[24] I define these components as follows:

Theory: Research to clarify and develop the theoretical frameworks used to explain and guide research on and actions to address social inequalities in health

Monitoring: Research to assess the magnitude of and to improve methods for routinely documenting social inequalities in health, including whether these injustices in health are increasing or decreasing over time

Etiology: Research to test hypotheses about the causes of social inequalities in the population distribution of (a) health status (disease, disability, death, and well-being), and (b) access to and provision of appropriate health care

Prevention: Research to develop, evaluate, and improve methods to assess (a) initiatives explicitly intended to address social inequalities in health, and (b) the beneficial and adverse health consequences of "non-health" policies and programs with social justice implications, including economic, trade, labor, housing, educational, transportation, agriculture, and military policies

For each component, I delineate broad principles and provide specific examples, recognizing that the work of developing specific hypotheses and analytical designs requires substantive and detailed knowledge conjoined with overarching ideas.

▨ THEORY: RESEARCH TO SHARPEN IDEAS, ANALYSIS, AND EXPLANATIONS

Why theory? Consider the model of determinants of population health—including social inequalities in health—shown in Figure 26–2. This model, centered on the distribution and level of population health, appeared in the U.S. federal report *Shaping a Health Statistics Vision for the 21st Century*,[25] with the express purpose of identifying the kinds of data that should be routinely obtained to permit monitoring and investigation of the public's health. Note its concern with context, time, and place and its attention to political, economic, social, cultural, physical, ecological, public health, and medical factors shaping population health. Its inclusion of these myriad determinants and its concern with injustice is not accidental but rather is structured by its explicit reliance on theories of population health.[2,18,26] This is what theory can do: It can provide insight into, and encourage us to test our ideas about the workings of, our world (and universe) by envisioning causal relationships between specified domains of phenomena, including links between social injustice and health, and suggesting ways to test whether the hypothesized relationships, in fact, exist.[2,17–19]

The ecosocial theory of disease distribution that I have been developing,[2,17,18,27] for example, calls attention to four constructs posited to be useful for determining "who and what drives population patterns of health, disease, and well-being, including social inequalities in health."[18] Aiding conceptualization of social injustices in health as biological expressions of social inequality, these constructs are as follows:

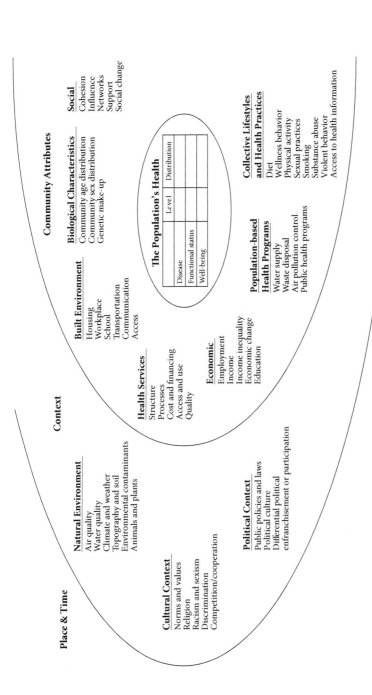

Place & Time

Context

Community Attributes

Natural Environment
Air quality
Water quality
Climate and weather
Topography and soil
Environmental contaminants
Animals and plants

Cultural Context
Norms and values
Religion
Racism and sexism
Discrimination
Competition/cooperation

Political Context
Public policies and laws
Political culture
Differential political
enfranchisement or participation

Health Services
Structure
Processes
Cost and financing
Access and use
Quality

Economic
Employment
Income
Income inequality
Economic change
Education

Built Environment
Housing
Workplace
School
Transportation
Communication
Access

**Population-based
Health Programs**
Water supply
Waste disposal
Air pollution control
Public health programs

Biological Characteristics
Community age distribution
Community sex distribution
Genetic make-up

Social
Cohesion
Influence
Networks
Support
Social change

**Collective Lifestyles
and Health Practices**
Diet
Wellness behavior
Physical activity
Sexual practices
Smoking
Substance abuse
Violent behavior
Access to health information

The Population's Health

	Level	Distribution
Disease		
Functional status		
Well-being		

Figure 26–2 Determinants of population health. (*Source:* U.S. Department of Health and Human Services Data Council, Centers for Disease Control and Prevention, National Center for Health Statistics, National Committee on Vital and Health Statistics. Shaping a health statistics vision for the 21st century: Final report. Washington, DC: National Center for Health Statistics, 2003.)

Embodiment, referring to how we literally incorporate, biologically, the material and social world in which we live

Pathways of embodiment, referring to how processes of embodiment are shaped simultaneously by histories of societal arrangements of power and property and by constraints and possibilities of our evolved biology, including gene expression—not just gene frequency

Cumulative interplay of exposure, susceptibility, and resistance across the life course, referring to the importance of timing and accumulation of, and responses to, embodied exposures

Accountability and agency, referring not only to the institutions and persons responsible for generating or perpetuating social inequalities in health, but also to the public health researchers for the theories used to explain or ignore these injustices

By using such a theory, one can begin systematically to select, for example, among determinants presented in Figure 26–2 to diagram diverse pathways of embodiment conceivably leading to social disparities in health and to discern whether additional determinants should be included. This is because theory enables perception of gaps, rather than drawing on only what has already been documented.[2]

Ecosocial theory, however, is only one of several theories of disease distribution that explicitly links issues of social justice and public health with others. Although it is beyond the scope of this chapter to explicate these theories (see references 2 and 18 for a review of the principal theories used in social epidemiology), others include the social production of disease, political economy of health, and health and human rights—all of which importantly emphasize societal determinants, but tend to leave biology relatively opaque.[2-5,18,28-30] Additional more biologically or psychologically oriented theories not inherently focused on social injustice, but nevertheless often drawn on in research concerned with social inequalities in health, include life course perspective, human and social ecology, social psychology, and various psychosocial theories focused on health behaviors.[2,31,32]

Also germane are frameworks explicitly focused on social justice and social change but not inherently concerned with health, including critical social theory, feminism, anti-racist theories, post-colonialism, post-structuralism, Marxist theories, and theories of justice.[2,3,29,30,33-38] Critical issues raised by these latter theories include defining (and debating) definitions of "social justice," "social injustice," "equity," and "inequity,"[2,29,30,34-38] all constructs highly relevant to the claims that social injustice in health exists and that social justice is the foundation of public health.[2,3,5,24,28,33] (See Chapter 1.) Although these diverse ideas are beyond the scope of this chapter to elaborate, at issue are fundamental notions of (a) distributive and procedural justice; (b) the constellation of indivisible social, economic, political, civil, and cultural rights core to a human rights framework; and (c) the actions of states plus private and public institutions to oppose or condone exploitation and to protect, promote, or violate human rights.[28-30,34-38] (See Chapter 22.)

Yet to date, little systematic research has been conducted on similarities, differences, and deficiencies of these diverse contemporary theories that explicitly—and all too often implicitly—inform research on social injustice and health.[2,38] Indeed, given the dominance of the biomedical paradigm and its positivist emphasis on individual "lifestyles" and faulty genes,[2,3,18,28,38,39] many public health researchers are often untrained in theories of disease distribution, let alone theories of justice. They are thus unaware of their potential usefulness for sharpening not only research questions, but also the design, analysis, and interpretation of public health investigations, interventions, and evaluations. Contemporary scholarship in science studies, however, highlights that advances in scientific understanding are achieved more often through refinement—and replacement—of concepts and ways of thinking, rather than by novel discoveries per se.[2,17,40] Research on characterizing and improving theories for social justice and public health is thus well warranted—and sorely needed, precisely because it is rarely explicitly funded.

▪ MONITORING: RESEARCH TO DOCUMENT THE EXTENT OF, AND TRENDS IN, SOCIAL INEQUALITIES IN HEALTH

Research to improve monitoring of social inequalities in health is likewise urgently required.[2,25,41–45] Without routine monitoring, it is not possible to assess the extent of these injustices in public health, whether they are becoming worse or diminishing over time, or their relationship to changes in their presumed societal determinants.

A prerequisite for tracking health outcomes and their determinants, however, is having a functioning public health monitoring infrastructure.[16,25,28,41,42,45] This entails systems that (a) can accurately and comprehensively document incident and/or prevalent cases (plus ensure confidentiality of this information), and (b) have access to relevant denominator data (such as from the census) to compute the desired rates. Also important is the capacity to link to data on relevant societal determinants of health, as suggested in Figure 26–2. Accomplishing any of these tasks is difficult—and even more difficult when public health agencies lack funds to provide essential services. Thus, in addition to generating social disparities in health, social injustice further compounds the problem by reducing the resources required to monitor its adverse effects on population health.[2,16,45]

Three types of research involving monitoring and social injustices in health are thus needed:

Research on the categories used to classify and the methods used to enumerate societal groups whose differential rates and risks constitute evidence of social injustice in health. At issue is how these categories are conceptualized and operationalized (such as regarding class, race/ethnicity, gender, sexuality, nationality, immigrant status, and disability),[2,37,42,45,46] plus problems with misclassification and biased ascertainment. Underscoring the need for research on these issues is, for example, one recent methodological study demonstrating how misclassification and the undercount together led to serious understatement of U.S. mortality rates in the 1980s among American Indians and Asian and Pacific Islanders compared with white Americans[47]; 30 years later, these problems continue to impair data accuracy and distort understanding of inequitable burdens of morbidity and mortality.[48–51]

Research on contextual data to augment public health monitoring data gathered on individuals to permit linkage to relevant data that cannot be reduced to individual-level characteristics. The need for such inquiry is suggested by results of the *Public Health Disparities Geocoding Project* on socioeconomic and racial/ethnic health inequalities in the United States, which found that choice and level of area-based socioeconomic measures matter—with the census tract poverty measure most sensitive to expected socioeconomic gradients in health, while ZIP code–level measures often missed, and in some cases reversed, these gradients.[52,53]

Research on the measures used to compare health status across societal groups, regarding both the choice of outcomes (such as debates over whether to use such summary measures as disability-adjusted life years [DALYs][28,54,55]) and the type of contrast (such as relative versus absolute risk, or comparing only the extremes versus the full distribution).[43–45,56] Indicating the need for such research are studies demonstrating, for example, that while women may, on average, have longer life expectancy than men, they often have the same or fewer years of *healthy* life expectancy,[57] and that the magnitude of socioeconomic inequalities in health among women is less than that among men if absolute risks are compared, but is similar if relative risks are compared.[58]

Together, these diverse examples suggest that the use of different methods can lead to very different understandings of who disproportionately endures burdens of ill health. If the impact of injustice on health is to be accurately assessed, context-specific research on diverse approaches to monitoring social disparities in health is essential.

▨ ETIOLOGY: INVESTIGATING THE DETERMINANTS OF, AND DETERRENTS TO, SOCIAL INEQUALITIES IN HEALTH STATUS AND HEALTH CARE

Although theory can provide critical insight into connections between injustice and health and monitoring can provide evidence of social disparities in health, etiologic research is required to determine if hypothesized determinants, in fact, explain the actual population distribution of health and social inequalities in health—over time and both within and between societies.[2]

■ CRITICAL QUESTIONS FOR RESEARCH ON SOCIAL JUSTICE AND PUBLIC HEALTH

Questions linking social injustice to population patterns of health, disease, and well-being are distinguished by their emphasis on societal accountability—for both the injustice at issue and its rectification. To show that poverty and ill health are causally connected due to constraints imposed by structural inequality rather than individual failure—that is, a social justice versus victim-blaming explanation[2-5,59,60]—requires evidence, not just ideological debate.

Three theoretically driven overarching questions useful for explicitly articulating issues of accountability and agency can thus be useful for guiding etiologic research on social injustice and health. Some of these questions and their derivatives have been examined in public health research, but many have not, suggesting that much remains to be done.[2-5,18,27-30,60-63] These questions are as follows:

How does prioritizing capital accumulation over human need and ecosystem sustainability affect health status and health care? At issue are neoliberal economic policies, injurious workplace organization and exposure to occupational hazards, inadequate pay scales, environmental pollution, unaffordable housing, privatization of health care, costly pharmaceuticals, and rampant commodification of virtually every human activity, need, and desire.

What is the public health impact of state policies enforcing these priorities? Included are policies that govern (a) regulation or deregulation of corporations, the real estate industry, the insurance industry, and interest rates; (b) enactment or repeal (or enforcement or neglect) of tax codes, trade agreements, labor laws, and environmental laws; (c) absolute and relative levels of spending on social and health programs compared with prison systems and the military; and (d) diplomatic relations with, economic domination of, and even invasion of other countries.

What are the impacts of impoverishment and violation of economic, social, political, civil, and cultural rights, singularly and combined, on population distributions of health and health care? For example, what are the health consequences of: experiencing economic and non-economic forms of racial discrimination; being sexually or physically abused by a family member or intimate partner or on account of belonging to a sexual minority (such as lesbian, gay, bisexual, transgender, or transsexual); or experiencing unjust repression and violence at the hands of agents of the state or paramilitary groups?

Although these questions importantly focus on societal determinants of health, they nevertheless offer little guidance on how to move from these determinants to their manifestation in population inequities in health. To the extent that evidence is needed on magnitude of harm caused, let alone mechanisms by which harm is caused (including to refute explanations embracing only individualized "risk factors"), more specificity is required.

▪ REFINING THE RESEARCH QUESTION:
AN ECOSOCIAL APPROACH

One way to develop a systematic approach to refining research questions addressing links between injustice and population health is perhaps to consider key socially structured and biologically contingent pathways by which inequality can become embodied, across the life course, as delineated using ecosocial theory.[2,17,18,27] These pathways—potentially multilevel and multitemporal—involve adverse exposure to:

Economic and social deprivation

Toxic substances, pathogens, and hazardous conditions

Discrimination and other socially inflicted trauma (mental, physical, and sexual, directly experienced or witnessed, from verbal threats to violent acts)

Targeted marketing of commodities that can harm health, such as "junk food" and psychoactive substances (alcohol, tobacco, and other licit and illicit drugs)

Inadequate or degrading medical care

Degradation of ecosystems, including as linked to systematic alienation of indigenous populations from their lands and corresponding traditional economies

Also relevant are health consequences of people's responses to being subjected to these structural, ecological, institutional, and interpersonal manifestations of inequality. These responses—each with their own set of potential health impacts—can range from internalized oppression and harmful use of psychoactive substances to reflective coping, active resistance, and community organizing to rectify inequity and promote human rights, social justice, and ecologically sustainable economies.

Translating these general concerns into specific research questions requires rigorously elaborating relevant hypotheses, generating valid study designs, and choosing or, if necessary, developing apt measures and analytic methods. In each and every case, scrupulous attention must be paid to issues of:

Etiologic period (time from exposure to when the outcome is manifested)

Type, level, and timing of measurement of the exposure(s), outcome(s), and other covariates

Specificity (or not) of the exposure–outcome relationship

Historical trends in the occurrence of the exposures and outcomes under study

Moreover, if current and changing patterns of population health and social inequalities in health are to be explained, then attention to the specifics of changing exposures—and not just "inequality" per se—is clearly warranted.[2,4,18,61]

Exemplifying why conceptual and operational clarity is critical is research that demonstrates what happens if the relevant social groups or exposures are misspecified. For example, measure social class only at the individual, rather than household level, and key trends in social inequalities in women's health will be missed.[64,65] Measure economic resources only in adulthood, not in childhood, and the cumulative impact of economic deprivation will remain invisible.[31,64,66] Measure household resources, but ignore neighborhood or regional economic conditions, and important contextual determinants will be missed.[52,53,67-69] Measure racial/ethnic identity, but ignore direct and indirect measures of racial discrimination, and the toll of racism on health will remain unknown.[9,70-78] Measure sex, gender, and sexuality, but omit data on current and past histories of sexual and/or gendered violence, and explanations of somatic and mental health will be incomplete.[27,70,79,80]

▧ CASE EXAMPLE: EXCESS HYPERTENSION AMONG AFRICAN AMERICANS

How might this way of thinking be used to generate specific research questions? Consider, as one example, the case of excess rates of hypertension among the U.S. black population compared with not only the U.S. white population but also other populations of West African descent, whether in West Africa, the Caribbean, or elsewhere, reflecting histories of the intercontinental slave trade and contemporary migration.[70-78,81] Research illuminating the impact of injustice on population distributions of hypertension—conceptualized as a biological expression of racial inequality[70,72,82]—could fruitfully be historical, international, contemporary, and local.[70-78,82-86]

To offer one approach to concretizing such a broad research agenda, Figure 26–3 illustrates a selection of possible hypotheses relevant to investigating injustice in relation to black–white disparities in blood pressure among working-age adults, generated using the list of pathways prompted by an ecosocial perspective.[2,17,70-72] These pathways, conjoining social and biological phenomena, explicitly involve structural, ecological, institutional, and interpersonal expressions of inequality, experienced and embodied across the life course. Thus, as diagrammed, conditions such as economic deprivation and racial discrimination can increase the risk of hypertension via pathways involving lead exposure, damaged kidneys, excessive body mass index, unmanaged hypertension due to lack of access to adequate health care, and increased allostatic load[70,72,81-91]—with the last of these defined as *"the wear and tear of the body and brain resulting from chronic overactivity or inactivity of physiological systems that are normally involved in adaptation to environmental challenge"* (italics in original).[89] To investigate any of these hypotheses would require adequate measures of both exposures and outcomes, plus numerous covariates. Highlighting the need for both methodological and etiologic research, moreover, the necessity for rigorous methodological research for developing, say, valid self-report measures of racial discrimination,[70-78,91] or of the body burden of lead,[88] cannot be minimized.

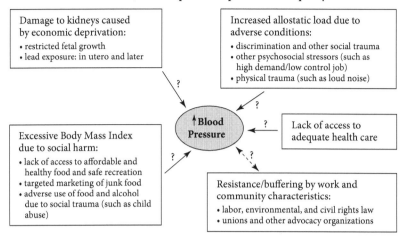

Figure 26–3 Case example: Social inequalities in the population distribution of hypertension—Selected hypotheses that could be systematically explored, involving multilevel pathways of embodiment across the life course. (*Source:* References 70,72,86–91.)

Clearly, no one study could ever realistically address even the restricted set of pathways proposed in Figure 26–3. The point is not that a focus on injustice means any given investigation should measure "everything"—that would be unrealistic and absurd. Instead, the aim should be to use relevant theories concerned with social inequalities in health to consider systematically the choice of hypotheses, study design, measured variables, and unmeasured covariates likely to be important, as well as potential confounders and possibilities of selection bias.[2] Equally key is identifying whose input would be helpful in sorting out these questions. Depending on the study hypothesis and sources of data, valuable input can likely be gained from academic researchers, public health practitioners, policymakers, and global, national, and community-based advocacy organizations, including members of groups whose experiences of inequality led them to bear the burden of the particular health problem under study.[2–5,28–30,33,60] By situating the knowledge and conduct of any given investigation within its broader societal context,[2,18,40] odds are that researchers will be better positioned to understand and convey the meanings and limitations of their study results.

▦ **PREVENTION: RESEARCH TO DEVELOP, EVALUATE, AND IMPROVE METHODS TO ASSESS THE HEALTH IMPACT OF PROGRAMS AND POLICIES INVOLVING ISSUES OF SOCIAL JUSTICE**

The content of the questions for prevention research differ from those of etiologic research, but when it comes to addressing links between injustice and health, some common principles apply. These principles include not only conceptualizing relevant pathways at multiple levels, in relation to relevant time frames, but also asking who gains from as well as who is harmed by injustice.[2-5,27,33,45,59-63] If social injustice were simply a matter of ignorance, increasing knowledge would be sufficient to render the world more equitable—yet many of those firmly holding on to power and privilege are highly educated persons. Indeed, buffered by their privilege, those with power have no need to recognize—and are instead more likely to deny—the harms caused by types of injustice from which they benefit. Underscoring how a hallmark of privilege is that which one can afford to ignore, persons who are white, for example, are protected from the everyday realities of racial discrimination that people of color experience—just as men are protected from the everyday realities of gender discrimination that women experience, just as heterosexual persons are protected from the everyday realities of anti-gay discrimination, or "native-born" persons are protected from the everyday realities of anti-immigrant discrimination. A corollary is that if it were easy to challenge privilege and rectify injustice, the world would already be a very different place.

Research on prevention and social inequalities in health tends to focus on two distinct topics: (a) prevention, health promotion, and advocacy explicitly focused on health, and (b) the health impact of policies and programs originating outside of public health.[28,33,45] Typically, research on designing, implementing, and evaluating explicitly health-oriented interventions is organized around social units whose physical and social conditions reflect (and generate) broader social inequities, such as workplaces, schools, and communities.[32,33,45,69,92] Examples include research on promoting workers' health by simultaneously addressing occupational hazards and health behaviors, increasing access to clean water, reducing exposure to ambient and indoor air pollutants (including cigarette smoke), increasing safer sex and condom use, reducing harm associated with use of licit and illicit drugs, and increasing access to health services.[33,45,92]

Also relevant is research to develop vaccines to prevent, and pharmacological agents to treat, the myriad infectious and parasitic diseases that disproportionately affect impoverished populations globally.[93-95] Research likewise is needed to develop more options for safe, effective, affordable, and user-friendly contraceptives, including barrier methods to curtail the spread of sexually transmitted infections.[96,97] Recommending this type of research in no way contradicts understandable concerns regarding commonplace and often-hyped suggestions that technological "magic bullets," improved health care, and public health programs can by themselves improve health without addressing the social injustices that create social disparities in health.[2-5,28] As the historical record and contemporary work make clear, however, the development of potentially life-saving technologies, therapies, and health interventions is nevertheless one component of a critical research agenda for social justice and public health; neglecting these concerns can lead to what has been termed "public health nihilism"[98] and fail to close gaps created by elite research programs that have long ignored "unprofitable" diseases that especially affect those bearing the brunt of social injustices in health.

Moreover, although diverse kinds of public health interventions can ethically be randomized among or between members of a designated community (such as the type of prevention message that is used), others cannot (such as the provision of clean water). One implication is that the randomized clinical trial (RCT) paradigm cannot be the sole standard for evidence on what makes a difference for addressing social disparities in health. This is because the RCT design cannot be used for critical determinants that can be changed, but cannot be randomized.[99] For this reason, research to evaluate the successes—and failures—of advocacy initiatives designed not for "research" but to improve people's lives[27,28,33,45,60] is also critically needed.

Also necessary is prevention-oriented research on the impact of policies and programs that affect health, but were not explicitly conceived or implemented in relation to public health concerns. Examples include policies on taxation, trade, labor, immigration, transportation, urban development, education, housing, and antipoverty programs, among others. Although concerns about the impact of such "non-health" policies on population health are not new, new attention to the promise of research on this topic for prevention of social inequalities in health is coalescing under the rubric of *health impact assessment* (HIA).[100-103] The conduct of HIAs could potentially (a) enhance recognition of societal determinants of health and of intersectoral responsibility for health, and (b) call attention to how "non-health" policies and programs have the potential to reduce—or exacerbate—social inequalities in health.[2-5,45,60-63,100-103] Even as HIA offers promise as a new avenue of prevention research, promoting links between social justice and health, important questions remain about both the process and its possible pitfalls, including feasibility and costs of generating valid estimates of likely health impacts.[101,102]

▓ CONCLUSION

Clearly, many questions can be asked about the links between social injustice and health. Determining whether such research should be conducted, and which types of questions should be prioritized, necessitates paying critical attention to principles of social justice and human rights. Concern for these principles is essential, from the first glimmers of a research idea all the way through to creating the study team, designing the study, getting it funded, collecting the data, testing hypotheses, and interpreting and disseminating results. It likewise necessitates collective strategizing to ensure that both public and private sponsors forthrightly fund research on social injustice and health. Suggesting this is possible are the myriad efforts that led to the requirement, issued in 2003, that every institute at the U.S. National Institutes of Health develop a strategic plan to address health disparities.[104]

The conceptual and methodological rigor required—and developed—for research linking social justice and public health refutes the oft-asserted conservative canard that advocacy and rigorous science are incompatible.[105-107] Instead, given the lives at stake, research tackling social inequities in health has the responsibility to use the best knowledge and methods available.[2-5,23,60,61] It is this hard-won knowledge, secured by dedicated and inspired effort to investigate determinants of and remedies for social inequalities in health, that public health researchers can uniquely bring to the proverbial table—one contribution among many to create a more just, caring, and sustainable world.

▪ REFERENCES

1. Lecumberri B. Brazil's Helder Camara, champion of poor, dies at 90. Agence France Presse, August 28, 1999. Available at http://www.hartford-hwp.com/archives/42/084.html. Accessed on April 28, 2012.

2. Krieger N. Epidemiology and the people's health: Theory and context. New York: Oxford University Press, 2011.

3. Navarro V, ed. The political economy of social inequalities: Consequences for health and quality of life. Amityville, NY: Baywood Publishing Company, 2002.

4. Kunitz SJ. The health of populations: General theories and particular realities. New York: Oxford University Press, 2006.

5. Tesh SN. Hidden arguments: Political ideology and disease prevention policy. New Brunswick, NJ: Rutgers University Press, 1988.

6. Kluger R. Ashes to ashes: America's hundred-year cigarette war, the public health, and the unabashed triumph of Philip Morris. New York: Alfred A. Knopf, 1996.

7. Brandt AM. The cigarette century: The rise, fall, and deadly persistence of the product that defined America. New York: Basic Books, 2007.

8. Thornton J. Pandora's poison: Chlorine, health, and a new environmental strategy. Cambridge, MA: MIT Press, 2000.

9. Krieger N. Does racism harm health? Did child abuse exist before 1962?—On explicit questions, critical science, and current controversies: An ecosocial perspective. *Am J Public Health* 2003;93:194–199.

10. Kaufman JS, Cooper RS. Seeking causal explanations in social epidemiology. *Am J Epidemiol* 1999;150:113–120.

11. Lynch JW, Davey Smith G, Kaplan GA, et al. Income inequality and mortality: Importance to health of individual incomes, psychological environment, or material conditions. *BMJ* 2000;320:1200–1204.

12. Marmot M, Wilkinson RG. Psychosocial and material pathways in the relation between income and health: A response to Lynch et al. *BMJ* 2001;322:1233–1236.

13. Leigh A, Jencks C. Inequality and mortality: Long-run evidence from a panel of countries. *J Health Econ* 2007;26:1–24.

14. Wilkinson RG, Pickett K. The spirit level: Why more equal societies almost always do better. London: Allen Lane, 2009.

15. Goldthorpe JH. Analysing social inequality: A critique of two recent contributions from economics and epidemiology. *Eur Sociol Rev* 2010;26:731–744.

16. Krieger N. The making of public health data: Paradigms, politics, and policy. *J Public Health Policy* 1992;13:412–427.
17. Krieger N. Epidemiology and the web of causation: Has anyone seen the spider? *Soc Sci Med* 1994;39:887–903.
18. Krieger N. Theories for social epidemiology in the 21st century: An ecosocial perspective. *Int J Epidemiol* 2001;30:668–677.
19. Haraway DJ. Situated knowledge: The science question in feminism and the privilege of partial perspective. In: Haraway DJ. *Simians, cyborgs and women: The reinvention of nature.* New York: Routledge Press, 1991:183–201.
20. Stellman SD, Resnicow K. Tobacco smoking, cancer and social class. In: Kogevinas M, Pearce N, Susser M, Boffetta P, eds. Social inequalities and cancer. (IARC scientific publication no. 138). Lyon, France: International Agency for Research on Cancer, 1997: 229–250.
21. Kevles DJ. In the name of eugenics: Genetics and the uses of human heredity. Cambridge, MA: Harvard University Press, 1995.
22. Sclar ED. Homelessness and housing policy: A game of musical chairs. *Am J Public Health* 1990;80:1039–1040.
23. Schwartz S, Carpenter KM. The right answer to the wrong question: Consequences of type III error for public health research. *Am J Public Health* 1999;89:1175–1180.
24. Krieger N, Birn AE. A vision of social justice as the foundation of public health: Commemorating 150 years of the Spirit of 1848. *Am J Public Health* 1998;88:1603–1606.
25. U.S. Department of Health and Human Services Data Council, Centers for Disease Control and Prevention, National Center for Health Statistics, National Committee on Vital and Health Statistics. Shaping a health statistics vision for the 21st century: Final report. Washington, DC: National Center for Health Statistics, 2003.
26. Krieger N. Ladders, pyramids, and champagne: The iconography of health inequities. *J Epidemiol Commun Health* 2008;62:1098–1104.
27. Krieger N, ed. Embodying inequality: Epidemiologic perspectives. Amityville, NY: Baywood Publishing, 2004.
28. Birn AE, Pillay Y, Holtz TM. Textbook of international health: Global health in a dynamic world. 3rd ed. New York: Oxford University Press, 2009.
29. Gruskin S, Tarantola D. Health and human rights. In: Detels R, McEwen J, Beaglehole R, et al., eds. The Oxford textbook of public health. 4th ed. New York: Oxford University Press, 2001:311–335.
30. Gruskin S, Mills EJ, Tarantola D. Health and human rights 1: History, principles, and practice of health and human rights. *Lancet* 2007;370:449–455.
31. Kuh DH, Ben-Shlomo Y, eds. A lifecourse approach to chronic disease epidemiology. 2nd ed. Oxford, UK: Oxford University Press, 2004.
32. Schneiderman N, Speers MA, Silva JM, et al., eds. Integrating behavioral and social sciences with public health. Washington, DC: American Psychological Association, 2001.
33. Wallerstein N, Duran B. The conceptual, historical, and practice roots of community-based participatory research. In: Minkler M, Wallerstein N, eds. Community-based participatory research for health. San Francisco, CA: Jossey-Bass, 2003:27–52.
34. Doyal L, Gough I. A theory of human need. New York: Guilford Press, 1991.
35. Miller D. Principles of social justice. Cambridge, MA.: Harvard University Press, 1999.
36. Venkatapuram S. Health justice. Cambridge, UK: Polity Press, 2011.

37. Grusky DB, Szelenyi S, eds. Inequality reader: Contemporary and foundational readings in class, race, and gender. 2nd ed. Boulder, CO: Westview Press, 2011.

38. Solar O, Irwin A. A conceptual framework for action on the social determinants of health. Social Determinants of Health Discussion Paper 2 (Policy and Practice). Geneva: World Health Organization, 2010. Available at http://www.who.int/sdhconference/resources/ConceptualframeworkforactiononSDH_eng.pdf. Accessed on March 11, 2013.

39. Lock M, Gordon D, eds. Biomedicine examined. Dordrecht, the Netherlands: Kluwer Academic Publishers, 1988.

40. Rosenberg CE, Golden J, eds. Framing disease: Studies in cultural history. New Brunswick, NJ: Rutgers University Press, 1992.

41. Krieger N, Chen JT, Ebel G. Can we monitor socioeconomic inequalities in health? A survey of U.S. health departments' data collection and reporting practices. *Public Health Rep* 1997;112:481–491.

42. ver Ploeg M, Perrin E, eds. Eliminating health disparities: Measurement and data needs. Washington, DC: National Academies Press, 2004.

43. Keppel K, Pamuk E, Lynch J, et al. Methodological issues in measuring health disparities. Hyattsville, MD: National Center for Health Statistics, 2005. (Vital and health statistics, series 2: data evaluation and methods research, no. 141). Available at http://www.cdc.gov/nchs/data/series/sr_02/sr02_141.pdf. Accessed on April 29, 2012.

44. Harper S, Lynch J. Measuring health inequalities. In: Oakes JM, Kaufman JS, eds. Methods in social epidemiology. San Francisco, CA: Jossey-Bass, 2006:134–168.

45. World Health Organization, CSDH. Closing the gap in a generation: Health equity through action on the social determinants of health. Final report of the Commission on Social Determinants of Health. Geneva: World Health Organization, 2008. Available at http://www.who.int/social_determinants/thecommission/finalreport/en/index.html. Accessed on April 29, 2012.

46. Krieger N. A glossary for social epidemiology. *J Epidemiol Commun Health* 2001;55:693–700.

47. Rosenberg HM, Maurer JD, Sorlie PD, et al. Quality of death rates by race and Hispanic origin: A summary of current research, 1999. *Vital Health Stat 2* 1999;Sep:1–13.

48. Arias E, Schauman WS, Eschbach K, et al. The validity of race and Hispanic origin reporting on death certificates in the United States. *Vital Health Stat 2* 2008;148:1–23.

49. Noymer A, Penner AM, Saperstein AM. Cause of death affects racial classification on death certificates. *PLoS One* 2011;6(1):e15812.

50. Espey DK, Wiggins CL, Jim MA, et al. Methods for improving cancer surveillance data in American Indian and Alaska Native populations. *Cancer* 2008;113(5 Suppl):1120–1130.

51. Gomez SL, Glaser SL. Misclassification of race/ethnicity in a population-based cancer registry (United States). *Cancer Causes Control* 2006;17:771–781.

52. Krieger N, Chen JT, Waterman PD, et al. Painting a truer picture of U.S. socioeconomic and racial/ethnic health inequalities: The Public Health Disparities Geocoding Project. *Am J Public Health* 2005;95:312–323.

53. Krieger N, Waterman PD, Chen JT, et al. The Public Health Disparities Geocoding Project Monograph. Initially launched 2004, with materials added subsequently. Available at http://www.hsph.harvard.edu/thegeocodingproject. Accessed on April 28, 2012.

54. Ezzati M, Lopez AD, Rodgers A, et al. Selected major risk factors and global and regional burden of disease. *Lancet* 2002;360:1347–1360.

55. Reidpath DD, Allotey PA, Kouame A, et al. Measuring health in a vacuum: Examining the disability weight of the DALY. *Health Policy Plan* 2003;18:351–356.

56. Wagstaff A, Paci P, van Doorslaer E. On the measurement of inequalities in health. *Soc Sci Med* 1991;33:545–557.

57. Mathers CD, Murray CJL, Lopez AD, et al. Global patterns of health life expectancy for older women. *J Women's Aging* 2002;14:99–117.

58. Mustard CA, Etches J. Gender differences in socioeconomic inequality in mortality. *J Epidemiol Commun Health* 2003;57:974–980.

59. Crawford R. You are dangerous to your health: The ideology and politics of victim blaming. *Int J Health Services* 1977;7:663–680.

60. Hofrichter R, ed. Health and social justice: Politics, ideology and inequity in the distribution of disease—A public health reader. San Francisco, CA: Jossey-Bass, 2003.

61. Davey Smith G, ed. Health inequalities: Lifecourse approaches. Bristol, UK: University of Bristol Policy Press, 2003.

62. Beckfield J, Krieger N. Epi + demos + cracy: A critical review of empirical research linking political systems and priorities to the magnitude of health inequities. *Epidemiol Rev* 2009;31:152–177.

63. Krieger N, Alegría M, Almeida-Filho N, et al. Who, and what, causes health inequities? Reflections on emerging debates from an exploratory Latin American/North American workshop. *J Epidemiol Commun Health* 2010;64:747–749.

64. Krieger N, Williams D, Moss N. Measuring social class in U.S. public health research: Concepts, methodologies and guidelines. *Annu Rev Public Health* 1997;18:341–378.

65. Cooper H. Investigating socio-economic explanations for gender and ethnic inequalities in health. *Soc Sci Med* 2002;54:693–706.

66. Graham H. Building an inter-disciplinary science of health inequalities: The example of lifecourse research. *Soc Sci Med* 2002;55:2005–2016.

67. O'Campo P. Invited commentary: Advancing theory and methods for multilevel models of residential neighborhoods and health. *Am J Epidemiol* 2003;157:9–13.

68. Macintyre S, Ellaway A, Cummins S. Place effects on health: How can we conceptualise, operationalise and measure them? *Soc Sci Med* 2002;55:125–139.

69. Kawachi I, Berkman LF, eds. Neighborhoods and health. New York: Oxford University Press, 2003.

70. Krieger N. Discrimination and health. In: Berkman L, Kawachi I, eds. Social epidemiology. New York: Oxford University Press, 2000:36–75.

71. Krieger N. Methods for the scientific study of discrimination and health: from societal injustice to embodied inequality—An ecosocial approach. *Am J Public Health* 2012;102:936–945.

72. Krieger N. The science and epidemiology of racism and health: Racial/ethnic categories, biological expressions of racism, and the embodiment of inequality—An ecosocial perspective. In Whitmarsh I, Jones DS, eds. What's the use of race? Genetics and difference in forensics, medicine, and scientific research. Cambridge, MA: MIT Press, 2010:225–255.

73. National Research Council. Measuring racial discrimination. Panel on Methods for Assessing Discrimination. Blank RM, Dabady M, Citro CF, eds. Committee on National Statistics, Division of Behavioral and Social Sciences and Education. Washington, DC: The National Academies Press, 2004.

74. Gee GC, Walsemann KM, Brondolo E. A life course perspective on how racism may be related to health inequities. *Am J Public Health* 2012;102:967–974.

75. Williams DR, Mohammed SA. Discrimination and racial disparities in health: Evidence and needed research. *J Behav Med* 2009;32:20–47.

76. Mays VM, Cochran SD, Barnes NW. Race, race-based discrimination, and health outcomes among African Americans. *Ann Rev Psychol* 2007;58:201–225.

77. Paradies Y. A systematic review of empirical research on self-reported racism and health. *Int J Epidemiol* 2006;35:888–901.

78. National Institutes of Health. Conference: The Science of Research on Discrimination and Health. Bethesda, MD, February 2–4, 2011. Available at http://healthservices.cancer.gov/areas/disparities/conference.html. Accessed on April 29, 2012.

79. Krug E, Dahlberg L, Mercy J, et al, eds. World report on violence and health. Geneva: World Health Organization, 2002.

80. Doyal L. What makes women sick? Gender and the political economy of health. New Brunswick, NJ: Rutgers University Press, 1995.

81. Cruikshank JK, Mbanya JC, Wilks R, et al. Sick genes, sick individuals or sick populations with chronic disease? The emergence of diabetes and high blood pressure in African-origin populations. *Int J Epidemiol* 2001;30:111–117.

82. Krieger N. Refiguring "race": Epidemiology, racialized biology, and biological expressions of race relations. *Int J Health Serv* 2000;30:211–216.

83. Krieger N, Sidney S. Racial discrimination and blood pressure: The CARDIA study of young black and white adults. *Am J Public Health* 1996;86:1370–1378.

84. Gravlee CC. How race becomes biology: Embodiment of social inequality. *Am J Phys Anthropol* 2009;139:47–57.

85. Elliott P. High blood pressure in the community. In: Bulpitt CJ, ed. Handbook of hypertension, vol. 20: Epidemiology of hypertension. Amsterdam, the Netherlands: Elsevier, 2000:1–18.

86. Brondolo E, Love EE, Pencille M, et al. Racism and hypertension: A review of the empirical evidence and implications for clinical practice. *Am J Hypertens* 2011;24:518–529.

87. Lopes AA, Port FK. The low birth weight hypothesis as a plausible explanation for the black/white differences in hypertension, non-insulin-dependent diabetes, and end-stage renal disease. *Am J Kidney Dis* 1995;25:350–356.

88. Vupputuri S, He J, Munter P, et al. Blood lead level is associated with elevated blood pressure in blacks. *Hypertension* 2003;41:463–468.

89. McEwen BS. Stress, adaptation, and disease: Allostasis and allostatic load. *Ann NY Acad Sci* 1998;840:33–44.

90. McEwen BS, Tucker P. Critical biological pathways for chronic psychosocial stress and research opportunities to advance the consideration of stress in chemical risk assessment. *Am J Public Health* 2011;101(Suppl 1):S131–S139.

91. Krieger N, Waterman PD, Kosheleva A, et al. Exposing racial discrimination: Implicit & explicit measures—The My Body, My Story study of 1005 U.S.-born black & white community health center members. *PLoS ONE* 2011;6(11):e27636. doi:10.1371/journal.pone.0027636.

92. Sorensen G, Emmons K, Stoddard A, et al. Do social influences contribute to occupational differences in smoking behavior? *Am J Health Promot* 2002;16:135–141.

93. Trouiller P, Olliaro P, Torreele E, et al. Drug development for neglected diseases: A deficient market and a public-health policy failure. *Lancet* 2002;359:2188–2194.

94. Musselwhite LW, Maciag K, Lankowski A, et al. First Universities Allied for Essential Medicines (UAEM) Neglected Diseases and Innovation Symposium. *Am J Trop Med Hyg* 2012;86:65–74.

95. World Health Organization on behalf of the Special Programme for Research and Training in Tropical Diseases (TDR). Global report for research on infectious diseases of poverty. Geneva, Switzerland: World Health Organization, 2012. Available at http://www.who.int/tdr/stewardship/global_report/en/. Accessed on April 29, 2012.

96. Reaves ND. Unresolved issues in contraceptive health policy. *Health Care Women Int* 2002;23:854–860.

97. Rowlands S. New technologies in contraception. *BJOG* 2009;116:230–239.

98. Fairchild A, Oppenheimer G. Public health nihilism vs. pragmatism: History, politics, and the control of tuberculosis. *Am J Public Health* 1998;88:1105–1117.

99. Davey Smith G, Ebrahim S, Frankel S. How policy informs the evidence: "Evidence based" thinking can lead to debased policy making. *BMJ* 2001;322:184–185.

100. Scott-Samuel A. Health impact assessment: An idea whose time has come. *BMJ* 1996;313:183–184.

101. Krieger N, Northridge M, Gruskin S, et al. Assessing health impact assessment: Multidisciplinary and international perspectives. *J Epidemiol Commun Health* 2003;57:659–662.

102. Dannenberg AL, Bhatia R, Cole BL, et al. Growing the field of health impact assessment in the United States: An agenda for research and practice. *Am J Public Health* 2006;96:262–270.

103. Mindell JS, Boltong A, Forde I. A review of health impact assessment frameworks. *Public Health* 2008;122:1177–1187.

104. National Center on Minority Health and Health Disparities. NIH strategic plan and budget to reduce and ultimately eliminate health disparities. FY 2002. Washington, DC: National Institutes of Health, U.S. Department of Health and Human Services, 2003.

105. Savitz DA, Poole C, Miller WC. Reassessing the role of epidemiology in public health. *Am J Public Health* 1999;89:1158–1161.

106. Rothman KJ, Adami H-O, Trichopolous D. Should the mission of epidemiology include the eradication of poverty? *Lancet* 1998;352:810–813.

107. Satel SL. PC, M.D.: How political correctness is corrupting medicine. New York: Basic Books, 2000.

108. Smedley BD, Stith AY, Nelson AR, eds. Unequal treatment: Confronting racial and ethnic disparities in health care. Committee on Understanding and Eliminating Racial and Ethnic Disparities in Health Care, Board on Health Sciences Policy, Institute of Medicine. Washington, DC: National Academies Press, 2003.

109. Erwin K. Interpreting the evidence: Competing paradigms and the emergence of lesbian and gay suicide as a "social fact." *Int J Health Serv* 1993;23:437–453.

110. Herrell R, Goldberg J, True WR, et al. Sexual orientation and suicidality: A co-twin control study in adult men. *Arch Gen Psychiatry* 1999;56:867–874.

111. Verduin P, Agarwal S, Waltman S. Solutions to obesity: Perspectives from the food industry. *Am J Clin Nutr* 2005;82:259S–261S.

112. Nestle M. Food politics: How the food industry influences nutrition and health. Berkeley, CA: University of California Press, 2002.

27

Protecting Human Rights Through International and National Law

■ PETER WEISS AND HENRY A. FREEDMAN

■ **INTRODUCTION**

International and national law can play a critical role in protecting human rights, and thereby in reducing social injustice, because law is the primary system through which the national and international communities seek to enforce social norms. Human rights are not a creation of the 20th century. Antigone, in Sophocles' play of that name from the fifth century B.C.E., defies a royal decree forbidding the burial of her brother Polyneices by relying on "the unwritten and unfailing laws of heaven" whose "life is not of today or yesterday, but from all time."[1] (See also Chapter 22.)

The notion of a supreme law that confers on individuals rights transcending those found in the codes of laws of their nations is a constant theme running through the writings of all major cultures for the past 2500 years. Heaven as the source of rights came gradually to be complemented by nature—hence the reference to "the laws of nature and of nature's God," which precedes the definition of the *inalienable rights* ("life, liberty, and the pursuit of happiness") in the U.S. Declaration of Independence of 1776. The fundamental law of the United States, the Constitution, signed in 1789, and the Bill of Rights (the first 10 Amendments to the Constitution), adopted in 1791, imposed few positive obligations on the government—and imposed no obligations related to economic or social rights.

The codification of international human rights began about the same time, with the branch of human rights law dealing with the obligations of combatants, known as *humanitarian law*—or by its Latin name, *jus in bello*. These obligations of omission and commission created, if only indirectly, concomitant rights in the people and institutions to be protected. In 1782, the United States and Prussia signed a treaty of amity and commerce, which provided that, should war break out between them, all women and children, scholars of every faculty, cultivators of the earth, artisans, manufacturers and fishermen, unarmed and inhabiting unfortified towns, villages or places, and, in general, all others whose occupations were for the common subsistence and benefit of mankind should be allowed to continue their respective employment and should not be "molested."[2] This treaty embodied the principle—increasingly ignored over the 20th century—that civilians are not legitimate targets in war.[3] (Parties to a conflict must always distinguish between civilians and combatants; attacks must not be directed against civilians.) This principle constituted the basis of subsequent international treaties, including the Hague Conventions of 1899 and 1907 and the Geneva Conventions of 1949.[4]

Meanwhile, in the United States, constitutional amendments following the Civil War (1861–1865) prohibited slavery and provided that no state shall "deprive any person of life, liberty, or property, without due process of law; nor deny to any person within its jurisdiction the equal protection of the laws."[5] These provisions have proven to be critical in securing certain social and economic rights; these provisions, however, do not affirmatively provide for these rights.

Because of the federal structure of the United States, each of the 50 states is also an important source of rights. However, only the constitution of New York State ensures that the assistance, care, and support for needy people are public concerns and must be provided by the state, and that protection and promotion of state residents are state responsibilities. Other states either have no provision for economic and social rights or have limited provisions that are easily satisfied.

The United Nations Charter, which came into force in 1945, constitutes a treaty binding on all of its original and future members. It states, at the start of the preamble, "We the Peoples of the United Nations" commit ourselves to "save succeeding generations from the scourge of war." In its second paragraph, it extends this commitment to reaffirming "faith in fundamental human rights, in the dignity and worth of the human person, in the equal rights of men and women." And a key purpose of the United Nations, as stated in the Charter, is "promoting and encouraging respect for human rights."[6]

■ INTERNATIONAL LAW

The United Nations Charter is like a *matryoshka,* a Russian nesting doll, producing document after document of greater particularity, but of smaller scope, than its predecessor. Thus, in 1948, under the leadership of Eleanor Roosevelt and with the approval of the United States, the United Nations adopted the first comprehensive, nonmilitary code of human rights, the Universal Declaration of Human Rights (UDHR). The UDHR contains articles addressing economic, social, and cultural rights. These rights include social security, education, and a standard of living adequate for health and well-being, ensuring adequate food, clothing, housing, and medical care, and necessary social services.[7] Mothers and children, whether born in or out of wedlock, are entitled to special care and assistance.

In 1956, two covenants—the International Covenant on Economic, Social and Cultural Rights (ICESCR)[8] and the International Covenant on Civil and Political Rights (ICCPR)[9]—provided greater detail on the rights described in the UDHR, and made nations who signed these covenants responsible for recognizing and implementing these rights. These nations, therefore, are required to (a) recognize the right to safe and healthy working conditions, (b) punish employers who employ children and young persons in harmful work, and (c) recognize "the right of everyone to the enjoyment of the highest attainable standard of physical and mental health." In order to achieve the highest attainable standard of health, these nations agree to reduce infant mortality; improve environmental and industrial hygiene; prevent, treat, and control epidemic, endemic, occupational, and other types of diseases; and ensure access of sick people to medical services. Ensuring access to medical services, which could be interpreted as a mandate for universal health care, may explain why the United States has never ratified ICESCR—although it finally ratified ICCPR in 1982. The United States, however, as a member of the World Health Organization (WHO), has accepted the WHO principle that "the enjoyment of the highest attainable standard of health is one of the fundamental rights of every human being."[10]

Another important source of national socioeconomic obligations is the Charter of the Organization of American States,[11] ratified by the United States in 1951. By its terms, member states pledge themselves "to accelerate their economic and social development" and to achieve "equitable distribution of national income...modernization of rural life, protection of [people's] potential through the extension and application of modern medical science, proper nutrition...adequate housing for all sectors of the population, and urban conditions that offer the opportunity for a healthful, productive, and full life."

The framers of the UDHR and the two covenants did not make a distinction between two sets of human rights. In identical preambles to the two covenants, they declared that there are two sets of rights that are completely interdependent and could only be achieved together: (a) civil and political rights; and (b) economic, social, and cultural rights. Unfortunately, many judges, policymakers, and academics have made a distinction between these two sets of rights. For example, during the Cold War, the capitalist Western bloc countries generally regarded the ICCPR rights as real and enforceable and the ICESCR as "aspirational" and unenforceable; in contrast, socialist Eastern bloc countries took the opposite view. The view of Western countries now prevails throughout most of the world. However, even the implementation of ICCPR leaves much to be desired. Indeed, it is fair to say that, especially in the United States and allied countries in the North Atlantic Treaty Organization, civil and political rights have become less secure since the terrorist attacks of 2001.

The time is ripe to transform the right to health and other social and economic rights from abstract concepts into legally enforceable instruments. Many courts, especially those in the United States, still refuse to treat ICESCR as "real." They adhere to the thought that economic, social, and cultural rights can only be progressively implemented as resources become available—ignoring that government resources are allocated by politicians according to their own values and priorities. But this is not true for other countries. The "case law" page of ESCR-Net lists about 150 recent legal cases from various countries and some international and regional human-rights organizations that address such economic, social, and cultural rights as social security, health, housing, and education. Decisions in these cases were made on the basis of ICESCR and national constitutions.

The *Grootboom* case, for example, was decided by the Constitutional Court of South Africa in 2000.[12] It involved an appeal by a community of squatters for assistance from the provincial and municipal authorities, based on sections of the South African Constitution that address the right to housing and children's right to basic shelter. The Constitutional Court ordered, for all of the squatters' households, construction and operation of permanent toilets, installation and operation of water taps, and provision of building material up to a value of 760 rands (US$130).

Based on the precedent of this case, the Constitutional Court of South Africa, in a 2001 case (*Treatment Action Campaign v. Minister of Health*) affirmed an order by a lower court to provide the retroviral drug nevirapine to all HIV-positive pregnant women in South Africa, probably saving tens of thousands of lives.[13] In 2011, slum dwellers in South Africa won a case in the Constitutional Court, which declared unconstitutional the section of the Slums Act (1936) that authorized the eviction of slum dwellers before suitable alternate housing could be found for them.

Cases from other countries involving social justice and public health have included the following:

- In *Maria Isabel Chamorro Santamaria et al. v. the Ministry of the Economy and the National Treasury,* the Supreme Court of Costa Rica decided that the national treasury had sufficient funds to provide the plaintiffs with the social services that had previously been denied them.[14]
- In *Paschim Banga Khet Samity v. State of West Bengal,* a case brought by a plaintiff who fell off a train and was denied emergency medical treatment in six government hospitals, the Supreme Court of India awarded compensation to the plaintiff and issued a detailed set of orders to the state government designed to improve the availability of medical services in West Bengal.
- In *Jorge Odir Miranda Cortez v. El Salvador,* the Inter-American Commission for Human Rights affirmed the right to health in the American Convention on Human Rights. It also requested the government of El Salvador to immediately supply retroviral medication to the plaintiffs with HIV/AIDS, a request that was later given the force of law by the Supreme Court of El Salvador.
- In *Shehla Zia v. Wapda PLD,* the Supreme Court of Pakistan, following the precedent set by the Supreme Court of India of accepting direct petitions from citizens who considered their human rights violated, stated that it lacked the expertise to decide whether a proposed power station would constitute a serious health hazard. However, it ordered the government to establish a commission of internationally recognized scientists to evaluate the petitioners' claim.

The best source for cases dealing with health is the table of cases in *The Right to Health in International Law* by John Tobin.[15] He states that most countries still lack immediately enforceable rights to health and health care, but that progress toward this long-term goal has begun. One example of the use of international norms to achieve this progress is the 2011 case of *Alyne da Silva Pimentel v. Brazil.* There the UN Committee on the Convention on the Elimination of All Forms of Discrimination Against Women (CEDAW) held the government of Brazil liable for the preventable death of a woman who hemorrhaged for 4 days in a public hospital after having had an abortion.[16]

In addition to national and regional tribunals, such as the Inter-American Commission and Court for Human Rights or the European Court of Human Rights, questions of humanitarian law concerning social injustice are subject to litigation in international tribunals. The International Court of Justice (ICJ) did so in the case brought by Nicaragua against the United States in 1984 concerning the activities of the U.S.-sponsored contras. In 1996, in its advisory opinion on the legality of the threat or use of nuclear weapons in the "nuclear weapons case," the ICJ held that "a threat or use of nuclear weapons should be compatible with the requirements of the international law applicable in armed conflict, particularly those of the principles and rules of international humanitarian law."[17] The ICJ refused to take the nuclear weapons case at the request of the World Health Assembly, but did take it at the request of the United Nations General Assembly. Cases involving violation of human rights or humanitarian law rarely come before the ICJ. However, in 2012, in *Belgium v. Senegal*, it unanimously ordered Senegal to either try Hissène Habré, the former dictator of Chad who had sought asylum in Senegal, or, under the principle of universal jurisdiction, extradite him to Belgium, where he had been indicted for genocide and crimes against humanity.

By contrast, the International Criminal Court (ICC), which was established in 2002, is likely to eventually have a docket addressing the principles of international humanitarian law to which the ICJ referred in the nuclear weapons case. The jurisdiction of the ICC is currently limited to "the crime of genocide, war crimes, and crimes against humanity."[18]

■ NATIONAL LAW IN THE UNITED STATES

Because social and economic rights are not mentioned in the U.S. Constitution, progressive forces have sought to address social justice and human rights issues through federal and state legislation. Two of the most significant developments at the federal level have been the 1935 Social Security Act (SSA) and the 2010 Patient Protection and Affordable Care Act (ACA).

Income Security

Until the Great Depression of the 1930s, the federal government played little role in providing economic or social protection, leaving such matters to the states. The SSA, sponsored by President Franklin D. Roosevelt, created federal retirement and survivor's benefits (disability benefits were added later) and the unemployment insurance program. While these benefits were based on earnings history and contributions, rather than current economic need, they have played a critical role for over 75 years in keeping millions of Americans out of poverty.

The SSA also provided matching funds for state welfare programs for older people and families with dependent children—largely for families missing one parent—with eligibility based on current financial need. In 1935, the U.S. Congress was dominated by Southern senators. To ensure that the federally supported needs-based programs would not promote a civil rights agenda, states were granted enormous discretion in setting eligibility and benefits. (In 1974, the federal government assumed responsibility for the needs-based cash assistance programs for older people and people with disabilities, now called the Supplemental Security Income [SSI] program.) As time passed, administration of these federally funded and state-operated needs-based programs was often permeated by arbitrary decision-making and racial discrimination. In more recent years, Congress and many state legislatures have stripped legal rights from many needs-based social welfare programs, narrowed eligibility criteria, and made application for programs and compliance with program requirements more difficult.

Nevertheless, creative lawyering in the late 1960s brought about profound changes in welfare programs through U.S. Supreme Court cases that established a legal "entitlement" to assistance.[19] In *Goldberg v. Kelly*, which continues to be good law today, the Court said welfare benefits could not be terminated unless advance notice was given and an opportunity for an in-person hearing provided. The Court adopted the argument raised by progressive lawyers and scholars that government benefits created with explicit eligibility conditions were a form of property (often called a "statutory entitlement") that could not be taken away without due process of law. This transformed state welfare administration, reducing arbitrary decision-making and increasing accountability. Still, bureaucracies were large and complex, social and political hostility to poor people was too great, and the ability of welfare recipients to assert and defend their rights too hampered for complete rationality and fairness to be achieved.

During the 1980s and 1990s, needs-based income security programs came under increasing attack, with charges that they nourished antisocial behavior and long-term impoverishment. Unfortunately, much of the public—including many poor people—have believed that poverty and other social ills are the sole responsibility of the individual, not the consequence of economic forces or government policy. One major trend was replacing federally created individual entitlements with block grants to the states, devolving to state and local authorities the power to set standards and rules.

In 1996, federal legislation replaced the 1935 federal/state Aid to Families with Dependent Children program with the block-grant Temporary Assistance to Needy Families (TANF) program, giving each state a fixed sum of money to use to provide aid and services to low-income families. The law stated explicitly that the benefits were not entitlements. This legislation gave the states far greater discretion, but imposed rigorous work requirements.

At first, TANF rolls decreased because of a growing economy, much harsher eligibility requirements, and services to assist people to get jobs. As unemployment and poverty increased in approximately 2008, TANF rolls did not rise to meet increased need. Fortunately, as poverty has grown, the food stamp program (now the Supplemental Nutrition Assistance Program, or SNAP), created in the 1960s as an entitlement paying for certain food purchases, has been able to grow. In addition, the Earned Income Tax Credit provides additional cash through the income tax system to low-wage workers. Unfortunately, both programs are now under sustained attack in Congress.

Although significant progress is being made in many other areas of human rights, as discussed below, poverty, with its severe impact on health and opportunity for children to thrive, has been growing in recent years—especially among racial and ethnic minorities and single mothers and their children.

Health Care

The United States has lagged behind most other countries in recognizing health care as a fundamental human right. The first major national steps in providing care were taken in 1965, when Congress created both (a) Medicare, a fully federally funded health-care program for older people and people with disabilities eligible for Social Security benefits, and (b) Medicaid, a state and federal program to fund health care for certain needy families, older people, and people with disabilities. In these programs, the government does not provide health care directly, as it does for veterans, but pays health care providers according to set rates.

After failed attempts over the several decades to attain more-universal health care, Congress took the next major step when it narrowly passed the Affordable Care Act (ACA) in 2010 following ferocious debate, complicated legislative maneuvers, an ambitious grassroots campaign, and intense lobbying by the insurance industry, drug companies, and hospitals and health care providers. The Act provides inducements for employers to provide health insurance, creates exchanges where people are able to shop for insurance if they are not covered at work, and provides subsidies to moderate-income families to ease the cost of purchasing health insurance. Insurance companies are barred from denying coverage because of pre-existing conditions and must spend most of the premiums collected on providing health care. These are all significant improvements.

Two key components of the ACA were challenged before the U.S. Supreme Court: (a) individuals will be penalized if they do not have insurance (the "individual mandate"), and (b) states will be provided significant funding to provide Medicaid to most people with income below 133 percent of the poverty line. In a major decision in 2012, the Supreme Court upheld the individual mandate by a 5–4 vote but, most unfortunately, also held that states could not be required to expand their Medicaid programs. Several Republican state governors have said they will not expand their Medicaid programs, raising the possibility that millions of low-income Americans will still not be covered. (See also Chapter 12.)

Other Rights and Benefits

Many states have constitutional provisions ensuring rights to public education, and lawyers have had some success in forcing states to address severe under-funding of education in local school districts. Nevertheless, the combination of tax cuts and state constitutional provisions forbidding budget deficits is making it difficult for public officials to provide adequately for education, much less other social needs not mentioned in state constitutions.

Greater legal success has been achieved in promoting civil rights. The U.S. Supreme Court declared racial segregation in education to be unconstitutional in 1954. Congress passed legislation prohibiting racial segregation in employment, transportation, housing, and many other areas, and profound changes have occurred in U.S. society as a result. Unfortunately, segregation in housing and education has persisted in much of the United States, persons of color are still far more likely to be poor, and conservatives have been successful in getting the courts to retreat on achieving student body integration and diversity in recent years. (See also Chapter 3.)

Constitutional decisions and legislation have also barred many forms of discrimination against women, and women have truly taken a far more significant role in business, politics, and sports than they have had before. Debate over reproductive rights persists, with only a narrow U.S. Supreme Court majority upholding a woman's right to abortion, while social forces and restrictive legislation have made the availability of abortion much more limited. During 2012, major battles erupted over mandated access to contraception coverage under the ACA. (See Chapter 4.)

Much progress has been made in eliminating various forms of discrimination on the basis of sexual orientation, with gay marriage now legal in several states and endorsed by President Barack Obama. Many other states, however, have amended their constitutions to prohibit same-sex marriage. (See Chapter 7.)

The rights of persons with disabilities have been recognized by Congress, with the result that public facilities and programs are far more accessible to persons with disabilities and employers are required to make reasonable accommodations for disabilities. (See Chapter 8.)

Undocumented immigrants continue to face hostility and pressure for deportation, but, in 2012, President Obama announced that young people who had grown up in the United States and who were pursuing school or military service would not be deported. In addition, in 2012, the Supreme Court affirmed that the federal government has responsibility for regulating immigration, and it struck down parts of an Arizona law that (a) made it a crime for undocumented immigrants to seek employment in Arizona, and (b) authorized police officers to make warrantless arrests of anyone they had probable cause to believe had committed a deportable offense. However, the Court upheld the Arizona law's central provision that required state law enforcement officers to demand immigration papers from anyone stopped, detained, or arrested whom they reasonably suspected was in the United States without authorization.[20] (See Box 22–1 in Chapter 22.)

Rights are meaningful only if there are courts to enforce them and lawyers to assert them, and there are reasons to be concerned about both at the present time. During the past two decades, a bare majority of the U.S. Supreme Court has issued a series of decisions imposing increased barriers to asserting claims of individual rights, especially against government officials and major corporations.

At the same time, there are far too few lawyers available to enforce social rights. While the Supreme Court has found a constitutional due process right to counsel in criminal cases, no equivalent right has been found for most civil cases.

Publicly funded civil legal aid has focused on defending individuals in the marketplace and in their dealings with government agencies. The privately supported legal aid societies in the early 20th century provided limited assistance in individual cases. An entirely new approach—law reform to end poverty—was articulated in the 1960s, when the federal legal services program was created as a part of President Lyndon Johnson's War on Poverty.

Federal funds, distributed since 1976 by the Legal Services Corporation, were used largely to establish local offices. A variety of national offices that focused on a specific area of the law, such as the National Center for Law and Economic Justice and the National Health Law Program, were also created and fulfilled their role of developing the legal theories and bringing cases that have made a mark on the legal landscape. Because much of this work at the national and local levels challenged powerful economic interests, especially large food growers and government bureaucracies, the legal services program was controversial from the outset. In 1995, power in Congress shifted sharply to the political right. Funding was slashed. Programs were barred from bringing high-impact class action lawsuits, providing representation to non-citizens, and using privately raised money for work that could not be performed with federal funds.

There is, however, a rich history of civil liberties and civil rights lawyering that has made a profound difference in U.S. society. Privately supported groups, such as the Center for Constitutional Rights, the American Civil Liberties Union, the NAACP Legal Defense Fund, and other groups with an ethnic, women's, or sexual-orientation focus, have had a major impact. Individual lawyers have joined together to defend rights in relatively radical membership groups, such as the National Lawyers Guild. Mainstream bar associations, including the American Bar Association, have become increasingly involved in many fights for civil liberties and civil rights. Because so many legal rights organizations are reliant almost entirely on private contributions, they can maintain their impact and independence only if foundations and individuals are willing to continue their financial support. In addition, the passage of federal and state antidiscrimination laws has brought government lawyers into court to enforce rights.

■ AN AGENDA FOR ACTION

As with every other social goal, the path to its achievement must include at least three elements: education, advocacy, and litigation.

An International Agenda

Education

Two WHO publications are helpful. *25 Questions & Answers on Health & Human Rights* describes human rights, the right to health, the rights-based approach to health, and how poor countries with resource limitations can be held to the same standards as rich countries. *The Right to Health* is a comic book for primary school students. The United Nations Human Rights Council (www.unhrc.org) provides information about human rights issues through a wide range of publications.

Advocacy

WHO's program to fulfill rights has three objectives: (a) to support governments in integrating a human rights–based approach to health development, (b) to strengthen WHO's capacity to integrate a human rights–based approach in its work, and (c) to advance the right to health in international law and international development processes.[21] There is much that health workers can do to promote this program, either by working with WHO or by undertaking their own projects. In 2003, the Food and Agriculture Organization (FAO) established an Intergovernmental Working Group "to elaborate a set of voluntary guidelines to support the progressive realization of the right to adequate food."[22] The guidelines were never adopted by FAO, but in 2011 Wikileaks published a set of documents showing that this was due to the opposition by the United States.[23]

Civil society organizations are increasingly active in promoting international economic and social rights, as illustrated by the following examples:

- Africa Action (www.africaaction.org), established by a coalition of three leading Africa advocacy groups based in the United States, has campaigned for "Africa's Right to Health" and other economic and social rights.
- The Center for Economic and Social Rights (www.cesr.org) implements projects that challenge economic injustice as a violation of international human rights law.

- The Kensington Welfare Rights Union (www.kwru.org) makes creative use of international law and nonviolent protests to advance economic and social rights.

One of the most underutilized human rights resources is the group of *special rapporteurs*, special representatives and independent experts operating under the aegis of the United Nations Human Rights Council. These experts are generally highly receptive to working with civil society organizations. They address a great variety of subjects, including physical and mental health, housing, food, human trafficking, violence against women, safe drinking water, and toxic waste.

Much can be accomplished by civil society organizations lobbying international organizations to hold governments accountable. For example, two human rights groups investigating psychiatric hospitals in Latin America reported dismal conditions in hospitals in Guatemala to the Inter-American Commission on Human Rights, which issued an official protest to the Guatemalan government.[24]

In March 2013, on the 10th anniversary of the start of the Iraq War, the Center for Constitutional Rights and other organizations filed a case with the Inter-American Commission on Human Rights, demanding accountability and reparations from the United States for the human rights violations and adverse health consequences caused by the War.[25]

Health professionals and their organizations can play major roles in protecting human rights. For example, health professionals have played major roles in documenting and preventing torture. (See Box 27–1.)

Litigation

There has been some litigation to address international human rights. For example, the Center for Constitutional Rights (www.ccr-ny.org) has pioneered the use of international human rights in domestic courts since it helped to bring about the 1980 landmark decision in *Filártiga v. Peña-Irala* under the Alien Tort Claims Act. A longtime advocate for economic and social rights, it has consistently used international law in litigation. A European offshoot of CCR, the European Center for Constitutional and Human Rights (www.ecchr.de) has emerged as one of the leading international organizations advocating and litigating for human rights, including social and economic rights. Founded in Berlin in 2007, it has more than 100 partner organizations.

An Agenda for the United States

As in the international arena, improvement in social and economic rights will require education, advocacy, and litigation by an unprecedented number of people. The forces seeking to turn back the clock and restrict wealth and well-being to the few have been setting the agenda and growing more powerful, but united efforts by caring people can change this situation.

BOX 27-1 ■ **Preventing Torture**

Leonard S. Rubenstein and Vincent Iacopino

Torture has been practiced throughout human history as a form of punishment, in the mistaken belief that torture can provide access to the truth or can intimidate or control individuals and entire populations. Today, torture and ill-treatment are practiced in more than half of the world's countries.

Torture is defined in the United Nations Convention Against Torture as "any act by which severe pain or suffering, whether physical or mental, is intentionally inflicted on a person"[1] by or with the acquiescence or approval of an agent of the state for purposes such as the obtaining of a confession, intimidation or coercion, or discrimination. The Convention also prohibits the use of cruel, inhuman, and degrading treatment or punishment—which is encompassed in the discussion in this box. Torture is used by police, members of paramilitary groups, and military personnel. While physical torture remains common, psychological torture has been increasingly employed, especially by governments that seek to avoid physical evidence of torture.

The prevention of torture is enormously challenging, given the barriers to legal investigation and prosecution. The persistence of torture and the extraordinary power it permits perpetrators to exercise over individuals—and communities—requires multifaceted prevention strategies. These include the following:

- Establishing and reinforcing norms through law
- Developing capacities for effective legal investigation and adjudication, engaging civil society as well as law enforcement and security officials in discussions about torture and its prevention
- Maintaining strict rules to govern the behavior of police, prison, jail, and security officers, including prohibiting secret detention and use of evidence obtained by torture and introducing safeguards in detention and interrogation
- Training these officers on how to avoid using torture
- Assuring access to prisoners and detainees by family members, lawyers, and medical personnel
- Assuring accountability for perpetrators and reparations for victims
- Monitoring places of detention[2]

During the past 20 years, the international community has considerably strengthened mechanisms to prevent torture. Most notably, in 1987, an international treaty, the Convention Against Torture and Other Cruel, Inhuman and Degrading Treatment or Punishment, entered into force.[1] Its key provisions include requirements for governments to criminalize torture under domestic law, prosecute perpetrators, and provide civil remedies for victims. States parties to the Convention periodically are reviewed by a United Nations committee to assess compliance. However, noncompliance is widespread in police stations, prisons, and other detention facilities throughout the world. For example, between 2000 and 2010, the U.S. military and Central Intelligence Agency engaged in systematic torture of detainees who had been captured in Afghanistan, Iraq, Pakistan, and elsewhere and who were thought to be supporting terrorism.

To strengthen compliance with the convention, the UN General Assembly adopted the Optional Protocol to the Convention Against Torture, which provides strict monitoring requirements for places of detention.[3] It requires states to agree to visits by international monitors from the UN Subcommittee on the Prevention of Torture. Because of the practical limitations of international monitoring—the subcommittee has the resources to visit only three countries a year—the Optional Protocol has a second and innovative requirement: States must create a domestic monitoring mechanism that has unrestricted access, including through unannounced visits, to all places where people are deprived of liberty. As of April 2013, 68 states had ratified the Optional Protocol and 72 states had signed it—although the United States had neither ratified nor signed it.

Health professionals often have knowledge and skills to provide care for survivors of torture—and also to document evidence of torture, which is critically important for judicial proceedings as well as human-rights investigations and monitoring. Health professionals were instrumental in developing the first international guidelines for medico-legal documentation of torture, which are contained in the United Nations' *Manual on the Effective Investigation and Documentation of Torture and other Cruel, Inhuman or Degrading Treatment or Punishment* (the Istanbul Protocol). It includes relevant legal standards and detailed guidelines for comprehensive forensic medical evaluations. It also contains minimum standards, known as the Istanbul Principles, to ensure the effective documentation of torture by states.[4,5]

The Istanbul Principles have been recognized by UN agencies and human rights compliance entities. Medical experts in court cases in which torture is alleged also rely on the Principles.

Health professionals have helped implement the Istanbul Protocol standards in many countries. National human rights agencies and civil society organizations, however, have not adequately incorporated the Principles into their work. An international consortium of health professionals is working with the United Nations High Commissioner for Human Rights to develop a global plan of action of the Istanbul Protocol standards by individual nations for the effective investigation and documentation of torture.

Box References

1. Office of the United Nations High Commissioner for Human Rights. Convention Against Torture and Other Cruel, Inhuman or Degrading Treatment or Punishment, June 26, 1987. Available at http://www2.ohchr.org/english/law/cat.htm. Accessed on August 20, 2012.
2. Amnesty International. Amnesty International's 12-Point Programme for the Prevention of Torture and other Cruel, Inhuman or Degrading Treatment or Punishment by Agents of the State, April 21, 2005. Available at http://www.amnesty.org/en/library/info/ACT40/001/2005/en. Accessed on August 20, 2012.
3. Office of the United Nations High Commissioner for Human Rights. Optional Protocol to the Convention Against Torture and other Cruel, Inhuman or Degrading Treatment or Punishment, June 22, 2006. Available at http://www2.ohchr.org/english/law/cat-one.htm. Accessed on August 20, 2012.
4. International Rehabilitation Council for Torture Victims. Model curriculum on the effective medical documentation of torture and ill-treatment. Available at http://phrtoolkits.org/toolkits/istanbul-protocol-model-medical-curriculum. Accessed on August 7, 2012.
5. Office of the United Nations High Commissioner for Human Rights. Istanbul Protocol. Geneva: OHCHR, 2004. Available at www.ohchr.org/Documents/Publications/training8Rev1en.pdf. Accessed on August 7, 2012.

Education

Fortunately, for those seeking to educate themselves on issues of health care rights and the broad range of economic and social justice issues, the challenge is choosing among the many resources available. Despite the rapidly evolving political and economic climate, updated information is available on the websites of many organizations. Among the excellent websites designed to support those advocating for progressive improvements in policy at either the federal or state level are those of the Center on Budget Policies and Priorities, the Coalition on Human Needs, the Center for Community Change, and the Sargent Shriver National Center on Poverty Law. Websites with a particular focus on health advocacy information include those of Families USA and the National Health Law Program. Other groups have focused on issues of race, such as the Poverty and Race Research Action Council and the Applied Research Center. Some websites are more neutral, focusing on academic and government reports and data; the website of the Urban Institute is an excellent starting point for social welfare information. Concerned persons can therefore educate themselves quickly, but the challenge is how to make change happen. There is much that can be done.

Advocacy

Advocacy organizations and coalitions are working in most states and in Washington, DC, advocating that elected officials and legislators preserve and improve health-care rights and other vital rights. These organizations and coalitions need volunteers and they need funds; many of the organizations cited in the "Education" section above can provide relevant information. Many parts of the faith community have been steadfast advocates for social and economic justice. Useful entry points for a wealth of leads on various issues and campaigns are the National Council of Churches, Catholic Charities USA, and the Religious Action Center of Reform Judaism. For more information on grassroots organizing concerning social justice, one can consult the Center for Community Change and the Applied Research Center.

Organizers in low-income communities are increasingly focusing on voter mobilization in recognition of the critical role played by elected officials. Conservative groups have greatly increased "voter suppression" (deterring people from voting). Good sources for voter mobilization can be found at Demos and the Brennan Center. Anyone can write letters to elected officials and the editors of newspapers and magazines about policies currently being discussed or debated.

Another critical area for advocacy efforts is to stop the U.S. Supreme Court and lower federal courts from weakening federal laws that protect rights. Many civil rights lawyers and academics have launched ambitious campaigns to alert the public to the dangers of judicial law-making that erases rights-creating legislation, and to take action to restore the federal courts as a bastion of individual rights. For information, consult the Alliance for Justice.

Litigation

Energetic and creative enforcement of critical laws and constitutional requirements is needed in many areas, such as current entitlements in benefit programs
such as Medicaid and SNAP (food stamps); federal and state laws protecting
wages, working conditions, and the right to organize; laws prohibiting discrimination on the basis of race, ethnicity, sex, citizenship, sexual orientation, and
disability; and the Constitution's due process clause. Such advocacy will help
many individuals, promote rationality and fairness in decision-making, and
educate the public and the judiciary about the needs to enforce those rights
and challenge prejudice and stereotypes.

There are far too few lawyers available to enforce these rights. While the federal
government provides limited financial support for civil legal-aid services for poor
people through the Legal Services Corporation, the restrictions on that program
have limited its ability to enforce these rights on a broad scale. Concerned people
can search out organizations pursuing matters of the most interest to them and
volunteer time, especially if they are legally trained. And people can contribute
financially. In addition, they can become engaged politically, at the local, state,
and federal levels, to oppose the right's relentless attack on public funding for civil
legal services.

■ CONCLUSION

For a variety of reasons, including the decline in civil liberties following the
terrorist attacks of 2001 and the triumph of free-market capitalism over social-
ism and social democracy, the pursuit of human rights has fallen on bad times.
However, the enforcement of economic, social, and cultural rights is beginning
to take root in the United States and some other countries. In the United States,
it is beginning to permeate civil society, and, eventually, it will enter into political and judicial life. Enforceable economic, social, and cultural rights represent
the only sure bulwark against social injustice. Lawyers must go to court, victims
of social injustice must take to the streets, and activists must lobby their elected
representatives. These are the paths for fighting social injustice and achieving
human rights.

■ REFERENCES

1. Encyclopedia Britannica. Great books of the Western world, vol. 5. Chicago: William
   Benton, 1952:135.
2. Friedman L, ed. The law of war: A documentary history. New York: Random House,
   1972:150.
3. Gnaedinger A, Director-General of the International Committee of the Red Cross.
   The protection of civilians in armed conflict. Statement to the United Nations Security

Council, December 10, 2002. Available at http://www.colombiaun.org/English/Security%20Council/Colombia%20Non%20Permanent%20Member/Documents%202002-2001/Statements%202002/statement_10dec_02.html. Accessed October 16, 2012.

4. International Committee of the Red Cross. ICRC Rule 1. Available at http://www.icrc.org/customary-ihl/eng/docs/v1_rul_rule1. Accessed on December 3, 2012.

5. U.S. Constitution, Amendments XIII and XIV.

6. United Nations. Charter of the United Nations. Available at http://www.un.org/en/documents/charter/. Accessed October 16, 2012.

7. United Nations. Universal Declaration of Human Rights. Available at http://www.un.org/en/documents/udhr/index.shtml. Accessed October 16, 2012.

8. Office of the High Commissioner of Human Rights. International Covenant on Economic, Social and Cultural Rights. Available at http://www2.ohchr.org/english/law/cescr.htm. Accessed October 16, 2012.

9. Office of the High Commissioner of Human Rights. International Covenant on Civil and Political Rights. Available at http://www2.ohchr.org/english/law/ccpr.htm. Accessed October 16, 2012.

10. WHO. Constitution of the World Health Organization. Available at http://www.who.int/governance/eb/who_constitution_en.pdf. Accessed October 16, 2012.

11. OAS. Charter of the Organization of American States (A-41). 1948. Available at http://www.oas.org/dil/treaties_A-41_Charter_of_the_Organization_of_American_States.htm. Accessed December 3, 2012.

12. Constitutional Court of South Africa—CCT 38/00. Grootboom v. Government of the Republic of South Africa and others. 2000. Available at http://www.saflii.org/za/cases/ZACC/2000/14.pdf. Accessed October 16, 2012.

13. Constitutional Court of South Africa—CCT 08/02. Minister of Health and Others v Treatment Action Campaign and Others. 2002. Available at http://www.saflii.org/za/cases/ZACC/2002/14.pdf. Accessed October 16, 2012.

14. International Network for Economic, Social and Cultural Rights. Caselaw database. Available at http://www.escrnet.org/caselaw. Accessed December 3, 2012.

15. Tobin JW. The right to health in international law. New York: Oxford University Press, 2011.

16. Mack J. In a first, UN holds Brazil accountable for maternal death under CEDAW. August 23, 2011. Available at http://msmagazine.com/blog/blog/2011/08/23/in-a-first-un-holds-brazil-accountable-for-maternal-death-under-cedaw/. Accessed December 3, 2012.

17. International Court of Justice. Legality of the threat or use of nuclear weapons, general list no. 95, Advisory Opinion of July 8, 1996, par. 105(D). Available at http://www.icj-cij.org/docket/index.php?sum=498&code=unan&p1=3&p2=4&case=95&k=e1&p3=5. Accessed October 16, 2012.

18. ICC. Rome Statute of the International Criminal Court. Available at http://untreaty.un.org/cod/icc/index.html. Accessed October 16, 2012.

19. *King v. Smith*, 392 US 309 (1968) (statute upon which the decision was based was repealed in 1996) and *Goldberg v. Kelly*, 397 U.S. 254 (1970).

20. U.S. Supreme Court. *Arizona v. United States*, 567 US __(2012). Available at http://www.supremecourt.gov/opinions/11pdf/11-182b5e1.pdf. Accessed November 19, 2012.

21. World Health Organization. 25 questions & answers on health & human rights. Health and human rights publication series no. 1. Geneva: WHO; July 2002. Available at

http://www.who.int/hhr/information/25%20Questions%20and%20Answers%20on%20
Health%20and%20Human%20Rights.pdf. Accessed October 16, 2012.

22. Food and Agriculture Organization. Intergovernmental working group for the elabora-
tion of a set of voluntary guidelines to support the progressive realization of the right
to adequate food in the context of national food security. Report of the Chair, October
2003. Available at http://www.fao.org/docrep/MEETING/007/j0838e.htm. Accessed
December 3, 2012.

23. Wikileaks. FAO Right to Food working group: Report of first session, April 1, 2003.
Available at http://www.cablegatesearch.net/cable.php?id=03ROME1380. Accessed
December 3, 2012.

24. Archibold RC. Guatemala: Commission calls for patient protection. *New York Times,*
November 30, 2012, p. A8.

25. Center for Constitutional Rights. U.S. Veterans, Iraqi Organizations Demand Justice
for U.S.-led Decade of War in Iraq, March 19, 2013. Available at: http://ccrjustice.org/
newsroom/press-releases/u.s.-veterans%2C-iraqi-organizations-demand-justice-u.s.-
led-decade-of-war-iraq. Accessed March 25, 2013.

28 Learning from the Social Movements of the 1960s

■ OLIVER FEIN AND CHARLOTTE PHILLIPS

▨ INTRODUCTION

Social movements occur when a critical mass of ordinary people mobilizes to exert collective power to address injustice in society. Examples of these movements in the United States have included the civil rights movement, the student movement, the anti-war movement, the women's movement, and the gay rights movement. The basic properties of these movements are "collective challenges, based on common purposes and social solidarities, in sustained (often contentious) interaction with elites, opponents and authorities."[1] This chapter will explore how these five social movements, all of which began or grew during the 1960s, impacted social injustice and public health.

Social movements have had—and will continue to have—a powerful impact on medicine and public health, motivating and energizing health workers to address social injustice. Although their roots were more than 50 years ago, each of these five social movements profoundly influenced the careers and the specific work of many health workers. It is therefore illuminating to review them in some detail to better understand how social movements can help achieve social justice and improve public health.

▨ THE CIVIL RIGHTS MOVEMENT

The bus boycott in Montgomery, Alabama, in 1955, protesting racial segregation on its public transportation system, and the sit-ins at a lunch counter at a Woolworth store in Greensboro, North Carolina, in February 1960, were early signs of a growing social movement to protest racial segregation. In the South, doctors' offices and hospitals were segregated—with separate entrances for black and white people. Most black physicians in the South could not treat their patients when they were hospitalized because they were not granted hospital admitting privileges in institutions controlled by "whites-only" medical societies.

In response to an urgent request of civil rights workers in Mississippi, the Medical Committee for Human Rights (MCHR) was established in the summer of 1964. Over 100 volunteer physicians, nurses, dentists, psychologists, and social workers provided emergency first aid, arranged medical care and hospitalization for ill or injured civil rights volunteers, visited jails, and participated in civil rights rallies. Perhaps even more important, MCHR provided a presence of sympathetic health workers in a hostile environment. In the summer of 1965, MCHR expanded its work to Alabama and Louisiana. Chapters in the North developed local programs, including screening clinics. Over the next decade, MCHR continued to provide support for civil rights workers and addressed underlying inequalities of segregated health care.

▓ THE STUDENT MOVEMENT

The civil rights movement was a powerful catalyst for the student movement. The aforementioned Greensboro sit-ins were student-led. In 1960, both the Student Non-violent Coordinating Committee (SNCC), an organization of African American students in the South, and Students for a Democratic Society (SDS) were founded.[2] SDS was a leading organization in the student activist movement in the 1960s. In 1962, SDS paid homage to the civil rights movement in its Port Huron statement: "As we grew (up)...our comfort was penetrated by events too troubling to dismiss .... (T)he permeating and victimizing fact of human degradation, symbolized by the Southern struggle against racial bigotry, compelled most of us from silence to activism."[3] SDS called for participatory democracy.

> The bridge to political power...will be built through genuine cooperation, locally, nationally and internationally, between a new left of young people and an awakening community of allies...As students for a democratic society, we are committed to stimulating this kind of social movement, this kind of vision and program in campus and community across the country.[3]

In 1963, SDS launched its Economic Research and Action Project (ERAP)[4] with community-organizing projects in large cities in the North, focused on building community-based organizations in low-income white communities that could ally with civil rights activists in black communities. ERAP projects organized unemployed people to demand "jobs or income NOW!" and welfare recipients to demand dignity, respect, and adequate benefits. In Cleveland, students and recent college graduates lived in a poor white Appalachian community, where they engaged in door-to-door organizing and developed projects such as a community theater, where local artists were encouraged to perform. White and black welfare mothers in Cleveland collaborated and formed the impetus for welfare rights organizing at the national level.

The Student Health Organization

During the 1960s, activist students who had participated in progressive organizations in college began to enroll in medical, nursing, public health, and other health professional schools. In 1965, 65 health professional students met in

Chicago to form the Student Health Organization (SHO)[5]—united by a strong commitment to community service for people in poverty. The federal government's Office of Economic Opportunity sponsored three SHO summer projects in 1966, six in 1967, and nine in 1968. At its height, more than 3000 students from 40 different schools participated in SHO.[6]

Its commitment to community service and participatory democracy was heavily influenced by the civil rights movement's emphasis on accountability to communities and community control.[7] Working in the community, students participating in service projects were confronted with the obligation to make their projects accountable to community organizations—easier said than done.

A controversy developed in the Bronx in 1968, when community groups began to question the role of these student service projects. They raised questions such as: "Were the well-intentioned student service projects being hijacked by academic medical centers, using federal money to assuage community demands for changes in these centers?" In other words, were SHO and its summer projects "making the community safe for the medical center?" Perhaps, some community leaders argued, students should turn their attention to making changes within the academic medical centers where they were being trained. Perhaps students should be challenging the two-class care system at many academic centers, where low-income people from the community were treated in open wards with 12 to 16 beds, in contrast to middle- and upper-class people who were treated in private and semi-private rooms. These community leaders asserted that students should be working "to make the medical center safe for the community." SHO was so shaken by this controversy that, in 1967, Stanford medical students returned some of their federal funds, and, in 1968, Albert Einstein medical students refused to accept any federal funds.

The Health Policy Advisory Center

At about the same time, one of SDS's founders launched the Health Policy Advisory Center (Health-PAC), a New Left think tank on health and medicine. It published a monthly bulletin, which provided a forum on community health initiatives in New York and analyses of the changing U.S. health care system.[8] In 1970, Health-PAC published *The American Health Empire: Power, Profits and Politics,* a book demonstrating that the U.S. health care "non-system" of private solo practitioners, non-profit hospitals, and for-profit health insurance companies was actually an organized "system"—the *Medical-Industrial Complex.*[6] In this book, Health-PAC documented that the boards of some academic medical centers in New York City included presidents of companies that sold their medications, medical supplies, and other products to these medical centers for a profit. Health-PAC concluded that "the most obvious function of the American medical system, other than patient care, is profit-making. When it comes to making money the health industry is an extraordinarily well-organized and efficient machine."[6]

Health-PAC's analysis dovetailed with the student movement's increasing focus, by 1970, on academic medical centers. In the early 1960s, students had focused on the American Medical Association (AMA) as the bastion of resistance to change in medicine in the United States. The AMA had long opposed national health insurance—one of the reasons that President Franklin D. Roosevelt did not include access to health insurance in the New Deal reforms. In 1965, the AMA spent over $5 million in a failed attempt to defeat Medicare. The Student American Medical Association (SAMA) mirrored the AMA's policies—one of the reasons that progressive students created SHO as an alternative. By 1970, supported by the Health-PAC analysis and by their experience in community health work, medical students across the nation focused on the corporate sector in health care, especially academic medical centers. For example, in Cleveland, medical students protested plans to have separate waiting rooms for privately insured patients and publicly insured patients in an ambulatory-care building under construction. They succeeded in getting the plans changed to joint waiting rooms for both groups of patients.

Community Control and the Lincoln Collective

One manifestation of this convergence of political analysis and community awareness was the Lincoln Hospital Pediatric Collective. Lincoln Hospital, a public hospital located in one of the nation's poorest urban communities, was in the South Bronx in New York. Founded in 1839 as a home for runaway slaves, it was so antiquated that in the 1960s it made its own electricity—producing direct current, not alternating current! Although affiliated with Albert Einstein College of Medicine ("Einstein"), it had been unable to attract any U.S. medical school graduates to its residency programs before 1968. In 1969, two U.S. graduates entered Lincoln's pediatric residency program. One of them, who had been active in SHO, recruited several pediatric residents from Jacobi Hospital in the North Bronx to do rotations at Lincoln. Together, they recruited other student and resident activists. In 1970, 18 first-year, five second-year, and six third-year residents arrived at Lincoln and established the Lincoln Hospital Pediatric Collective.[9] (At the same time, the residency program in social pediatrics was established at Montefiore Medical Center in the North Bronx[10]—also designed to train pediatricians to practice medicine in underserved, disadvantaged communities.)

Previously, Lincoln had been a hotbed of community-worker activism in mental health. Einstein had established a federally-funded community mental health center that was training community residents as mental health workers. In 1967 and 1968, these community health workers demanded a greater role in operating the center. In 1969, 150 of them, self-described as the Health Revolutionary Unity Movement (HRUM), seized control of Lincoln's Mental Health Center for 2 weeks. They replaced professional administrators with nonprofessionals—most of whom lived in the community. They chose the tactic of an occupation and "work-in" rather than a strike. Their main goal was improving services, not making economic demands.[6] HRUM declared its 10-point program, seeking community-worker control of health institutions, free health services, increased preventive services, and open admission to medical schools for minority students. After the arrest of 23 mental health workers and intense negotiations, the top administrators of the Mental Health Center were reassigned, and workers were told that they could elect an internal board to administer the Center.

The Pediatric Collective recruited as its initial members students and residents who had participated in the social movements of the 1960s and had chosen professional training to develop skills that would be useful long-term in a broad-based movement for a better world. Members of the Collective aimed to resist the negative influences of "professionalization" by having a critical mass of colleagues with a shared perspective and by building on the energy of other activist movements.[11] Aware of the major impact that social injustice has on public health and experienced in community and political organizing to challenge social injustice, Collective members transformed the residency training program and hospital services, including expansion of services beyond the walls of the hospital.

In its first year, the Lincoln Collective reached out to the Black Panther Party and the Young Lords Party. Both were developing "free clinic" programs as part of their community-organizing work. Collective members volunteered to provide medical services in these free clinics, in the hopes of supporting the overall political program of these groups.[12] In its second year, the Department of Pediatrics was approached by a group of community health workers, employed by the City Health Department, who had organized themselves into the Community Medical Corps, and requested technical assistance and training so that they could make door–to-door visits to perform skin tests for tuberculosis, blood tests for anemia and lead poisoning, and immunizations. (Many of these community health workers enrolled in community colleges and became public health workers; several ultimately became physicians and nurses.)

Meanwhile, inside the hospital, the Collective initiated many reforms to improve patient care that have since become standard practice in U.S. residency training programs today. For example, the Collective created continuity of outpatient care by ensuring that each patient saw the same resident on every visit to the clinic. It initiated a "night float" system that improved resident staffing at night and enabled on-call residents to get more sleep—a change that immediately and dramatically improved the quality of patient care. The Collective also led an initiative to appoint parents from the community to the selection committee for pediatric residents.

In 1971, the Collective program spread to the residency program in internal medicine, which adopted many similar innovations. What is notable is that the residents themselves, not staff physicians or faculty members, initiated these reforms. The reforms continued although the Collective gradually disbanded as many of its graduates moved on from Lincoln to work elsewhere. Social movements of the

1960s had empowered young physicians and also developed the context in which social change was possible.

What happened to these physicians who had been guided and energized by the social movements of the 1960s? Some members of the Collective remained at Lincoln as faculty members, a few for many years. The residency program in social pediatrics at Montefiore and similar programs in medicine and family medicine at Montefiore continue up to the present time. Some graduates of the Lincoln and Montefiore programs have practiced in inner-city and rural health centers as well as community and public hospitals. Others have worked in academic medical centers, making them more socially accountable. Still others have played significant roles in the U.S. Public Health Service and the community health center movement.

Poverty and Health Care: Physicians for a National Health Program

In 1986, health activists who were working in poor communities throughout the United States convened a conference in New Hampshire to discuss innovations in the health care delivery system for poor people. Despite Medicare and Medicaid, the number of uninsured people in the United States was continuing to increase by almost one million annually. Participants in the conference proposed a national health program based on a single-payer system similar to Canada's—providing universal coverage through a government-sponsored health care program like Medicare. This proposal led to the establishment of Physicians for a National Health Program (PNHP). In 1989, PNHP's proposal for reforming the U.S. health care system was published as the lead article in *The New England Journal of Medicine*.[13] (See Box 12–1 in Chapter 12.)

Since its founding, PNHP has grown to 18,000 members, with active chapters in 33 states.[14] It has advocated for universal coverage through a single-payer financing system—an improved and expanded version of "Medicare for All." Many of its leaders had participated in the social movements of the 1960s.

PNHP has documented the consequences of not having health insurance— 45,000 deaths in the United States annually.[15] And PNHP has demonstrated that, if the United States transformed its multi-payer, for-profit, private health insurance system to a single-payer system, it would save $400 billion annually.[16] This could provide adequate coverage for all 50 million uninsured and 89 million underinsured residents of the United States, without increasing the percentage of the gross domestic product spent on health. Although there still is no mass social movement for single-payer health care in the United States,[17] both the number and the size of groups demanding change have been increasing. For example, Healthcare-NOW! is a grassroots coalition with affiliated groups in 48 states.[18] The California Nurses Association (CNA) and National Nurses United (NNU) have become major forces within the labor movement for a single-payer system.[19]

In addition, as of 2012, 590 union organizations in 49 states had endorsed HR676, the Expanded and Improved Medicare-for-All Act that had been introduced in the House of Representatives, with 77 co-sponsors.[20]

▪ THE ANTI-WAR MOVEMENT

War has long been recognized as a major threat to public health. (See Box 17–1 in Chapter 17.) Broad social movements opposing war have been part of the U.S. experience since World War I, although groups with pacifist beliefs—both religious and secular—have existed since the 1600s.[21]

The movement opposing the Vietnam War grew from a relatively small group in late 1964 into a national antiwar movement. The first national demonstration opposing the Vietnam War was organized by Students for a Democratic Society in April 1965.[22] Growing resistance to the war within the military spread via "GI Coffeehouses," established by antiwar activists near army training bases. These venues offered social space and psychological support to service members who began to question the political and moral rationales for the war.[23] Physicians, nurses, and other health workers supported the anti-war movement in a variety of ways, such as offering counseling on draft resistance to young people facing military service and providing a medical presence at demonstrations. Widespread opposition to the Vietnam War influenced Congress to ultimately stop funding the war.

Movement leaders questioned the ethics of the military's using medical techniques for its own purposes.[24] Howard Levy, a dermatologist who was assigned to train Green Berets in basic medical techniques, refused to do so when he realized that these techniques would be used in programs to pacify Vietnamese villages. As a result, he was ultimately court-martialed and imprisoned for over 2 years.[25]

During the Vietnam War, all male graduates of medical schools were required to serve in the military. As opposition to the war grew, the Medical Resistance Union, a loose-knit organization, coalesced around a pledge signed by over 800 medical students, stating that they would not serve in the military. Upon graduation many of these students enrolled in the U.S. Public Health Service as an alternative to military service. Some applied for conscientious-objector status, claiming that military service even in a non-combatant role would contribute to the war effort by treating wounded soldiers who would then return to the battlefield. Some physicians and other health professionals emigrated to Canada to avoid military service.

Physicians for Social Responsibility (PSR) was founded in 1961. Its goal was to end the threat of nuclear war by educating the public and policymakers about the risks of nuclear weapons and advocating their abolition.[26] In the 1980s, a popular movement with nearly one million participants advocated the abolition of nuclear weapons. At a major demonstration in New York in 1982, participants proclaimed that nuclear weapons pose unacceptable risks for civilization.[27] The Peace Caucus affiliated with the American Public Health Association (APHA), established in 1986, demonstrated at the nuclear weapons test site in Nevada to end the development of nuclear weapons. It continues to sponsor programs on the health consequences of war at APHA annual meetings.[28] The 2011 tsunami disaster at Fukushima, Japan, has emphasized the need for joining the movement against nuclear weapons with the movement advocating an end to nuclear power. The entrenchment of the military-industrial complex in the U.S. economy siphons resources needed to address health and other human needs. Militarism in various insidious forms adversely affects our entire society. Locally based groups, such as Brooklyn For Peace,[29] offer opportunities to connect issues and respond actively. United for Peace and Justice is a national coalition of such locally based groups.[30]

■ THE WOMEN'S MOVEMENT

The women's movement, considered one of the most inclusive social movements, has had a profound impact on women's health.[31] (See Chapter 4.) Growing awareness by women of the ways they were considered as less than equal to men, even after they had achieved the right to vote, led to formation of consciousness-raising groups involving women from all socioeconomic backgrounds. Health issues became a major focus of the women's movement, given that health issues are inherently women's issues and most health workers are female.[32] Reflecting the strength of the movement and that "feminism is a multi-issue movement,"[33] organizations developed to demand changes in policies affecting women and improvements in health services and research in areas specific to women. Women also asserted themselves in such groups as the Boston Women's Health Book Collective, which published in the early 1970s the first of many editions of *Our Bodies, Ourselves*.[34] (See Box 4–1 in Chapter 4.) In 1973, *Witches, Midwives, and Nurses: A History of Women Healers* was published, reflecting concerns about medical professionals' claiming areas that had previously been controlled by women who were caring for other women, based on their own experiences and understanding.[35] In spite of the tremendous advance in access to abortion services achieved by the *Roe v. Wade* decision in 1973, there is a continuing need for ongoing social action and political pressure to maintain this important right for women.

Lasting effects of the women's movement on health care are reflected in medical education. In the 1960s, 10 percent or fewer medical students were women. The prevailing attitude that a medical career was too difficult for women, especially if they intended to have children, did not encourage women to apply to medical school. Explicit and implicit admission policies were stacked against acceptance of women applicants. Today, in contrast, more than half of students at many medical schools are women. Reforms in medical school curricula now require inclusion of topics specifically addressing women's issues. The introduction of "trained patients" to teach physical exam techniques arose primarily from women's refusal to tolerate continued exploitation of female patients for the purposes of medical education.

■ THE GAY RIGHTS MOVEMENT

Before the 1960s, the primary thrust of the gay rights movement was attaining civil rights for homosexuals, such as non-discriminatory employment practices. Influenced by the civil rights movement, gay activists became more visible in the late 1960s. In 1969, 3 days of riots resulting from a police raid on the Stonewall Inn, a gay bar in New York City, marked the birth of a more activist gay rights movement. By 1987, over 600,000 people had marched in Washington to demand equality for the lesbian, gay, bisexual, and transgender (LGBT) community. (See Chapter 7.)

With the spread of the AIDS epidemic in the 1980s, organizing within the LGBT community intensified.[36] Service organizations, such as the Gay Men's Health Crisis (GMHC) in New York City, were established to provide access to health care and social services for AIDS patients. Activist political advocacy was initiated, in 1987, by the AIDS Coalition To Unleash Power (ACT-UP). Through the use of direct, nonviolent actions, ACT-UP activists succeeded in changing the system. They challenged drug prices established by the pharmaceutical industry for AZT (azidothymidine) by chaining themselves to the "very important person" (VIP) balcony at the New York Stock Exchange. They shut down the Food and Drug Administration (FDA) in Washington for a day, protesting restrictive experimental research protocols. They demonstrated at St. Patrick's Cathedral in New York City to protest the Catholic archdiocese's stand against "safe-sex" education and condom distribution in the public schools. ACT-UP's activism resulted in pharmaceutical companies' lowering their prices for HIV drugs and the FDA's releasing experimental AIDS drugs early. By 2000, when effective AIDS treatments were widely available, ACT-UP broadened its advocacy focus to include universal access to health care, since many people living with AIDS lacked health insurance. In 2007, ACT-UP/New York, together with PNHP and Healthcare-NOW!, sponsored the first demonstration in which patients and doctors committed civil disobedience together and were arrested demanding single-payer national health insurance for all.[37,38] (See Chapter 13.)

■ NEW SOCIAL MOVEMENTS

Income and wealth disparities in the United States are growing.[39] During the past 30 years, income of people in the bottom 90 percent has grown by only 15 percent, while the income of those in the top 1 percent has increased almost 150 percent.[40] In response to these increasing disparities, the Occupy Movement was born. (See Box 28–1.) Occupy Wall Street (OWS) has been the most publicized part of the movement.[41] Health care activists mobilized by the movement established Health Care for the 99%, with members from Healthcare-NOW!, PNHP, NNU, and other organizations participating in and supporting the OWS demonstrators. In New York City, Health Care for the 99% supported the health care tent at the site of the OWS occupation, conducted a free influenza

BOX 28-1 ■ The Occupy Wall Street Movement

Arthur M. Chen and Peggy Saika

Occupy Wall Street (OWS), also known as the Occupy Movement, is a grassroots movement whose primary concern is to right the unfair policies and structures of the "1 percent"—the wealthy class, large corporations, and the global financial system—that disproportionately favor the rich while undermining a more democratic society that would lift up the other 99 percent. Begun in September 2011, OWS has drawn national attention to the inequalities between the wealthy 1 percent and the mainstream 99 percent and has inspired many similar protests.

What started with a handful of protestors in New York City has blossomed into an international movement for a more fair and more just society—a movement that is inclusive, horizontally led, and democratically modeled. Its process is a large part of its message. The success of OWS has been fueled by the global economic recession, participation by "tech-savvy" activists, robust use of social networking, and mobilization of social-justice activists and organizations. It has been enhanced by people's deep sense of uncertainty and powerlessness about many issues concerning jobs, housing, health care, poverty, student debt, climate change, and the military-industrial complex. OWS has inspired activists and others impacted by economic and social conditions to work together to restore a more equitable distribution of income and wealth and to strengthen vital programs and services.

Understanding these concerns and learning lessons from the "Arab Spring," OWS is using the Internet to create opportunities for connection and solidarity, knowledge-sharing, and participation in local, regional, national, and international events and initiatives.

The official website of the original OWS occupation and the New York City General Assembly is www.nycga.net. It works to organize and set the vision for the OWS movement.

"Occupy Wall Street News," an app for smart phones, and "The Occupied Wall Street Journal," an OWS affinity group at occupiedmedia.us, collect news about the Occupy Movement from the United States and other countries.

The website interoccupy.net seeks to "foster communication between individuals, Working Groups, and local General Assemblies," using modern conference-call technology to host large-scale weekly calls. Subgroups include www.occupyourhomes. org, an "issue hub" that supports Americans who fight foreclosure on their homes, and www.WomenOccupy.org, an "identity hub" that works to aggregate and create resources for women and those committed to confronting patriarchy, heterosexism, and transphobia.

The website www.strikedebt.org, a collaboration between Strike Debt and OWS, provides strategies for fighting credit-card, medical, student, housing, and municipal debt.

Health Care for the 99% (www.owshealthcare.wordpress.com) and Doctors for the 99% (www.doctorsforthe99.org), view health care as a human right. They aim to challenge for-profit health care while addressing the social determinants of health.

Many other unaffiliated sites promote outreach and further engagement, education, and mobilization of the public. For example, www.occupytogether.org promotes community organizing, mobilization, and direct action to "curb the domination of big business within their local communities." The sites www.occupy.

net and www.OccupyWallSt.org provide technical tools and support work. Website www.openspaceworld.com/users_guide.htm recreates a modern version of the town hall meetings, where participants listen and respond to proposals generated by work groups.

As of March 15, 2013, OWS had recorded over 1041 occupations in the United States and 1498 in over 70 countries and all continents. (See www.directory.occupy. net.) Each occupation built a local base of activists that has since functioned autonomously, but in solidarity and communication with national and global efforts. Increased local awareness and policy changes can serve as precursors to national proposals and legislation. For example, in 2012, spurred by an OWS campaign, the New York City Council passed a resolution opposing the U.S. Supreme Court's ruling in *Citizens United v. Federal Election Commission*, which granted corporations the rights of natural persons regarding the expenditure of corporate money to influence the electoral process.

OWS has had a profound impact on public discourse regarding the economic system's failures—blaming the influence of the wealthy class (the 1 percent) for the income inequality and hardships of the middle class. A national survey in 2011 found that 66 percent of respondents believed that there were "very strong" or "strong" conflicts between rich and poor people—a 19 percent increase from 2 years before.[1] A subsequent survey showed that, by a two-to-one margin, respondents favored a tax increase on higher incomes to make the system more fair.[2]

It is not known if OWS will affect major sustainable change in national policy. A national working group of OWS in 2012 listed the following 12 issues as representing its future vision: clean water, air, and food; free education for all; no war; sustainable human society; a culture of direct democracy; free universal health care; local food production, community gardens, and permaculture agriculture; economic equality; localized economies; a world where basic needs are met; the military-industrial complex destroyed and military spending slashed; and an economic system based not on profits, but mutual aid and meeting all human needs.

By evoking a simple and clear distinction between the "1 percent" and the "99 percent," the OWS movement has created a target to direct people's frustration and anguish due to failed economic policies. Catalyzing systemic and sustainable transformation will require enormous collaboration, coordination, and support among activists on many issues and from many sectors of society. It will also require massive public engagement and direct action to lessen the influence of the 1 percent with the greatest wealth, while maximizing opportunities for public debate and expression of the public will.

Box References

1. Morin R. Rising share of Americans see conflict between rich and poor. January 11, 2012. Available at http://www.pewsocialtrends.org/2012/01/11/rising-share-of-americans-see-conflict-between-rich-and-poor/. Accessed on August 27, 2012.
2. PEW Research Center. Raising taxes on rich seen as good for economy, fairness. July 16, 2012. Available at http://www.people-press.org/2012/07/16/raising-taxes-on-rich-seen-as-good-for-economy-fairness/. Accessed on August 27, 2012.

vaccination campaign, and advocated for universal access to health care at the OWS mass demonstrations.

Other current social movements are focused on immigrants' rights, prisoners' rights, and environmental challenges—all of which have direct implications for health and offer opportunities for health professionals and students at health professions schools to participate.

▓ CONCLUSION

The impact of social movements on social injustice in medical care and public health has been profound. Even though there has been no social movement directed explicitly at reforming the medical and public health systems, a review of the social movements of the 1960s demonstrates the multiple ways in which social injustice in medical care and public health were challenged by social movements. The civil rights movement led to the desegregation of hospitals in the South, the emphasis on community control of health facilities and community health centers, and the focus on minority admissions programs in medical schools. The student movement changed the professional aspirations of many health professional students, and led them to community involvement and ultimately to challenge academic health centers to include community service among their traditional missions of research, education, and patient care. Health professional involvement in the antiwar movement contributed to the end of the Vietnam War and continues to challenge the siphoning of millions of dollars from public health and medical care into the military. It also calls attention to the threat of nuclear war and the risks of nuclear power. The women's movement brought a new focus on women's health issues and contributed to the rise in gender equality in medical education. The gay rights movement and the AIDS activist movement have led to dramatic changes in the treatment of LGBT patients and patients with HIV/AIDS.

What have we learned from these movements? The most striking lesson is that, for transformative change to occur, a social movement is necessary. Since so much remains to be done before we achieve a just society in which everybody can develop their full potential, we must continue to work to establish a social movement with the energy and passion of the social movements of the 1960s. In addition, the experiences of the 1960s teach us the significance of the leadership of young people. With the growing inequality of income and wealth in the United States and heavy reliance on private, for-profit health insurance for access to health care, a worthy goal for a new civil rights movement would be a single-payer health care system with universal access.

▓ REFERENCES

1. Tarrow SG. Power in movement: Social movements and contentious politics. Cambridge, UK: Cambridge University Press, 2011.
2. Sale K. SDS. New York: Random House, 1973.

3. Hayden T. The Port Huron statement. New York: Thunder's Mouth Press, 2005:45–168.

4. Frost J. Interracial movement of the poor: Community organizing and the New Left in the 1960s. New York: New York University Press, 2001.

5. Hoffman LM. The politics of knowledge: Activist movements in medicine and planning. Albany, NY: State University of New York Press, 1989:57–66.

6. Ehrenreich B, Ehrenreich J.The American Health Empire: Power, profits, and politics. A Report from the Health Policy Advisory Center (Health-PAC). New York: Random House, 1970.

7. Weisberg IS. Cleveland Student Health Project—1968—Final report. National Technical Information Service, U.S. Department of Commerce. 1968.

8. Health/PAC Archives (1968–1994). Available at http://www.healthpacbulletin.org/. Accessed December 19, 2012.

9. Dittmer J. The good doctors: The medical committee for human rights and the struggle for social justice in health care. New York: Bloomsbury Press, 2009:6.

10. Montefiore Medical Center. Social pediatrics residency program. Available at http://www.montefiore.org/social-pediatrics-residency-program. Accessed August 31, 2012.

11. Mullan F. White coat, clenched fist: The political education of an American physician. New York: Macmillan Publishing Company, 1976.

12. Nelson, A. Body and soul: The Black Panther Party and the fight against medical discrimination. Minneapolis, MN: University of Minnesota Press, 2011.

13. Himmelstein DU, Woolhandler S. A national health program for the United States: A physicians' proposal. *N Engl J Med* 1989;320:102–108.

14. Physicians for a National Health Program. Available at http://www.pnhp.org/about/about-pnhp. Accessed August 31, 2012.

15. Wilper A, Woolhandler S, Lasser K, et al. Health insurance and mortality in U.S. adults. *Am J Public Health* 2009;99:2289–2295.

16. Woolhandler S, Campbell T, Himmelstein DU. Cost of health care administration in the United States and Canada. *N Engl J Med* 2003;349:768.

17. Hoffman B. Health care reform and social movements in the United States. *Am J Public Health* 2003;93:75–83.

18. Healthcare-NOW! Available at http://www.healthcare-now.org/. Accessed August 31, 2012.

19. National Nurses United. Available at http://www.nationalnursesunited.org/. Accessed August 31, 2012.

20. Unions for Single Payer Health Care. Available at http://unionsforsinglepayer.org/. Accessed August 31, 2012.

21. Cooney R, Michalowski H. Power of the people: Active nonviolence in the United States. Philadelphia: New Society Publishers, 1987.

22. Garvy H. Rebels with a cause. Los Gatos, CA: Shire Press, 2007:44–50.

23. Sir! No Sir! Available at http://www.sirnosir.com/. Accessed August 31, 2012.

24. Levy H. The military medicinemen. In: Ehrenreich J, ed. The cultural crisis of modern medicine. New York: Monthly Review Press, 1978:287–300.

25. Levy H, Miller D. Going to jail: The political prisoner. New York: Grove Press, 1971.

26. Physicians for Social Responsibility. Available at http://www.psr.org/. Accessed August 31, 2012.

27. Warburg J, Lowe D. You can't hug with nuclear arms! An Institute for Policy Studies book. Dobbs Ferry, NY: Morgan and Morgan, 1982.

28. American Public Health Association. Peace caucus. Available at http://www.apha.org/membergroups/caucuses/CaucusDescriptions.htm. Accessed August 31, 2012.

29. Brooklyn For Peace. Available at http://www.brooklynpeace.org/. Accessed August 31, 2012.

30. United for Peace and Justice. Available at http://www.unitedforpeace.org/. Accessed August 31, 2012.

31. Morgan R. Sisterhood is forever: The women's anthology for a new millennium. New York: Washington Square Press, 2003:xv.

32. Reverby S. Health: women's work. In: Kotelchuk D, ed. Prognosis negative: Crisis in the health care system. New York: Vintage Books, 1976:170.

33. Smeal E. The art of building feminist institutions to last. In: Morgan R. Sisterhood is forever: The women's anthology for a new millennium. New York: Washington Square Press, 2003:542.

34. Boston Women's Health Book Collective. Our bodies, ourselves. New York: Simon and Schuster, 1973.

35. Ehrenreich B, English D. Witches, midwives, and nurses: A history of women healers. New York: Feminist Press, 2010.

36. Crimp D. AIDS demographics. New York: Bay Press, 1990.

37. Boyle A. ACT-UP letter, March 29, 2007 (personal communication).

38. Straube T. Rally to reform health care ends in "deaths." New York Blade, March 30, 2007:1.

39. Moss NE. Socioeconomic disparities in health in the United States: An agenda for action. In: Hofrichter R, ed. Health and social justice: Politics, ideology, and inequity in the distribution of disease. San Francisco: Jossey-Bass, 2003:502.

40. Stiglitz JE. The price of inequality: How today's divided society endangers our future. New York: W.W. Norton, 2012:8.

41. Taylor A, Cessen K, eds. Occupy! Scenes from occupied America. London: Verso, 2011.

29 Promoting Equitable and Sustainable Human Development

■ RICHARD JOLLY

■ INTRODUCTION

Progress towards social justice in public health requires actions to reduce the extremes of social injustice on a far wider scale—well beyond health and health services—within each country and globally. The level of economic inequalities have never been greater than at present, especially in income gaps between the poorest and the richest people. Globally, the richest 20 percent of people receive more than 70 percent of all income, while the poorest 20 percent receive only 2 percent. The richest 61 million people receive the same amount of income as the poorest 3.5 billion.[1] Within most rich and poor countries, the levels of income inequality are currently at record levels. The global and national dimensions of inequality present major challenges for reducing health inequities, a commitment declared at the World Conference on Social Determinants of Health in 2011.

Structural inequalities of power, income, and living standards have long been present throughout the world. And power and income inequalities among countries have increased over the past two centuries. In 1820, for example, average income of the United States and Great Britain was estimated to be about three times that of India and China. Since then, the gap in average income between the richest and poorest countries has substantially increased. By 1870, the gap was seven-fold. By 1913, 11-fold. By 1950, 35-fold. By the late 1990s, more than 70-fold.[24] Even these estimates of the gap understate income disparities between the richest and the poorest countries.

The gap in average income between the richest and poorest countries reflects a global framework of social injustice that impedes reduction of poverty. Progress toward greater social justice will lay the foundation for further economic and social development. But substantially reducing global inequalities will require broader and more fundamental actions than those that are now present on the global agenda. Yet there are important reasons for keeping them alive as visions of future realistic challenges.

Reducing social injustice and achieving equity in public health are not utopian dreams. Globally, there have been major improvements in health and public health over the past 50 years, including unprecedented decreases in the child (under-5) mortality rate in all regions of the world, and, despite HIV/AIDS, increases in life expectancy. There have also been advances in many related areas: assertion of human rights, commitment to goals for reducing poverty, development of affordable strategies for improving living standards, and, in many countries, demonstration that pursuing these advances can be practical politics.

The possibilities for human progress have also been demonstrated in decreases in the infant mortality rate, expansion of school enrollments and adult literacy, and advances in the status and empowerment of women and girls in most low-income countries. These improvements over the past 50 years have generally exceeded the achievements of countries now in the high-income category when they were in the early stages of their development or long periods of economic and social advancement. For example, all but 26 low-income countries now have an infant mortality rate below 100 per 1000 live births—a rate achieved only by Norway by 1900.[2] By 2010, over 90 developing countries had achieved child (under-5) mortality rates below 70, the level reached by the United States and the United Kingdom in about 1940.[3]

These advances are models for what can be done—not monuments to goals that have been universally achieved. Given the unprecedented levels of wealth and income, the wide gaps between the potential and actual achievements in public health are scandalous. So are the wide gaps in other major measures of the human condition—especially given the unprecedented levels of public awareness of these disparities.

Globally, social injustices represent not only violations of human rights, but also missed opportunities on a large scale. These injustices signify failures of government obligations to enable their citizens—especially children—to achieve the highest possible standard of health. And, they represent failures of international cooperation by high-income countries to assist low-income countries in advancing health and education—a responsibility that they assumed in signing the Convention on the Rights of the Child.

This chapter explores the broader economic and political issues in ending these social injustices. It analyses the broader economic and social challenges of moving towards greater justice in public health, especially emphasizing actions that low-income countries can take. And it considers priorities for necessary support by high-income countries. It concludes with a discussion of priorities for all countries for sustainable human development.

▪ ECONOMIC AND SOCIAL REQUIREMENTS FOR GREATER JUSTICE IN PUBLIC HEALTH

Most people in the health sector—physicians, public health workers, policymakers, patients, and others—recognize the need for broad economic and social action to achieve greater justice in public health. Action should not be limited to changes in medical care, such as ensuring public or private financing for hospitals, greater access to low-cost pharmaceuticals, or support for medical research and technological advancements. Action needs to include, but must go beyond, improved access to basic education, clean water, and adequate sanitation. It must include policies and action for general economic advances combined with action to reduce poverty and achieve greater social justice—as has occurred in countries such as Malaysia, Tunisia, Botswana, Mauritius, Sri Lanka, China, Korea, Vietnam, Cuba, Costa Rica, and Barbados.

Economic growth has played a part in these advances. Initially, these countries were poor and lacked the household, community, and government resources necessary for progress in public health. Economic growth alone, however, was not sufficient to bring about this progress. Changes were also needed in economic and social structures, laws and institutions, and norms and practices that helped lay the foundation for advances in social justice and public health. Economic growth combined with structural and institutional change requires three priority strategies:

- "Pro-poor" economic growth—economic growth where benefits are widely distributed and where poor people attain increasing shares of these benefits over time
- Social policies that incorporate strong legal and political commitments to social justice and greater equity, beginning with commitments to education and health for all
- Long-term measures for economic and environmental sustainability, essential for ensuring equity and social justice for future generations

Implementing such strategies is challenging. Most of the countries mentioned above made substantial progress using these strategies. (Cuba is an exception, because its remarkable improvements in public health were achieved with little, if any, economic growth.) In Africa, Botswana, Mauritius, and Tunisia stand out as impressive examples of human and social success.[4-6] (Tragically, the surge in HIV/AIDS set back much of this progress.)

In Asia, China, South Korea, Malaysia, Sri Lanka, Vietnam, and the Indian states of Kerala and Tamil Nadu have combined accelerated economic growth with policies and institutional changes to reduce poverty, malnutrition, and other major causes of ill health.[7] Beginning in the 1950s and 1960s, South Korea and Taiwan combined economic growth with redistributive measures, and demonstrated commitments to public health and education for all. The progress in South Korea and Taiwan illustrates how long-term, sustained economic growth can be achieved using policy instruments that differ sharply from the neoliberalism, which has been strongly promoted by the World Bank and the International Monetary Fund since 1980.

In Latin America and the Caribbean, Costa Rica has, for more than 50 years, combined a strong commitment to democracy with policies for public health and universal education. Its constitution, adopted in 1949, prevents it from having an army, saving the country billions of dollars each year on military expenditures and enabling it to spend much more on health and education than most other countries in Latin America and the Caribbean. Not surprisingly, Costa Rica has some of the best economic and social indicators in the region. Barbados and Cuba are other countries in the region that have achieved high levels of social development and equality relative to their per-capita income.

▓ MYTHS ABOUT THE COSTS OF EQUITY AND SOCIAL JUSTICE

The experiences of these countries help dispel various myths. One myth is that equity is associated with high costs in terms of economic efficiency—therefore, in low-income countries, achievement of equity must be abandoned or postponed. The early experiences of South Korea, Malaysia, Mauritius, Taiwan, and Tunisia demonstrate that this is a false dichotomy. Skillfully pursued, equity and social justice can contribute positively to economic growth, productivity, and efficiency.

A second myth is that there is a trade-off between economic development and human rights. Here, the experiences of these and other countries is less clear. There is no strong evidence of such a trade-off, but there is also no strong evidence that support for human rights always enhances economic development. Rather, as the Nobel Laureate Amartya Sen has asserted, human rights and expanded freedoms are both integral parts of development.[5,8,9] Development should therefore be pursued in ways that are consistent with human rights and that further their attainment.

A third myth is that social justice, human goals, and human development are luxuries that must wait until countries become rich enough to afford them. This myth is contradicted by the experiences of the economically successful countries already described. Achieving human development—and pursuing public health and education for all—depend more on setting clear priorities than on having large amounts of national resources. Although availability of resources depends partly on the level of a country's development, the commitment to achieve health and education for all need not wait until the highest possible standards can be achieved. The experiences of some successful countries, such as Sri Lanka in eradicating malaria in the late 1940s, demonstrate that early progress toward public health is possible—and that this progress helps lay the foundation for further economic and social progress.

▓ PLACING PEOPLE AT THE CENTER OF DEVELOPMENT

A requirement for achieving social justice is placing people at the center of development. People need to be empowered to take charge of their own lives and their own health, so development strategy must focus on strengthening human capabilities through education and provision of opportunities for people to earn adequate income. Access to health services, safe water, and basic sanitation are also necessary for strengthening capabilities. Many well-intentioned projects in health, water supply, agricultural production, and education fail because people have not been put at the center of planning or implementation. This explains why development projects often end with rusting water pumps, abandoned plows, or tractors captured by interest groups that have seized most of the benefits and left most of the local people with little incentive to support and continue the projects.

Much has been learned about practical ways to achieve participatory people-centered approaches to human development. Using the framework of human development, a methodology has been developed and applied in many countries. Over 140 countries have prepared national human development reports, analyzing the situations and needs of their populations and planning policy development.[10]

Human development focuses on development as "the strengthening of human capabilities and the expansion of human choices, to enable people to live the lives they have reason to value."[11] The essential capabilities are defined by reference to human rights and by concerns for social justice and equity between women and men, between girls and boys, and among ethnic, religious, geographic, and other groups within countries—and equity between present and future generations.

The impact of this human development approach has been reinforced, nationally and internationally, by the use of human development indices. These have been designed to shift attention from the narrowness and inadequacies of mainly using economic indicators, such as a country's gross national product (GNP), as a measure of national progress and health and well-being. Instead of GNP, one can use the *Human Development Index* (HDI), an indicator by which the United Nations Development Programme (UNDP) assesses almost all countries annually. The HDI combines data on longevity, knowledge, and access to income for a reasonable standard of living. Longevity is measured by life expectancy. Knowledge is measured by the mean number of years of education. Income for a reasonable standard of living is measured by a modified measure of a per-capita income that gives greatest weight to income up to approximately the world average and relatively less weight to levels of income above this level.

There have been other indicators of human development, such as the *Gender Development Index*, which applied the HDI only to females, and the *Gender Empowerment Measure*, which measured the proportion of women in a country's leadership in government, business, science, and technology.

■ MULTIDIMENSIONAL INDICATORS OF POVERTY AND INEQUALITIES

The *Multidimensional Poverty Index* (MPI), which uses household data, is an indicator of deprivation. It is based on the proportion of households failing to reach minimum standards of education, health, access to clean water, improved sanitation, and use of modern fuels, and three other parameters. For example, a household is considered deprived in education if it has no member with at least 5 years of education or if it has one or more children not attending school (up to grade 8). In health, a household is treated as deprived if it has someone who is malnourished or if one or more children have died. A household's MPI is its composite score in all the areas. Because it focuses on households and specific areas of deprivation, the MPI is a better measure of deprivation than one based on national averages. The MPI is also more meaningful in low-income countries than definitions of poverty based on the proportion of individuals falling below some income level, such as $1.25 or $2.00 per day—which can be an almost meaningless measure for poor people in rural areas or peri-urban slums.

Social justice, however, is not only a matter of poverty, but also a matter of inequality and inequity. The annual *Human Development Report* by UNDP has always recognized this reality and, therefore, now includes the *Inequality-adjusted Human Development Index* (I-HDI), which combines measures of longevity, education, and living standards—all of which are adjusted for inequality. In any country, if longevity, education, or income were equal throughout the entire population, then its I-HDI would equal its HDI. But, when inequalities exist, the inequality-adjusted measures of longevity, education, and income are discounted according to the degrees of inequality in each of these indicators. The extent to which I-HDI or its components are discounted indicates the extent to which inequality in a country decreases human development.

Table 29-1 provides estimates of losses in HDI due to inequality and social injustice—23 percent globally and 13 to 35 percent in various regions of the world. Almost certainly these are underestimates of the losses attributable to inequalities; for example, they do not consider overlaps in which inequality in one area is likely to be associated with inequality in another.[12]

TABLE 29-1 *Impact of Inequality on Levels of Human Development: Losses in Human Development Index Due to Reduced Life Expectancy, Education, and Income (by Percentage), 2010*

World Regions	Overall Loss in HDI	Loss to Life Expectancy Through Inequality	Loss to Education Through Inequality	Loss to Income Index Through Inequality
Arab States	26%	18%	41%	18%
East Asia and the Pacific	21%	14%	22%	27%
South Asia	28%	27%	41%	15%
Latin America and the Caribbean	26%	13%	23%	39%
Sub-Saharan Africa	35%	39%	36%	28%
Europe and Central Asia	13%	12%	11%	16%
Least Developed Countries	32%	35%	37%	25%
Small Island States	28%	19%	30%	36%
Global Totals	23%	19%	26%	23%

(*Source:* United Nations Development Programme. Human Development Report 2011: Sustainability and equity: A better future for all, technical notes. New York: Oxford University Press, 2011.)

Of great concern, socially excluded groups of poor people are not included in the progress of most countries. In addition to economic deficits associated with poverty, these people often face a variety of types of discrimination—related to race, ethnicity, gender, caste, and occasionally language or religion. Each type of discrimination interacts with other types, and tending to reinforce the impact of all the types of discrimination. Groups of these excluded people are often residentially concentrated in disadvantaged locations, which contributes to their political exclusion.[13]

▪ WHAT NEEDS TO BE DONE

Economic and social inequalities often constrain the adoption of policies and actions in public health, or prevent otherwise good policies from taking full effect. This section therefore focuses on key economic priorities for action—nationally, regionally, and internationally.

Although all public health workers do not need to be expert in economic matters, those committed to reducing social injustice need to have a general sense of the types of economic policies that will contribute to their goals and will therefore deserve their support.

Making Equity an Economic Priority

Reduction of inequalities requires a broad range of national actions in such areas as salary structures, minimum wages, taxes, and public expenditures. Necessary actions relate to both the public and private sectors. Although the political influence of those with power and wealth often limits what may be possible in the short run, experience shows that constraints are less over the long run. Knowledge of what other countries are doing or have achieved often opens the door to a bolder vision and bolder actions in one's own country.

Brazil, Thailand, Argentina, Chile, Malaysia, Bolivia, and a dozen other countries have taken substantive action in recent years to reduce inequalities. This has usually required strong political leadership in such areas as these:

- Fiscal policy, while usually aimed at balancing budgets, has also involved progressive public expenditure policies in key areas such as public health, education, and social protection
- Expansionary fiscal elements to create jobs
- Minimum-wage legislation to raise the economic status of low-income people
- Policies to increase access for poorer groups to secondary and higher education
- Social protection measures involving cash transfers to poor families, often made conditional on their children's attending school and mothers' attending health clinics
- Increased taxation as a share of national resources, often by increasing the taxes on oil and mineral exports[14]

Policies like these are in sharp contrast to the cutbacks and restraints of the austerity policies adopted by many European countries since the economic crisis that began in 2008—and, to a lesser extent, with U.S. government policies since then. These austerity policies have been justified on the basis of "there being no alternative," given high levels of accumulated debt or threats and pressures from financial markets.

Both arguments have been strongly used in the United Kingdom by the coalition government, where, in 2010, debt as a percentage of GNP was high (76 percent) —although less than in Germany, France, Japan, and the United States. Claiming there were no alternatives, the coalition government made major cuts to public expenditures, reductions strongly denounced as self-defeating and poverty-creating by Keynesian and other progressive economists.[15,16]

The existence of alternatives in line with social justice can be illustrated from the experience of the United Kingdom after World War II. In 1945, public debt as a percentage of GNP was over 220 percent—three times the proportion in 2010. But high levels of debt did not prevent the UK government then from establishing the National Health Service, a national pension scheme, and many other programs of social justice. The UK government adopted all these while pursuing full-employment policies that kept unemployment well below 3 percent for 25 years. The UK government also kept income inequality well below levels present earlier in the 20th century—and far below those of today. Public debt was not neglected, but was gradually reduced over the long term—rather than slashing social programs and thereby increasing poverty.

The experiences of many countries in Latin America and sub-Saharan Africa in the 1980s and 1990s illustrate many of the negative lessons of policies of extreme austerity. To cope with accumulated debt and a global recession, many of these countries were required to adopt policies of structural adjustment as a condition of obtaining international support from the International Monetary Fund and the World Bank. Almost always this involved reducing support for education and for health and other social services, thereby increasing inequality and social injustice. Julius Nyerere, the President of Tanzania, challenged orthodoxy by asking: "Must we starve our children to pay our debts?"

The results were serious human and economic failures. Structural adjustment had a devastating impact on economic growth and social services. Between 1980 and 2000, per-capita income in Latin America increased slowly, much less than in the 1960s and 1970s. In sub-Saharan Africa it actually decreased—by 15 percent.[17]

All of this experience has demonstrated the need to combine measures of economic growth with measures to promote social justice and measures to reduce inequality—a strategy known as *redistribution with growth* (RWG).[18] Under RWG, a proportion of the additional income of those who are better-off is transferred each year, by taxation or other measures, to increases in social investment, education, and health services for poor people, thereby improving their production and productivity over the long term.

Providing International Support

Although national action is at the heart of diminishing social injustice, international action is also needed. Many proposals for stronger international action have been made in recent years, notably to the United Nations by the "Stiglitz Commission" during the global economic crisis in 2009.[19]

The starting point for the Commission was the belief that, in a globalized world, "a global crisis demands a global response." Despite a succession of international and regional meetings, international action has been weak in restoring growth globally and limited in its concerns and objectives. Sustainability and reduction of global inequalities, present in rhetoric, have almost been absent from operational objectives. And as the global economy has slowed, the annual cost of failure to act effectively has been at least $1 trillion in lost production since 2011.

The Stiglitz Commission recommended global action to coordinate recovery as well as regional and international action to address employment, equality, and environmental sustainability. The Commission also recommended action to strengthen the international system, by (a) restoring the position of the United Nations in global economic and social management, (b) reforming the governance structure of the International Monetary Fund and the World Bank, and (c) exploring the fundamental changes needed for achieving stability, sustainability, and equity. The Commission also explored creating a global reserve system, mechanisms to diminish causes of economic instability, and methods for preventing accumulation of sovereign debt. These changes can help reduce extremes of economic inequality, especially as it impacts low-income countries. International non-governmental organizations and foundations have important roles to play in promoting equitable and sustainable human development (Box 29–1 and Box 29–2).

Using the Millennium Development Goals to Reduce Poverty

Although many may consider international action for poverty reduction little more than a fantasy, facts show otherwise. In 2000, 147 heads of state and senior representatives of another 30 countries at the Millennium Summit, convened at the United Nations, took a major step towards generating global commitment and action toward the reduction of poverty. These national leaders agreed to the Millennium Declaration and eight Millennium Development Goals (MDGs), focused on a halving of the proportion of people in poverty in all countries by the year 2015.[20] The first seven MDGs are as follows:

- Goal 1—Eradication of extreme poverty and hunger by 2015, halving between 1990 and 2015 the proportion of people with incomes below $1 per day and the proportion of people who suffer from hunger.

(Text continues on page 528.)

BOX 29-1 ■ The Roles of International Non-Governmental Organizations in Promoting Equitable and Sustainable Human Development

Raymond C. Offenheiser and Porter McConnell

International non-governmental organizations (INGOs) operate in a field where good intentions have sometimes had unintended negative consequences. But INGOs have a constructive role to play in fighting poverty and inequality, specifically by strengthening a country's ability to care for its own—which is the best way to achieve long-term results from aid. Achieving sustainable health results, for example, depends upon a country's having a functioning health care system.[1] Too often, diseases like polio that were nearly eradicated have reappeared after global "big push" programs because these programs did not support the emergence of permanently sustainable health systems to vaccinate against and treat diseases.

Development occurs through a "compact" between people and their governments: Citizens pay taxes and demand public goods, and governments, in turn, provide services like roads and health care that can enable equitable growth. Aid can strengthen this compact in a country, but it can also weaken it. As Freddie Ssengooba of Makerere University in Uganda has stated: "Citizens need to be able to hold their governments accountable, and, when donors bypass ministries of health and set up parallel HIV and AIDS programs, citizens give the credit or blame to donors, not their own [governments]."[2] INGOs can control for this by supporting citizens in holding their governments accountable, and helping to strengthen their governments' capacity to deliver.

How INGOs Can Help Promote Health and Development

There are four ways that INGOs can contribute to health and development in low-income countries: solidarity, capacity building, piloting a new approach, and service delivery in humanitarian situations.

Solidarity

INGOs can play a supporting role for local civil society groups, which can advocate directly to their governments about their own priorities. Because citizens are the people who are most personally invested in their country's health and well-being, they are the most effective advocates. INGOs can play a key role in advocacy if an advocacy movement's leaders are local NGOs. In Malawi, for example, Oxfam supported civil society groups that were monitoring the *stockouts** of essential medicines at regional clinics that were caused by mismanagement or theft. By recruiting citizens to report these stockouts when they occurred, a civil society campaign was able to reduce the stockout rate from 70 percent in 2008 to 25 percent in 2009.[3]

Capacity Building

INGOs can help build the capacity of local groups to improve their communities—as long as the capacity building is driven by local demand. For example, Save the Children has been the prime recipient of a large grant from the U.S. Agency

---

* A *stockout* is defined as a situation in which the demand or requirement for an item cannot be fulfilled from the current inventory.

for International Development (USAID) for a project to help small-scale farmers gain access to markets. AGEXPORT, a Guatemalan consortium of food exporters, had been a sub-grantee. After 5 years of capacity building from Save the Children, AGEXPORT took the lead in implementing the project, with Save the Children then serving in an advisory role.[4] AGEXPORT is likely to manage the next project itself.

Piloting a New Approach

As the chief *duty bearer*,* a country's government is ultimately responsible for delivering essential services to its citizens. But INGOs can pilot new approaches for governments to adopt and then bring to scale. The Horn of Africa Risk Transfer for Adaptation (HARITA) project in Ethiopia illustrates how an INGO can pilot a new approach. Rural farmers in Ethiopia needed crop insurance to order to adapt to climate change. In response to their request, Oxfam and its local partner, the Relief Society of Tigray, paid for their crop insurance in exchange for the farmers' providing labor on community projects. To bring this *insurance-for-work* concept to scale, the Ethiopian government integrated it into its nationwide Productive Safety Net Program, enabling HARITA to reach over 40 villages.[5] This pilot approach was successful because it built on local ingenuity, rather than supplanting it.

Service Delivery in Humanitarian Situations

In humanitarian emergencies or other critical situations, governments may either be unwilling or unable to provide necessary services and may request temporary external assistance critical to saving lives. However, this approach cannot provide long-term solutions. And it can create parallel systems that siphon talent from local agencies and organizations, making it more difficult for them to build long-term capacity. Therefore, this role for INGOs should be limited to short-term assistance in humanitarian relief situations, in which they work closely with local agencies and organizations.

Conclusion

Ultimately, development is about the relationship between people and their governments. INGOs, however, can help strengthen this relationship and help people around the world lift themselves and their communities out of poverty.

Box References

1. Fryatt R, Mills A, Nordstrom A. Financing of health systems to achieve the health Millennium Development Goals in low-income countries. *Lancet* 2010;375:419–426.
2. Ssengooba F. Uganda: How long will we depend on the U.S. for HIV money? Allafrica.com, online edition, January 5, 2010. Available at http://allafrica.com/stories/201001060660.html. Accessed on August 24, 2012.
3. Mazengera S. Missing medicines in Malawi: Campaigning against stock-outs of essential drugs. Local Governance and Community Action Programme Insights Series, May 30, 2012. Available at http://policy-practice.oxfam.org.uk/publications/missing-medicines-in-malawi-campaigning-against-stock-outs-of-essential-drugs-226732.Accessed on August 24, 2012.
4. Cardenas C. Moving local organizations into the driver's seat. July 18, 2012. Available at http://savethechildren.typepad.com/blog/2012/07/moving-local-organizations-into-the-drivers-seat.html. Accessed on August 27, 2012.
5. Oxfam America. What Oxfam is doing. 2012. Available at http://www.oxfamamerica.org/issues/insurance/what-oxfam-is- doing/?searchterm=harita. Accessed on August 27, 2012.

* A *duty bearer*, which is often the state, assures that it meets its obligations under international law to respect, protect, and fulfill people's rights.

BOX 29-2 ■ The Roles of Foundations in Promoting Equitable
and Sustainable Human Development

Mark Sidel

The challenges of promoting equitable and sustainable human development are primarily the work of citizens, social movements, and governments. But others can contribute, too, and in many countries private foundations—indigenous and external—have played a role in these difficult and complex processes.

Often governments are ill-equipped, or unwilling, to utilize the "best practices" that we now know are crucial for equitable and sustainable development. Governments often play important roles in promoting inequality, rather than in redressing it. For example, they often violate rights rather than protect them, and they often support initiatives that benefit business and wealthy people, rather than supporting economic growth policies that support poor people.

Private foundations can play an important role in (a) providing alternatives to these policies and programs, and (b) promoting citizen-based initiatives in development and health that challenge business-oriented policies, while being linked to government programs. For example, in China and Vietnam, significant programs are promoting development and economic growth. However, these programs often involve clashes between policies that strengthen business and private wealth and those that promote poor people and social justice. In countries like these where the development agenda is based largely on economic growth, private foundations—especially those based outside these countries—often provide the only major sustained support for policies that benefit poor people and initiatives that promote social justice.

In China and Vietnam, external foundations have helped to pioneer new models of citizen initiatives in health policy, environmental advocacy, and social justice aimed at primary health care, HIV/AIDS treatment and prevention, environmental health, reproductive health, and tobacco control. In countries where governments have supported traditional health and development programs, external foundations, such as the Ford Foundation, the Bill & Melinda Gates Foundation, the William J. Clinton Foundation, and the China Medical Board, have supported grassroots initiatives oriented to poor people and linked them to the government's development of health policy. These external foundations have also supported new approaches to public policy in health, economics, and other areas that support a greater voice for citizens, sustained public expenditures, a continued significant role for government-operated (rather than privatized) health care, and primary health care and prevention programs (rather than highly-specialized tertiary care facilities).

External—and domestic—foundations that are focused on equitable development can be especially important in countries like China and Vietnam, where other forms of external assistance are beginning to wane. As these countries and others move toward "middle-income status," many multilateral and bilateral aid organizations that are focused on equitable development are moving their work to poorer countries—as indeed they should. As they move away, governments of countries like China and Vietnam may be left without alternatives to growth-focused policies. As a result, citizens of these countries who are focused on public participation and grassroots initiatives that support poor people may be left without the moral and financial support to sustain their work. In these situations, external foundations can play an even more important role as incubators of new ideas and supporters of new approaches.

Over time, external foundations will eventually also leave, and domestic foundations will ideally support citizens' initiatives and policies that support poor people—as is now beginning to happen in countries like China and Vietnam. But the road ahead may be difficult if the leaders of major domestic foundations come from business backgrounds and they are not concerned about equitable development. External foundations can therefore also play important roles in orienting domestic foundations to equitable policy and social justice.

There are limits to what foundations can do. For example, they cannot sustain a human rights agenda in countries where government support is absent or inadequate. But they can—and do—facilitate and support the development of fresh approaches to health, environment, and economic policies that can promote equitable and sustainable development and social justice.

- Goal 2—Achievement of universal primary education, by ensuring that, by 2015, girls and boys in all countries can complete a full cycle of basic primary education.
- Goal 3—Promotion of gender equality and empowerment of women, by eliminating gender disparities in primary and secondary education, preferably by 2005, and at all levels of education by 2010.
- Goal 4—Reduction of child mortality by two-thirds of its 1990 level by 2015.
- Goal 5—Improvement of maternal and reproductive health, including the reduction of the maternal mortality ratio of 1990 by three-fourths by 2015.
- Goal 6—To combat HIV/AIDS, malaria, and other diseases by halting, by 2015, in each country the rise in HIV/AIDS and to begin to reverse its spread, and to halt, by 2015, the rise and to begin to reverse the spread of malaria and other major diseases.
- Goal 7—To ensure environmental sustainability by integrating principles of sustainable development into country policies and programs and to reverse the loss of environmental resources; to halve by 2015 the proportion of people without access to safe drinking water and adequate sanitation; and to achieve by 2020 a significant improvement in the lives of at least a 100 million slum dwellers.[6] (See Table 21–7 in Chapter 21.)

Progress towards the MDGs is being monitored by the United Nations. By 2012, progress was considerable, sometimes exceeding the targets, especially in Asia and Latin America, but less so in sub-Saharan Africa and the 48 least-developed countries, landlocked countries, and small island states.[21] Progress has included the following:

- Extreme poverty has been decreasing in every region, and the target for global poverty reduction was met in 2010.
- The proportion of people without access to improved sources of water has been halved. Between 1990 and 2010, two million people gained access to improved water sources.

- Significant improvements have occurred in the lives of 200 million slum dwellers, exceeding the 2020 target, with the *proportion* of urban residents in developing countries living in slums declining from 39 percent in 2000 to 33 percent in 2010. However, the *numbers* of people living in slums has continued to increase.
- Many countries have made significant progress toward universal primary education, with parity already achieved between girls and boys.
- Under-5 child deaths have decreased from 12 million in 1990 to 6.9 million in 2011.
- Access to treatment for HIV has increased in all regions for a global total of 6.5 million HIV patients in treatment. Progress is on track to halting the spread of tuberculosis, raising expectations that the tuberculosis mortality rate may be halved by 2015. And the number of malaria deaths globally has declined.[22]

Less progress has, however, been made in the following areas:

- Reducing maternal mortality
- Access to improved water supplies in rural areas
- Hunger (Almost one-third of children under age 5 in South Asia were underweight in 2010.)
- Access to adequate sanitation (Half of the population in developing countries still lacks improved sanitation facilities.)[22]

In addition, inequality and the global economic crisis have been detracting from progress in achieving the MDGs. In high-income countries, austerity programs have cut back health and education programs and are contributing to increased poverty and unemployment.

Within most countries, progress toward the MDGs has been least and slowest for disadvantaged and marginalized groups, notably girls and women. United Nations Secretary-General Ban Ki-Moon summarized progress and also the remaining challenge that is closely linked to social justice: "The MDGs have helped lift millions of people out of poverty, save countless children's lives and ensure that they attend school.... At the same time, we still have a long way to go in empowering women and girls, promoting sustainable development, and protecting the most vulnerable."

Initiating Actions Toward Social Justice

In spite of progress toward the MDGs, four actions still stand out as priorities for greater social justice in most developing countries:

1. Shifting the focus in accelerating and monitoring progress to equity, by providing the most marginalized and poorest groups with adequate education, health care, access to water, and other services

2. Decentralizing approaches to ensure greater participation of all communities, especially to ensure that the people affected by inequality and social injustice can guide action and outcomes in relation to their own perceptions of needs

3. Setting budget priorities and providing adequate resources to support action toward achieving the MDGs

4. Reducing corruption and conflict to ensure that resources allocated in support of the MDGs are not captured or diverted by those with power or wealth

Ensuring Supportive Actions by High-Income Countries

The role of developed countries is important in assisting or facilitating developing countries in making progress towards the MDGs. This also is a role shrouded in confusion and myths. One myth is that the developed countries can do little—and need do little. A second myth is that the public sector (the government) can do little and the private sector can do whatever is important. A third myth is that the main role of developed countries is to provide aid, and, with aid, developing countries would have the resources to accelerate action toward the MDGs; and, without aid, the task would be impossible for many developing countries, especially the poorest.

All three myths have grains of truth, but all three are oversimplified and not completely accurate. In fact, developed countries and their economies are of enormous importance for the economic and social future of developing countries, especially for accelerating progress towards the MDGs. Most important is the role of developed countries in enabling—or obstructing—creation of a supportive environment that makes possible trade, investment flows on fair conditions, debt relief for heavily indebted developing countries, access to technology, and development assistance on fair and reasonable conditions—especially for the poorest and least-developed countries.

Goal 8 of the MDGs—the only goal without quantification or time-bound targets—calls for strengthening of "a global partnership for development," which lists seven priority actions for high-income developed countries:

- Further developing an open, rule-based, predictable, non-discriminatory trading and financial system, nationally and internationally
- Addressing the special needs of the 48 least-developed countries, with tariff-free and quota-free access for exports, enhanced programs for debt relief and cancellation of official bilateral debt, and more-generous aid for countries committed to poverty reduction
- Addressing the special needs of landlocked and small-island developing countries
- Dealing comprehensively with the debt problems of developing countries by national and international measures designed to make the debt sustainable in the long term

- Developing and implementing strategies for decent and productive work for youth
- Providing access to affordable essential drugs in developing countries, in cooperation with pharmaceutical companies
- Making available the benefits of new technologies, especially information and communication technologies, in cooperation with the private sector[23]

Implementing these priority actions would do much to enable most developing countries to accelerate their overall economic and social advance and, as part of this, to accelerate their progress toward the MDGs. Such actions would represent a significant shift from policies pursued by the leading developed countries in recent years.

Past experience does not encourage optimism for achieving Goal 8. Goals for aid, trade, and debt relief established in a series of global conferences over the past four decades have generally not been achieved. For example, commitments to open markets in developed countries to imports from developing countries have generally not been honored.

Nevertheless, several significant initiatives have followed from the Millennium Summit of 2000—offering hope that international action to reduce poverty can be successful:

- Most countries have publicly committed to the achievement of the MDGs.
- The World Bank, the International Monetary Fund, and United Nations agencies have established new mechanisms for cooperating to support the reduction of poverty.
- There has been renewed commitment to overseas development assistance by some countries, especially in Europe. Until 2010, five European countries had been, for many years, fulfilling the overseas development assistance target recommended by the United Nations—0.7 percent of GDP—and six others had committed to achieving this target by 2015. Because of the global economic crisis, however, overseas development assistance decreased in 16 of the 24 DAC donor countries (developing countries that are members of the Development Assistance Committee of the Organization for Economic Co-operation and Development).

Since 2000, the global economy has been rapidly changing, with the center of economic gravity and power shifting towards the East and the South. Emerging countries, especially Brazil, Russia, India, China, and South Africa, have been rapidly increasing their national income, wealth, and economic influence. They have also been pioneering new approaches to economic development—and demonstrating the possibility of accelerated economic development. In many ways, they provide models on how to accelerate development in other countries. And other countries have benefited from growing trade and investments.

▓ CONCLUSION

As a global society, the challenge we face has been well expressed by historian David Landes:

> The old division of the world into two power blocs, East and West, has subsided. Now the big challenge and threat is the gap in wealth and health that separates rich and poor. These are often styled North and South, because the division is geographic; but a more accurate signifier would be the West and the Rest, because the division is also historical. Here is the greatest single problem and danger facing the world in the Third Millennium.[25]

Substantially reducing social injustice on a global scale requires fundamental actions, most of which are not yet politically acceptable in high-income countries. It is gratifying to recognize the achievements in recent decades to improve human health and well-being. However, substantially reducing social injustice will require action beyond the health sector—especially in economic and social policy, nationally and internationally. Health workers need to understand this challenge—and advocate for, and participate in, broader actions to reduce social injustice.

▓ REFERENCES

1. Ortiz I, Cummins M. Global inequality: Beyond the bottom billion. A rapid review of income distribution in 141 countries. Social and Economic Policy Working Paper. New York: UNICEF, 2011.
2. Mitchell BR. European historical statistics, 1750–1970. London: Macmillan, 1978.
3. UNICEF. State of the World's Children, 2010. Oxford, UK: Oxford University Press, 2012:88–91.
4. United Nations Development Programme. Human Development Report, 1997. New York: Oxford University Press, 1997. Available at http://hdr.undp.org/en/reports/global/hdr1997/. Accessed on August 30, 2012.
5. United Nations Development Programme. Human Development Report 2000: Human rights and human development. New York: Oxford University Press, 2000. Available at http://hdr.undp.org/en/reports/global/hdr2000/. Accessed on August 30, 2012.
6. United Nations Development Programme. Human Development Report 2003: Millennium development goals: A compact among nations to end human poverty. New York: Oxford University Press, 2003. Available at http://hdr.undp.org/en/reports/global/hdr2003/. Accessed on August 30, 2012.
7. Mehrotra S, Jolly R. Development with a human face: Experiences in social achievement and economic growth. Oxford, UK: Clarendon Press, 1997.
8. Sen A. Development as freedom. New York: Random House, 1999.
9. Sen A. The idea of justice. London: Allen Lane, 2009.
10. United Nations Development Programme. Human Development Report. Available at: www.hdr.undp.org. Accessed March 11, 2013.
11. United Nations Development Programme. Human Development Report 2011: Sustainability and equity: A better future for all. New York: Oxford University Press,

2011:1–2. Available at http://hdr.undp.org/en/reports/global/hdr2011/. Accessed on August 30, 2012.

12. United Nations Development Programme. Human Development Report 2011: Sustainability and equity: A better future for all, technical notes. New York: Oxford University Press, 2011:170. Available at http://hdr.undp.org/en/reports/global/hdr2011/. Accessed on August 30, 2012.

13. Kabeer N. Can the MDGs provide a pathway to social justice? The challenge of intersecting inequalities. New York: United Nations Development Programme, 2010:6. Available at http://www.ids.ac.uk/files/dmfile/MDGreportwebsiteu2WC.pdf. Accessed on August 30, 2012.

14. Cornia GA, Martorano B. Democracy, the new left and income distribution in Latin America over the last decade. In: V Fitzgerald, J Heyer, R Thorp, eds. Overcoming the persistence of inequality and poverty. Basingstoke, UK: Palgrave and Macmillan, 2011:172–199.

15. Krugman P. End this depression now. New York: W.W. Norton, 2012.

16. Stiglitz J. The price of inequality: The avoidable causes and invisible costs of inequality. New York: W.W. Norton, 2012.

17. Weisbrot M, Naiman R, Kim J. The emperor has no growth: Declining economic growth rates in the era of globalization. Washington, DC: Center for Economic and Policy Research, 2001.

18. Chenery HB et al. Redistribution with growth. London: Oxford University Press, 1974.

19. United Nations. Report of the Commission of Experts of the President of the General Assembly on Reforms of the International Monetary and Financial System. September 21, 2009. New York: United Nations, 2009. Available at http://www.un.org/ga/econcrisissummit/docs/Final Report_CoE.pdf. Accessed on August 30, 2012.

20. UN General Assembly. United Nations Millennium Declaration and the Millennium Development Goals. Available at www.un.org/millennium/summit. Accessed on August 30, 2012.

21. United Nations. The Millennium Development Goals Report 2010. New York: United Nations, 2010. Available at http://mdgs.un.org/unsd/mdg/Resources/Static/Products/Progress2010/MDG_Report_2010_En_low%20res.pdf. Accessed on August 30, 2012.

22. United Nations. The Millennium Development Goals Report 2012. New York: United Nations, 2012. Available at http://mdgs.un.org/unsd/mdg/Resources/Static/Products/Progress2012/English2012.pdf. Accessed on August 30, 2012.

23. United Nations Development Programme. Human Development Report 1999. New York: Oxford University Press, 1999:38. Available at http://hdr.undp.org/en/media/HDR_1999_EN.pdf. Accessed on August 30, 2012.

24. World Bank. World Development Report, 2003: Sustainable development in a dynamic world: Transforming institutions, growth and quality of life. New York: Oxford University Press, 2002:183. Available at http://www-wds.worldbank.org/servlet/WDSContentServer/WDSP/IB/2002/09/06/000094946_02082404015955/Rendered/PDF/multi0page.pdf. Accessed on August 30, 2012.

25. Landes D. The wealth and poverty of nations: Why some are so rich and some so poor. New York: W.W. Norton, 1999.

SOME ORGANIZATIONS ADDRESSING SOCIAL INJUSTICE

American Civil Liberties Union (ACLU)

125 Broad Street, 18th Floor
New York, NY 10004
Tel.: 212-549-2500
Website: www.aclu.org
Works daily in courts, legislatures, and communities to defend and preserve the individual rights and liberties guaranteed to every person in the United States under the Constitution and federal laws.

American Public Health Association (APHA)

800 I Street, NW
Washington, DC 20001–3701
Tel.: 202-777-2742
Website: www.apha.org
The oldest and largest organization of public health professionals in the world, representing more than 50,000 members from over 50 occupations in public health. Brings together health service providers, administrators, teachers, researchers, and other health workers for professional exchange, study, and action. Actively serves the public, APHA members, and the field of public health through its scientific and practice programs, publications, annual meeting, awards program, educational services, and advocacy work.

Amnesty International

1 Easton Street
London WC1X 0DW
United Kingdom
Tel.: 44 20 7413 5500
Website: www.amnesty.org

Amnesty International USA

322 Eighth Avenue
New York, NY 10001–4808
Tel.: 212-807-8400
Website: www.amnestyusa.org
Global movement of people who campaign to end grave abuses of human rights. Its vision is for every person to enjoy all the rights enshrined in the Universal Declaration of Human Rights and other international human rights standards.

Center on Budget and Policy Priorities

820 First Street, NE, Suite 510
Washington, DC 20002
Tel.: 202-408-1080
Website: www.cbpp.org
Conducts research and analysis to help shape public debates over proposed budget and tax policies and to help ensure that policymakers consider the needs of low-income families and individuals in these debates. Also develops policy options to alleviate poverty.

Center for Constitutional Rights (CCR)

666 Broadway, 7th Floor
New York, NY 10012
Phone: 212-614-6464
Website: www.ccrjustice.org
Dedicated to advancing and protecting the rights guaranteed by the U.S. Constitution and the Universal Declaration of Human Rights.

Center for Defense Information (CDI)

1779 Massachusetts Avenue, NW
Washington, DC 20036–2019
Tel.: 202-332-0600
Website: www.cdi.org
Operating under the aegis of the World Security Institute, it is
composed of academics and high-ranking retired U.S. military officers who conduct critical analyses of U.S. defense and security policy.

Center for Economic and Social Rights (CESR)

162 Montague Street, 3rd floor
Brooklyn, NY 11201
Tel.: 718-237-9145
Website: www.cesr.org
Promotes the universal rights of every human being to housing, education, health, food, water, work, and other economic, social, and cultural rights essential to human dignity.

Center for Policy Analysis on Trade and Health (CPATH)

P.O. Box 29586
San Francisco, CA 94129
Tel.: 415-922-6204
Website: www.cpath.org
Brings a public health voice to the debate on trade and sustainable development. Conducts research, policy analysis, and advocacy for protecting and improving

the health of individuals, communities, and populations; for expanding access to health-related services; and for advancing global economic policies that are democratic, sustainable, and socially just.

Center for Reproductive Rights (CRR)

120 Wall Street
New York, NY 10005
Tel.: 917-637-3600
Website: www.reproductiverights.org
Advances reproductive freedom as a fundamental human right that all governments are legally obligated to protect, respect, and fulfill.

Children's Defense Fund (CDF)

25 E Street, NW
Washington, DC 20001
Tel.: 800-233-1200
Website: www.childrensdefense.org
Champions policies and programs that lift children out of poverty, protect them from abuse and neglect, and ensure their access to health care, quality education, and a moral and spiritual foundation.

Council for a Livable World (CLW)

322 4th Street, NE
Washington, DC 20002
Tel.: 202-543-4100
Website: www.clw.org
Advocates for reducing the danger of nuclear weapons and increasing national security.

Disability Rights International

1666 Connecticut Avenue, NW, Suite 325
Washington, DC 20009
Tel.: 202-296-0800
Website: www.disabilityrightsintl.org
Promotes the human rights and full participation in society of people with disabilities globally.

Disabled Peoples International

214 Montreal Road, Suite 402
Ottawa, Ontario
Canada K1L 8L8
Tel.: 613-563-2091
Website: www.dpi.org
Raises awareness about persons with disabilities as embodied in the Convention on the Rights of Persons with Disabilities (CRPD) and other human rights treaties. Creates and promotes an environment for sustainable development.

Doctors for Global Health (DGH)

P.O. Box 1761
Decatur, GA 30031
Tel.: 404-377-3566
Website: www.dghonline.org
Promotes health, education, art, and other human rights throughout the world. Funds and supports local projects. Educates and advocates for policies that promote justice and peace.

Federation of American Scientists (FAS)

1725 DeSales Street, NW, Suite 600
Washington, DC 20036-4413
Tel.: 202-546-3300
Website: www.fas.org
Provides rigorous, objective, evidence-based analysis, and practical policy recommendations on national and international security issues connected to applied science and technology. Educates policymakers, the public, the news media, and the next generation of scientists, engineers, and global leaders about the urgent need for creating a more secure and better world.

Francis X. Bagnaud (FXB) Center for Health and Human Rights

Harvard School of Public Health
651 Huntington Avenue, 7th Floor
Boston, MA 02115
Tel.: 617-432-0656
Website: www.harvardfxbcenter.org/index.php
Works to protect and promote the rights and well-being of children, adolescents, and their families in extreme circumstances globally. Conducts and supports research, teaching, advocacy, and targeted action.

Gay Men's Health Crisis

446 West 33rd Street
New York, NY 10001–2601
Tel.: 800-243-7692
Website: www.gmhc.org
Provides HIV/AIDS prevention, care, and advocacy. Works to end the AIDS epidemic and uplift the lives of all affected.

Global Lawyers and Physicians for Human Rights

Department of Health Law, Bioethics and Human Rights
Boston University School of Public Health
715 Albany Street
Boston, MA 02118
Tel.: 617-638-4626
Website: http://www.globallawyersandphysicians.org/
Works at the local, national, and international level through collaboration and partnerships for global implementation of the health-related provisions of the Universal Declaration of Human Rights and the Covenants on Civil and Political Rights and Economic, Social, and Cultural Rights, with a focus on health and human rights, patient rights, and human experimentation.

Healthy Communities Institute

2054 University Avenue, Suite 600
Berkeley, CA 94704
Tel.: 866-499-6423
Website: www.healthycommunitiesinstitute.com/international-foundation/
Facilitates linkages among people, issues, and resources in order to support development of Healthy Cities initiatives.

Hesperian Health Guides

1919 Addison Street, Suite 304
Berkeley, CA 94704
Tel.: 510-845-1447
Website: www.hesperian.org
Promotes health and self-determination in poor communities globally by making health information accessible. Produces publications that are written simply and include many illustrations so people with little formal education can understand, apply, and share medical information.

Human Rights Watch

350 Fifth Avenue, 34th Floor
New York, NY 10118–3299
Tel.: 212-290-4700
Website: www.hrw.org
Defends and protects human rights. Stands with victims and activists to prevent discrimination, uphold political freedom, protect people from inhumane conduct during wartime, and bring offenders to justice.

International Disability Alliance

245 Park Avenue, 39th Floor
New York, NY 10167
Tel: 212-672-1614
Website: www.internationaldisabilityalliance.org/en
Advances the human rights of persons with disabilities as a united voice of organizations of persons with disabilities, utilizing the Convention on the Rights of Persons with Disabilities and other human rights instruments.

International Physicians for the Prevention of Nuclear War (IPPNW)

66–70 Union Square, #204
Somerville, MA 02143
Tel.: 617-440-1733
Website: www.ippnw.org
Global federation of national medical organizations in 62 countries dedicated to the common goal of creating a more powerful and secure world that is freed from the threat of nuclear annihilation.

Lambda Legal

120 Wall Street, 19th Floor
New York, NY 10005–3904
Tel.: 212-809-8585
Website: www.lambdalegal.org
National organization committed to achieving full recognition of the civil rights of lesbians, gay men, bisexuals, transgendered people, and people with HIV/AIDS through impact litigation, education, and public policy work.

Medact (IPPNW/United Kingdom)

The Grayston Center
28 Charles Square
London N1 6HT
United Kingdom
Tel.: 44 20 7324 4739
Website: www.medact.org
Undertakes education, research, and advocacy on the health implications of conflict, development, and environmental change.

National Center for Law and Economic Justice

275 Seventh Avenue, Suite 1506
New York, NY 10001–6708
Tel.: 212-633-6967
Website: www.nclej.org
Advances economic justice throughout the United States, secures systemic reform in the delivery of income support and related human services, and safeguards important legal and constitutional rights.

National Center for Lesbian Rights (NCLR)

870 Market Street, Suite 570
San Francisco, CA 94102
Tel.: 415-392-6257
Website: www.nclrights.org
Advances the rights and safety of lesbians and their families through litigation, public policy advocacy, free legal advice and counseling, and public education. Provides representation and resources to gay men and to bisexual and transgender individuals on key issues that also advance lesbian rights.

National Centre for Social Research

35 Northampton Square
London EC1 0AX
United Kingdom
Tel.: (44 20) 7250 1866
Website: www.natcen.ac.uk
Designs, performs, and analyzes research studies in social and public policy.

National Coalition for the Homeless

2201 P Street, NW
Washington, DC 20037
Tel.: 202-462-4822
Website: www.nationalhomeless.org
With a mission to end homelessness, it works on issues of housing justice, economic justice, health care justice, and civil rights. Its programs focus on public education, policy advocacy, and grassroots organizing.

National Coalition for LGBT Health

1325 Massachusetts Avenue, NW, Suite 705
Washington, DC 20005
Tel.: 202-558-6828
Website: www.lgbthealth.net
Advocates for changes in public-sector and private-sector policies, laws, and regulations regarding LGBT health and related issues. Increases resources to expand culturally competent health and social services delivery to a diverse and inclusive LGBT population. Builds and disseminates knowledge regarding the LGBT population's health status, access to and utilization of health care, and other health-related information.

National Economic and Social Rights Initiative

4233 Chestnut Street
Philadelphia, PA 19104 and
90 John Street, Suite 308
New York, NY 10038
Tel.: 212-253-1710
Website: www.nesri.org
In partnership with communities, works to build a broad movement for economic and social rights, including health, housing, education, and work with dignity.

National Gay and Lesbian Task Force

1325 Massachusetts Avenue, NW, Suite 600
Washington, DC 20005
Tel.: 202-393-5177
Website: www.ngltf.org
Builds the grassroots power of the LGBT community by training activists, equipping state and local organizations with the skills needed to organize broad-based campaigns to defeat anti-LGBT referenda and advance pro-LGBT legislation, and building organizational capacity.

National Senior Citizens Law Center

1444 Eye Street, NW Suite 1100
Washington, DC 20005
Tel.: 202-289-6976
Website: www.nsclc.org
Protects the rights of low-income older adults through advocacy, litigation, and the education and counseling of local advocates.

Office of the United Nations High Commissioner for Human Rights

Palais Wilson
52 rue des Pâquis
CH-1201 Geneva, Switzerland
Tel.: (41 22) 917 9220
Website: www.ohchr.org
Represents the world's commitment to universal ideals of human dignity. Promotes and protects all human rights.

Open Society Foundations

224 West 57th Street
New York, NY 10019
Tel.: 212-548-0600
Website: www.opensocietyfoundations.org
Helps protect and improve the lives of people in marginalized communities throughout the world.

Oxfam America

226 Causeway Street, 5th Floor
Boston, MA 02111
Tel.: 617-482-1211
Website: www.oxfamamerica.org

Oxfam Great Britain

Oxfam House
John Smith Drive Cowley
Oxford OX4 2JY
United Kingdom
Tel.: (44 18) 6547 3727
Website: www.oxfam.org.uk

Works to build a future free from the injustice of poverty. Works directly with communities and seeks to influence the powerful to ensure that poor people can improve their lives and livelihoods and have a say in decisions that affect them.

Pan American Health Organization (PAHO)
WHO Regional Office for the Americas
525 Twenty-third Street, NW
Washington, DC 20037
Tel.: 202-974-3000
Website: www.paho.org
It operates the Equity, Health and Human Development listserv (www.paho.org/english/dd/ikm/eq-list.htm), which shares public health information of international significance that enables policymakers, researchers, and practitioners to improve health, especially among disadvantaged populations.

Partners in Health
888 Commonwealth Avenue, 3rd Floor
Boston, MA 02115
Tel.: 617-998-8922
Website: www.pih.org
Provides direct health care services and performs research and advocacy activities for sick and poor people.

Physicians for Global Survival (IPPNW/Canada)
30 Cleary Avenue, Suite 10
Ottawa, Ontario K2A 4A1
Canada
Tel.: 613-233-1982
Website: www.pgs.ca
Educates and advocates for the abolition of nuclear weapons, the prevention of war, and the promotion of nonviolent means of conflict resolution and social justice.

Physicians for Human Rights (PHR)
Two Arrow Street, Suite 301
Cambridge, MA 02138
Tel.: 617-301-4200
Website: www.phrusa.org
Uses medicine and science to stop mass atrocities and human rights violations against individuals. Uses investigations and expertise to advocate for the prevention of individual or small-scale acts of violence from becoming mass atrocities, to protect internationally guaranteed rights of individuals and civilian populations, and to prosecute those who violate human rights.

Physicians for a National Health Program (PNHP)

29 East Madison, Suite 602
Chicago, IL 60602
Tel.: 312-782-6006
Website: www.pnhp.org
Advocates for a universal, comprehensive single-payer national health program in the United States.

Physicians for Social Responsibility (PSR) (IPPNW/USA)

1111 14th Street, NW, Suite 700
Washington, DC, 20005
Tel.: 202-667-4260
Website: www.psr.org
Works to prevent nuclear war and proliferation of nuclear weapons and to slow, stop, and reverse global warming and toxic degradation of the environment.

Rehabilitation International

25 East 21st Street
New York, NY 10010
Tel.: 212-420-1500
Website: http://www.riglobal.org/
Works to improve the quality of life of people with disabilities.

Spirit of 1848 Listserv

Website: www.spiritof1848.org/listserv.htm
An e-mail community that serves an activist network of people concerned about social inequalities in health by posting information on social justice and public health.

UCL Institute of Health Equity

Marmot Review Secretariat
Department for Epidemiology and Public Health
University College London
1–19 Torrington Place
London WC1E 7HB
United Kingdom
Tel: (44 20) 7679 8259

Website: http://www.instituteofhealthequity.org
Works to reduce inequalities in health. Seeks to increase health equity through action on the social determinants of health, specifically in the following four areas: influencing global, national, and local policies; advising on and learning from practice; building an evidence base; and building capacity.

United Nations Children's Fund (UNICEF)
3 United Nations Plaza
New York, NY 10017
Tel.: 212-326-7025
Website: www.unicef.org
Supports health and survival of children and advocates for the realization of the rights of every child.

Union of Concerned Scientists (UCS)
2 Brattle Square
Cambridge, MA 02138
Tel.: 617-547-5552
Website: www.ucsusa.org
Works for a healthy environment and a safer world. Develops innovative, practical solutions and secures responsible changes in government policy, corporate practices, and consumer choices.

United Nations Educational, Scientific and Cultural Organization (UNESCO)
7 Place de Fontenoy
75352 Paris 07 SP
France
Tel.: (33 1) 45 68 10 00
Website: www.unesco.org
Contributes to the building of peace, the eradication of poverty, sustainable development, and intercultural dialogue through education, the sciences, culture, communication, and information.

USC Program on Global Health and Human Rights
USC Institute for Global Health
2001 Soto Street (SSB), Floor 3
Los Angeles, CA 90032
Tel.: 323-865-0419
Website: globalhealth.usc.edu
Develops practical and effective responses to global public health challenges through the innovative application of human rights concepts and methods in research, policy, capacity building, development of tools for analysis, and monitoring and evaluation.

WITNESS
80 Hanson Place, Floor 5
Brooklyn, NY 11217
Tel.: 718-783-2000
Website: www.witness.org
Brings attention to human rights abuses. Empowers human rights defenders to use video to fight injustice, and to transform personal stories of abuse into powerful tools that can pressure those in power and those with power to act.

World Health Organization (WHO)
Avenue Appia 20
1211 Geneva 27
Switzerland
Tel.: (41 22) 791 21 11
Website: www.who.int
The specialized United Nations agency for health, it provides leadership on global health matters, shapes the health research agenda, sets norms and standards, articulates evidence-based policy options, provides technical support to countries, and monitors and assesses health trends.

■ INDEX

Printed in Great Britain
by Amazon

"An invaluable primer on how inequity breeds ill health. It should be widely read by policymakers and practitioners looking for a passionate and scholarly review of societal changes that would avert enormous suffering."

— *THE NEW ENGLAND JOURNAL OF MEDICINE* REVIEW OF THE FIRST EDITION OF *SOCIAL INJUSTICE AND PUBLIC HEALTH*

This completely revised and updated second edition is a comprehensive, evidence-based resource on the relationship of social injustice to public health. Its 78 contributors are experts in public health, human rights, medicine, nursing, law, social sciences, and other disciplines. This highly readable and thoroughly referenced book documents the adverse effects of social injustice on specific population groups and specific aspects of public health. In addition, it makes many recommendations for reducing social injustice and its health consequences.

Social Injustice and Public Health is the definitive resource for practitioners, policymakers, and others seeking to better understand and address the social determinants of health. Physicians, nurses, other health professionals, human rights activists, sociologists, lawyers, and others—as well as their academic institutions, agencies, and organizations—will find this book to be informative and useful.

BARRY S. LEVY, MD, MPH, is an Adjunct Professor of Public Health at Tufts University School of Medicine and a past president of the American Public Health Association (APHA). He has had extensive experience in public health practice, education, research, and consulting, both in the United States and 20 other countries. He has written numerous articles and book chapters on a wide range of public health subjects and has co-edited 16 other books, including, with Dr. Sidel, two editions of *War and Public Health* and two editions of *Terrorism and Public Health*.

VICTOR W. SIDEL, MD, is Distinguished University Professor of Social Medicine Emeritus at Montefiore Medical Center and Albert Einstein College of Medicine, and an Adjunct Professor of Public Health at Weill Cornell Medical College. He is also a past president of APHA and has been active in Physicians for a National Health Program (PNHP). He was a founder of Physicians for Social Responsibility (PSR) and of the International Physicians for the Prevention of Nuclear War (IPPNW), which received the 1985 Nobel Peace Prize.

OXFORD
UNIVERSITY PRESS

www.oup.com

ISBN 978-0-19-993922-0

9 780199 939220

90000